AFRICAN HOLISTIC HEALTH

Llaila O. Afrika

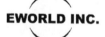

EWORLD INC.

Buffalo, New York
14208
eeworldinc@yahoo.com

Also by Dr. Afrika

The Gullah People
Nutricide

AFRICAN HOLISTIC HEALTH

Llaila O. Afrika

REVISED AND EXPANDED 7TH EDITION

- Disease Remedies
- Wholistic Sex Laws
- AIDS & Herpes Treatments
- Cocaine Detox
- Foods to Avoid
- Recipes
- Relationships
- Self Diagnosis
- Complete Remedy Guide for:
    - Herbs
    - Amino Acids
    - Homeopathics
    - Vitamins and Minerals

EWORLD INC.

EWORLD INC.
Buffalo, New York 14208
eeworldinc@yahoo.com

Graphic Design & Production:
Krystal Jackson
konakeka@comcast.net

Cover Design:
Llaila O. Afrika

Cover Illustration:
John "Kofi" Bedward

Other Illustrations:
Llaila O. Afrika

ISBN 978-1-61759-031-3

Formally published by
A&B Publishers Group
Brooklyn, New York
ISBN 978-1-881316-82-4

11 12 13 14   6 5 4 3 2 1
Manufactured and Printed in the United States

To my family, friends and Ancestors

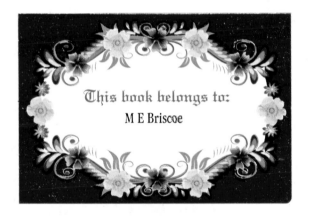

This book belongs to:

M E Briscoe

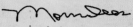

Contents

*Abscesses, Abrasion/Cuts, Aches, Anemia, Poor Appetite, Appendicitis,
Arthritis, Asthma, Backache, Bed Wetting, Bladder, Bleeding, Blood
Circulation, Blood Cleaner, Blood Impurities, Bowel, Breasts,
Bronchitis, Burns, Childbirth, Chills, Colds/Flu/Fever, Convulsion,
Corns/Calluses, Coughs, Cramps, Dandruff, Diabetes, Dizziness,
Eczema, Epilepsy, Eyes, Fainting, Fever, Gallstones, Gangrene,
Gargle, Gas, Genitals, Glandular Organs, Goiter, Gonorrhea, Hair,
Halitosis, Hay Fever, Heart, Heartburn, Hemorrhoids, Headache,
Hemorrhages, Hernia, High or Low Blood Pressure, Hips, Hypnotics,
Hysteria, Influenza, Inflammation, Insomnia, Impotence, Kidney
Problems, Laxative, Leukorrhea, Liver Bile, Liver Problems, Low
Back Pain, Menstruation, Mental Illness, Mucus, Muscle Spasms,
Nausea, Nose Bleed, Pancreas, Paralysis, Pneumonia, Prostate,
Sexual Excess, Skin Eruptions, Skin Eruptions, Spleen .....Problems,
Stomach, Swellings, Syphilis, Throat, Thyroid, Toothache, Tumors,
Tuberculosis, Spleen Problems, Ulcers, Urine, Varicose Veins*

*Allergy/Hay Fever, Boils/Bumps, Broken Bones, Bruises, Burns, Colds,
Colic, Constipation, Cuts, Diarrhea, Earache, Eye Injuries, Fever,
Headache, Indigestion, Menstruation, Motion Sickness, Physical
Trauma, Shock, Sunburn, Teething*

*Athlete's Foot, Bedbugs, Bedwetting, Bleeding, Candles, Cataracts,
Chapped Lips, Cigarette Smoke, Corns, Dandruff, Deodorant,
Disinfectant, Dizziness, Dog Bite, Eye Drops, Falling Hair, Flea
Repellent, Foot Cooler, Foot Warmer, Gas, Gout, Gray Hair, Hair
Rinse, Hair Oil, Hay Fever, Insect Repellent, Itchy Skin, Mildew,
Mildew Stains, Natural Contraceptives, Natural Hair Relaxer, No
Taste or Smell, Rats, Red Eyes, Refrigerator Freshener, Ringworm,
Rinse Water, Skin Oil, Split Fingernails, Swollen and Baggy Eyes,
Tension and Anxiety, Tired Feet, Warts, Whiten Teeth, Worms,
Wrinkles, Lotion, Lips, Facial Mask, Dry Skin Cleanser, Facial
Vegetable Pack*

   *Aloe/Aloe Vera, Agrimony, Basil, Boga Bark, Calumba, Chamomile,
   Camphor, Cinnamon, Celery, Clove, Coriander, Cumin, Eucalyptus,
   Fennel, Frankincense, Gotu Kola, Herbane, Henna, Horsetail, Hyssop,
   Kola Nuts, Licorice, Lime, Mandrake, Marshmallow, Marjoram, Mastic,
   Myrrh, Olive Oil, Oranges, Opopanax, Parsley, Papaya, Peppermint,
   Peony, Periwinkle, Plantain, Pineapple, Pyrethrum,Rose, Saffron, Sage,
   Sandalwood, Squil, Tragacant*

Introduction

Physician Heal Thyself!

This axiom is the foundation upon which the original African Medical system was founded.

Let us explore two major systems of healing before we investigate what this axiom really implies.

The African Healing Arts were extraordinary because all physical, mental and spiritual phenomena were studied, understood, practiced and taught to its entire society whereas, the European Healing Arts were kept secret from the European masses and applied as the European physicians saw fit.

Legal statutes had to be erected within the European civil structure to insure and maintain an ethics of medical standards. The Europeans studied, practiced, and taught their Healing Arts only to physicians and primarily from its mundane aspect. Their understanding of science and nature was only understood through their perception of their basic physical senses (vision, taste, touch, hearing, and smell).

The European physicians used their physical senses as their barometer for acquiring information that became the foundation upon which all diagnoses and prescriptions were based.

Dr. Afrika has succinctly and accurately explained in his book African holistic Health the neglect of the European medical system to teach its practitioners how to develop their higher senses to assist in gaining a deeper understanding of and an accurate alignment with Nature.

This lack of alignment and understanding of the profoundness of nature stimulated the practitioners of the European medical Arts to create Pseudo-Technologies such as radios, Televisions, X-Ray machines, Laser detection and projection devices, to assist in healing themselves.

The failure of the Europeans to understand the subtleties of Light, which is "The life Force Energy", has caused much suffering and death among people throughout the world.

Before the occurrence of the decline of the consciousness of the African Healer, the ancestral teachers of the African Healing Arts understood and taught its practitioners that:

1. All things in Nature were related.
2. All Matter in Nature originated from "The One Divine Source."
3. All creation was related and similar, but each living organism was original and unique.
4. All life and matter was created for a specific purpose and for a specific divine reason.

The African Healing Arts required all of its practitioners to undergo an intense study of "Self" and to understand how one's self was unique, yet related to the whole, and to be able to identify one's divine "Life Purpose."

The Ancient African society required all of its citizens to identify themselves just as the practitioners of its healing arts were required to, through the ubiquitous "Rites of Passage Ceremonies."

The most unique property of the Ancient African Societies was their Melanin content. Our Ancient African Ancestors were well aware of the complete bands of life forces composing the entire Electromagnetic spectrum. Through their Melanin they were capable of perceiving and interacting with television waves, radio waves, cosmic, laser, X-rays, etc.

Through their activated Melanin they perceived visions of the far and near past, present, and future projected upon their mind the same way that images are projected to us today through our TVs through their "Neuro-Melanin." They were able to hear conversations afar and converse with people afar using radio waves perceived and transmitted through their Neuro-Melanin. Melanin has the capacity to resonate and respond to all frequencies of the electromagnetic spectrum.

Our Ancient African ancestors understood that all frequencies of light had to be transduced (funneled) through Melanin before it could be applied directly to the physical body.

Light as it exists in this dimension is a vast expression of forces, which is responsible for creating all physical and subtle phenomena in our world.

Light is the unified collection of "Photons." Photons are the smallest measurable units of the life force energy.

As the motion and speed of photons vary, the character of the light changes, as does its activity. TV waves, micro-waves, radio waves, cosmic waves, x-rays etc., are all forms of the life force energy acting in unique ways, simply because of the difference of the speed and motion the photons within each band are exhibiting at any particular time.

The frequency are rate of movement of life force (light) relative to our Conscious Awareness, determines our ability to perceive to one, three or all bands of light (life force) which, is part collectively known as the Electromagnetic spectrum.

The amount of Melanin contained within one's body establishes innately the potential of an individual to perceive and interact with Melanin. However the mind set of the individual determines if one can consciously perceive or interact and manipulate the multiple frequencies of the Electromagnetic spectrum.

An individual with minimal Melanin content but with a focused and receptive mind set to a particular frequency of light, can perceive and interact with a particular band of light more successfully than a deeply melaninated person who is absolutely unaware of light and its effects relative to him or her. A good example of this was the ability of Madame Currie a "Melanin recessive" woman scientist to emission from Radium without the use of a machine she was able to perceive this intuitively. However because she was "Melanin Recessive," her physical body was not an adequate transducer and neutralizer of this frequency of light, therefore she died of radiation exposure. Radium was a well-known medical remedy in our ancient healing system for certain diseases. Our Ancient African healers were aware of the energy it emitted and handled it appropriately. They were "Melanin Dominant" and could handle such energy with proper training, therefore not creating health hazardous to their patients or themselves. All frequencies of light beyond the "Visible Spectrum" cannot be applied directly to humans without grave consequences to our health. However if these frequencies are passed through a natural transducer and equalizer before they are applied to humans, the light becomes a healing agent as opposed to being hazardous.

The African healers realized that the body of the Melanin dominant healer was a "Natural transducer and equalizer" for all forms of light. One of the major and prolonged areas of study for the African Healer was to understand the various bands of light and how to transduce or channel them through their body of a natural tool correctly, so as to affect a spontaneous cure for the ill.

With the colonization of Africa and the refusal of Africans and their descendants to acknowledge their melanin, allowed the tenets of the European Healing arts to dominate the world's present health care institutions and establish the standards for our present medical educational system. Through the use of Pseudo-technologies the present medical system is exposing its sick to pure frequencies of light without the proper human transduction systems, causing more disease and increased rates of death.

As we prepare to move into the twenty-first century. Much about the hidden natural phenomena of this planet will be revealed. Each species of life must be functional and active within the dominion of its divine purpose.

Africans as the innate and natural transducer for the healing forces of light are unconsciously and silently abdicating their divine purpose for existing. Africans and their descendants are the Natural Healers of this planet. They must begin to use their natural healing agent...Light, to remove the morbid disease factor that has begun to take over earth.

African Holistic Health, written by Dr. Llaila O. Afrika is our first intense primer to awaken us from our deep sleep. It Reviews and explains the major healing techniques and principles, which if studied by continental and American Africans and their descendants, will quite definitely begin to awaken the dormant genes within our cells that contain the ancient knowledge of how to use light properly. It will also reveal to us how to redevelop the appropriate technology, which will affect immediate cure instead of disease.

Melanin Dominant Humans of the world, Physicians, Heal thyself and take your proper place within our society of true Gods and Goddesses.

Lovingly and with light,
Jewel Pookrum, M.D., Ph.D.

Foreword

In this book, I have given the foundation of African holistic health, diet and dis-ease treatment. However, the treatments given have incorporated many conflicting systems because Black folks are at many different stages of treatment awareness.

In this book, terms "Wholistic" and "Holistic" are used interchange-able because they both represent the spirit, mind and body. Dis-ease and dis-ease are used interchangeably. When the body is not "at-ease," it is at "dis-ease," which means that the spirit, mind and body are ill. In orthodox medicine, disease usually means physical illness. In this book, the words European tribes or Europeans refer to a mixture of Caucasian ethnic groups that are called French, Spanish, Scandinavian, English, Dutch, Italians, Mongolians, Goks, Barbarians, Franks, Russians, Portuguese, Prussians, Bravians, etc. The ethnic groups have common rituals and ceremonies— a common ethic.

African holistics (ethnomedicine) is too vast a science and art to cover in one book. Therefore, this book is but a brief introduction to the cultural language called health. In my attempt to be brief, many valuable concepts had to be reduced and modified. Modifications were done with the utmost scrutiny and with the realization that thousands of years of African health wisdom and African historical ignorance cannot be erased with any book. This book is largely a response to the many questions asked by people during my nutritional counseling and at my lectures. It represents my intense desire to provide African-centered health information for Black children. Furthermore, it represents the frustration and despair I have suffered in my attempts to get precise African-centered information on the subject of African holistic health. My frustration was caused by Black folks and scientists not understanding African science and art. I had to labor to filter out the overwhelming abundance of science propaganda, White racism, Caucasian culturally biased, contaminated and distorted dysinformation in order to get to the fiber of the cultural language of the Ma'at science and art of healing. Aside from this, writing requires an understanding of how to use nouns and verbs with clarity. Writing demands a "writing style." A writing style is personal and demands knowing yourself and being truthful to yourself. I have used the written word to look at a past, a present and a future in such a way that a path to freedom can be spelled out emotionally and spiritually. I guess this is why this book has been emotionally expensive for me to write. I had to be a science griot. When I lecture, I have to be a performing artist griot. Telling a story, be it fiction (novel, poetry) or scientific drains your silence, focus and emotional fire. I was blessed in this writing because I was not alone, the Ma'at ancestors helped me to keep the fire of freedom alive.

I have had tremendous help from my family, children, wife, ancestors and friends. I have had to struggle against those who worked to stop this book from being written and published. I have had to struggle against my own ignorance, dysfunctionality and slavery trauma. I had to unlearn and re-learn. Writing this book reminded me of high school. I barely escaped (graduated) because subjects did not make sense to me. Later in my life, I discovered the science of herbology. It was when sciences were applied to a living thing and culture they began to make sense to me. Eventually, I began to write in order to share our African living sciences with you. However, I am still learning and I wish I was as smart as people think I am. This book is my humble attempt to share with you. This book is written solely to fill the void concerning African holistics and it is written to empower everyone to share the light that God created. This light is called a healthy spirit, mind and body—holistic health. The beauty of holistic diagnosis and treatments is that they work despite the position that our ignorance has put us in.

About the Author

Llaila (La-ee-la) Afrika (Ah-Free-kah) is a health consultant, certified Addictionologist, Accupuncturist, Metaphysician, Massage Therapist, Herbalist, historian, writer, lecturer, teacher, Medical Astrologist and naturopath. Llaila specializes in ethnomedicine, which is the usage of disease remedies and diagnosis based upon the biochemistry of a race. He believes that each of his clients (children to elderly) have been among his teachers and is fully indebted to them. Llaila uses a common sense approach to health. He has military and civilian work experience as a psychotherapist and nurse. Llaila has dropped out of colleges in America and attended health schools and seminars in America and Europe. He says his formal caucasian education was "culturally abrasive" and was "academically indigestible." He is self taught and dedicated to educating African people. Llaila believes a healthy body is the temple for building a healthy race. He lectures on over 70 different topics.

For lectures, workshops, classes, books, CDs, DVDs, audios and videos, contact:

A&B Publishers Group
1000 Atlantic Avenue
Brooklyn, New York
11238

Seduced by Ignorance
and Research

Research should be used to find the art and science of a subject in order to find out the facts. However, research as used by Caucasians has other meanings.

Caucasians have an over abundance of research projects and institutions and devote large sums of money to them. When you research any subject it means that you lack knowledge about the subject. In other words, you are ignorant of the subject. In this case, we have a civilization (European) that is ignorant.

African civilization did not and has not lacked knowledge. Ancient Africa was the first civilization that used its vast knowledge base to holistically master technology and medicine. The major problem that the Caucasians have with African functional research is that it is holistic. It is written by using words as structural, mental and spiritual symbolism called homonyms. The African spiritually based organic rhythmic conceptualized science is difficult for Caucasians to comprehend. Caucasians have devised a way to acculturate, translate and fragment African science so that they can understand it. They call this fragmented translation "Research." They use non-holistic laboratory studies, statistics and experiments to understand African holistic functional research. It is obvious that the Pyramids took functional research established over 5,000 years before they were built. In other words, the research era in Africa was over and only products of past research appear such as the Pyramids of Giza. The functional research for holistic medicine was arrived at long before the ancient text (papyrus) was written.

Written documents are evidence that African functional research was done holistically. The Turin papyrus is 54,000 years old (11th to 12th Dynasties). The 12th to 13th Dynasties include the Ramesseum papyrus and the Kahun papyrus. These papyri reveal high levels of holism. The 19th Dynasty has the Chester papyrus and the Berlin papyrus, which has functional research. The Ebers and Edwin Smith papyri are full text, comprehensive and are used more and more by holistic medical scholars.

The creation and introduction of medical terms is African. These papyri and other writings gave the world these terms: kidney, saliva, dura mater, sarrow, testicles, buccal cavity esophagus, brain, throat, tongue, bile urine, uterus, vulva, stomach, ear, intestines, trachea, lung, spinal cord, heart, eye, disease, rectum diaphragm, labia, vagina, perspiration, liver, gall bladder, baldness, muscle, cerebrospinal fluid, spleen, air, obesity, bone, abdomen and many other terms. This indicates that pre-historical research was done and knowledge was obtained by Africans.

The constant demand of Caucasians for scientific proofs, statistics, research rituals and ceremonies and documentation is their search for a ritual and ceremony that allows them to get knowledge. Once the knowledge is translated and applied in a scientific way, Caucasians label the research "modern" or a "recent discovery." This word, "modern" is the new word for stolen information and makes you forget that the research was already done by Africans. Most of the Caucasian research is redecorated knowledge that was raped from Africa. They use chemical acrobatic laboratory rituals and ceremonies to disguise the rape. Their science is a form of information colonialization of science, White Supremacy and cultural bias. The Caucasians have discovered science in the same way that they discovered America. They invaded the ancient African Egyptian science knowledge, raped, pillaged and burned ancient African textbooks. They call African science primitive, then take that same science, give it a new name and call it a modern discovery. They seduce themselves into believing that gynecology, ophthalmology and other medical sciences are modern when in fact, Athotis, the son of Mena (circa 3,000 BC), wrote an encyclopedia of medicine that included these subjects. To compound this ignorance, non-Holistic, White racist historians such as Diodorus, Strabo, Herodotus and Monetho personally reported on the research of ancient Africa. However, this fact is ignored by "modern" day Caucasian scientists and historians. These cultural spies (historians) helped to create the present historical ignorance. Caucasians in search of knowledge have invented a new ignorance called "research" and have become seduced by their own ignorance.

Research institutions and projects are not simply operating in the quest of truth and knowledge. Research is funded and politically manipulated by the monies of the Drug and Junk Food companies and the military. Research has become a business that operates to stay in business. It operates similar to the automobile business. Each year, they produce a new model car (i.e., unproven new technology or research finding) in order to increase profits. For example, the United States of America is not a country. It is a business. Slavery was not a crime. It was a business. When chattel (chains) slavery ended, the ownership of the non-chattel slavery business was transferred from individual slave masters to the United States as slave master. It was a larger business (United States) taking over smaller businesses. The word "Emancipation" means transfer of ownership. Slaves were emancipated, not freed. The profit from non-chattel slavery is a perpetual economic inheritance, the same as the profits from research and profits of the disease industry. Diseases such as AIDS and Cancer are no longer diseases. They are businesses. The research and disease business are the new Slave Masters and the consumer is the slave. It is a continuation of slavery (African knowledge and health slavery). People are seduced into believing that research is pure and an honest branch of science. It is not and will not ever be that. It is a business. A pure science cannot come from society sick with White Supremacy psychosis. You cannot get a straight piece of wood (pure science) from a crooked tree (White Supremacy). Science is a language of White Supremacy. Research has to be evaluated based upon Ma'at holistics and African-centeredness before it can be African acculturated and used.

An African-centered scientist must use African-centered research in its fullness in order to recover, sustain and maintain the health of our race. African health practitioners and teachers should use Ma'at culture and holistic health practices as part of their lives. The disease treatment methods and healing practices use African rituals and ceremonies that perpetuate the culture. Culture provides the language that enables you to spiritually, mentally, emotionally and physically modify a health treatment method (make it so-called modern). The rationale (cause/effect) for disease has to mirror culture. Disease, as explained and defined by African peoples is based upon a mixture of the past, present, future and ancestors. Research into African Ma'at healings and healers reveals and defines truth.

An illness occurs when an individual's wellness changes from the culture's normal standard to a state that cannot adapt or conform to wellness. Normal or ill health standards have to be consistent with and reflect the culture. Wellness cannot be based upon an assumed truth. Truth is people and people are culture. Truth is not an abstract idea or a scientific laboratory experiment generated concept. Truth is an agent of a culture. Healers are agents of a culture. If the African healers mix and accept an alien culture's wisdom (Caucasian), certification and accreditation then African healing science and art becomes diluted and alien to Africans. An African that changes any aspect of an African healing modality is performing a delicate surgery. One slip of the cultural surgical knife (error) can cause African culture to become colonialized and/or diseased. Making a change in treatment is like digging a well for water. You have to dig deep into African cultural soil to reach an underground stream of fresh water—a new African healing modality. Ma'at guided research is a way to dig into African healing systems. However, Caucasian research methods are controlled by the political, economic and military industrial motives of the funding source. In many cases, their research outcomes are dictated to their scientists as well as research and data altered in order to satisfy the economic sponsor. This makes the research itself dubious. It is essentially not about discovering truth but discovering more power over the minds and bodies of the consumer. It is a research that uses scientific language to seduce you into a state of ignorance called knowledge, facts and proofs = dysinformation. In order to clearly understand science as culture, you must first examine the quality of day-to-day life of the children, elders and parents. If the people are abusive, exploiters, violent and deceitful, then their science will be abusive and deceitful. Science is people. People are science. A science cannot be more advanced, perfect, or purer than the people that created it. Therefore, the research done by a Caucasian scientist is merely another reflection of the Caucasian people's behavior, morality and ignorance. Health research decorates Caucasians primitiveness with science language and seduces them into more ignorance. Caucasians search or research for something that is not lost or they are always discovering something that has already been found (discovered), i.e., Caucasians believe they discovered America—a land already occupied and found by Indians.

Black folks should not blindly accept Caucasian research. They must scrutinize it for truth, evaluate it based upon Ma'at and translate it. The key to making an evaluation is to attach people (culture) to the subject. Music, mathematics, religion, biology, chemistry, words, art and research is people (culture). These subjects have to be directly connected to people in order to understand the subject. For example, words such as "snack food" is not merely a food item, it is people in another form. The ancient Caucasians (cave dwellers and those too uncivilized to live in caves) had food shortages due to famines and the Ice Age. Consequently, they stole food from each other in order to survive, they snatched food—snack food. The words "snack food" reflects people, people (culture) make research valid and alive. Their research is their culture and satisfies the needs of their culture. Caucasian research was not and is not done to benefit or serve African peoples.

RACES OF HUMANS

Races are classified based upon Melanin content of the body.

RATED	COLOR	RACE
6(Highest)	Black, Blue/Black (Highest Melanin Content)	Africans (Melanin is Selenium Centered)
5	Black/Brown, Brown	Native Indians (Mexicans, Malaysians, etc.)
4	Brown, Red	Native Americans, Japanese
2 and 3	Yellow, Mixed, Mixed Brown	Orientals
1(Lowest)	White	Caucasians (Melanin is Sulphur Centered)

The Caucasians' medical research was used to set norm values, calibrate machines and measuring devices based upon their science mythology (theories), cultural norms and the biochemistry of the White race. The Caucasian rate themselves as the race with the least melanin, vitamin and mineral content. When a Black person's blood chemistry is at the Caucasian normal (healthy) level, they are subclinically sick.

Health standards are based upon the Caucasians as well as medical laboratory, normal values, daily recommended allowance of vitamins and minerals, therapeutic dosages of herbs and drugs, baby's formulas, disease reactions, human growth and development schedule, and brain activity, Their psychology is based upon mythological people (Greek fairy tale, Oedipus).

The Overlooked Revolution

There is an overlooked revolution in Black worldwide culture. Socially, Black people have protested, marched, rebelled, voted, sang, and cried for a revolution for Black Nationalism, freedom, justice, self-identity, self-destiny, equality and the reaffirmation of African medical treatment concepts. Today, Blacks are totally enslaved by another culture's (Caucasian) diet and medical system. They have become a Black Nation of Nutritional Uncle Toms who are denied the Human Right to practice their culture's medicine (i.e., denied insurance coverage for herb and folk medicine). An African health practitioner is denied the legal right to practice and is considered unscientific.

The Africanization of Caucasian culture has occurred in Black culture. For example, Africanization of English has resulted in the Negro Dialect, Africanized European music resulted in jazz, Africanized religious music resulted in Gospel, the Africanization of the waltz resulted in the jitterbug and the impact of this African thrust has caused Black (African) Studies in colleges. The reclaiming of African clothes and garments, hairstyles (cornrows), languages, names, and history has demonstrated the extent of the social revolution. Yet one major step has been overlooked in this process: the reclaiming of African herbal medicine and a natural whole foods diet and lifestyle.

Wholistic thinking is the key to understanding Caucasian cultural bias and White racism as applied to diet and medicine. Wholism means that everything (i.e., air, water, fire, earth, electricity, colors, metal) has a form (physical body), intelligence, and spirit energy state. This wholistic concept was a part of African cultures that existed before the Sahara Lake became the Sahara Desert. In any case, European cultural bias and racism has contaminated and distorted African medical and dietary writings. In fact, all Chinese, Japanese, and Hindu cultures and their forms of yoga, meditation, exercise, diagnosis, and treatments are biased in that they accentuate their own cultural frame of reference and disregard that the source of their science and art is Africa. African civilization (frame of reference) was built on a Ma'at approach to natural foods, wellness, diet and herbal medicine. Blacks who accept Caucasian science as the only true science are whitewashed. Black folks who do not use their own culture's healing art and science are addicted to Caucasian culture. They are accepting the fact that African culture produced calculus, psychology, bureaucracy, biology, medicine, astronomy, algebra, architecture, alchemy and anatomy while at the same time emotionally rejecting the African wholistic diet and medical art and science. They are practicing self-hatred on subconscious levels and ignoring the obvious facts on a conscious level.

The medical writings of Imhotep (Egyptian God of Medicine) are the oldest medical documents written. Imhotep's books were stolen from Africa and are presently at Karl Marx University in Leipzig, Germany. Imhotep wrote over ten volumes on holistic treatments, diets, and foods over 2,000 years before Hippocrates (European father of medicine) was born. Part of Imhotep's principles appear in *The Canon of Medicine*—medical books written by a Black Muslim, named Avicenna, who used Islamic culture. He and another Black Muslim, named Rhazes, influenced European medicine. In fact, Rhazes wrote about a hundred medical books that utilized natural foods, herbal remedies, and diets. All major European medical schools used his books extensively in the 15th and 16th centuries. Of course, the aforementioned works are distorted and contaminated by the Islamic culture of the authors and racist biases of the European translators. Nonetheless, the African wholistic natural foods and herbal concepts were clearly in their works.

Europeans' cultures and science use good (drug medicine) against evil (bacteria, virus) fragmentation or the so-called analytical concept. In other words, they separated the mind, the body and the spirit. Caucasians treat the mind in a psychiatric clinic; the spirit in a church, and the body in a hospital while African science includes the spirit, mind and body, present, past and future as a whole—wholistically. In fact, orthodox Caucasian science does not include the spirit's affect upon the body, mind, diet, wellness or disease. Caucasians do not see culture as the foundation for the healing art and science.

Culture creates the individual and family. It provides the rewards, punishments, and values for an individual's emotional, mental, physical and spiritual personality. Culture serves the individual and individual serves culture. An individual's healing art and science serves their culture. A wholistc foods or medicine book written from a Chinese, Japanese or Caucasian cultural perspective is unacceptable to Black folks' cultural needs. There is not one institution (science, medicine, mathematics, physics, chemistry) in Caucasian culture, which has not become wet with White racism from soaking in over 3,000 years of White Supremacy. Caucasians wholistic health and medicine needs White Supremacy detoxification and therapy. Many obvious facts point to the need to abandon Caucasian culture's wholism other than the Predatory White Supremacy Psychosis involved (*see* White Racism Addiction).

The mindset of Caucasians with Predatory Militaristic White Supremacy Psychosis is a thought process in which the Caucasian believes good and evil are tools to use to manipulate and control Africans. Evil is created and maintained to control good; good is created only to control evil. Within good, there is evil and within evil, there is good. Good and evil are mixed together as one. Evil (slavery) is rewarded with good (wealth). Good (wealth) is punished with evil (embezzling, robbery, stealing of money, etc.). Good is used to terrorize (forcing the Caucasian rules and laws upon Africans) and then bad (racial profiling, racism,discrimination, etc.) is forced upon Africans for following Caucasian good (rules and laws). Africans must keep in mind that you do not protest, vote, demonstrate or march to get rid of a mental illness (psychosis). Mental illnesses require therapy. When Blacks do not believe psychotherapy is needed to treat Caucasians with the psychosis, it indicates that the African has Co-Dependent Addiction to White Supremacy Psychosis. Africans cannot overlook China's mental illness, called Heroin Addiction, which was treated successfully. The mentally ill either got treatment or were killed. Needless to say, they were 100% successful in solving the mental illness (drug) problem. Britain forced Heroin on China, which resulted in the 1839 Opium War.

Blacks have specific biochemical, nutritional and dietary needs. These nutritional needs arise because Blacks are Melanin dominant and have specific bodily differences as compared to less Melaninated races. For example, over 70% of Black people (worldwide) cannot digest cattle milk. In addition, the intestinal florae (bacteria, virus, fungus and yeast) that naturally live in Black people's intestines are unique to Blacks. Subsequently, Blacks assimilate food in the intestines differently as Melanin improves the efficiency of carbohydrate digestion. Despite centuries of eating a non-AFrican diet and living in Caucasian controlled countries outside of Africa, the Africans intestinal florae remains the same as it was in their ancestors' stomachs 2,000 years ago in Africa. Melanin (black color pigment) is obviously most abundant (dominate) in Blacks. This melanin aids in protecting Blacks from the ultraviolet rays of the sun. It also increases the speed and storage of nerve and brain messages. Africans have the largest mid-brain and have more harmony between the left and right hemispheres of the brain, more fast twitch muscles, and the highest amount of vitamins and minerals in the body as compared to other races. The Black woman's vagina is longer, the minor lips of the vagina are larger and breastmilk has higher nutrients as compared to women of other races. The Black woman's birth canal is the most efficient and sealed tighter. Black people's blood crystallizes differently from Caucasians' blood. These are some of the many reasons why Blacks have a unique biochemical, nutritional, medical and dietary need (*See* Anatomy Chart).

Traditional African Diet

Fiber...................... 8 times higher than Caucasian processed food diet
Sodium.................... ⅛th of processed food diet
Calcium.................... 7 times higher than processed food diet
Phosphorus................. 5-8 times higher than processed food diet
Vitamins.................... Higher levels of water and fat-soluble vitamins
Sunlight.................... 80% more sunlight stimulation for the Pineal Organ (so-called gland)
Water...................... 90% higher water intake
Vegetables and Fruit...... 85% higher and organic
Meat...................... 15% organic animal flesh (includes insects) was eaten during cultural and health decline
Breastmilk................. Cow's milk is indigestible, causes colds, allergies, diseases and mood swings

Milk

	Human	Cow (Not for Humans)
Protein-total %	1.0 to 1.5	3.5 to 4.0
Casein %	50	82
(main protein in cow's milk)		
Whey %	60	18
(watery part of milk contains lactose,		
vitamins, minerals, lactalbumin, fat)		
Calcium-phosphoric ratio	2:1	1.2:1
Vitamin A (per liter)	1,898	1,025
Niacin (mg. per liter)	1,470	940
Vitamin (mg. per liter)	43	11
Reaction in the body	alkaline	acid

MEDICINE

European orthodox medicine (synthetic drugs and surgery) is based upon predatory military logic and is organized to treat symptoms in a triage method. African medicine is organized wholistically to treat the spiritual, mental and physical causes of dis-ease. For instance, the body tries to maintain adaptability (which means adjusting holistically). Whenever the body is overloaded (biochemically imbalanced), it tries to get rid of the toxic (imbalanced) state. It uses urine and bowel movements to keep it free of toxins. If the urine and bowels fail to eliminate toxins, then the skin is used for a bowel movement (bumps, acne, blackheads, herpes, rashes, measles, smallpox, etc.). If this fails to cleanse the body, then the lungs and nasal cavities are used to get rid of toxins (sinuses, running nose, bronchitis, catarrh). The body uses a warning signal such as a headache to notify you of a toxic state. In African wholistic medicine, the cause of the toxic state would be treated with massage, acupuncture, aromatherapy, herbs and a cleansing diet. European medicine stops or suppresses the symptoms of disease with aspirin, cough suppressants, antihistamines, etc. This causes the body to remain toxic and these toxins cause dis-ease. The symptom treating system keeps the individual in a disease state. This causes Blacks' health to be exploited by diseases for economic profits.

DIET

The contemporary junk food and fast food diet is based upon denatured, highly refined, processed, genetically altered and synthetically chemicalized non-foods. This modern stuff looks like food, tastes like food, smells like food, but amounts to chemical waste (junk food) and a type of synthetic dirt.

The most damaging criminals in the modern diet are bleached white flour and white sugar. Bleached flour is constipating because it has no fiber (non-digestible roughage). Fiber allows food to exercise and cleans the digestive organs and leaves the body at a normal rapid rate. Bleached white flour is robbed of over twenty-two vitamins and minerals. White sugar has no fiber, no nutrients and increases the sugar level in the body beyond its natural level, which results in nutrient deprivation, diabetes, high blood pressure, nerve and brain damage, kidney failure and eye deterioration. Fried foods are non digestible, constipating, and partially used by the body. The combination of these foods with edible drugs such as preservatives, additives and dyes results in behavior control and chemical warfare upon the health. It is common knowledge that chemicals (drugs, aspirin, depressants, amphetamines) influence behavior and alters moods. The eating of these chemicals indirectly causes robotized nutritional slavery (limits the range of thoughts and wellness).

African coprolite (fossil food and feces) studies reveal a natural diet in Africans. The scientific analysis of coprolites verifies that Africans ate whole foods, bee pollen, herbs, nuts, vast variety of raw vegetables, and some cooked foods. Ancient fossilized African foods in no way resemble modern foods. Eating a processed food diet is against life and against the African culture.

African Empires, civilizations, music, art, philosophy, science, medicine and culture is built upon wholistic foods and medicine (*see* music, science and psychology chart). Blacks who eat a modern diet are being oppressed and enslaved by Caucasians through their stomachs. This dietary enslavement results in dis-eases, constipation and bodily destruction. Eating this modern junk food (chemical waste) results in the abandonment of Black acculturated diet and African cultural castration. Any social cry of Reparation, Human Rights and Black Liberation by a nation of constipated Blacks is a cultural joke. Blacks must revolutionize their diets and stop eating fast foods and eat slow foods (whole, unprocessed). There are no people who are free if they are controlled by another people's foods. Blacks must reclaim control of their stomachs and see African culture and Ma'at in the diet.

African wholistics is still a part of Black culture. Wholism in Black culture is based upon "concept." Concept is the inclusion of every part of a picture. For example, Black "concept." thinking (whole picture or story) when applied to health, as well as language, is evident. Blacks use the word "bad" and it has many meanings based upon the particular story (concept) in which it is used. "Bad" can mean fine, excellent, expensive, intelligent, sex and terrible. It takes its meaning from the context of the whole picture (story). However, Caucasian cultures' health, as well as language, is negatively analytical (meaning divide, good vs. evil, fragment, isolate). Subsequently, bad means bad and the further conjugation (i.e., badder, baddest) of the word are degrees of being bad.

European wholistics is not inherently concept-oriented. It is fragmented. Subsequently, it can analyze the nutritional worth of herbs and foods, not the intelligence of an herb or the spiritual use or purpose of the herb. They isolate a dangerous chemical or nutrients of a herb and then conclude that the entire mixture of healing nutrients in the herb are dangerous. Furthermore, anything that cannot be done in a so-called scientific laboratory (analysis) does not exist. Often when Caucasian scientists mention African wholistic herbal use (a science of herbs over 10,000 years old), it is negatively called unscientific, voodoo, witchcraft, mysticism or cultural ignorance. This is Caucasian cultural bias and White racism. Actually, African-centered wholistic health, herbal medicine, healers and whole food diet utilize the total energies of the plants (spiritual, intellectual, nutrient) rather than the partial nutrient values. So, it followed that a whole (unprocessed) plant treated a whole person. The primary differences between European and African wholistic health is in the concept and analytical (fragmentation) approach. African wholism never divided, isolated a nutrient or fragmented a plant to understand its personality. Plant personalities are very specific properties associated with a particular plant. A "plant personality" causes it to treat, heat or cool a particular part of the body or organ. It also affects the speed or slowness of its use in the body. Each plant or treatment has a ritual and ceremony associated with the plant's cycle, the time of day it is picked, and the day of the week it is prepared. The zodiac sign, deity and/or the personality of the plant, patient, healer or dis-ease has to be given attention, primarily, because wellness or dis-ease represents a spiritual, mental and physical part of the culture. The culture dictates that the herb, as well as the person taking the herb, are in communion with God. Plant personality dictated the choice of plant (herb) to use in disease treatment. Isolating an herb's nutrient or chemical is like having two blind people describe an elephant—the one at the tail says the elephant is skinny, and the one at the foot describes the elephant as tall with a shell (toe nails). Isolating an herb's nutrient or chemical destroys its wholistic value and destroys the healing effect of its characteristics (plant personality).

The choice is simple. Blacks who accept another culture's definition of health, healing, medicine and food are enslaved by that culture via their stomachs. These nutritional slaves can be seen smoking tobacco and marijuana cigarettes (the lighting of them turns them into a synthetic chemical, a non-food which destroys the oxygenation of blood, produces poor quality sperm), using synthetic drugs, drinking sodas (a synthetic chemicalized liquid sugar), eating white sugar products (i.e., candies, pastries—which produce low and high blood sugar and sugar addiction), bleached white flour (produces vitamin deficiency and cancer), drinking alcohol (destroys brain cells), and eating denatured fast foods. These nutritional Uncle Toms and dietary slaves produce children who eat like Caucasians. They are slaves by African wholistic definition and Caucasoid Blacks. The "overlooked revolution" or Africanization of Black health (African-centered art and science of health) can no longer be overlooked!

MA'AT PRINCIPLES OF DIET

Use these principles as your diet guidelines. If you are hungry and have a craving for sweets, junk foods, fattening foods, alcohol, snack foods, etc., evaluate your emotions and reasons for craving and relate them to Ma'at principles. Question your emotions (feelings) and reasons based upon Ma'at.

Truth	Am I really hungry? Am I medicating emotions with junk foods/alcohol? Does my body need nourishment? Am I being a slave to my taste buds? Am I treating food as if it is a "slave" and my eating it as "the slave master"?
Justice	Does my choice of food give nutritional justice to my body or does it nutritionally starve my body?
Righteousness	Is the food good for God's Temple (my body)? Is there a healthy snack I can eat instead of junk?
Harmony	How does eating junk food serve my body and benefit my wellness?
Balance	Does eating this food maintain my biochemical balance or does it cause a negative drain of energy?
Order	Does the food follow the correct order (amount) of nutrients? (6 grains, 5 fruits or vegetables, 2 proteins – vegetable/meat, 8-10 glasses of water?)
Propriety	Is the food adding to my wellness and helping me to eliminate or decrease my intake of packaged, processed, synthetic, foods, dead animal flesh, cloned, hybridized, chemical-laced preservatives?
Compassion	Do I accept that my wellness adds to the health of my race and serves Ma'at or do I feel deprived when I do not eat junk foods?
Reciprocity	Am I using food to commit suicide, to punish myself, or to maintain low self-esteem or am I using it to reward myself? Does this food ultimately cause disease or wellness?

EAT SNACKS AND DYSFUNCTIONALITY
(UNHEALTHY EMOTIONS AND/OR LIFESTYLES)

The tendency to like types of foods or snacks can indicate emotional problems. The food industry makes food that will appeal to the dysfunctional feelings, emotions and lifestyle of oppressed Africans. The industry uses psychologists to help create emotions and feelings for food and to connect subconscious desires to food. Oppressed African consumers tend to medicate (pacify) their feelings with sugar and salt. It is no accident that Blacks are largest consumers of salty potato chips and have the highest diabetes rate. Caucasian oppression makes Black folks dysfunctional and then Caucasians profit from the dysfunctionality via snack foods. Aside from this, no animal, insect or plant eats snacks. They eat to satisfy hunger, not to medicate emotions. The following is a partial list of foods and emotions. There are many different combinations of snack foods that cover many types of subconscious desires to be healthy.

SNACK FOOD GROUPS

Type	Emotional Addictive Factor
Bready	Relieves feelings of insecurity and soothes dissatisfaction
Chewy	Relieves tension/stress and need to slow down and unwind
Creamy	Helps satisfy need to be nurtured and comforted
Crunchy	Helps release anxiety and social pressure caused by cultural abrasion (white control)
Salty	Redirects anger, frustration, violence
Sugary	Helps satisfy the need to give and/or receive love

MEDICINES, MACHINES AND IGNORANCE

The orthodox medical field (non-wholistic, non-natural) relies on machines and so-called technology. These modern machines, technology and gadgets are presumed to improve the human capacity to diagnose and treat the body. Similarly, it is assumed humans lack the ability to diagnose at the level of modern machines (i.e., computers). An examination of ancient medical theory, diagnosis and treatment can help to dissolve this modern primitive medical addiction to machines.

The history of medicine and medical treatments is well-defined. In fact, pre-Egyptian medical science was constructed by the same Black scientific intelligence that constructed calculus, nutrition, algebra, astronomy, physics and ecology. These natural wholistic scientific treatments, which used no contemporary fuel driven machines, gadgets or technology, are documented in the African "Eber Papyrus" (1500 B.C.), *Canon of Medicine* by Avicenna and the *Medical Papyrus of Amen-Hotep* (written over 2,000 years before Hippocrates' birth). Additionally, the Chinese *Pen Tsao* (around 1000 B.C.) further documents the scientific analysis of dis-ease states without machines. *The Yellow Emperor Classic of Chinese Medicine* also used looking touching and smell for diagnosis.

Contemporary medical technology is not an advancement in medicine, it indicates the failure of Caucasian medical science and is a sign of ignorance. Technology cannot replace the human ability, diagnose dis-ease by looking, touching and smell and perform treatments without drugs.

Ancient health practitioners taught the patient about herbs and healing. They instructed the patient on how to achieve higher wellness on a spiritual, mental and physical level. The medicine man was used as a human technology for the culture. Each individual was taught that all senses were active (Male Principle) and passive (Female Principle) and all dis-eases were active and passive and taught the spiritual and mental causes of disease.

The life (existence) of human beings is a combination of the past, present, future, ancestors, physical, mental, and spiritual. Each of these factors of life was sublimely analyzed. Consequently, an imbalance (disease) in any factor of life represented an imbalance in other factors. The African health practitioner had to first develop their own human detection sensitivity capacities by using Ma'at before they could treat the dis-eased individual. The healer used sight, music, touch, hearing, dance, smell, food, rituals and ceremonies as diagnostic and healing instruments. Therefore, electrical and fuel driven machines, gadgets and so-called modern technology were not needed. The healer had dis-ease detection intelligences on many levels and realized that Ma'at diagnostic wisdom is inherent in individuals, not machines. The machines used helped the healer diagnose, machines did not diagnose. It was wisdom of the manifested (physical) and unmanifested (spiritual) that guided the medicine men/women (healers).

Healers were guided in treatment by the wisdom that all organs are related to each other, in that the human developed as an undifferentiated mass (egg) in which all organs and organ systems were connected together (*see* the Chart Organ Regions). The organs began to specialize in function (i.e., lungs for breathing, etc.). However, they never lost their inherent connection to the whole body (*see* Acupressure Chart). In fact, every cell in the body possesses the genetic code (fingerprint of the body). Therefore, any part of the body can be used to analyze another part or organ. The internal organs have nerve endings in the feet, hands, head, teeth, tongue, etc. All organs in the body are connected (related) to each other, similar to the telephone systems in the world. The knowledge of the interrelatedness of bodily organs and parts combined with the healers' ability to use their body as a gadget, machine, technology and instrument for diagnosing and treating disease put the African healer on the highest level of science.

A fuel driven machine, gadget or technology does not possess wisdom or Ma'at. A machine, be it a bullet or a bomb, will kill an infant child or an enemy. Particles of metals or plastics do not possess wisdom, power or knowledge or Ma'at. A sophisticated computerized medical testing machine does not reflect the wholistic intelligence of humans. These machines reflect the interaction of particles of metal. No machine possesses more knowledge than its maker. No modern fuel (electrical) driven machine possesses the wisdom of Ma'at and power of the unmanifested (spirituality) of humans. A healer that relies totally on machines is reflecting ignorance and a lack of African-centered spiritual and psychic training.

Ancient African medicine was founded upon wholistic spirituality and Ma'at. This pre-Egyptian medical science is between 20,000 and 100,000 years old. In fact, it is the oldest medicinal science on this planet. The Westcar Papyrus (1550 B.C.) of the 18th Dynasty has stories from the early empires, which date before the Great Pyramid, and they make reference to priest/herbalist doctors of King Khufu (Cheops) of the 4th Dynasty (3800 B.C.). Most importantly, Herataf, son of King Khufu, mentions a surgeon named TET. African medicine used the full scope and capacities of wholistic calculus and other sciences. The realization that the spiritual fueled human body is an advanced technological instrument for diagnostic and treatment purposes was well known. The Caucasians with the lowest Melanin content can only understand between twenty-five to forty percent of the astronomy, magnetism and other mathematical concepts required to build the Great Pyramids in Africa. The Caucasians' limited understanding of the African mathematical concepts has resulted in the invention of the so-called modern machines of computers, spaceships, automobiles and nuclear bombs. The other seventy-five percent of the African astrology, health science and mathematics is beyond the scope of the Caucasian thought process. The African Rhind mathematical papyrus (1650 B.C.) is the oldest text on mathematics and it reveals that the remaining seventy-five percent of mathematics the ancient medical scientist used has not been interpreted. It can be seen that the ancient African scientist had the mathematical capacity to build machines of any type. Obviously, their advanced biochemistry and use of the body as a technological instrument is yet to be explained or understood.

Machines (modern gadgets) do not possess wisdom or Ma'at. Machines such as computers will send checks to dead people and death notices to live people. A thermometer will register the human temperature at 98.6 degrees. However, a thermometer cannot register (indicate) whether the temperament of the body temperature is moist, wet, dry, hot, earth, air, fire or water. The energy projected from the eyes is measured, identified as active (Male) or passive (Female) and classified by the temperament system. Eye-projected energy can be felt. An individual can feel another person staring at them while their back is turned away from the person. This is an example of the registering of eye energy upon the back. Ancient medical practitioners developed their ability to measure, identify and classify eye energy.

Wholistic abilities gave the medial scientist vast sublime resources for the diagnosis of dis-ease states and treatments. Each disease, organ and hormone has a sublime odor. Each organ produces a specific odor whether in a state of health or dis-eased. These odors were classified as sweet, bitter, salty, pungent, sour, active, passive, earth, water, air, fire and ethereal. Energy projected by the ears, pulse, nose, breath, hair and skin were diagnosed and classified. These are but a few of the sublime human abilities a medial practitioner developed and utilized in dis-ease detection and treatment.

The non-wholistic thinkers are trying to copy wholistic human abilities with machines. Machines can only use coarse energy (electrical, nuclear, gas, etc.) while humans can use fine mental, spiritual, emotional and physical energy. Humans are not limited to one energy input. Humans can use all energy (psychic, emotional, spiritual) to diagnose and treat disease. A wholistic diagnosis of a wholistic human, gives a wholistic treatment. No machine, gadget or technology can wholistically perform this "unless it relies on the fuel of the human mind, spirit, emotion and body." *The House of Light* by Paul Ghaliounegve has further information.

Caucasian non-wholistic medicine (i.e., European) is using fragmentation and predatory military logic to duplicate African wholistic non-fuel driven machine medicine. Caucasian culture, medical science and civilization has failed to substitute electrical and fuel driven machines for human ability. This failure is reflected in the overabundance of Caucasian physical dis-eases, cultural psychosis (social wars) and spiritual failures (individuals profess belief in God and yet steal, lie, murder and kill for a particular government or self). It will continue to fail because Caucasian culture uses failure to manipulate and control people.

Ancient African wholistic health science produced many healing instruments. These Ma'at instruments required the usage of higher developed psychic and spiritual energy for their proper use. The names of these instruments have been distorted and acculturated by Europeans. Many of these healing and diagnostic devices are labeled as toys and games.

The games of "chess" and "checkers" are extracted from an African divination and healing device call Draughts. This device looks exactly like chess except the so-called playing board has 27 squares, which are laid out, in 3 rows of squares with 9 columns. Each column of nine squares represents the nine energy forces (Chakras) of the individual respectively; nine columns for the body, nine for the mind and nine for the spirit. The so-called playing pieces were placed in a Terra Cotta Bowl or cloth bag and mixed by shaking. Next, the pieces were removed (without looking) and placed on the board from right to left. The pieces have meanings similarly to "tarot cards." These divining statues (pieces) once placed on the board were read to diagnose the illness, social problem, emotional issues and prescribe treatment.

"Bowling" is an African healing and diagnostic and divination instrument mistaken for a game. Actually, it is the pyramidal and divining egg device. The so-called pins (chakras) were placed in a pyramid shape, each pin representing an organ, fate as well as spiritual, mental, emotional and social state. The divining egg (bowling ball) was programmed with the aura of the patient (a witness of cloth or hair was used). Then the ball was rolled to strike the pins. Next, the healer would read the pins based upon how they fell, the direction they lay in and according to astrology and what matrix they formed. Finally, the healer would then program the ball (egg) and strike the pins (chakras) in order to change fate or find a remedy.

The "sliding board" is actually the African "negative gravity ionic device." This instrument usually had an electromagnetically charged board and 12 (or 24) magnet charged steps. These steps (chakra planes) were used to recharge the positive chakra while the board was used to stimulate the pineal gland and increase circulation to the brain. The patient would slide down the board head first and/or feet first according to the type treatment of necessitated.

The "swing" is another ill-named African healing instrument. The horizontal bar would support the swing; this bar would be suspended and attached to vertical support posts (three posts), which were arranged in a pyramid shape. The posts and the horizontal bar would be charge by magnets. Thus, the patient would swing through the electromagnetic force field; the alpha-gamma rays and the pyramidal energy field would cause a polarization of energies on a psychic and physical level. This is a Pendulum Pyramidal Healing Device.

The "see-saw" or African Electromagnetic Adjustable Alignment Board is an ancient healing device. It was arranged in a circular sphere according to the organ being treated (*see* Eye Chart). The alpha ray energy angular wave were used. The board was placed on a pyramid pivot with crystals or metals (*see* Crystal and Metal Charts) as a counterbalance for the dis-eased patient. Then, the patient would be caused to "see-saw" according to the rhythm vibrations (*see* Music Chart) of the dis-eased organ. This would result in polarization of the dis-eased organ. The internal organ vibration adjustments caused by the electromagnetic force field of board, pyramid, crystal and ionic wave force excited the healing care.

The above ancient African instruments are but a few of the many found in fossil remains, tombs and drawings. In the book *Supersensonics* by Christopher Hill, healing devices are scientifically explained and validated to function. A wholistic Ma'at life with higher human training was required for a healer to operate them. European invaders and grave robbers (archaeologists) believed the devices were toys and games. They can only use instruments that they can understand and validate by their science (primitive cartoon logic). *Magnetism and Its Effects on the Living System* by A. Davis and W. Rawls, Jr. can be used to further understand these devices.

African science is complex and yet based on the physiology of the body and taught systematically.

THE DECK OF CARDS

The Caucasians have reduced the deck of cards to a play toy. They are African in origin and had the symbolism of Egyptian Tarot cards and African astrology and spirituality. The cards were used to teach astrology, astronomy, mathematics, divining, spirituality and to diagnose and treat diseases.

A deck of cards has...

| *Two Colors* | Red and black; active and passive; positive and negative; Male Principle and Female Principle; Masculine Signs (Aries, Gemini, Leo, Libra, |

	Sagittarius, Aquarius and Feminine Signs (Taurus, Cancer, Virgo, Scorpio, Capricorn, Pisces).
Four Suits	Hearts, Clubs, Diamonds, Spades; the four elements (fire, water, air, earth); the four seasons.
Twelve Court Cards	Kings, Queens, Jacks; the twelve months of the year.
52 Cards	The 52 weeks of the year.
13 Cards in each Suit	The 12 signs of the zodiac and the sun; the body of Osiris that was cut into 13 pieces (dis-membered, so we must re-member).
Values of Numbers	Seven and nine. The *number seven (7)* is the center of each suit. Ancients believe there were seven planets. They are heavenly forces (seven planets) that symbolize Chakras; Ma'at and the Seven Halls of Osiris. There are seven days to a week. The *number nine (9)* as the last single number. The Cycle of experience; the number that includes all planets; and is the highest digit. After nine, there is "0" and the sequence starts over with "1." There are nine holes in the body (umbilical navel hole is closed).
The Joker	The "remnant of days" beyond the logical seven times fifty-two, to total our required 365¼ days for the Sun's travel in the solar year. This is more fully explained in the *Mystic Text Book.*
	The Joker is the "highest" symbol in the deck. Usually pictured as fate in a fools clothes. It is rejected or "played wild" in Caucasian card games. Its true significance is identical with that of the "0" or "Fool Card," in Egyptian Tarot. It also symbolizes "1" day that is part of the 365¼ day solar year. It is the spiritual element that completes the earth's existence (365 days).

Basic Characteristics of Personality or Disease

Fire Sign	Hearts = Aries, Leo, Sagittarius
Earth Sign	Spades = Taurus, Virgo, Capricorn
Air Sign	Diamonds = Gemini, Libra, Aquarius
Water Sign	Clubs = Cancer, Scorpio, Pisces

Quality of Personality or Disease

Cardinal (Outgoing, initiators, aggressive, illness) = Aries (Hearts), Cancer (Club), Libra (Diamond), Capricorn (Spade).

Fixed (resist change, originators, severe disease) = Taurus (Spade), Leo (Hearts), Scorpio (Club), Aquarius (Diamond)

Mutable (flexible, versatile, healing is fast) = Gemini (Diamond), Virgo (Spade) Sagittarius (Heart), Pisces (Club)

Suits of Cards
The order corresponds to the Seasons: Hearts, Clubs, Diamonds, Spades or Spring, Summer, Harvest, Winter.

THE MYSTERY SYSTEM

The medical practitioners of Africa received formal education by being initiated in the mystery system. A medical student was selected for initiation just as students are selected for college via scores and personality profiles. The students (initiates) could participate in their education on a general educational level call Exoteric learning or on a higher level called Esoteric.

The mystery system has seven degree (levels or steps) of learning before completion. The first degree educates you in the coarse or base aspects of medicine and is known as Pastorphoros. This system is not confined to medicine and includes all known and unknown sciences. However, the initiate could be educated for a specific area (major) or talent or a combination of areas (majors). In any case, upon competition of the first degree the student advances to the Neocoros degree, which focuses on the structural energy of medicines such as the energy of shapes (squares, pyramids, triangles, obelisks). Then, the Melanophoros degree is studied whereby the student learns the energy forces of non-polarized energy such as the Melanin-DNA energy state, which is created between the death and life state.

In the Kistophorus degree, the student learns how to will the inherent law of plants, crystals metals, colors, magnets, music, etc. In the fifth degree of Balahate, the student learns the science of nature and interactions of alchemic laws. In the sixth degree of Astronomos, the student learns cycles, astrology and the manipulations of the cosmic forces and their reaction in the cells, thoughts, biochemistry, organs, bones, emotions, vitamins and minerals in the body and on the galaxy. In the seventh degree of the Propheta the student learns all the secrets of the higher mystery system and becomes a god (Master, Ph.D.). Interesting to note, the word god is not meant in the European orthodox sense. In African culture, if a chicken had offspring (children) they were called chickens and if God had children (man) they could be called gods. The title of god was earned via the mystery system and the application of Ma'at in the daily life. The course completion could take up to 13 years or more (a combination of high school and college). Today, the course has to be adapted, reduced and translated and put in a language conducive for the social condition Africans are in (White Supremacy). It has to be used as technology for African liberation.

The selection of a student into esoteric mystery system would take from two to three years. Hippocrates spent at the most extreme estimate two years or less in Africa. His knowledge of medicine would have been the esoteric or a general mystery system course. In other words, Greek and Caucasian medicine is based upon the first books (first degree) of African medical science. Yet, with this limited knowledge, Hippocrates cured approximately 3,000 people in his lifetime. He did not know blood circulated in the body. He used the books stolen from Africa along with the information taught by the Priest/Monk health practitioners of the Escalypius Temple cult.

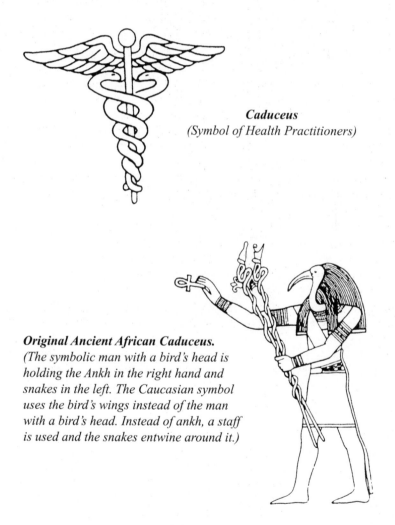

Caduceus
(Symbol of Health Practitioners)

Original Ancient African Caduceus.
(The symbolic man with a bird's head is holding the Ankh in the right hand and snakes in the left. The Caucasian symbol uses the bird's wings instead of the man with a bird's head. Instead of ankh, a staff is used and the snakes entwine around it.)

Section I

Dis-ease
Treatment
and Health

ABCESS

Abscess is the accumulation of pus in a particular part of the body due to infection. An abscess can be externally or internally. They lead to bacterial infection. The infected area becomes swollen, inflamed, and tender. Intermittent fever and chills can be a result of Abscess. Abscess can be in the brain, lungs, abdominal wall, gastrointestinal tract, teeth, gums, ears, tonsils, sinuses, breasts, kidneys, prostate gland, etc.

Supplement	Suggested Dosage	Remarks
Zinc	80 mg., daily in divided doses.	Use for infections.
Garlic capsules	2 capsules 3 times daily.	A natural antibiotic.
Vitamin A	Begin with 100,000 IU for the first 5 days, decrease to 50,000 IU for the next 5 days. Then decrease again to 25,000 IU.	Combats infection.
Vitamin E	400-600 IU.	Good for circulation and increases oxygen in cells.
Germanium	100 mg., daily.	Builds the immune system
MSM	1,000-2,000 mg.	Skin diseases of all types.
VitaminC with Bioflavonoids	6,000-10,000 mg., in daily divided doses.	Aids tissue repair and immunity.
Multiple Vitamins and Minerals	As directed.	Aids healing.
Digestive Enzyme	As directed.	Breaks down waste.

AMINO ACIDS

Lysine	1,000 mg., daily.	Used for infection.

HERBS

Burdock Root, Chaparral, Dandelion Root, Echinacea, Red Clover, Thuja, Yellow Greens.

FOODS
(Eaten Whole or Juiced. Use Proper Food Combining)

Cabbage, Corn, Dandelion Greens, Figs, Lemon.

HOMEOPATHIC

Pyrogenium 7	5 gr., every 24 hours.	Aids excretion of pus.
Hepar Sulphur 7	5 gr., every 48 hours.	Expels pus.

TISSUE SALTS

Ferr. Phos. and Kali. Mur.	Alternate hourly.	Enhances skin cleansing.

ACNE

Acne is a skin inflammation. A sebaceous gland, in each hair follicle produces oil that lubricates the skin. Some of the oil becomes trapped and bacteria grow, which inflames the skin. Adolescents have acne because the sebaceous glands are stimulated by an imbalance of the male hormone at puberty or fermenting food (constipation) in the digestive tract, synthetic chemicals or sex hormones and steroids in the food.

Blackheads form when sebum combines with skin pigments and clogs the pores. When scales under the skin become filled with sebum, white heads appear. White heads can spread under the skin, and rupture, which spreads the inflammation.

Supplement	Suggested Dosage	Remarks
Chromium	200-400 mcg.	Helps reduce infections of the skin.
Lecithin	1 capsule before meals.	Helps use essential fatty acids.
Primrose Oil	As directed.	Helps healing.
Unsaturated Fatty Acids	1 tbsp. cold-pressed or take in capsule form.	Repairs damaged cells.
Zinc Gluconate	30-80 mg., daily.	Heals tissue and combats scarring.
Vitamin A and E	100,000 IU Vitamin A and 400 Vitamin E.	Protective of epithelial (skin) tissue.
Chlorophyll (liquid or tablets)	As directed.	Purifies blood and prevents infections.
Hydrochloric Acid (HCL) with Digestive Enzymes	Take with meals.	Caution: Those with ulcers should not take digestive enzymes containing HCL.
Niacin	100 mg., 3 times daily with meals.	Increase blood flow to the skin.
Vitamin B Complex (high potency) with extra B$_6$ and Pantothenic Acid	50 mg., 3 times daily.	Builds healthy skin tone.
Vitamin C with Bioflavonoids	3,000-5,000 mg., daily in divided doses.	Improves immunity.
MSM	1,000-3,000 mg.	Fights skin diseases.

AMINO ACIDS

Lysine	1,000 mg., daily.	Combats infection and skin disease.

HERBS

Burdock Root, Dandelion Root, Echinacea, English Walnut, Marigold, Wild Strawberry.

FOOD

Cabbage, Corn, Dandelion Greens, Lemon, Soybeans.

HOMEOPATHIC

Calcarea Phosphorica and Pulsatilla 7	2 gr.	Promotes healthy skin.
Kali Bromatum 4	2 gr., alternate days and at night.	Maintains healthy skin

Homeopathic Crème, Crème Homeodora		Cleanses skin.

TISSUE SALTS

Ferr. Phos. and Nat. Phos.	Alternate.	Inflammation.
Calc. Phos. and Silicea	Alternate.	Stabilizes tissue.

ADRENAL GLAND EXHAUSTION

The adrenal glands are small glands. There is one on top of each kidney. The gland secretes hormones and can be exhausted owing to states of stress (emotional, mental, physical), hyperactivity, disease, oppression, under-nutrition, crisis, microwave usage, anger, violence, fights (verbal/physical), drugs, radiation, synthetic chemicals, etc. The adrenal has two parts the Medulla (Male Principle), which secretes norepinephrine and adrenaline, they increases metabolism in order to adapt to stress and the Cortex (Female Principle), which adjusts natural sugar metabolism and regulates levels of steroid hormones (aldosterone, estrogen, DHEA, testosterone, progesterone).

Supplements	Suggested Dosage	Remarks
Panthothenic Acid	500-2,000 mg., daily.	Regulates stress hormones.
CoEnzyme Q$_{10}$	30 mg., 3 times daily.	Helps regulate glands.
Vitamin B-Complex	100 mg., daily.	Anti-stress.
Germanium	100-300 mg., daily.	Cleanses glands.
Vitamin C or	3,000 mg., daily.	Protects nervous system.
Ester C	1,500 mg., daily.	
Evening Primrose	4 to 6 capsules daily.	Reduces stress & irritability
Potassium	99 mg., daily.	Helps stablilze nerves.
Zinc	50 mg.	Enhances glandular function.
Vanadyl Sulfate	100 mg.	Regulates energy level.
Manganese	10-50 mg.	Useful for nerves, hormones and sex glands.

GLANDULARS

Adrenal	As directed	Nourishes adrenal glands.

AMINO ACIDS

Tyrosine	500 mg., daily.	Relieves stress.

ADRENAL STRESS AND DISEASE

The adrenal glands are triangular-shaped organs that sit on the top of each kidney. The gland has two sections. The outer section is responsible for the production of cortisone. The medulla or central section secretes adrenaline.

The adrenal cortex helps to maintain electrolyte, salt and water balance. It is also involved in the metabolism of carbohydrates and the regulation of blood sugar. The cortex produces a sex hormone similar to that secreted by the testes.

The Medulla of the adrenal gland produces the hormone epinephrine, (adrenaline). It is used when the organs inside the body are stressed and whenever you are under emotional, mental and/or spiritual stress. The type of stress and duration of stress, such as social stress (job, marriage, family, money), emotional stress (low self esteem, racism) spiritual stress (conflict with life's purpose) and disease stress (High Blood pressure, drugs) can increase the aging of the internal organs and make you old. One has to be nutritionally able to endure stressors or else the stress will cause a disease. Adrenaline speeds up the rate of metabolism in order to help the body cope with stressful situations and stressful diseases.

The health of the adrenal glands can be impaired due to extensive use of cortisone therapy for non-endocrine diseases, such as arthritis and asthma. Excessive or long-term use of cortisone drugs causes deterioration or shrinkage of the adrenal gland. Adrenocortical failure can be caused by pituitary disease and tuberculosis.

When the adrenal cortex is under-active, it can cause Addison's disease. Discoloration and darkening of the skin is common in Addison's disease. There may be discoloration of knees, vagina, mouth, elbows, scars, skin folds, and creases in the palms. There may be dark vertical lines on the fingernail and darker hair. There may be a decrease in body hair (i.e., under the arms), a loss of appetite, mood swings, dizziness or fainting, fatigue, an inability to cope with stress and nausea. The individual can be cold all the time.

Cushing's syndrome is caused by an overactive adrenal cortex. Those with this disease can be heavy in the buttocks, abdomen, and face, and have skinny limbs. Muscular weakness and deterioration of muscle mass are typical of this syndrome. Dark spots may appear on the face, and the eyelids may be swollen. There is an increased growth of body hair. Women may grow mustaches and beards. A "Cushinoid" appearance is frequently present with excessive or prolonged cortisone use. People with Cushing's get illnesses easily and have poor healing ability. Cushing's causes thin skin, stretch marks and bruising.

The symptoms of Adrenal function problems are dizziness, weakness, lethargy, allergies, headaches, blood sugar problems, food cravings, weakness and forgetfulness. A normal systolic (top number) blood pressure is approximately 10 mm higher (150) when you are standing than when you are lying down. To test adrenal function, compare two blood pressure readings—one while lying down and one while standing. Rest for five minutes, lying down before taking the reading. Stand up and then take the blood pressure. If the blood pressure is lower after standing, this can indicate reduced adrenal gland function. The degree to which the blood pressure drops is proportionate to the degree of hypo-adrenalism (under active adrenals).

Supplement	Suggested Dosage	Remarks
Pantothenic Acid (Vitamin B$_5$)	100 mg., 3 times daily	The adrenal glands function with Pantothenic Acid.
Vitamin B Complex	100 mg., twice daily	Improves adrenal function.
Vitamin C	4,000 to 10,000 mg., daily in divided doses.	Helps glands to function.
Chlorophyll	As directed	Purifies blood and increases oxygen to cells.
Coenzyme Q$_{10}$	60 mg., daily	Carries oxygen to all glands.
Germanium	100 mg., daily	Improves immunity.
Multiple Vitamin and Mineral Complex with Beta-Carotene	15,000 IU daily	Activates immunity.
Copper	3 mg., daily.	Activates immunity.
Zinc	50 mg., daily.	Activates immunity.

GLANDULARS

Raw Spleen Tissue and Pituitary Glandulars.	As directed	Enhances the healing process.
Raw Adrenal extract or tablets	As directed.	Helps build and repair the adrenal glands.
Liver (Organic)	As directed.	Nourishes the Liver.

AMINO ACIDS

L-Tyrosine	1,000 mg., on empty stomach.	Relieves adrenal gland stress.

HERBS

American Sanicle, Barberry, Bear's Garlic, Black Cohosh, Blue Cohosh, Blue Vervain, Boneset, Chervil, Cleavers, Ergot, European Mistletoe, Garden Violet, Garlic, Hawthorn, Onion, Parsley, Rue, Scotch Broom, Skullcap, Storksbill, Wild Black Cherry.

FOOD

Barley, Broccoli, Cantaloupe, Carrots, Cauliflower, Celery, Cranberries, Cucumbers, Endives, Garlic, Guavas, Jackfruit, Jujube, Kumquats, Nectarines, Oranges, Parsley, Peaches, Pears, Peppers, Pineapple, Raspberries, Spinach, Squash (Summer), Strawberries, Tangerines, tomatoes, Turnip Greens.

HOMEOPATHIC

Rhus. Tox. 9 (Poison Oak)	5 gr., every 48 hours.	Used for skin disease.
Ignatia 7 and Cocculus 7	2 gr. Alternate, take in the a.m.	Expels cellular waste.
Arnica 8	5 gr., every 48 hours.	Promotes healing.

TISSUE SALTS

Kali. Phos.	Daily.	Helps expel pus.
Ferr. Phos. and Silicea	As directed or twice daily.	Cleanses and heals skin.

AIDS
(ACQUIRED IMMUNE DEFICIENCY SYNDROME)

For further information, see AIDS-A-Black Un-Dis-ease.

Supplement	Suggested Dosage	Remarks
Multimineral (high potency) with Omit Zinc plus	50 mg., daily.	Hypoallergenic form is best. iron supplements if fever is present.
Copper	3 mg., daily.	
Garlic Tablets	2 capsules with meals 3 times daily	Antibiotic and blood purifier.
Germanium	200 mcg daily.	Improves interferon and cell oxygen supply.
Protein Supplement (Free from amino acids)	As directed.	Protein in this form is digested.
Selenium	200 mcg daily.	Destroys free radicals.
Vitamin B Complex plus B_{12} and B_6 (pyridoxine)	100 mg., 3 times daily in tablet form under doctor's supervision.	Helps the nervous system and brain function.
Vitamin C plus Bioflavonoids	10,000 mg., in divided doses throughout the day.	Use buffered, powdered ascorbic acid.
Vitamin A	50,000 IU daily.	Reduce dosage if known to have liver disease, and use caution if using pill form.
Vitamin E	200 IU daily, increasing to 800 IU.	Emulsified form is readily and rapidly assimilated. Vitamins A and E destroy purities and help immune function.
Acidophilus	3 times daily. Take a high-powered form.	Supplies bacteria for intestinal tract.
Coenzymes Q_{10}	100 mg., daily.	Enhances immune system.
Essential Fatty Acids	As directed.	Unsaturated fatty acids such as Primrose Oil, Black Currant Oil, Salmon Oil and Linseed Oil are vital.
Proteolytic Enzymes	6 tablets between meals.	Aids digestion.
Quercetin plus Bromelin	As directed.	Decreases reactions to certain foods, pollens and other allergens.
Digestive Enzyme Formula	Take with meals.	Aids digestion.
RNA-DNA Complex	As directed.	Builds healthy tissue.

GLANDULARS

Raw Thymus plus multiglandulars, including Spleen	As directed.	Strengthens glands.

AMINO ACIDS

L-Carnitine, L-Cysteine,	As directed on label.	Improves immune function.

| L-Methionine and L-Ornithine | Take on an empty stomach. with 500 mg., Vitamin C. and 50 mg., Vitamin B_6. | Ornithine should not be used by children. |
| Lysine | 500 mg. | Infection. |

HERBS
Burdock, Chaparral, Comfrey, Dandelion Root, Echinacea, Elecampane, Gingko, Ginseng, Goldenseal, Milk Thistle, Pau D'Arco, Pleurisy, Red Clover, St. John's Wort, Saw Palmetto, Suma, Yohimbe (women should combine Yohimbe with Damiana).

FOOD
Beet Greens, Broccoli, Cauliflower, Dandelion Greens, Dates, Figs, Guava, Kale, Lemon, Mustard Greens Peaches, Pears, Rice, Rye, Turnip Greens.

HOMEOPATHIC

| Bryonia 9 | 5 gr., every 48 hours. | Maintains skin moisture. |
| Aestus P.C. and Calcarea Carbonica 7 | 2 gr., alternate. | Restores skin vitality. |

TISSUE SALTS

Nat. Mur. and Kali. Phos	Twice daily.	Stabilizes nutrients.
Silicea	Daily.	Heals tissue.
Ferr. Phos. and Kali. Mur.	Alternate.	Increases nutrients' absorption.

AGING

Aging is a natural process of all living organisms. Disease does not come with old age. There are old people with diseases. The body's utilization of and absorption of vitamins, minerals, amino acids and digestive enzymes decreases with age. The body wears out.

Supplement	Suggested Dosage	Remarks
Multiple Vitamin and Mineral with trace minerals		Vital nutrients.
Vitamin A	25,000 IU daily.	Protects and heals tissue.
Beta-Carotene	15,000 IU daily.	Prevents disesase.
Selenium	200 mg., daily.	Stops free radical damage.
Calcium Asporate or Chelate	1,500 mg., daily.	Helps to prevent bone loss and good for normal heart function.
Magnesium	75 mg., daily	Good for heart, nerves, lungs and depression
Vitamin D	600-1,000 mg., daily.	Stabilizes bones and nerves.
Coenzyme Q_{10}	100-200 mg.	Helps circulation. Improves cellular oxygenation.
Lecithin	1tbsp. with meals or 4-6 capsules daily.	Enhances brain function and memory. Protects nervous system cells and emulsifies fat.

Nutritional Brewer's Yeast	Start with ½ tsp and work up.	A source of B Vitamins.
Germanium	60 mg., twice daily.	An antioxidant and immune system enhancer.
Lactobacillus Bulgaricus	As directed.	Enhances liver function and digestion.
Digestive enzymes (with meals)	After meals, as directed.	Aids digestion. For ulcers, avoid enzymes with HCL.
Vegetable Protein (Soy free powder)	As directed.	Vital for health.
RNA-DNA	As directed.	Should not be used if you have elevated serum uric acid because you may have gout. Helps build healthy cells.
Vitamin C plus Bioflavonoids	4,000-10,000 mg., daily in divided doses.	An antioxidant and immune system enhancer.
Vitamin E	Start with 200 IU. Slowly increase dosage to 800 IU daily.	Helps utilize oxygen and aids vitality.

GLANDULARS

Raw Thymus	500 mg., daily.	Stimulates the immune system.

AMINO ACIDS

L-Methionine	500 mg., twice daily on an empty stomach.	Helps build tissue and aids liver.
L-Carnitine	500 mg., twice daily on an empty stomach.	Aids heart and use of fatty acids.
L-Cysteine	500 mg., twice daily on an empty stomach.	Maintains skin texture and glucose usage.
Tyrosine	500 mg., twice daily on an empty stomach.	Brain function.

HERBS

Alfalfa, Bilberry, Burdock, Echinacea, Fo-Ti, Ginseng, Goldenseal, Hawthorn, Milk Thistle, St. John's Wort, Sassafras, Suma.

FOOD

Fresh vegetables, fruits and whole grains of all types.

HOMEOPATHIC

Baryta Carbonica and Aurum	As directed.	Aids metabolism, colds and irritability.

TISSUE SALTS

Silicea and Calc. Flour.	Both twice daily.	Strengthens bones and skin.

ALCOHOLISM
(ALCOHOL ADDICTION)

Alcoholism (alcohol addiction) means that a person will go through physical withdrawal if they stop drinking alcohol. Alcohol addiction is a mental, physical and spiritual dependency, with many negative repercussions that affect marriage, parenting, jobs, relationships, sexuality and can cause violent episodes. Alcoholism causes many emotional problems aside from low self-esteem, self-hatred and denial of the reality of your life. Alcohol is a socially approved poison that people are taught to want and drink, it can lead to a holistic craving.

Alcohol causes the liver to get inflamed (hepatitis) then the liver gets hard (cirrhosis) and finally it is destroyed. Drinking alcohol damages all cells, tissue, nerves, organs and bones and kills brain cells. Drinking gradually causes the liver to lose its ability to produce digestive enzymes, metabolize oil soluble Vitamins A, D, E and K, neutralize toxins, store energy (glycogen) and absorb fats and proteins. Alcohol is a legally approved recreational drug. Alcohol consumption in the form of beer, wine and whiskey is anti-health and anti-life. Men and women that intend to have children should not drink because alcohol causes birth defects. Pregnant women must not drink.

Supplement	Suggested Dosage	Remarks
Multiple Vitamin and Mineral with Selenium	200 mcg daily.	Selenium is an important trace mineral that builds immune function.
Niacinamide	200-1,000 mg., daily.	
Lecithin (Choline and Inositol)	1 capsule or 1 tbsp. before meals.	Enhances brain function. Helps correct fatty liver degeneration.
Choline Complex, Acetyl Complex or Phosphatidyl	As directed on label	Reduces fatty liver damage and enhances liver function.
Vitamin A-D-E	25,000 IU Vitamin A; 400 IU Vitamin D; 400-1,2000 IU Vitamin E.	Vitamins A, D and E are poorly absorbed when the liver is damaged.
Vitamin C with Bioflavonoids	3,000-10,000 mg., daily.	Increases healing in divided doses potential.
Calcium	2,000 mg., daily.	Has a sedative effect and calms nerves.
Magnesium	1,000 mg., 3 times daily.	Deficiency due to alcohol abuse.
Pantothenic Acid (B$_5$)	100 mg., 3 times daily.	
Thiamine (B$_1$)	200 mg., 3 times daily.	Alcoholics are deficient in B vitamins, especially B$_1$.
Vitamin B-Complex	50-100 mg.	Nourishes nervous system.
Essential fatty acids (Primrose Oil)	2 capsules with meals.	A good source of essential fatty acids.
Vegetable Protein (Soy free powder)	As directed on label.	Amino acids in proteins aid in withdrawal and are needed for brain and liver function. Protein is necessary for generation of liver cells.
Maxidophilus or Megadophilus Bulgaricum I. B.	As directed on label.	Needed for proper or digestion. Aids the damaged liver.

| Vanadium and Chromium | As directed on label. | Reduces craving for sweets. |

GLANDULARS

Raw Brain	As directed.	Helps repair brain cells.
Raw Duodenum	As directed.	Aids digestion.
Raw Liver	As directed.	Aids digestion.
Raw Pancreas	As directed.	Aids digestion.

AMINO ACIDS

L-Cysteine	Take on an empty stomach. Work up to 1 gr., daily.	Protects against effects of alcohol.
L-Glutamine	Take 3 gr., with vitamin B_6 (pyridoxine) on an empty stomach.	Decreases craving for alcohol. Good for depression and memory.
L-Methionine	Must be taken on an empty stomach and is best taken with small amounts of Vitamins B_6 and C.	Detoxifies liver and prevents fatty acid buildup.

HERBS

Dandelion Root, Echinacea, Feverfew, Goldenseal, Kudzu, Milk Thistle, Nerve Root, Passion Flower, Quassia, Thyme.

FOOD

Broccoli, Brussels Sprouts, Collard Greens, Dandelion Greens, Kale, Mustard Greens, Okra, Oranges, Peaches, Pears, Quince, Raw Peanuts, Turnip Greens.

HOMEOPATHIC

Nux. Vomica 8 and Spiritus Quercus Glandium 7	As directed.	Used for addictions.
Stramonium 7	5 gr.	Craving.
Ethyl Alcohol 7	2 gr., 1 hour before party or event that has alcohol.	Curbs alcohol craving.
Paullinia	2 gr., half-hour before event that has alcohol.	Reduces craving.

TISSUE SALTS

Silicea	As directed.	Heals nerves and tissue.
Kali. Sulph.	As directed.	Normalizes tissue.
Nat. Mur.	As directed.	Helps reduce moodiness.
Kali. Phos.	As directed.	Nerves, shakes.

ALLERGIES

An allergy is the inability of the body to handle a substance that is not normally harmful. The substance that causes the allergic response is called an *allergen*. The problem with allergens is whether they are organic and/or *absent of synthetic chemicals*. The allergens causes the body *to reach* its threshold (tolerance) of synthetic chemicals, resulting in allergies. Within the body, synthetic chemicals are mixed, creating *another synthetic* that causes allergic reactions. The synthetic chemicals can be *reacting upon* each other, causing allergic reactions. The allergic person may be a host to synthetics at war with each other. Allergic reactions to synthetics in foods are a natural response and not disease reactions. The *Food Industry* and *Drug Industry* do not blame themselves for the allergy causing chemicals that they have made. Food and Drug industries let the public believe that an evil allergen has created the allergy problem instead of the synthetic foods. Every response of the body is its attempt to defend itself.

The accumulation of synthetic toxic chemicals in the air, water, soil, and food can trigger an allergic response. The allergen is merely the straw that broke the camel's back (a trigger agent).

The body makes and stores chemicals from the food, air, water and soil Each change in emotions, thought and spirit causes a different ratio of chemicals, fats, hormones, vitamins and minerals. A change in ratios plus the change brought on by what has been eaten can cause an allergic response. In any case, a true test of food allergies is best after a fast and a colonic irrigation. The *organic* food eaten after this and the body's reaction to it could be called an allergy.

When you eliminate so-called *allergic foods* from your diet, you are also decreasing the nutrients you need. A decrease in nutrients weakens the body and makes you more susceptible to allergies.

Any substance can cause an allergy. The common allergens are molds, grass pollen, lanolin (sheep fat), common drugs (aspirin, penicillin), vaccinations, insect bites and stings, metals (nickel, etc.), dust, animal hair, foods (shellfish, strawberries, eggs), white sugar, milk, beef, bananas, caffeine, tomatoes, white rice, wheat, oats, citrus fruits, processed and refined chemicalized foods) and additives (sulfur dioxide, benzoic acid, annatto, BHT-BHA, vanillin, monosodium glutamate, eucalyptol, benzyldehyde, F, D, and C Yellow #5 dyes). Added to this, allergens can cause mental illness, violent outbursts, mood swings, schizophrenia, hallucinations, eczema, hay fever, hives, asthma, headaches, heart palpitations, upset stomachs, diarrhea, itching, swelling, etc.

Supplements	Suggested	Dosage Remarks
Multiple Vitamin and Minerals	As directed.	Use hypoallergenic product.
Potassium	99 mg., daily.	Aids adrenal gland function.
Vegetable Protein Supplement	As directed.	Vegetable protein is easily absorbed and assimilated by the body.
Vitamin B-Complex	100 mg., daily and up.	
Pantothenic Acid (B_5) and B_{12})	100 mg., 3 times daily.	
Vitamin C with Bioflavonoids	2,000 mg., and up, 3 times daily	Enhances immune function.
Bee Pollen (raw crude pollen)	2 tsp. daily, or take in capsule form, beginning with a few granules at a time.	Builds up a resistance to pollen.
Vitamins B_6 (Pyridoxine) and C	50 mg., each daily.	Essential for immunity.
Manganese Chelate	2-10 mg.	Essential for nerve, gland and sex organs.

Vegetarian Acidophilus	As directed.	Take on an empty stomach for easier access into the small intestine.
Calcium	1,500 – 2,000 mg., daily.	Reduces stress.
Magnesium	750 mg., daily.	
Bromelin	Take with meals.	Those with ulcers should take a brand without hydrochloric acid (HCL).
Beta Carotene	1,500 IU daily.	Stimulates immune response.
Quercitin	500 mg., twice daily.	A co-bioactive bioflavonoid that builds immunity and decreases reactions to certain foods, pollens, and other allergens.
Vitamin A	10,000 IU daily.	Vital for proper immune function.
Vitamin D	600 IU daily.	Vital in calcium metabolism.
Vitamin E	600 IU daily.	Necessary for proper immune function.
Zinc	50 mg., daily.	Enhances immune function.
Coenzyme Q_{10}	100 mg., daily.	Aids cellular oxygenation and immune function.
Germanium	60 mg., daily.	Enhances immune response.

GLANDULARS

Raw Adrenal, Raw Thymus, and Raw Spleen	500 mg., each, twice daily.	Stimulates immune function.

AMINO ACIDS

L-Tyrosine and L-Cysteine	500 mg., each on empty stomach daily.	Vitamins B_6 and C aid in assimilation.

HERBS

Burdock, Centaury, Cubeb, Dandelion, Eyebright, Fringe Tree, Goldenseal (those with ragweed should avoid), Milk Thistle, Papaya, Phytolacca, Skunk Cabbage.

FOODS

Organic fruits and vegetables as much as possible. Eat what can be tolerated.

HOMEOPATHIC

Kali Iodatum 7, Allium Cepa 7 and Naphthalinum 7	2 gr., once a day.	Relieves symptoms.

TISSUE SALTS

Kali. Mur.	As directed.	Eczema like.
Ferr. Phos.		Hot, dry throat and temperature.
Ferr. Phos. and Nat. Mur.	As directed.	Hay Fever and running nose.

A book such as *Allergies* by Graham-Bonnalie is a useful guide.

ALZHEIMER'S DISEASE/SENILE DEMENTIA

In Alzheimer's Disease or Senile Dementia, the memory and abstract thinking is deteriorated. In Alzheimer's, there is a loss of the ability to communicate and focus on ideas, people or situations. There are wide mood and thought swings, with a loss of where you are and what date and time it is. It causes the inability to recognize family and/or friends. There can be incontinence of bowel movements and bladder (needs to wear a diaper). In the later stages, the individual's health slowly deteriorates until they are incapacitated. The untreated person usually will die within five years.

The brain has physical changes. In the brain's memory center (Hippocampus), the nerve fibers are tangled. This stops messages from being carry to and from the brain. Many times, a series of unnoticed and notice strokes cause Alzheimer's. The arteries leading to the brain can get hard (arteriosclerosis) and/or clogged with waste (atherosclerosis) as well as the veins (varicose), which can lead to Alzheimer's. A nutritional imbalance caused by a junk food diet affects the body and the brain resulting in deficiencies of Potassium, Zinc, Boron, Vitamin B Complex, especially B_{12} and Selenium. These deficiencies have been noted from autopsies of Alzheimer victims. These victims also had high quantities of Aluminum, Silicon, Sulfur, Bromine and Calcium in the brain. These can cause a high conductance of electricity that wears out the covering of the nerves, reducing their efficiency to carry information. Other diseases such as hypothyroidism, syphilis, brain tumors, as well as blood clots to the brain and drugs can cause an Alzheimer's reaction. A child that has been breastfed and eats natural foods will more than likely never become a victim of this modern dis-ease.

Supplement	Suggested Dosage	Remarks
Niacinamide	300 mg.	Dilates vessels, which increases nutrients to the brain.
Magnesium	500 mg.	Aids transmission of nerve impulse.
Potassium	99 mg.	Aids nervous system and electrochemical impulses.
Zinc	50 mg.	Enhances electrical transmission.
Manganese	2 mg.	Increases health of nerves.
Selenium	200 mcg. daily.	Improves nerve function.
Vanadium	100 mg., daily.	Provides energy to brain.
Boron	3 mg., daily.	Stabilizes nerves.
Vitamin B Complex	100 mg.	Enhances brain function.
Vitamin B_6	50 mg.	Helps in the digestion of food.
Vitamin B_{12}	1,000 mg.	Helps nerves and brain function.

Vitamin C with Bioflavonoids	6,000-10,000 IU daily, in divided doses.	Aids immune function and increases energy levels.
Vitamin E	Start at 400 IU daily and increase to 800 IU.	Facilities transport oxygen to the brain cells.
Coenzyme Q_{10}	200 mg., daily.	Carries oxygen to cells and helps in generating cellular energy.
Germanium	200 mg., daily.	Aids immune function.
Kelp	5 tablets daily.	Supplies trace minerals.
Vegetable Protein Powder (Soy free)	As directed.	Enhances brain function and tissue repair.
RNA-DNA	200 mg., RNA; 100 mg., DNA.	The brain's cellular building blocks.

GLANDULARS

Parathyroid	As directed.	Aid electrical flow.
Pituitary	As directed.	Stimulates energy to tissues.

AMINO ACIDS

Glutamine	2,000 mg., daily.	Restores memory, repairs brain cells.
Taurine	1,000 mg.	Nerve transmission and anticonvulsant.
GABA	750 mg.	Helps control behavior.
Glycine	500-1,000 mg.	Anti-anxiety.

HERBS

Butcher's Broom, Gingko, Ginseng, Gotu Kola, St. John's Wort.

FOODS

Almond, Avocado, Barley, Beans, Beets, Brazil Nuts, Cabbage, Collard Greens, Corn, Eggplant, Lettuce, Peas, Raw Peanuts, Rye, Turnip Greens, Turnips.

HOMEOPATHIC

Kali. Phosphoricum	2 gr., in the mornings.	Mental fatigue and function.
Anacardium and Cocculus	As directed.	Anxiety and nerviousness.
Lycopodium (Club Moss)7	5 gr., Sundays upon awakening.	Anxiety and aggressiveness.
BarytaCarbonxica 9	5 gr., Thursdays upon awakening.	Moodiness.

TISSUE SALTS

Kali. Phos. and Mag. Phos.	Daily For nerves.
Silicea	Daily.

ANEMIA

Anemia is the reduced number of circulating red blood cells, hemoglobin and volume in the blood. It is not a dis-ease, but a symptom of various diseases. The disease may develop slowly and the person may adjust to it and function with irritability, loss of appetite, constipation, problems concentrating and headaches. The noticeable symptoms are drowsiness, slight fever, pale fingernail beds, dizziness, sore tongue, angina pectoris, loss of sexual interest, fast heartbeats, menstruation may stop, indigestion, paleness under the eyelid, depression and weakness.

Anemia can be caused by hormonal disorders, liver damage, radiation, ulcers, drugs, surgery, hemorrhoids, heavy bleeding during menstruation or between menstruation cycles, infections, diverticular disease, thyroid disorders, bone marrow disease, rheumatoid arthritis and/or repeated pregnancies.

Supplements	Suggested Dosage	Remarks
Iron (Vegetable Source)	15-65 mg.	Easily absorbed.
Liquid Iron (Vegetable Source)	2 tsp. daily.	Easily absorbed.
Manganese	As directed.	Converts to Iron.
Blackstrap Molasses	1 tbsp. twice daily for adults; for children and babies, add 1 tsp to vegetable milk.	Has iron and essential B Vitamins
Brewer's Yeast	As directed on label.	Rich in basic nutrients.
Copper plus	2 mg., daily.	Copper is used in red blood cell production.
Zinc	30 mg., daily.	
Raw Spleen Concentrate	As directed.	
Vitamin A plus	10,000 IU daily.	Vital for blood cells.
Beta-Carotene	15,000 IU daily.	
Vitamin E emulsion	700 IU daily or take in capsule form.	Take emulsion for easier assimilation Helps utilize red blood cells.
Folic acid	800 mcg., twice daily.	For red blood cell formation.
Biotin	300 mcg., twice daily.	
Vitamin B_{12}	2,000 mcg., 3 times daily. Injections are the most effective or take in sublingual form.	Essential in red blood cell production.
Vitamin B complex with	50 mg., of each 3 times daily.	Pantothenic acid and
extra Pantothenic acid (B_5) and	100 mg., 3 times daily.	Pyridoxine build red blood
Vitamin B_6 (Pyridoxine)	50 mg., 3 times daily.	cells.
Vitamin C	3,000-10,000 mg., daily.	Needed for iron absorption.
Betaine Hydrochloride	After meals.	Helps assimilate Iron and B_{12}.

GLANDULARS

Raw Liver	500 mg., twice daily.	Aids red blood cell production.

AMINO ACIDS

Methione	As directed.	Cleanses liver.

HERBS

Alfalfa, Barberry, Comfrey, Dandelion, Elecampane, Milk Thistle, Mullein, Nettle, Oregon Grape, Red Raspberry, St. John's Wort, Thyme.

FOODS

Apples, Apricots, Beets, Blackberries, Blueberries, Broccoli, Cabbage, Cauliflower, Cherries, Collards, Currants, Dandelion Greens, Dates, Endive, Figs, Grapefruit, Guava, Kale, Macadamia Nuts, Mustard Greens, Peppers, Turnip Greens, Raisins.

HOMEOPATHIC

China 4	As directed.	Used for skin diseases.

TISSUE SALTS

Ferr. Phos.	As directed.	Essential for iron anemia.

A book such as *Overcoming Anemia,* by Gregory Hall is a useful resource.

APPETITE (POOR)

Mental, emotional and spiritual factors such as suppressed anger, self-hatred, guilt, depression, episodes of White Racism, negative spiritual energy, being sick, stress, boredom, undefined Slavery Trauma feelings, nutrition deficiencies, legal and illegal drug use, an illness, toxins from the environment (air, water, chemicals) and fumes from chemicals in buildings (school, where you work, etc.) and/or being poor can lead to a poor appetite. The sight of food can cause an undernourished person to lose their appetite. A person switching from junk food to healthy food may lose their appetite because the taste of whole foods is different. Past arguments or negative feelings and/or behaviors at a previous meal can cause recurrent bad moods and loss of appetite. The appetite can be stimulated with a pleasant eating environment and eye appealing and good tasting food and the elimination of factors causing a poor appetite.

Supplement	Suggested Dosage	Remarks
Multiple Vitamin and Mineral	As directed.	Necessary nutrients.
Vitamin A	25,000 IU daily.	Cleanses and protects.
Calcium	1,500 mg., daily.	Helps maintain healthy digestive tract.
Magnesium	750 mg., daily.	Aids digestion.
Vitamin B Complex	100 mg., or more daily.	Relieves stress. Increases appetite.
Zinc	80 mg., daily.	Increases appetite and the taste of foods.
Copper	3 mg., daily.	Needed to balance Zinc level.
Vitamin B_1	10-25 mg.	Stimulates appetite.
Vitamin B_2	10-100 mg.	Stimulates appetite.
Nutritional Brewer's Yeast	Start with ½ tsp.	Improves the appetite.
Vegetable Protein Powder (Soy Free)	As directed.	Helps tissue. Acts as an appetite stimulant.

GLANDULARS

Raw Pancreas, Raw Liver		Aids digestion.

AMINO ACIDS

Histidine	1,000-2,000 mg.	Aids stimulation.

Arginine	500-1,000 mg.	Increases use of energy and thus improves appetite.

HERBS

Alfalfa, Allspice, Anise, Artichoke, Caraway, Celery, Coriander, Cardamom, Dill, Goldenseal, Thyme, Milk Thistle, Parsley, Plum, Rosemary, Savory, Tarragon, Wormwood.

FOOD

Apricots, Asparagus, Beet Greens, Broccoli, Cabbage, Cantaloupe, Carrots, Corn, Dandelion Greens, Kale, Lettuce, Mustard Greens, Oranges, Papaya, Peas, Yams, Turnip Greens.

HOMEOPATHIC

Wheat, Barley, Oats	1st Centesimal 10 drops before every meal.	Helps stimulate appetite.
Lycopodium 7	5 gr., every 10 days.	Aids loss of appetite

TISSUE SALTS

Calc. Fluor.	As directed.	Nourish digestive organs and glands.
Nat. Phos. and Kali Sulph.	Alternate.	Aids digestion and appetite problems.

ARTERIOSCLEROSIS/ATHEROSCLEROSIS

Arteriosclerosis (artery, sclero = hard) is the thickening, hardening and loss of flexibility of the arteries. There can be an accumulation of Calcium on the inside wall of the artery. Atherosclerosis is the accumulation of fatty substances, carbohydrates, fibrous tissue, blood and blood products in the artery. Both conditions are completely avoidable and related to eating junk foods. Both conditions cause the artery to narrow, which reduces the blood supply to cells, tissues, organs and bones. This causes high blood pressure, cells starve (ischemia), arteries get blocked, which results in heart attacks (myocardial infarction), strokes (cerebrovascular accidents), coronary disease (angina), and death. Toxic metal from public drinking water, copper and/or aluminum plumbing (lead), and cooking utensils, lead-glazed ceramics, polluted air, etc. can deposit on the artery walls causing them to get hard.

Narrowed arteries can cause legs to feel heavy and/or painful while walking with the symptoms stopping when you sit down. The symptoms vary based upon the location. There can be weakness, numbness, aching muscles, cramp-like sensations, fatigue, pain and coldness in areas such legs, ankles, thighs, hips, etc. It can affect the hearing, vision and sex organs.

If there are narrowed arteries in the legs, there will be a weak pulse felt behind the knee, on the top of the foot and/or the inner part of the ankle.

Supplement	Suggested Dosage	Remarks
Niacinamide	500 mg., 3 times daily.	Dilates and increases blood flow.

Lecithin	1 tbsp or 2 capsules with meals.	Dissolves fat.
Vegetarian Multiple Vitamin and Mineral		Vital nutrients.
Choline	500-10,000 mg.	Lowers lipid (fat) content of blood.
Calcium	1,500 mg., daily.	Use chelate or asporotate.
Magnesium	750 mg., daily.	
L-Methionine and L-Cysteine	500 mg., each, daily.	Should be taken on an empty stomach. Take with Vitamin C or with Vitamin B_6
	for easier assimilation.	
Unsaturated Fatty Acids	As directed.	Makes blood slippery. Aids circulation.
Vitamin B Complex	100 mg., 3 times daily.	B vitamins work better as a complex. Niacin (B_3) dilates the small arteries (arteri-
oles).		
Zinc Chelate	50 mg., daily.	Helps cleansing and healing.
Copper Chelate	3 mg., daily.	
Coenzyme Q_{10}	100 mg., daily.	Enhances tissue oxygenation.
Germanium	200 mg., daily.	Lowers cholesterol and aids cellular oxygenation. Vitamin
C (buffered)	6,000-10,000 mg., in daily divided doses.	Helps cleanse arteries.
Garlic tablets	As directed.	Has an effect on lipids (fat).
Multidigestive Enzymes	Take with meals.	Aids in proper digestion.
Proteolytic Enzymes	Take between meals.	Helps in destroying free radicals. Aids digestive function.
Selenium	200 mcg daily.	Enhances Vitamin E usage.
Vitamin A and E Vitamin A:	25,000 IU;	Increase slowly. Helps get rid of cellular waste accumulation.
	Vitamin E: 400-1,000 IU.	

GLANDULARS

Raw Liver	As directed.	Helps absorb nutrients and detoxifies.

AMINO ACIDS

Histidine	1,000-2,000 mg.	Dilates arteries. Increases blood flow.
Arginine	500-1,000 mg.	Fat metabolizer.
Carnitine	1,000-2,000 mg.	Useful in circulatory disorders.

HERBS

Artichoke, Cayenne, Chickweed, Currants, Gotu Kola, Hawthorn, Horsetail, Hyssop, Nutmeg, Shepherd's Purse.

FOODS

Asparagus, Beans, Beets, Blackberries, Cantaloupe, Carrots, Cherries, Collard Greens, Cucumbers, Dandelion Greens, Dulse, Endives, Gooseberries, Grapefruit, Kale, Mustard Greens, Okra, Oranges, parsley, Pineapple, Pomegranate, Pumpkins, Quince, Rhubarb, Spinach, Strawberries, Sunflower Seeds, Tangerines, Turnips, Wheat.

HOMEOPATHIC

Baryta Carbonica and Aurum Mettallicum 7	2 gr., alternate and take in the a.m.	Used for cleansing vascular system.
Cupressus 7 and Kali Iodatum 7	2 gr., alternate and take in the p.m.	Helps cleanse and dialite vessels.

TISSUE SALTS

Silica	Daily.	Dissolves waste.
Kali. Sulph.	As directed.	Oxygen deficient tissue.
Mag. Phos.	As directed.	Oxygen deficient tissue.
Nat. Phos.	As directed.	Emulsifies waste.

ARTHRITIS

Arthritis is a dis-ease reaction and a symptom of a dis-ease. It is an inflammation caused by crystallized toxic waste from a constipating diet and earth mineral deposits in the joints. The presence of arthritis can mean that the body is not dissolving and flushing out deposits of toxins or earth minerals. The waste deposits can collect in the tissues and muscles. The body immobilizes (stops) any part of the body that needs repairs. For example, a sprained wrist becomes stiff and a strained muscle becomes stiff (called nature's cast). An injured part of the body remains sore or stiff until it is repaired. If repairs are not made then that part becomes permanently stiff (calcified) or immobilized. The crystalized waste in the joints and/or tissue can rub against each other causing inflammation. Arthritis is waste in the bone joints while rheumatism is waste in the muscles.

Supplements	Suggested Dosage	Remarks
Vitamin C with Bioflavanoids	3,000-10,000 mg., daily in divided doses	Powerful free radical destroyer.
Calcium-Magnesium	2,000-10,000 mg.	Stabilizes bone.
Bromelain	500 mg.	Anti-inflammatory.
Potassium	50-80 mcg.	Soothes nerves.
Vitamin B	60-100 mg.	Anti-stress.
Vitamin B_6	50 mg.	Nerve pain.
Vitamin E	10,000 IU.	Strengthens nerves and muscles, heals tissue
Multiple Vitamin and Mineral	As directed.	Essential nutrients.
Brewer's Yeast	As directed.	Anti-stress.
MSM	1,000-2,000 mg.	Used fro inflammation and pain.
Panthothenic Acid	1,000 mg.	Promotes healing.
Niacinamide	50-100 mg.	Used for stress, pain, skin and cramps.
Zinc	15-50 mg.	Heals tissue.
Copper	1-8 mg.	Heals skin, muscle and bones.
Manganese	2-10 mg.	Used for hormone function and protects tissue.

GLANDULARS

Raw Adrenal	As directed.	Reduces symptoms.
Raw Pancreas	As directed.	Stimulates cleansing.
Raw Liver	As directed.	Dissolves waste between bones.

AMINO ACIDS

Clucosamine and Chondroitin	2,000 mg., twice daily.	Used for inflammation and pain. Heals tissue.
Cysteine	As directed.	Rids bones and muscles of waste.

HERBS

Bladderwrack, Buckthorn, Burdock, Chaparral, Cornsilk, Devil's Claw, Orris, Peppermint, Poke Berries, Ragwort, Sassafras, Slippery Elm.

FOODS

Aloe Vera, Carrots, Celery, Cherry Juice, Grape Leaves, Kiwi, Pineapple, Red Beets, Raw Potatoes, Yucca.

HOMEOPATHIC

Ferr. Phos.	As directed.	Helps prevent inflammation.
Kali. Mur.	As directed.	Gets rid of waste in muscle and bone.
Silicea	As directed.	Heals tissue.
Calc. Flour.	As directed.	Protects bones and muscles.

Additional information can be found in *Overcoming Arthritis and Other Rheumatic Diseases* by M. Warmbrand and *Nature Cure for Arthritis* by H. Clement.

TREATMENT

Oil Pack

Arnica oil, yarrow, oil, castor oil, ginger oil, camphor oil for rubbing on the area. To make an oil pack, put 2 tablespoons of each oil in a pan. Heat the oil slowly, pour water on top of the oil (to prevent evaporation); heat until oil simmers. Pour off water, then dip flannel cloth in oil. Use enough cloth to wrap affected parts. If more oil is needed use more castor oil. After dipping flannel cloth in oil, place it on affected part (rub affected part with camphor oil first). Cover the flannel cloth with plastic and place a heating pad over the part. Keep heating pad on for at least 1 hour.

Poultice

To make a poultice, use 2 tablespoons ginger root, 2 tablespoons horseradish, 1 tablespoon Orris Root, 3 tablespoons slippery elm powder and 1 teaspoon red cayenne pepper. Mix herbs together and place in a bowl. Use the measurement of 1 tablespoon to 1 cup of water or 1 ounce herbs to 20 ounces of water.

Add hot water and mix herbs together until it forms into a paste. Spread the herb paste on a white cotton cloth (the cloth should be the size to cover joint). Wrap the cloth with a plastic sheet. Then wrap a dry towel over the plastic sheet. Leave poultice on joint for at least one hour or until poultice becomes painful.

ASTHMA
(CONGESTED LUNGS)

Asthma is a disease reaction caused by a trigger (allergen, emotions, stressors) and over-stimulation of the nerve. The tissue of the lungs (bronchial tubes) gets small (constrict) and hold more mucous than air. This makes breathing difficult (labored). The mucous accumulation results in the lungs getting inflamed and swollen, which further reduces the air supply. In response to this, the lungs constrict in order to squeeze out the mucous. This starts the asthma cycle of constriction, inflammation, swelling and then constriction. The pulse is fast because of a low air supply. The asthmatic breathes fast because they are too alkaline, then breathes slow because they are too acidic, which causes another cycle of fast breathing because they are too alkaline.

The body needs excessive (large quantities) amounts of air in order to burn (break down) toxins, white sugar, alcohol, synthetic chemicals and allergens that irritate the lungs; causing fluid to form in order to protect the membranes. This excessive work makes the lungs tired and causes dis-eases and dis-ease reactions.

Asthma, like all other dis-eases and dis-ease reactions, is wholistic (combined spirit, mind/emotions and body). Therefore, it requires a wholistic cure.

Contra-indicated foods that should be avoided are animal flesh, cow's milk, alcohol, cigarettes and all processed foods (junk foods).

Supplements	Suggested Dosage	Remarks
Vitamin A	10,000-50,000 IU.	Prevents infection.
Vitamin C	3,000-10,000 mg.	Strengthens and protects lungs.
Vitamin E	10,000 IU.	Thins mucus, heals tissue.
Vitamin B_6	50–80mg.	Relieves lung. stress.
Vitamin D	400 IU	Maintains healthy lungs and sinus.
Vitamin F	50 mcg.	Stimulates cell repair.
Bee Pollen Capsules	As directed.	Provides nourishment to tissue.
Magnesium Chloride	750-1000 mg.	Prevents lung problems.
Manganese	10-50 mg.	Helps repair cells.

| Garlic Capsules | As directed. | Prevents infection, thins mucus. |
| Panthothenic Acid | 5-50 mg. | Relieves stress. |

GLANDULARS

| Raw Adrenal, Raw Liver, Raw Heart, Raw Pancreas | As directed. | Relieves symptoms. |

AMINO ACIDS

| Tyrosine, Glutamine, | 1,000-2,000 mg. | Increases circulation. |
| Aspartic Acid | 1,000-2,000 mg. | Helps detoxify lungs. |

HERBS

Alfalfa, Anise, Arnica, Chamomile, Chickweed, Coltsfoot, Comfrey, Ginseng, Goldenseal, Horehound, Hyssop, Lobelia, Marjoram, Mullein, Myrrh.

FOODS

Brewer's Yeast, Celery, Cucumber, Garlic, Lecithin, Parsley, Stringbean Juice, Watercress.

HOMEOPATHIC

Mag. Phos.	As directed.	Cleanses tissue.
Kali. Mur.	As directed.	Helps cleanse lungs and sinus.
Nat. Sulph.	As directed.	Helps prevent infections.

TREATMENT

Vapor baths (or herbs added to vaporizer): add eucalyptus, camphor, wormwood, cudweed, ragwort. Boil 2 ounces of each herb in a quart of water, then use in vaporizer or bath. Additional information can be found in *Sinusitis, Bronchitis and Emphysema* by C. Quick.

ATHLETE'S FOOT

Athlete's foot (ringworm, dermatophytosis, tinea pedis) is a fungus (similar to mushrooms) that grows on the dead outer layers of skin (i.e., calluses). It is usually found between the toes. The fungus lives in warm and damp areas (poorly ventilated shoes), in floors around pool areas and in locker rooms. Good hygiene, drying between the toes and wearing cotton socks that can absorb moisture is a good prevention. Antibiotics, radiation and drugs can destroy the natural bacteria and fungus synergistic balance of the body, which increases fungus growth (Athlete's Foot). The typical symptoms are itching, burning, inflammation, blisters and scaling between toes and other areas of the foot.

A diet of eating sweets (white sugar, honey and maple syrup, etc.), yeast-containing foods (i.e., bread, etc.), alcoholic beverages, fermented foods (i.e., vinegar, soy sauce, beer, wine) and digestive problems can contribute to yeast infections, which can cause fungus growth.

Supplement	Suggested Dosage	Remarks
Garlic tablets	2 tablets, 3 times daily.	Odorless garlic. Aids in destroying fungus.
Zinc	50 mg., daily.	Inhibits fungus and stimulates the immune system.
Vegetarian Acidophilus	As directed.	Restores bacteria balance, which prevents fungus growth.
Methylsulfony-Methane (MSM)	1,000-2,000 mg.	Good for infection.
Germanium	100 mg., daily.	A good antioxidant and pain reliever.
Unsaturated Fatty Acids	As directed.	Supplies the essential fatty acids.
Vitamin A	50,000 IU daily for 1 month, then reduce to 25,000 IU.	Aids the healing of tissue and their immune system.
Vitamin B-Complex	As directed.	Use a yeast-free product.
Vitamin C (Buffered)	3,000-10,000 mg., 3 times daily in divided doses.	Decreases stress. Enhances immune function.
Selenium	50 – 200 mcg.	Enhances immunity.
Grape Seed Oil Capsules	As directed.	Helps destroy impurities.
Tea Tree Oil or Garlic Powder	Apply to the area.	Fights fungus.

GLANDULARS

Raw Thymus	As directed.	Stimulates immunity.
Raw Liver	As directed.	Helps destroy waste.

AMINO ACIDS

Lysine	1,000-2,000 mg.	Used for infections.
Glutathione	1,000-2,000 mg.	Enhances immunity.

HERBS

Black Walnut, Pau D'Arco.

FOOD

Carrots, Collard Greens, Corn, Dandelion Greens, Endives, Mustard Greens, Loquats, Parsley, Peaches, Pears, Quince, Turnip Greens, Yams.

HOMEOPATHIC

Mercurius Cyanatus 7	2 gr., in the a.m. and p.m.	Infections.
Canella 4	2 gr., midday and in the p.m.	Relieves symptoms.

TISSUE SALTS

Kali. Mur.	In the a.m., noon and p.m.	Eliminates impurities.
Kali. Sulph.	In the a.m., noon and p.m.	Helps prevent infections.
Nat. Phos.	In the a.m., noon and p.m.	Emulsifies waste.
Silicea	In the a.m., noon and p.m.	Heals tissue.

AUTISM

Autism (auto = self, ism = condition) is a syndrome that usually appears in childhood. The person seems to be withdrawn into themselves; tends to be alone; unable to coherently communicate to others; uses nonsense rhyming; is withdrawn; has repetitive play activities and will go into a rage if play is interrupted; lacks response to love, nurturing and affection; may beat on themselves or bite themselves and have episodes of hyperactivity. Basically, they cannot get out of their minds' ideations and you cannot get into their minds. They are emotionally locked into themselves and exclude reality. Their I.Q. tends to not be a factor as they test from low to high range.

Supplement	Suggested Dosage	Remarks
Multiple Vitamin and Mineral	As directed.	Vital nutrients.
Magnesium plus Calcium	1,000 mg., daily.	Helps normal brain and nervous system function.
Vitamin B Complex and Niacinamide	300 mg., daily .	Vital for normal brain and nervous system function.
Niacin (both B_3) and	50 mg., 3 times daily.	Increases nutrients to brain and nerves.
Vitamin B_5 (Pantothenic Acid)	500 mg., daily.	Combats stress.
Vitamin B_6 (Pyridoxine)	50 mg., 3 times daily.	A Vitamin B_6 deficiency has been linked to Autism. Take in higher amounts only if under professional care.
Potassium	5-50 mg.	Aids communication between mind and body.
RNA and DNA RNA,	200 mg., daily; DNA, 100 mg., daily.	Needed circulation and brain tissues.
Vitamin E	200-600 IU daily.	Aids circulation and brain function.
Choline	500-2,000 mg., daily.	Enhances brain function and blood circulation to the brain. Use under supervision.
Nutritional Brewer's Yeast	Start with ½ tsp. and work up slowly.	Helps a proper balance of the B Vitamins.
Vitamin C	3,000-10,000 mg., 3 times daily in divided doses.	A powerful free radical scavenger.
GLANDULARS		
Raw Brain	As directed.	Nutrients for nerve transmission.
Raw Adrenal	As directed.	Stimulates immunity.
AMINO ACIDS		
L-Glutamine	1,000-2,000 mg.	Aids normal brain function.
L-Phenylalanine	500-1,000 mg. with Vitamins B_6 and C.	Vital for normal brain function.
GABA	750 mg.	Helps control behavior. Used for anxiety, stress, epilepsy and tension.

HERBS

Feverfew, Gingko, Gotu Kola, Rosemary.

FOOD

Barley, Black Walnuts, Broccoli, Brazil Nuts, Collard Greens, Corn, Kale, Peas, Pecans, Potatoes, Raw Peanuts, Rice, Soy Beans, Tomatoes, Turnip Greens.

HOMEOPATHIC

Gelsemium (Jasmine)	As directed.	Used for skin problems, mood swings.
Kali. Phosphoricum	As directed.	Used for ental fatigue, tension.
Ignatia	As directed.	Used for mood swings, easily hurt feelings.

TISSUE SALTS

Kali. Phos. and Mag. Phos.	3 times daily.	Obsession with self.
Ferr. Phos.	Daily.	Nerve disorders.
Nat. Phos.	3 times daily.	Nervous withdrawal.

BACKACHE

Backaches and pains can be caused by poor postures, sleeping on a soft mattress, stress, incorrect lifting, improper walking techniques, slouching while sitting, improperly fitted shoes (designed for fashion not for wearing), a slipped disc, prostate disease, fibroid tumors, kidney and bladder disorders, rheumatism, bone disease, arthritis, abnormal curvature of the spine, varicose veins, arteriosclerosis, emotional problems, motor vehicle accidents, psychosomatic issues, muscle spasms, etc.

Supplement	Suggested Dosage	Remarks
Glucosamine Sulfate	1,000-2,000 mg. and tissue repair.	Used for pain, arthritis, bone
Multi-Mineral Complex	As directed.	Vital in muscle and bone metabolism.
Calcium	1,500–2,000 mg., daily.	Enhances assimilation. Use 3 different forms of Calcium (chelate, carbonate and asporatate).
Magnesium (Chelated form)	700–1,000 mg., daily.	
Boron	3 mg., daily.	Enhances calcium uptake, which is needed for bone and muscle repair. When healed, discontinue use unless over age 50.
Manganese Gluconate (Trace Mineral)	2 – 5 mg., daily.	Helps in healing cartilage and tissue in the neck and back.

Vitamin A	25,000 IU daily.	Aids in healing.
Vitamin E	400 – 800 IU daily.	Aids in healing.
Zinc	50 mg., daily.	
Silicon	3 times daily.	Enhances Calcium uptake. Horsetail is a good source of Silicon.
Vitamin B_{12} (Sublingual Form)	2,000 mg., daily.	Helps Calcium absorption.
Vitamin D	400-600 IU daily.	Enhances Calcium uptake.
Vegetable Protein (Soy free powder)	As directed.	Vital in bone and tissue repair.
Enzymes with Bromelin	2 tablets with meal.	Helps with digestion and relieves muscles.
Vitamin C with Bioflavonoids	3,000 – 10,000 mg., daily.	Helps the repair of tissues. Relieves tension in the back area.
Vitamin B Complex	Take 3 times daily.	Helps repair and relieve stress in the back muscles.
Vitamin B_6	2-200 mg.	For nerve pain.
Vitamin B_{12}	1,000 mcg.	Vital nutrient.

GLANDULARS

Raw Thymus	As directed	Stimulates repair.

AMINO ACIDS

Phenylalanine (DLPA)	Take daily, every other week. Follow label instructions.	Decreases pain. Do not use if pregnant, diabetic or have high blood pressure.

HERBS

Arnica, Boswellia, White Willow	Pain.
Feverfew	Nerve pain.
Burdock, Cat's Claw, Devil's Claw, Horsetail, Yucca	Cleanses bone joints, relieves pain.

FOOD

Barley, Black Walnut, Broccoli, Brussels Sprouts, Cauliflower, Collard Greens, Currants, Guava, Kale, Lemon, Orange, Peas, Pecans, Soy Beans, Spinach, Turnip Greens.

HOMEOPATHIC

Rus. Tox. 9	5 gr., as directed.	Spasms, pain.
Lachesis 7	As directed.	Spasms, pain.
Causticum 7	5 gr., as directed.	Spasms, pain.
Sedative P.C.	2 gr., 3 times daily.	Spasms, pain.

TISSUE SALTS

Silicea and Calc. Flour.	Both in the a.m. and p.m.	Arthritis, pain.
Kali. Sulph. and Mag. Phos.	Alternate.	Pain.
Kali. Phos.	3 times daily.	Pain.
Nat. Mur.	3 times daily.	Pain, spasm.

BAD BREATH
(HALITOSIS)

Bad Breath is the foul fumes from rotten food in the digestive tract caused by constipation. It can also be caused by Liver problems, tooth decay, inadequate protein digestion, foreign bacteria in the mouth, gum, throat or nose infection, indigestions, improper diet and/or food combining and inadequate dental care.

Supplement	Suggested Dosage	Remarks
Chlorophyll	1 tbsp. in juice, twice daily.	Green drinks are one of the best ways to combat bad breath. Chlorophyll can also
	be used as a mouth rinse—	
		1 tbsp. to ½ glass of water.
Fiber (Oat, Wheat or Rice Bran) or	1 tbsp. in juice on an empty stomach twice daily.	Do not take fiber at the same time that you take vitamins medications, because the fiber can absorb them.
Vitamin C	2,000 – 6,000 mg., daily.	Vital in healing mouth and gum disease in preventing bleeding gums. Rids the body of excess mucous and toxins that can cause bad breath.
Vitamin A	15,000 IU daily.	Needed for control of infection and in healing of the mouth.
Beta-carotene	10,000 IU daily.	
Vitamin B Complex	100 mg.	Vitamin B_6 is used for all enzyme systems in the
body.		
Vitamin B_6 (Pyridoxine)	50 mg.	Niacin dilates tiny capillaries for improved blood flow to infection sites.
Niacin (Pyridoxine)	50 mg.	
Niacin (B_3)	50 mg., 3 times daily.	
Garlic capsules	2 capsules with meals and at bedtime. bacteria in both the mouth	Garlic acts as a natural antibiotic, destroying foreign and colon.
Vegetarian Acidophilus	As directed.	Needed to replenish/restore "friendly" bacteria balance in "friendly"
	the colon. Insufficient	
bacteria balance dance of cause		and an overabun- harmful bacteria can bad breath.
Alfalfa tablets or liquid Chlorophyll	6 tablets daily or 1 tbsp liquid in juice or water, 3 times daily.	Chlorophyll cleanses the bloodstream and colon, which can be the site where bad breath begins.

GLANDULARS

Raw Liver	As directed.	Aids in digestion.
Raw Pancreas	As directed.	

AMINO ACIDS

Arginine	1,000-2,000 mg.	Helps digestion of food.

HERBS

Bennet, Caraway, Dill, Echinacea, Linden, Myrrh, Rosemary, Senna (laxative).

FOOD

Apricots, Artichoke, Asparagus, Avocado, Beet Greens, Blueberries, Cantaloupe, Cherries, Chestnuts, Cranberries, Endive, Figs, Grapes, Gooseberries, Jackfruit, Nectarines, Olives, Peaches, Pecans, Peppers, Plums, Quince, Raisins, Raspberries, Rhubarb, Squash, Tomatoes.

HOMEOPATHIC

Nux Vomica 8	2 gr., in the a.m.	Aids digestion.
Lycopodium 7	2 gr., at noon.	Increases movement of food.
Opium 7	2 gr., at in the a.m.	Helps stimulate metabolism.

TISSUE SALTS

Nat. Phos. and Nat. Mur.	3-200 x, alternate.	Helps moisturize cells, aiding food transient.

BED-WETTING

Bed-wetting usually refers to nocturnal (nighttime) incontinence or wetting the bed while sleeping. It can be caused by drinking fluids too late at night, small or weak bladders, smooth muscles weakness, a type of rheumatism, stress, fear, urinary tract infections, nutritional deficiencies, behavioral problems, emotional imbalances, allergies, fibroid tumors, prostate problems, diabetes, etc.

Supplement	Suggested Dosage	Remarks
Multiple Vitamin and Mineral Complex	As directed.	Helps supply all needed nutrients.
Vitamin B Complex	1,000-2,000 mg.	Strengthens nerves.
Potassium	As directed (99 mg., for children, 12 and older).	Helps to balance sodium.
Vitamin A	10,000-50,000 IU.	Vitamins A and E aid in normalizing bladder muscle function.
Vitamin E	100 IU daily for children, 6 – 12 years old; 600 IU daily for adults.	Aids bladder muscle function.
Zinc	10 mg., daily for children; 80 mg., daily for adults.	Helps to improve bladder function. Enhances the immune system.
Pumpkin Seed Oil Capsules	As directed.	

Calcium plus	500 mg., daily.	Dosage is for children 6 to
Magnesium	250 mg., daily	12 years old. Dosage must
		be adjusted for others.
Vegetable Protein Supplement	Follow label directions.	Helps to strengthen bladder
		muscle.

GLANDULARS

| Raw Kidney, | As directed. | Helps regulate urine flow. |
| Raw Prostate (men, boys). | As directed. | Helps control urination. |

AMINO ACIDS

Taurine	1,000-2,000 mg.	Helps nervous problems
		(i.e., epilepsy, fits).
Glutamine	500-2,000 mg.	Helps behavioral problems
		that may be a factor.

HERBS

Bearberry, Betony, Bistort, Cubeb*, Fennel, Hops, Horsetail, Juniper Berry, Milkweed, Oat, Pansy, Plantain, St. John's Wort, Uva Ursi* (* = diuretics. Give early during the day).

FOOD

Asparagus, Avocado, Beets, Cabbage, Celery, Dandelion Greens, Grapes, Mango, Olives, Radish, Raw Peanuts, Spinach, Squash, Strawberry, Watercress, Watermelon.

HOMEOPATHIC

Children:

Pulsatilla 7 and	2 gr., in the a.m.	Helps control urine flow.
Sulphur Iodatum 7		
Ferrum Phoshoricum 4	2 gr., in the p.m. and alternate.	Infections, skin problems.
and Equisetum 4		
China 7	2 gr., in the afternoon.	Helps stabilize bladder.

Adults:

Sepia 7 and Causticum 7	2 gr., in the a.m. and alternate.	Occurs after operation
		and/or childbirth.
Arnica 8 and Staphysagria 7	2 gr., in the a.m. and alternate.	After Diabetes, fright, etc.
Opium 7 and Gelsemium 7	2 gr., in the a.m. and alternate.	Helps regulate urine flow.

TISSUE SALTS

| Nat. Mur. And Nat. Phos. | Alternate. Take twice daily. | Helps normalize urine flow. |

BLADDER INFECTION
(CYSTITIS)

Bladder infections can cause an urgent need to urinate. Urination is usually frequent and painful. When the bladder is empty, there may still be a need to urinate. The urine may have a cloudy appearance and a foul unpleasant odor. Chlamydia can cause bladder problems. Bacterial infections (Escherichia coli) can cause a urinary tract infection. In women, bacteria from the anus can migrate to the vagina and uterus resulting in an infection. In children, a bladder infection can cause lower abdominal pain and the urine may give a burning sensation. The acid content of the urine can be raised with cranberry juice. This can help to retard bacterial growth. A kidney infection can result from inflammation of the bladder, Fibroid tumors, holding the urine in the bladder too long, and prostate problems. An enlarged or swollen prostate can block urine resulting in a bladder infection.

Supplement	Suggested Dosage	Remarks
Multiple Vitamin and Mineral	As directed.	For essential vitamins and minerals.
Vitamin A	10,000 IU daily.	Enhances the healing process and immune function.
Beta-Carotene	15,000 IU daily.	
Vitamin E	600 IU daily.	Fights infecting bacteria.
Zinc	50 mg., daily.	Vital in tissue repair and immunity.
Betaine Hydrochloride	1-2 tablets after each meal or snack with ½ glass of water.	Raises acid level of urine.
Garlic Capsules	2 capsules, 3 times daily.	Garlic is a natural antibiotic.
Carrot Acidophilus (Milk Free)	2 capsules, 3 times daily. Can use 1 tbsp. in 1 quart of warm water as a douche. If	associated with Vaginitis, alternate with apple cider vinegar. Balances bacteria level.
Vitamin C	4,000 – 5,000 mg., daily.	Creates an antibacterial effect through acidification of urine. Vital for immune function.
Vitamin B Complex	50 – 100 mg., twice daily.	High doses are necessary when antibiotics are used.
Calcium	1,500 mg., daily.	Reduces bladder irritability.
Magnesium	750 – 1,000 mg., daily.	Helps in the stress response when balanced with cal-
cium. infection.	MSM (Methylsulfonyl-Methane)	1,000-2,000 mg. Fights

GLANDULARS

Raw Kidney	As directed.	For infection.
Raw Thymus and Raw Pituitary	50 mg., twice daily.	Increases immunity.

AMINO ACIDS

Lysine	As directed.	For infection.
L-Cysteine	500 mg., twice daily on an empty stomach.	A potent detoxifier.

HERBS

Bearberry, Buchu, Burdock, Cubeb, Echinacea, Goldenseal, Juniper Berry, Marshmallow (increases acid of urine), Uva Ursi (increases acid of urine).

FOOD

Broccoli, Brussels Sprouts, Cauliflower, Celery, Collard Greens, Currants, Endive, Guava, Grapefruit, Kale, Lemons, Parsley, Peppers, Spinach, Tomatoes, Turnips, Watercress, Watermelon.

HOMEOPATHIC

Cystitis

Cantharis 4	2 gr., immediately.	Repeat for once or twice daily for 3 days.
Mercurius Corrosivus 4	2 gr., 1 hour later.	
Terebinthina 4	2 gr., 1 hour after Mercurius.	

TISSUE SALTS

Fer. Phos and Nat. Mur.	Alternate. Take 3 times daily.	Helps blood to rid body of toxins.

BOIL
(FURUNCLE)

A boil is a round pus-filled eruption that is tender to touch. A carbuncle occurs when boils erupt and spread the infection.

Boils begin when a small skin area swells, itches and becomes painful. Boils erupt abruptly and within a 24-hour period, they can become inflamed and filled with pus. A lymph gland close to the boil can get congested with waste and swell. Boils can occur on the face, buttocks, underarms and scalp. A hair follicle can get infected and inflamed, causing a boil. Boils can be caused by an infected wound, thyroid problems, stress, anger, a disease, drugs, junk foods, poor hygiene, toxic waste in the blood, constipation, bacteria and/or food allergies.

Supplement	Suggested Dosage	Remarks
Garlic Capsules	2 capsules, 3 times daily.	A natural antibiotic and good for immune function.
Vitamins A and E emulsion	Vitamin A—75,000 IU and Vitamin E – 600 IU daily for 1 month. Then 25,000 IU of Vitamin A and 600 IU of Vitamin E.	Vital for proper immune system function.
MSM (Methylsulfonyl-methane) tablets and/or lotion.	1,000-3,000 mg.	Fights infection.
Vitamin C	3,000 – 8,000 mg., daily in divided doses.	An anti-inflammatory and immune system stimulant.
Coenzyme Q$_{10}$	60 mg., daily.	Vital for oxygen utilization and immune function.
Chlorophyll	1 tbsp, 3 times daily.	Wheatgrass and Alfalfa are good sources. Needed to clean the blood.
Silicon tablets	10-40 mg.	Diseases inflammatory reaction.

Germanium	200 mg., daily.	Vital for immune system. Aids in cleansing the blood.
Proteolytic Enzymes	Twice daily on an empty stomach.	Improves the cleansing process at infection sites.
Kelp	6 tablets daily.	Needed for balanced minerals.
Multiple Mineral Complex	As directed.	Needed for balanced minerals.

GLANDULARS

| Raw Thymus | 500 mg., daily. | Aids the immune system. |

AMINO ACIDS

| Methione | 500-1,000 mg. | Good for eruptions, cysts, tumors, etc. |
| Lysine | 1,000-2,000 mg. | Good for infection. |

HERBS

Barberry, Black Walnut, Burdock, Calendula (Marigold), Chickweed, Comfrey, Dandelion Root, Echinacea, Goldenrod, Goldenseal, Horsetail, Indigo, Life Everlasting, Mullein, Nettle, Pau D'Arco, Periwinkle, Red Clover, Rose, Sarsaparilla, Sassafras, Stillingia, Thuja, White Oak Bark, Wormwood, Yellow Dock.

FOODS

Bananas, Black Radish, Currants, Onions.

HOMEOPATHIC

| Pyrogenium 7 | 2 gr., in the a.m. daily. | Helps cleanse skin. |
| Arsenicum Album 7 | 5 gr., in the p.m., every 2 days. | Rids skin of toxins. |

TISSUE SALTS

Ferr. Phos. and Kali. Mur.	Alternate, take every hour.	Aids the cleansing of tissue.
Silicea	Daily.	Skin disease remedy.
Calc. Sulph. and Nat. Sulph.	Alternate, take every 2 hours.	Not healing, fluid oozing out.
Kali. Phos.	Take hourly.	If fluid oozing out, has foul smell.

BREAST CANCER

The breast glands contains fatty tissue, milk ducts, lymph vessels and lobes, which rest on the chest muscles and intercoastal muscles of the ribs. The breasts are subject to the same diseases that affect all muscles (i.e., rheumatism, etc.), blood vessels (varicose) and hardening of the arteries. The lymph glands absorb impurities in the blood such as waste and cancer. Breasts can get impacted with waste and become inflamed and/or develop cysts as well as tumors. Cancerous malignant tumors of the breast are a leading cause of death. A breast lump that does not move freely may be cancerous. Lumps that move freely are usually non-cancerous.

There are various types of breast cancer. Cancer cells within ducts are called Intraductal Carcinoma. The cancer may not spread to surrounding tissue. Lobular (in the lobes), adenoid, tubal, medullary and cystosarcoma cancers are not the dominant types. The major type is infiltrating, ductal cancer. It spreads (infiltrates) to all surrounding tissue. Women become aware of cancer when a lump is found or a mammogram test indicates it. Cancer lumps are firm, usually painless, and never move or change texture or go away. A clear, bloody or yellow discharge from the nipple is usually a sign of cancer in non-pregnant women. Cancer can spread (migrate) to the nipples from another region of the breast. Cancer can cause itching, a rash, soreness and inflammation. In inflammatory cancer, the cancer tumors fill the blood vessels and lymph tissue. The skin becomes red, tender to touch and thickens. This cancer strikes quickly because it is constantly nourished by blood and lymph vessels.

Men are currently having an increase in breast cancer. They usually do not examine their nipples or the surrounding areas for lumps or changes. Therefore, the breast cancer is usually far advanced before it is medically detected.

Supplement	Suggested Dosage	Remark
Digestive Enzyme	Take with meals, as directed.	Helps digestion.
Multiple Vitamin and Mineral	Take with meals.	Vital nutrients.
Niacin (B$_2$)	100 mg., daily.	B Vitamins improve circulation, build red blood cells and help liver function.
Choline	500–1,000 mg., daily.	Increases nourishment to breast.
Calcium	2,000 mg., daily.	Stabilizes healthy tissue.
Magnesium	1,000 mg., daily.	Enhances cleansing.
Carnitine	500-4,000 mg.	Helps to protect the skin in post mastectomy and the x-ray treated patient.
Megadophilus (Milk free) or Maxidophilus or Primadophilus	As directed.	Provides an antibacterial effect on the body.
Vitamin A and Vitamin E	50,000 – 100,000 IU. Vitamin A daily for 10 days or for as long as on program. Start with 400 IU Vitamin E daily. Increase to 1,000 IU.	Vitamin A is essential to immunity. Vitamin E deficiency is associated with breast cancer. Vitamin E helps balance hormones.
Vitamin B	100 mg., 3 times daily.	B Vitamins are vital for normal cell division and function. Helps to reduce estrogen production.
Garlic Capsules	2 Capsules, 3 times daily.	Improves immune function.
Germanium	200 mg., daily.	Enhances immunity and cellular oxygenation. Inhibits cancer growth.
Proteolytic	2–6 tablets with meals.	Helps rid body of impurities.
Selenium	200 mg., daily.	Helps rid body of impurities.
Seaweed or Kelp	5 tablets daily.	For mineral balance.

Vitamin B_{12}	1,000 mg.	Prevents anemia, strengthens nerves.
Manganese	10-50 mg.	Converts to iron and prevents anemia.
Beta-carotene	10,000 units.	Rids body of impurities.
Coenzyme Q_{10}	100 mg., daily.	Improves cellular oxygenation.
MSM	1,000-2,000 mg.	Combats disease.
Vitamin C plus Bioflavonoids	5,000 – 10,000 mg., daily.	Combats cancer.

GLANDULARS

| Raw Glandular Complex | As directed. | Stimulates glandular function. |
| Raw Thymus | As directed. | Stimulates T-Lymphacyte thymus function. |

AMINO ACIDS

L-Cysteine	400-800 mg.	Rids body of impurities.
L-Methionine	500-2,000 mg.	Cleanses toxins.
L-Taurine	1,000-2,000 mg.	Provides a foundation for tissue and organ repair.
Arginine	500-2,000 mg.	Stimulates thymus.
Glutathione	500-3,000 mg.	Enhances immunity. Helps rid the body of impurities.

HERBS

Burdock Root, Chaparral, Dandelion Root, Echinacea, Goldenseal, Milkweed, Red Clover, Thuja.

FOOD

Artichoke, Beet Greens, Blackberries, Broccoli, Brussels Sprouts, Cauliflower, Cherries, Collard Greens, Endive, Figs, Garlic, Grapes, Kale, Kelp, Mustard Greens, Parsley, Pomegranate, Strawberries, Turnip Greens, Watercress, Yams.

HOMEOPATHIC

Thuja 9	As directed.	Fights abnormal tissue growth.
Conium 7 and Phytolacca	2 gr., Alternate days of use.	Cleanses glands.
Arsenicum	As directed.	Purifies blood.

TISSUE SALTS

Ferr. Phos.	6x or 3-200x, as directed.	Purifies tissue.
Silicea	12x or 3-200x, as directed.	Combats abnormal growth.
Kali. Mur.	12x or 3-200x, as directed.	Rids the body of waste.

BREAST SELF-EXAMINATION
(MEN AND WOMEN)

Examine your breasts each month at the same time. Do not examine the breasts before or during the menstrual cycle. Familiarize yourself with the normal feel of your breasts so that you can detect any changes or enlargement of a lump.

Stand and look into the mirror at your breasts. Raise your hands over your head, rub your breasts (men) or press them together (women). Notice the shape of your breasts. Place your hands on your hips, apply pressure to the breasts, and look for dimpling of the skin, nipples that seem to be out of position, differences in individual shape or thickening of the skin and nipple or red scaling.

Raise one arm above your head. With the other hand, firmly touch your breast beginning at the outer edge. Using a circular motion, gradually move toward the nipple. Examine the area between the nipple and the armpit, and feel the armpit. There are nodes in the armpit; which move freely and feel soft, and are not painful to the touch. Look for lumps that are hard and do not move. Cancers are usually attached to underlying muscles or the skin. Examine both sides of each breast.

Repeat Step 2 while lying on your back. Lumps are easily noticed while lying on your back. Squeeze each nipple gently to check for blood or a watery yellow or pink discharge.

BROKEN BONES (FRACTURES) AND BONE SPURS

A fracture is a broken bone. A bone still intact and yet cracked is called a hairline fracture. Bone fractures and bone spurs are caused by jumping up and down on asphalt, concrete and artificial turf while playing games (basketball, jumping rope), as well as running or constantly walking on hard surfaces. The concrete can be covered with floor tile or outdoor carpet and still cause bone spurs and/or fractures. Bone spurs are pointed and/or bump-like calcium deposit type bandaids that grow in response to bone trauma, neuritis, tendonitis, arthritis and/or alkalosis. Fractures and/or Spurs can develop because bone tissue becomes congested with waste, weakened or demineralized. Bones deteriorate and demineralize from consuming junk food, carbonated sodas, eating red meat, cow's milk, caffeine or drugs. A bone trauma, resulting in a fracture should be splinted or immobilized. There are two types of fractures, exposed and closed (skin intact). Do not attempt to reset the bone, as this requires skill and a sanitary procedure.

Supplement	Suggested Dosage	Remark
Glucosamine Sulfate	500 mg., 3 times daily.	Bone repair and pain.
Chondroitin	500 mg., 3 times daily.	Bone repair.
Calcium	1,000 – 2,000 mg., divided up.	Needed for proper bone repair.
Kelp	5 tablets daily after meals and at bedtime.	High in Calcium and minerals
Magnesium	1,000 mg., daily.	Gives strength to bones.
Mineral Complex and Trace Minerals	As directed.	Essential for repair of tissues.

Silicon	10-40 mg.	Vital for Calcium uptake and connective tissue repair. Springtime horsetail herb is a good source.
Vitamin D	400 – 1,000 IU daily.	Vital for Calcium absorption and repair.
Vegetable Protein (Soy Free Powder)	As directed.	Enhances healing.
Vitamin A	Start at 50,000 IU daily. Then drop to 25,000 IU daily.	Protein is not utilized without Vitamin A.
Zinc	80 mg., daily.	Aids tissue repair.
Octocosonal	3,000 mg., daily.	Enhances tissue repair.
Panthothenic Acid (B$_3$)	100 mg., 3 times daily.	Antistress vitamin. Helps vitamin utilization.
Potassium	99 mg., daily.	Helps to reduce swelling. Balances sodium.
Vitamin C with Bioflavonoids	3,000 – 6,000 mg., daily in divided doses.	Necessary in bone muscle trauma.
Proteolytic Enzymes	Take on an empty stomach between meals .	Reduces inflammation.
Betaine Hydrochloride	As directed.	Helps retain Calcium (May have to avoid if you have ulcers or history of heartburn).
Creatine	1,000-3,000 mg.	Builds tissue.

GLANDULARS

Mixed Bovine Neonatal Tissue	As directed.	Promotes healing.
Raw Liver	As directed.	Provides balanced B Vitamins and other needed vitamins and minerals.

AMINO ACIDS

Arginine	500-1,000 mg.	Increases healing ability.
Proline	1,000-3,000 mg.	Helps repair connective tissue (collagen).
Glutamine	1,000-2,000 mg.	Aids healing of tissue (ulcers).

HERBS

Alfalfa, Boneset, Calendula, Comfrey, Dandelion Root, Goldenseal, Horsetail, Nettle, Periwinkle, Plantain, Prickly Ash, Shepherd's Purse, White Oak Bark.

Heal Bone Spurs Arnica, Boswella*, Chamomile, White Willow, Arnica and Chamomile Soak in Tea Combination. Can also use extracts. *Can be taken orally for pain. Relieves pain.

FOOD

Currants, Grapefruit, Guava, Horse Radish, Kale, Lemons, Oranges, Parsley, Pistachios, Rice, Spinach, Tomatoes, Turnip Greens, Watercress, Wheat, White Yam.

HOMEOPATHIC

Closed Fracture

Arnica 8	2 gr., every 2 days .	Reduces pain.

Calcarsea Carbonica 7	2 gr., every day.	Heals tissue.
Symphytum 7	2 gr., every other hour.	Increases healing.
P.C.	2 gr., every other hour.	Pain sedative.

Open Fracture

Pyrogenium 7	5 gr., daily.	Open fracture.
Naja 4	2 gr., daily.	Take along with remedies for closed fracture.

TISSUE SALTS

Calc. Flour.	6x or 3-200x, 2-3 times daily.	Helps stabilize tissue.
Silicea	6x or 3-200x, every other day.	Strengthens tissue.
Kali. Mur.	6x or 3-200x, 3 times daily.	Increases healing.

BRONCHITIS

Bronchitis is the inflammation of the breathing tubes or obstruction of the bronchi (breathing tubes) that lead to the lungs. The inflammation and irritation causes constant coughing, mucous congestion, fever, sore throat, difficulty breathing and painful chest and back discomfort. Acute bronchitis follows upper respiratory tract infection such as influenza, which may cause pneumonia. Chronic bronchitis results from air pollution, radiation and smoke irritation of the lungs. It is not an infection. Allergies to food or chemicals may cause chronic bronchitis. The heart has to pump harder to keep an adequate volume of blood. This is due to a decrease of space available for the exchange of carbon dioxide for oxygen. The body accumulates waste and the muscles and bones get congested. This decreases oxygen to the brain and nerves and may cause fatigue and a vague sense of fear. The bodily fluids accumulate too much waste, stressing the kidney, liver and heart.

Supplement	Suggested Dosage	Remarks
Zinc	50 mg., daily.	Aids healing.
MSM tablets	1,000-2,000 mg.	Combats infections.
Vitamin A	Capsules 20,000 IU, twice daily for 1 month, dropping to 15,000 IU.	Aids healing of tissue and protection of all tissues.
Vitamin C	3,000 – 10,000 mg., daily in divided doses.	Combats infections. Aids healing.
Vitamin E	400 IU and up, twice daily.	Combine with Vitamin C. Essential for healing of tissues and improved breathing.
Chlorophyll tablets or liquid	3 times daily, as directed.	Helps absorb oxygen.
Garlic tablets	2 tablets with meals .	A natural antibiotic that reduces infection and detoxifies the body.
Vitamin B Complex	100 mg., 3 times daily.	Stimulates many enzymes. Needed for healing.
Calcium Chelate	1,000 mg., daily.	Essential for healing.
Magnesium	500 mg., daily.	

Coenzyme Q$_{10}$	60 mg., daily.	Enhances circulation and breathing.
Proteolytic Enzymes	Take between meals.	Necessary to reduce inflammation.
Beta-Carotene	15,000 IU daily.	Helps to protect the lung tissue.

GLANDULARS

Raw Thymus	As directed.

AMINO ACIDS

L-Arginine	2 gr., at bedtime with a small amount of L-Lysine.	Helps in liver detoxification. Essential for protein synthesis to aid in healing. Depresses elevated ammonia.
L-Cysteine	500 mg., twice daily .	Improves cellular immunity and contains needed sulfur.
L-Ornithine	500 mg., twice daily on an empty stomach.	For adults only. Not for children. Promotes and detoxifies ammonia.

HERBS

Betony, Cat's Claw, Chickweed, Coltsfoot, Comfrey, Elecampane, Eucalyptus, Horehound, Lungwort, Mullein, Pleurisy, Skunk Cabbage.

For Inflammation
Cat's Claw, Feverfew.

FOOD

Apricots, Asparagus, Beans, Beet Greens, Broccoli, Cabbage, Cantaloupe, Carrots, Corn, Dandelion Greens, Dates, Endive, Elderberry, Garlic, Kale, Leeks, Lettuce, Mustard Greens, Oranges, Papaya, Parsley, Pecans, Peaches, Peas, Pineapple, Plum, Spinach, Tangerines, Turnip Greens, Watercress.

HOMEOPATHIC

Acute

Phosphorus Triodatus 7	5 gr., once daily.	Reduces inflammation.
Bryonia 9	5 gr., once daily an hour after above.	Increases healing.
Ipecac 4	2 gr., every other hour.	Releases toxins.

In Babies

Same as above, plus Coccuc Cact 4	2 gr., between other remedies.	Helps purify tissue.

Chronic

Silicea 7 and Kali. Bichromicum 7	2 gr., in the morning. Alternate.	Heals inflamed tissue.
Senega 4	2 gr., before bed.	Reduces inflammation.

If Bronchitis includes Pulmonary Ephysema

Arsenicum Album 7	2 gr., in the evening, every other day.	Aids healing.

TISSUE SALTS

Reduces Fever

Ferr. Phos.	6x or 3-200x, every 30 minutes until fever is over.	
Ferr. Phos.	12x or 3-200x, 2 times daily (if no fever).	

Chronic

Nat. Mur.	12x or 3-200x, 3 times daily.	Heals illness.
Ferr. Phos.	12x or 3-200x, 3 times daily.	Purifies and heals.

Reduces Mucous Loose and Frothy

Nat. Mur.	12x or 3-200x, 3 times daily.	
Ferr. Phos.	12x or 3-200x, 2 times daily.	

Reduces Mucous Thick, White or Gray

Nat. Mur.	12x or 3-200x, 2 times daily.	
Ferr. Phos.	12x or 3-200x, 2 times daily.	

Chronic for a Long Time

Kali. Mur. or Kali Sulph.	As directed.	Heals illness.

BRUISING

The upper layer of the skin is not broken. The layer below the upper skin is traumatized and the tissue is slightly torn with dark discoloration, swelling and pain. If you easily bruise, it may be a sign of nutrient deficiency. Bruises can be related to Leukemia (blood cancer), Overweight, Anemia, Malnutrition, Drugs, Acidosis and/or Microwaves (weakened tissue below top layer). It can be an early sign of cancer.

Supplement	Suggested Dosage	Remarks
Glucosamine Sulfate	1,000-2,000 mg.	Helps heal.
Coenzyme Q_{10}	60 mg., daily.	Vital for construction and reconstruction of cells.
Vitamin K	50-80 mcg.	Helps heal tissue.
Alfalfa Tablets	5 tablets daily.	Supplies Vitamin K.
Vitamin C plus Bioflavonoids	3,000 – 10,000 mg., daily in divided doses.	Vital to prevent bruising.
Vitamin D	400 – 800 IU daily.	Aids in protecting the skin. Needed for blood cell formation.
Calcium	1,500 mg., daily.	Stabilizes and heals tissue.
Magnesium	750 mg., daily.	
Vitamin E	Start at 400 IU daily and increase slowly to 800 IU.	
Germanium	100 mg., daily.	Essential for circulation and boosts the immune system.
Iron	15-65 mcg.	Good iron supplement.
Vitamin B Complex plus Folic Acid	100 mg., twice daily.	Helps in protecting the tissue.

GLANDULARS

Raw Thymus	As directed.	Activates immunity.
Raw Liver	As directed.	Helps reduce toxicity.

AMINO ACIDS

Arginine	1,000-2,000 mg.	Accelerates healing.
Cysteine	400-800 mg.	Maintains skin integrity.

HERBS

Balm of Gilead, Calendula, Comfrey, Laurel, Life Everlasting, Lobelia, Nettle, Pennyroyal, St. John's Wort, Tansy, Witch Hazel, Wormwood.

FOOD

Collard Greens, Grapefruit, Guava, Horseradish, Kale, Lemons, Oranges, Spinach, Tomatoes, Turnip Greens, Watercress.

HOMEOPATHIC

Calendula M.T.	Apply to area.	Heals tissue.
Eau de Philae	After it dries, apply Homeodora.	Promotes healing.
Arnica 4 and Bellis Perennis 4	2 gr., 3 times daily.	Increases tissue strength.
China 4	2 gr., 2 times daily.	Gets rid of skin toxins.

TISSUE SALTS

Ferr. Phos.	3x or 6x or 3-200x as directed	Helps purify skin.

Bruise with inflammation

Kali. Mur.	3x or 6x or 3-200x as directed

Bruise with swelling

Calc. Flour.	Mix with a little water and apply to area. Also apply a bandage.

BRUXISM
(TOOTH GRINDING)

Bruxism is the sporadic, cyclical, and/or constant grinding of the teeth. It can occur during the day but usually happens at night while the person is asleep. The grinding can be unconscious and develops into an addiction. It is treated as an addiction and a psychosomatic, spiritual, nutritional and emotional problem. Grinding can cause the teeth to wear down, loosen and cause the gums to recede. Teeth can fall out or become damaged, requiring extraction. This disease is related to stress, sugar craving, nervousness, holding in feelings, hyperactivity, hypoglycemia, calcium and mineral deficiencies, adrenal stress as well as sensitivity to cold and/or heat.

Supplement	Suggested Dosage	Remarks
Potassium	100 mg., daily	Aids communication between brain and body.
Calcium and Magnesium	1,500 – 2,000 mg., daily; 750 mg., daily.	A deficiency is related to tooth grinding.

Pantothenic Acid (B₅)	500 mg., twice daily.	Decreases stress.
Lecithin	2 capsules with meals.	Helps provide coating for the nerves. Aids brain and nerve function.
Multiple Vitamin and Mineral	As directed.	Essential to reduce stress.
Vitamin B Complex	100 mg., twice daily.	High stress formula.
Zinc	50 mg., daily.	Helps to reduce stress.
Vitamin C	3,000 – 5,000 mg., daily.	Stimulates adrenal function, acting as an anti-stress vitamin.

GLANDULARS

Raw Adrenal	As directed.	Reduces stress.
Raw Brain	As directed.	Provides nutrients for brain.

AMINO ACIDS

Tyrosine	500-1,000 mg.	Reduces stress.
GABA	2,000-5,000 mg.	Acts as a tranquilizer.
Glycine	500-1,000 mg.	Anti-anxiety.
Taurine	500-2,000 mg.	Anti-convulsant.

HERBS

Catnip, Chamomile, Feverfew, Melissa, Passion Flower, Rosemary, Skullcap, St. John's Wort.

FOOD

Almonds, Avocado, Barley, Beets, Cabbage, Collard Greens, Dates, Eggplant, Kale, Mushrooms, Peas, Potatoes, Raw Peanuts, Rice, Soybeans, Tomatoes, Turnip Greens, White Yams.

HOMEOPATHIC

Sedative P.C.	2 gr., every other hour.	Relaxes tense muscles.
Strontium Iodatum 4	2 gr., twice daily.	Increases tissue flexibility.
Chamonilla 7 and Ignatia 7	2 gr., in the morning.	Alternate taking one every other day.

TISSUE SALTS

Kali. Phos.	12x or 3-200x, 3 times daily.	Helps reduce inflammation.
Nat. Phos.	12x or 3-200x, 3 times daily.	Reduces tension.
Mag. Phos.	12x or 3-200x, 3 times daily.	Reduces constant illnesses.
Silicea	12x or 3-200x, once a day.	Repairs damaged tissue.

BURNS

Burns are cooked tissue resulting from excessive heat from chemicals, fire, radioactive agents (radiation), and electricity. There are First Degree burns, which cook the outer skin (epidermis); Second Degree burns, which is superficial to deep partial thickness of skin (dermis), resulting in blisters and redness; and Third Degree burns in which the tissues of the muscles, nerves and blood vessels are cooked. The tissues are charred (like charcoal) or coagulated (like liquid plastic). A burn specialist usually has to treat Third Degree burns.

Supplement	Suggested Dosage	Remarks
MSM Tablets and Lotion	As directed.	For infection.
Zinc	As directed.	Increases healing for tissues.
Potassium	99 mg., daily.	Replaces Potassium that is lost due to burns.
Vegetable Protein (Soy Free Powder)	As directed.	Necessary for the healing of tissues. Free form amino acids are easily absorbed and assimilated by the body.
VitaminC plus Bioflavonoids	10,000 mg., daily and up.	Helps the healing process.
Vitamin E	600 – 1,600 IU, increasing slowly.	Needed for healing and to prevent scarring.
Calcium with Magnesium and Vitamin D	1,500 mg., daily; 750 mg., daily; 400 IU daily.	Calcium is necessary for protein structuring. Loss of body fluids increases the need for Magnesium. Vitamin D helps Calcium uptake.
Coenzyme Q_{10}	100 mg., daily.	Enhances circulation and healing of tissues.
Germanium	200 mg., daily.	Improves circulation and healing of tissue.
Betaine Hydrochloric Acid	As directed.	Helps to alkaline system, which promotes healing.
Selenium	200 mcg., daily.	Vital for tissue elasticity. Enhances protection at the cellular level.
Unsaturated Fatty Acids (Linseed and/or Primrose Oil)	As directed.	Helps stimulate tissue repair.
Vitamin A	100,000 IU daily for 1 month, then drop to 50,000 IU. End with 25,000 IU.	Necessary for tissue repair.
Creatine	1,000-2,000 mg.	Promotes tissue growth.

GLANDULARS

Raw Thymus	As directed.	Stimulates immunity.
Raw Pituitary	As directed.	Helps promote healthy tissue.
Raw Liver	As directed.	Aids skin healing.

AMINO ACIDS

Lysine	1,000 mg., twice daily.	Combats infection.
Arginine	500-1,000 mg.	Stimulates healing.
Cysteine	500-1,000 mg.	Enhances texture of skin.
Glutamine	2,000 mg.	Helps heal sores.

HERBS

Aloe, Burdock, Blackberry Leaves, Calendula, Goldenseal, Plantain, Poplar, St. John's Wort, Sumac, Witch Hazel. Pain Relief: White Oak Bark, Arnica, Boswella, White Willow.

FOOD

Grapefruit, Guava, Kale, Lemons, Lime, Orange, Parsley, Peppers, Spinach, Tomatoes, Turnip Greens, Watercress.

HOMEOPATHIC

Pyrogenium 7	5 gr., daily.	Tension and jaw pain.
Cantharis 4	2 gr., 2 times daily.	Releases tension.
Apply Eau de Philae or Calendula MT		Promotes healing.

TISSUE SALTS

Ferr. Phos. and Kali. Mur.	3x or 3-200x every hour.	Second and third degree burns: Take every 10 minutes.
Colloidial Silver	Apply to burnt tissue.	Heals tissue.

BURSITIS

Bursitis is the inflammation of the bursae. The suffix, "itis" at the end of a word means inflammation. Bursae are small liquid-filled cushion pads (sacs) that reduce friction and/or rubbing together of bones. Bursae are located in or near tendons, joints, bones and muscles. The inflammation of the bursae can be caused by junk food, calcium deposits, crystallized waste, and physical trauma (injury). There is usually tenderness, sensitivity or pain around the bursitis area. Bursitis usually occurs in the elbow (tennis elbow), hip, toe area (bunions), shoulder and/or wrist area (computer wrist).

Supplement	Suggested Dosage	Remarks
Vitamin A	100,000 IU daily for 1 month, then decrease to 50,000 IU daily for 2 weeks, and end with 25,000 IU daily.	Vital for tissue repair and the immune system.
Vitamin C plus Bioflavonoids	3,000 – 8,000 mg., daily in divided doses.	Decreases inflammation and enhances immunity.
Vitamin E	Start with 400 IU and increase slowly to 1,000 IU.	It is an anti-inflammatory.
Zinc	15-50 mg.	Aids tissue repair.
Calcium plus Magnesium	1,500 mg., daily; 750 mg., daily.	Stabilizes tissue.
Digestive Enzymes	2 tablets between meals.	Enhances anti-inflammatory process.
Coenzyme Q_{10}	60 mg., daily.	Improves circulation.
Germanium	100 mg., daily.	Improves immunity and reduces inflammation and pains.
Multiple Vitamin and Mineral	As directed.	Essential for tissue repair
Vitamin B Complex	100 mg., twice daily.	B Vitamins are vital for cellular repair.
Vitamin B_{12}	1,000 mcg in lozenges.	Necessary for proper digestion and absorption of foods. Good for nerve repair.

Vegetable Protein (Soy Free Powder)	As directed.	Free form amino acids are more readily available for use by the body.

GLANDULARS

Raw Thymus	As directed.	Stimulates immunity.
Raw Liver	As directed.	Helps neutralize toxins.

AMINO ACIDS

Arginine	500-1,000 mg.	Stimulates tissue repair.
Glutamine	1,000 mg., twice daily.	Repairs nerve cells.
Proline/Hydroxyproline	1,000-3,000 mg.	Repairs tissue.

HERBS

Arnica, Balm of Gilead, Borage, Coltsfoot, Comfrey, Echinacea, Fenugreek, Goldenseal, Mullein, Poke Root, Sarsaparilla, Tansy, Witch Hazel.

FOOD

Asparagus, Barley, Beans, Black Walnut, Brazil Nuts, Collard Greens, Cucumbers, Dandelion Greens, Endive, Kale, Mustard Greens, Okra, Parsley, Pecans, Potatoes, Raw Peanuts, Rice, Rye, Spinach, Turnip Greens, White Yam.

HOMEOPATHIC

Belladonna 4	2 gr., every 12 hours.	Relaxes muscles.
Arnica 8	2 gr., every 12 hours.	Reduces muscle tension.
Apis 6	2 gr., every 12 hours.	Combats tissue stress.
Apply Eau de Philae or Calendula M.T. to area.		Helps heal tissue.

TISSUE SALTS

Silicea and Calc. Flour.	30x or 3-200x, 3 times a day.	Reduces muscle stress.

CANCER

The word Cancer means crab and/or creeping sore. Cancer tissue and cells cover a broad spectrum of malignant (bad) neoplasms (new cells). There are over one hundred types of bad new cells (malignant neoplasm) classified as cancer. Each is believed to have a different cause. The Cancer theory (belief, best guess) supports each cause. The types of cancer are "carcinomas," which affect glands, skin, organs and mucous membrane skin; "lymphomas," which affect lymph glands and fluid; "sarcomas" which affect bones, muscles, connective tissue "leukemias" which affect blood.

Cancer cells and corpuscles have an over 60% decrease in oxygen levels. The specific cells grow excessively and corpuscles reproduce excessively. These cells and/or corpuscles cluster together (tumors) as well as travel throughout the body via the blood and lymph fluid. Cancer cells often travel to weak tissue and organs. For example, the actual cancer can be in the colon. The colon cancer cells can migrate (travel) to the lungs. An individual, with cancer, could be identified as having lung cancer when actually they have colon cancer cells in the lung tissue.

The major causes of cancer are the non-organic synthetic junk food diet, meat, eggs, dairy, synthetic toxic chemicals, under-nutrition physical, emotional and spiritual stressors; radiations, polluted air, water, soil and vegetables, drugs (legal and illegal), smoking marijuana and/or tobacco; medical examination procedures; computers; diabetes; synthetic chemicals in buildings and homes; airplanes, obesity, etc. Basically, cancers can be caused by anything that harms the immunity such as environmental factors and the diet.

There are "social" medical terms used to describe cancer that challenge your sanity. "Benign Cancer" means a mild, kind, gentle, non-threatening, to health cancer. Calling Cancer gentle and non-threatening does not stop it from being cancer. Cancer in "Remission" means asleep, laid aside— partly or wholly— sent back and not active, but resting cancer. If the cancer is resting, it does not stop from being a disease. Either you have cancer or you do not have cancer. If you have a car (cancer) and you park it (remission) or drive it mildly or in a kindly fashion (benign) it is still a car (cancer).

Cancer is a disease that has become a profit-making industry. As an industry, it must expand the medical signs and symptoms of cancers as well as the definition of cancer. This expands the market share (amount of people to buy treatments). This industry also expands its arsenal of treatments, such as drugs, research projects, chemotherapy and surgeries, which increases profits. Unfortunately, cancer is not a disease, but an industry.

Supplement	Suggested Dosage	Remarks
MSM	1,000-2,000 mg.	Helps purify the blood.
Zinc	15-50 mg.	Aids in building healthy tissue.
Beta-Carotene	10,000 units.	Essential antioxidant that destroys free radicals.
Coenzyme Q_{10}	100 mg., daily.	Gets more oxygen to cells.
Selenium	200 mcg.	Helps immunity and protein digestion.
Milk Free Maxidophilus, Megadophilus, or Primadophilus	As directed.	Improves antibacterial effect on the body.
Digestive Enzyme Formula	Take with meals, as directed.	Aids digestion.
Niacin, Folic Acid, and Choline	100 mg., daily; 500-1,000 mg., daily.	B vitamins that improve circulation, build red blood cells, and aid liver function.
PABA	Less than 400 IU daily.	Combats skin cancer.
Multiple Vitamin and Mineral	As directed.	Essential nutrients.
Calcium and Magnesium	2,000 mg., daily; 1,000 mg., daily.	
Potassium	100-500 mg.	Aids nerve communication.
Seaweed (Sea Vegetable)	5 tablets daily .	Helps maintain mineral balance.
Vitamin B_{12}	A sublingual form.	Prevents anemia.

Vitamin B Complex and Nutritional Brewer's Yeast	100 mg., daily. 3 times daily.	B vitamins are essential for cell division and function.
Vitamin C plus Bioflavonoids	5,000- 10,000 mg., daily, divided doses.	Powerful anticancer agent.
Multiple Trace Element	As directed.	Vital for normal cell division and function.
Garlic capsules	2 capsules, 3 times daily.	Improves immune function.
Germanium	200 mg., daily.	Enhances cellular oxygenation, deterring cancer growth. Aids in relieving pain and discom-
fort.		Stimulates immunity.
Proteolytic Enzymes	2 – 6 tablets with meals.	Essential free radical scavengers.

GLANDULARS

Raw Glandular Complex	As directed.	Enhances gland function.
Raw Thymus	As directed.	Stimulates T-Lymphacyte.
Raw Liver	As directed.	Helps purify blood.

AMINO ACIDS

Lysine	1,000 mg., twice daily.	Combats infections and toxins.
Carnitine	500-1,000 mg.	Combats oxygen radical damage and toxins.
L-Cysteine and L-Methionine	500-2,000 mg.	Gets rid of toxic substances. Protects the liver and other organs.
L-Taurine	100-2,000 mg.	Helps organ repair and builds healthy tissue.
Glutathione	1,000 mg., twice daily.	Enhances immunity.

HERBS

Apricot Pits, Burdock Root, Chaparral, Dandelion Root, Echinacea, Garlic, Goldenseal, Milk Thistle, Milk Thistle, Red Clover, Thuja.

FOOD

Apples, Artichoke, Asparagus, Blackberries, Blueberries, Broccoli, Brussels Sprouts, Cabbage, Cantaloupe, Cauliflower, Cabbage, Cherries, Currants, Dandelion Greens, Grapes, Lentils, Millet, Mustard Greens, Oat, Poke Greens, Pumpkin, Red Beans, Rye, Squash, Wheat, White Yams.

HOMEOPATHIC

Canella 4 and China 4	2 gr., every hour, alternate	Purifies tissue.
Thuja, Benzol, Phosphorus Triodatus, Chrysis, Ceanothus, Picric Acid, and Crotalus	As directed (Use any combination)	

TISSUE SALTS

Silicea, Kali. Sulph., Ferr. Phos.	12x or 3-200x, 3 times daily (Use any combination)	Causes tissue to release waste.

CANDIDA
(YEAST INFECTION)

Candida Albicans is a fungus overgrowth resulting in infection. It is a yeast-like fungus that normally lives in the digestive and genital tract. The fungus moves throughout the body by traveling with the blood and lymph fluid. The body normally maintains a balance of fungus, yeast and bacteria. This balance becomes disturbed by many factors such as white sugar, synthetic junk foods, drugs, antibiotics, allergies, chemotherapy, hypoglycemia, synthetic steroids, birth control pills, meat, synthetic underwear, diabetes, damp moldy places, dairy foods with yeast in them and fermented foods (i.e., vinegar, wine, beer) all of which can cause Candida.

Women tend to be most prone to this fungus infection. They erroneously call it a yeast infection. It can infect the vagina resulting in vaginitis. The most common symptom is a white cheesy-like discharge and itching. A pregnant women and/or a mother can pass the infection to their child. Fungus infection appears as red spots and white milk-like spots on the baby's tongue. Fungus infection of the throat is called Thrush. There are many names for fungus infection such as Athlete's Foot, Jock Itch, Diaper Rash, Ringworm, etc. There are many symptoms of it such as numb hands, legs or face; constipation; hyperthyroidism; diarrhea; abdominal pain; constant heart burn; nagging coughs; muscle and joint pain; canker sores; congestion; arthritis; hyperactivity; kidney and bladder infection; hypoglycemia; depression; colitis; etc. Many with Candida are highly sensitive to and cannot tolerate synthetic chemical odors, petroleum products, exhaust fumes, rubber and/or smoke from marijuana and tobacco.

A person with Candida disease should not eat fermented foods (beer, wine, vinegar, or cheese) white sugar, dried fruit, ham, alcohol, honey, high gluten grains (wheat, oats, rye, barley) bleached white flour, white rice, mushrooms, soy sauce, chocolate and yeast (used for baking) in foods. This requires reading the labels of foods and supplements very carefully in order to avoid yeast and fermented ingredients.

Supplement	Suggested Dosage	Remarks
Caprylic Acid	1st week: 1 tablet, twice daily. 2nd week: 2 tablets, twice daily.	Destroys fungus.
Grape Seed Oil	As directed.	Combats infection.
Garlic Capsules (Use Odorless)	2 capsules, 3 times daily.	Garlic inhibits the infecting organism. Garlic suppositories also effectively treat Candida vaginitis.
Multiple Vitamin and Mineral (Yeast Free)	Daily, as directed.	Vital nutrients for proper immune function.
Maxidophilus (Milk Free) or Megadophilus	As directed.	

Omega Oils, Flaxseed Oil, Primrose Oil	1,000-3,000 mg.	A vital essential fatty acid.
Coenzyme Q_{10}	100 mg., daily.	Enhances tissue oxygenation.
Vitamin B Complex (Yeast Free)	100 mg., daily.	Faulty absorption is common in candidiasis.
Vitamin B_{12} Lozenges	1 Lozenge (2,000 mcg) under the tongue 3 times daily, taken between meals.	Vital for digestion. Needed for metabolism of carbohydrates, fats, and proteins. Candida prevents the absorption of nutrients from the intestinal tract.
Germanium	100 – 200 mg., daily.	Enhances tissue oxygenation.
Vegetable Protein (Soy Free Powder)	As directed.	Helps build healthy tissue and balances the flora.

GLANDULARS

Raw Thymus	As directed.	Stimulates immunity.
Raw Liver	As directed.	Helps remove toxins.

AMINO ACIDS

L-Cysteine	500 mg., on empty stomach, twice daily.	An antioxidant and free radical destroyer.

HERBS

Clove Tea, Grape Seed Oil, Pau D'Arco, Uva Ursi.

FOOD

Fresh Cranberries or Raw Cranberry Juice.

HOMEOPATHIC

Mercuris Cyanatus 7	2 gr., once daily.	Stops infection.
Canella 4	2 gr., 2 times daily.	Use for infection.
Borax 7	2 gr., once daily.	Fights infection.

TISSUE SALTS

Kali. Phos. and Nat. Sulph.	6x or 3-200x, 3 times daily.	Reduces skin irritation.
Nat. Phos.	6x or 3-200x, 3 times daily.	Removes weaste from tissue.
Silicea	6x or 3-200x, 3 times daily.	Reduces skin problems.

CHICKEN POX

Chicken Pox is a childhood disease caused by undernutrition, dairy products, junk foods and meats. When a child's body is in an undernutritional condition it creates a cleansing reaction called a disease (chicken pox). The duration of the undernutritional disease condition's subtle symptoms are erroneously called an incubation period. The disease condition gets worse and the toxins are released through the skin. At this point, the chicken pox disease is believed to be born (active period). The body's cleansing reaction to rid itself of toxins is given various names based upon the pox (bump) shape, color and size or whether the bump is filled with fluid (pustule). Waste leaving the body usually travels out the cell to the tissue and then to an organ (skin). This skin is used for cleansing. It is not the cause of the disease, it is merely used to help get rid of the disease. There are many diseases (cleansing reactions), which are classified as chicken pox such as mosquito bites, ivy/oak poison, mild small pox (amaas), etc. Any time there is a change in the body (i.e., mental, physical, spiritual) the ratio of vitamins, minerals, hormones, bacteria, yeast and fungus will change. A bacterial over-population due to a change in health state (disease) is blamed on the bacteria. The bacteria is victimized. It is present to eat waste caused by the undernutritional state of the body. Bacteria is not the creator of a disease. It is an opportunist.

The symptoms of chicken pox begin with a fever and headache. Within twenty-four to thirty-six hours after the fever starts, small round bumps will occur on the torso, face and body. The bumps develop a crust. The bumps will continue to appear in cycles for three to seven days or more. It is a self-limiting disease. Once the scabs appear, the crisis is over. However, the bumps are very itchy. Therefore, the child's fingernails have to be kept short and clean so that the skin will not get infected or be scarred due to scratching.

It is a medical belief that a disease goes to sleep (incubates) then wakes up and causes the disease.

Supplement	Suggested Dosage	Remarks
Vitamin A Capsules	20,000 IU capsules daily for 1 month, dropping to 15,000 IU daily.	Heals tissues and helps immunity.
Vitamin C		Combats infections. Helps reduce fevers.
MSM	1,000-2,000 mg.	Fights infections.
Beta-Carotene	15,000 IU daily.	Heals tissues.
Vitamin E	400 – 600 IU daily.	Destroys free radicals. Increases oxygen to cells.
Potassium	99 mg., daily.	Reduces fever. Helps healing process.
Zinc	80 mg., daily.	Helps skin to heal.
GLANDULARS		
Raw Thymus	As directed.	Stimulates T-Lymphocytes.
AMINO ACIDS		
Lysine	1,000-2,000 mg.	Combats infection.

HERBS

Chaparral, Chickweed, Goldenseal, Pau D'Arco, Pleurisy Root, Red Clover, Thuja, Yarrow .

FOOD

Apples, Beet Greens, Blackberries, Broccoli, Cabbage, Carrots, Cauliflower, Collard Greens, Corn, Dandelion Greens, Grapes, Kale, Lemons, Peaches, Pears, Plums, Romaine Lettuce, Tangerines, Turnip Greens, Watercress.

HOMEOPATHIC

Bufo 7 and Rhus. Tox 7	5 gr., once daily in the a.m. Alternate.	Purifies skin.
Belladonna 4	2 gr., once daily.	Helps release skin toxins.

TISSUE SALTS

Kali. Phos. and Nat. Mur.	6x or 3-200x, 3 times daily or children's dosage daily.	Fights skin disease.

CHLAMYDIA

Chlamydia is a collection of symptoms (diseases) that includes inflammation of the genitals, watery mucous discharge from sex organs, itching around inflamed areas, tumors (swelling) of the sex glands, painful sexual intercourse, difficulty in urinating, in men inflammation of the prostate and seminal vesicles and in women inflammation of the vagina and urethra. Basically, it is a "cold" (mucous discharge) and fever (inflammation) of the reproductive system and a type of arthritis. The heat (inflammation) expands the cells and tissue and helps liquefy waste. This allows fluid (mucous) to flush out the waste congestion of the genitals. A lost of water (mucous) results in dehydration and an electrolyte disturbance. The glands filter out waste and adjust fluids by adding to or taking nutrients (ionize). Glands that become swollen or develop tumors lose their protective ability and allow waste to pass into the blood stream. This dumping of waste causes stress on other organs and causes waste to collect in the joints (arthritis). Waste congested tissue deteriorates. The body heals the deteriorated tissue by knitting it together, resulting in an itching sensation.

If the disease is untreated, it can cause infertility. Many times, it goes untreated because approximately 70% of the women and 10 % of men do not have any Chlamydia symptoms.

Supplement	Suggested Dosage	Remarks
Vitamin C (buffered/acid free)	1,500 mg., 4 times daily.	Enhances healing.
Vitamin E	600 IU daily.	Increases energy.
MSM	1,000-2,000 mg.	Fights infections. Helps nourish sex organs. Has antibiotic qualities.
Garlic capsules	2 capsules, 3 times daily.	A natural antibiotic.
Zinc	50 mg., daily.	Helps heal tissue.
Beta-Carotene	As directed.	Vital for healing.
Coenzyme Q_{10}	60 mg., daily.	Increases oxygen to cells.

Germanium	200 mg., daily.	Helps deliver oxygen to the cells and the immune system.
Kelp	6 tablets daily.	Provides minerals needed for healing.
Multiple Vitamin and Mineral	As directed.	Vital for healing.
Digestive Enzymes	3 tablets between meals and at bedtime.	Has an anti-inflammatory action.

GLANDULARS

Raw Thymus	As directed.	Enhances healing.

AMINO ACIDS

Lysine	1,000-2,000 mg.	Combats infection.

HERBS

Burdock, Cat's Claw, Echinacea, Feverfew, Goldenseal, Pau D'Arco, Red Clover, Sanicle, Tansy, White Oak Bark.

FOOD

Asparagus, Beet Greens, Broccoli, Cabbage, Carrots, Corn, Dandelion Greens, Dates, Elderberry, Garlic, Kale, Leeks, Mustard Greens, Onions, Oranges, Papaya, Parsley, Peaches, Pineapple, Plums, Romaine Lettuce, Spinach, Tangerines, Turnip Greens, Watercress, Yams.

HOMEOPATHIC

Thuja 9	5 gr., every other day.	Stops skin disease.
Rhus Tox 9 and Arnica 8	2 gr., once daily. Alternate.	Detoxifies skin.
Apis 5 and Lycopodium 7	2 gr., once daily. Alternate.	Destroys skin toxins.

TISSUE SALTS

Ferr. Phos. and Kali. Mur.	12x or 3-200x, 3 times daily. Alternate.	Used for mucous. discharge, inflammation and swelling.

CHRONIC FATIGUE SYNDROME

Chronic Fatigue Syndrome (CFS) has symptoms of extreme fatigue, "tired of being tired," anxiety, depression, mood swings, aching joints and muscles, fever, swollen glands, loss of appetite, sore throat, headache, backache, memory loss, irritability, colds, flu, over sensitivity to heat, cold and light, digestive problems, spasms, yeast infections, sleeping disorders, low blood sugar and anemia. It is commonly blamed on a bacteria or a dead particle (virus). It is often misdiagnosed as a psychosomatic illness (it is all in your head) or hypochondria (need to complain about illness). CFG is erroneously associated with genital herpes, shingles and a mononucleosis type virus (dead cell particle), Epstein Barr Virus (EBV).

Extreme fatigue can be caused by an extreme lack of energy, which means lack of adequate oxygen, hydrogen, iron, iodine, calcium, etc. An extreme deficit of energy occurs when the carbohydrates are not properly metabolized by the pancreas and liver. Processed (denatured, synthetic) foods such as white sugar, bleached white flour and polished rice, drugs, salt (mined, sea salt, kelp, etc.) and fried foods weaken the pancreas and liver resulting in loss of energy (fatigue). A weak liver fails to store energy (glycogen), which means a lack of reserve energy. Lack of reserve energy causes the adrenal glands to become active. They burn out the low energy supply, resulting in a double fatigue (energy drain). Junk foods produce a small energy output and a large amount of energy-draining waste. Junk foods cause nutrient starvation, energy starvation and fatigue. Aside from this, processed (junk) foods dehydrate cells, tissues, organs and bones compounding the waste accumulation in the body. This also lowers the energy output and contributes to fatigue.

Drugs (legal or illegal), junk food, synthetic chemicals and excessive estrogen hormones in non-organic foods and junk foods cause digestion to be too fast or too slow, resulting in inadequate metabolism and a lack of energy. The highly acidic junk foods cause energy to be burnt up quicker than it can be replaced. Acidity ages the body, which further drains the body of energy. Extreme low energy causes cells to die before they can be replaced or moved out the body. Consequently, the dead cells (minerals salts) get impacted in veins cartilage, arteries, nerves, organs and bones. This causes an electrical drain, weak nerves, dehydration, electrolyte imbalance, rheumatism, arthritis, etc. Organ weakness or disease further depletes the energy level causing extreme fatigue.

An inadequate diet (junk food, non-organic foods), physiological weakness and brain drain deplete Melanin. This electromagnetic drain of Melanin energy throws the African in an energy crisis. The African without adequate amounts of Melanin to help extract nutrients from food becomes fatigued easily. With exhausted Melanin levels, the African cannot fight infection, stabilize immunity and metabolize carbohydrates, resulting in fatigue (spiritual, mental, physical).

Computers, radiation, appliances, electrically driven machines and toxic radiation drains the body of energy. An energy drain causes biochemical imbalances such as yeast infection, excessive fungus growth, food addiction, high blood pressure, diabetes, hyperactivity, boredom and improper sleep = fatigue.

Supplement	Suggested Dosage	Remarks
DHEA (Dehydroepiandostrone)	5-15 mg. (women); 10-30 mg. (men).	Stimulates energy.
Creatine	1,000-10,000 mg.	Promotes cellular energy release.
Pantothenic Acid	5-50 mg.	Enhances adrenal glands function.
Black Currant Oil	2 capsules with meals.	Contains GLA (Gamma-Linoleic Acid) and all of the essential fatty acids.
Ascorbic Acid with Bioflavonoids	5,000 – 10,000 mg., daily.	Promotes the growth of healthy cells.

Coenzyme Q$_{10}$	75 mg., daily.	Aids energy production.
Lecithin	1,000-3,000 mg.	Encourages energy production.
Choline	500-1,000 mg.	Stimulates energy.
Garlic Capsules	2 capsules with meals.	Helps protect energy production.
Germanium	200 mg., and up.	Helps deliver energy to cells.
Vegetable Protein (Soy Free Powder)	As directed.	For tissue and organ repair and energy utilization.
Vitamin B Complex	100 mg., 3 times daily.	Enhances energy levels.
Multiple Vitamin and Mineral	As directed.	Essential for energy production.
Beta-Carotene	15,000 IU daily.	Helps enhance immunity.
Calcium	1,500 mg., daily.	Stabilizes energy.
Magnesium	1,000 mg., daily.	Fights fatigue.
Potassium	99 mg., daily.	Helps transport nutrients.
Selenium	200 mcg., daily.	Reduces energy exhaustion.
Zinc	50 mg., daily.	Helps maintain energy.

GLANDULARS

Raw Thymus	As directed.	Builds immunity.
Raw Liver	As directed.	Excites energy.
Raw Spleen	As directed.	Regulates energy.
Raw Glandular Complex	As directed.	Enhances glands.

AMINO ACIDS

Phenylalanine	As directed.	Stimulates energy.
Tyrosine	As directed.	Stimulates energy.
Glutamine	As directed.	Enhances brain ability to get nutrients and memory.

HERBS

Burdock Root, Damiana, Dandelion Root, Echinacea, Fo-Ti, Ginseng, Goldenseal, Pau D'Arco, Schizandra, Sumac, Yohimbe.

FOOD

Apricots, Asparagus, Barley, Beans, Beet Greens, Brussels Sprouts, Cabbage, Cantaloupe, Carrots, Cauliflower, Collard Greens, Corn, Currants, Dandelion Greens, Endive, Grapefruit, Guava, Kale, Lemons, Mustard Greens, Oranges, Papaya, Peaches, Raw Peanuts, Pecans, Plums, Romaine Lettuce, Soy Beans, Spinach, Tomatoes, Yams.

HOMEOPATHIC

Ignatia 7 and Cocculus 7	2 gr., once daily. Alternate.	Stabilizes energy.
Bryonia 9 (Bryany)	5 gr., once daily.	Releases energy in cells.
China 4 (Cinchona)	2 gr., twice daily.	Hormonal energy stimulation.

TISSUE SALTS

Kali. Phos. and Nat. Phos.	3x or 3-200x.	Essential for metabolism and utilizing energy.

CHOLESTEROL (HIGH)

Cholesterol is fat crystals. It is used to make the skin (membrane) of cells, sex hormones, myelin, used in digestion and picks up oxygen for the cell. It is a natural part of the nerves, bile, brain, blood and liver. Approximately 80% of the body's cholesterol is made by the liver and the diet supplies 20%. High levels of cholesterol can block and/or clog the veins and arteries of the brain, sex organs, eyes, kidney, scalp (baldness) and extremities. The two types of cholesterol that most concern people is High Density Lipoproteins (HDL) and Low Density Lipoproteins (LDL). LDL can cause severe problems and disease. It is found in dairy products, milk, meat and heated oils (margarine, coconut, palm, and cotton seed oils). Excessive alcohol made by the pancreas from refined carbohydrates as well as coffee, steroids, sex hormones in eggs, dairy, fruits, vegetables and in meat, caffeineated tea, tobacco and alcohol drinks can raise cholesterol.

The tissue of the veins and arteries can get congested with mineral salts from cellular waste (dead cell particles), table salt and protein urea salts waste. Congested vessels lose their flexibility causing further vascular stiffness. This causes a suffocation of vascular cells and decreases blood supplies to organ tissue. Cholesterol is a slippery oily substance, which helps blood slip through the blood vessels in order to increase blood supplies to organs. The body's attempt to increase blood flow through the narrow vascular tubes is viewed as a cholesterol problem. Aside from this, blood with high amounts of Mineral Salt waste and cellular waste damages blood vessels. The Mineral Salts and cell waste scrape and scratch the inner walls of blood vessels and cholesterol sticks to the walls. This narrows the vessels, decreases circulation, and stiffens vascular tissues.

Cholesterol is increased in order to improve circulation. Cholesterol gives a "pinching" effect to the blood vessels. Blood vessels are similar to the plumbing pipes in a house or a water hose. Cholesterol "pinching" is similar to pinching a hose with your fingers in order to increase water pressure and water flow (volume). This pinching increase in blood volume elevates cholesterol, which further raises the cholesterol level.

Faulty metabolism caused by the liver being stressed by junk foods, oils (fried foods, oil in baked goods and condiments) and radiation elevates cholesterol. The stressed liver, pancreas and digestive system cannot utilize calcium, break down oils, supply vital oxygen to cells or produce enough strong bile (digestive fluid) to metabolize food elements. This causes cholesterol to form and become impacted within the tissue of the veins and arteries.

Waste impacted in the tissue and nerves causes them to sub-clinically overheat. The insulation (cholesterol-like myelin) around nerve bundles and fibers wears away due to excessive electrical charge and the overheating of nerves. Stress causes the nerves to fire off more, creating more electrical heat and wearing away the myelin resulting in elevated cholesterol in order to recoat the nerves. Raw nerves and nerves lacking adequate cholesterol coating can produce numbness, irritability, feelings of tension, hypersensitivity, exhaustion and tingling.

Supplement	Suggested Dosage	Remarks
Coenzyme Q_{10}	60 mg.	Enhances oxygenation of cells and circulation.
Corn, Rice and Wheat Brans and/or Guar Gum	As directed.	Helps to lower cholesterol and supply needed fiber.
Garlic Capsules	2 capsules, 3 times daily.	Lowers cholesterol levels.
Lecithin	2 capsules or 1 tbsp 3 times daily, before meals.	Lowers cholesterol.
Lipotropic	As directed.	Prevents accumulation of fats (cholesterol).
Unsaturated Fatty Acids (Black Currant, Flax or Sunflower Borage and/or Primrose Oils)	As directed.	Helps normalize cholesterol.
Choline	100-300 mg., 3 times daily.	Helps metabolize oils.
B Complex	100 mg.	Lowers cholesterol.
Thiamine	10-50 mg.	Lowers cholesterol.
Chromium	200 mcg., daily.	Necessary for cholesterol balance.
Proteolytic Enzymes	Take between meals	Helps digestion.
Selenium	200 mcg.	Selenium deficiency has been linked to heart disease.
Niacin (B3) or Niacinamide	500 mg., daily.	Lowers cholesterol.
Vitamin C plus Bioflavonoids	3,000–8,000 mg., daily in divided doses.	Lowers cholesterol.
Vitamin E	400-800 IU.	Improves circulation.

GLANDULARS

Raw Liver	As directed.	Helps lower cholesterol.

AMINO ACIDS

Carnitine	500-1,000 mg.	Emulsifies fat.
Taurine	1,000-2,000 mg.	Lowers fat and cholesterol.

HERBS

Cayenne, Fenugreek, Goldenseal, Green Tea, Guggulipids, Hawthorn Berries, Irish Moss.

FOOD

Blackberries, Blueberries, Cabbage, Carrots, Corn, Olives, Peas, Raw Peanuts, Tomatoes.

HOMEOPATHIC

Bile-stones 9	5 gr. Take once a month in the a.m.	Dissolves fats (cholesterol).
Podophyllum 4	2 gr. Take every other day in the a.m.	Reduces fat.
China 4	2 gr. Take daily, 30 minutes before lunch and dinner.	Stimulates metabolism of fats.

TISSUE SALTS

Kali. Mur. and Nat. Phos.	3x or 3-200x, twice daily. Alternate.	Helps reduce cholesterol level.
Calc. Phos. and Silicea	3x or 3-200x, twice daily. Alternate.	Aids fat emulsion.

CIRCULATION (POOR)

Poor circulation can be indicated by paleness of the fingernail, cold toes and/or fingers, dark purplish toes or fingers, coldness on the tip of the nose, numbness in the fingers and toes, tingling and/or burning sensation in the fingers and toes, the skin on the underside of the eyelids may appear pale, the sensation of feeling cold when people around say they are not cold, etc.

Poor circulation can be caused by hypertension, arteriosclerosis, stress, cardiovascular problems, Buerger's (tingling pins and needles to extremities), Raynauds (extremities hypersensitive to cold), diabetes, high blood pressure, junk food, meat, dairy, drugs, radiation, synthetic chemicals, etc. In poor circulation, the blood gets overloaded with waste (liquid manure) and becomes thick and slow to move (circulate). The blood is meant to be alkaline and not over acidic with liquid manure. Slightly acidic blood decreases the ability of cells, tissue and organs to get oxygen and nutrients. Acidic blood or body condition causes oxygen starvation in the body tissue and cells. Waste-filled blood causes too much electricity and heat to the nerves, muscles, bones, cartilage, and cells. Unhealthy blood causes the body to decrease oxygen and nutrients to the extremities (controlled by the sympathetic nerves) in an attempt to get more oxygen and nutrient to the parasympathetic trunk/torso. This energy diversion further deteriorates the organ systems, resulting in energy loss and increased aging. Poor circulation is reaction to a disease and not itself a disease. However, it eventually becomes a disease that produces its own effect. Acid waste from the tissues, organs, muscles and bones get dumped into the blood. This causes the blood to get alkaline minerals from the bones. The blood slightly increases its alkalinity in defense from the overly acid tissues. Slightly high alkaline blood holds more oxygen, which deteriorates blood and nutrients and bonds carbon dioxide and waste to it at a higher level. This type blood is starving for nutrients and starts a chain reaction of starving everything it comes in contact with. It is nutritionally poor blood; waste-filled blood and thick blood that is circulating and deteriorating veins and arteries, resulting in poor circulation. Poor circulation is an effect, not a cause.

Supplement	Suggested Dosage	Remarks
Calcium and Magnesium	1,500– 2,000 mg. 750 – 1,000 mg. after meals and at bedtime.	Normalizes blood thickness (viscosity) and strengthens the heart.
Coenzyme Q$_{10}$	100 mg., daily.	Aids circulation by putting more oxygen in blood.
Germanium	200 mg., daily.	Helps tissue oxygenation.

Chlorophyll	Liquid or pill form as directed.	Improves circulation and builds healthy cells.
Multiple Vitamin and Mineral	As directed.	Helps circulatory function.
Vitamin A and E	As directed.	Helps metabolism of fat (cholesterol) and gets oxygen to cells.
Vitamin B Complex	100 mg.	Improves circulation by metabolizing fat and cholesterol.
Garlic Capsules (Odorless)	2 capsules with meals.	Lowers cholesterol and blood pressure.
Vitamin C plus Bioflavonoids	5,000–10,000 mg., daily in divided doses.	Helps prevent blood clotting.
Vitamin B_6	2-200 mg.	Prevents numbness.
Niacinamide	50-100 mg.	Diabetes vessels and improves circulation.
Choline	100 mg., 3 times daily with meals.	Improves circulation and lowers cholesterol.
Lecithin	2 capsules, 3 times daily or 1 tbsp in dry form before meals.	Lecithin emulsifies (breaks up) fats.
Digestive Enzymes	As directed.	Aids digestion and circulation.
Zinc	50 mg., daily.	Necessary for immune function.
Niacin (B_3)	3 mg., daily.	Dilates vessels and improves circulation.
Proteolytic Enzymes	2 tablets between meals.	Helps to break down undigested food particles in the blood and colon.
Selenium	200 mcg daily.	Helps heart and circulation.

GLANDULARS

Raw Heart	As directed.	Improves circulation.
Raw Kidney	As directed.	Reduces waste in blood.
Raw Liver	As directed.	Helps filter waste out of blood.

AMINO ACIDS

Glutathione	500-3,000 mg.	Helps get rid of toxins in the blood and liver.
L-Carnitine	500 mg., twice daily.	Helps to remove fats and promotes circulation.

HERBS

Anise, Black Cohosh, Butcher's Broom, Cayenne, Gingko, Chickweed, Garlic, Ginger, Goldenseal, Hawthorn Berry, Horseradish, Horsetail, Hyssop, Licorice, Milk Thistle, Pleurisy, Shepherd's Purse, Wormwood.

FOOD

Cabbage, Corn, Dandelion Greens, Figs, Guava.

HOMEOPATHIC

Arsenicum Album 7	2 gr., daily.	Reduces waste in blood.

Baryta Carbonica 7 and Aurum Metallicum 7	2 gr., in the a.m. Alternate.	Increases circulation.
Cupressus 7 and Kali Iodatum 7	2 gr., in the p.m. Alternate.	Improves oxygen in blood.

TISSUE SALTS

Kali. Phos.	12x or 3-200x, 3 times daily.	Enhances circulation.
Silicea and Calc. Flour.	12x or 3-200x, 3 times daily.	Aid elasticity of blood.

COCAINE ADDICTION DETOX
(DETOXIFICATION)

Cocaine is a drug that is abused. It causes gradual damaging effects upon the body. The disease effects of cocaine may take several hours/years before they appear and then they are misdiagnosed as being caused by some bacteria, virus or germ. The Cocaine "high" is caused by its ability to stimulate an adrenaline rush. Adrenalin is secreted to speed up the defense reactions and to protect the body from Cocaine. The speed-type high, caused by Adrenalin is the reaction to the disease state caused by Cocaine. In other words, the person makes himself or herself sick and the sickness is called a "high." Cocaine poisons the body and endangers the brain and nervous system. The body's reaction to the toxic synthetic chemical is to rush energy to remove this poisonous chemical. The body's attempt to remove cocaine causes a temperature increase in organs. Thus, the toxic cocaine remains in the body. The Cocaine high causes a decrease of energy and blood circulation to the extremities such as the ears, toes, and fingers. The Cocaine causes a decreased energy state, which is erroneously called a "high." Cocaine users believe that feeling normal (good health) feels sick, so they make their body sick with Cocaine so they can feel good (healthy). Their mind and emotions are sick, not their body.

The detoxification of the body is a gradual process. It is suggested that detox should span over a two-to four-week period. The suggested remedies should be taken daily. Supplements with meals and amino acids between meals or on an empty stomach. For further information, a book such as *Getting off Cocaine* by M. Weiner, Ph.D. is suggested.

Supplements	Suggested Dosage	Remarks
Multiple Vitamin and Minerals	As directed.	Provides nutrients.
Digestive Enzyme	As directed.	Improves digestion.
Vitamin A	25,000 IU.	Strengthens tissue.
Beta Carotene	20,000 IU.	Enhances immunity.
Vitamin C (buffered)	10,000 mg.	Combats infection.
Vitamin E	25,000 IU.	Aids circulation and immunity.
Lecithin Capsules	1,000-4,000 mg.	Used for depression and nerves.
Garlic Capsules	2 capsules three times daily.	Purifies blood.

GABA	1,000-5,000 mg.	Stabilizes nerves.
Pantothenic Acid	5-50 mg.	Reduces stress.
Calcium	2,000 mg.	Calms nerves.
Magnesium	1,000 mg.	Nourishes nerves.
Lipoic Acid	100-200 mg.	Heals nerve damage.
Plant Sterolins	As directed.	Helps defend the tissue.

GLANDULARS

| Raw Adrenal, Raw Liver | As directed. | Relieves stress. Neutralizes drugs. |

AMINO ACIDS

Tyrosine	1,000 to 3,000 mg.	Daytime energizer.
Phenylalanine	1,000 to 3,000 mg.	Relieves stress and pain.
5HTP	500-2,000 mg.	Relaxes, rest, sleep.
Glutathionine	500-3,000 mg.	Removes toxins.
Glucosamine and Chondroitin	1,000 mg.	Heals tissue and relieves pain.

HERBS

Pau D'Arco, Echinacea, Gotu Kola, Goldenseal, Chaparral — Combine and drink in glass daily.

Stimulator

| Yohimbe and Ephedra | Daytime. | Combination is believed to be a natural type of "high" (Cocaine sensation). |

Nervousness

Valerian, Passion Flower, Skullcap, Catnip, Chamomile — Sleeping Aid.

FOODS

Raw fruits and fruit juices, fresh vegetables. If animal flesh is eaten, it must be baked or broiled without added oil. Use raw almond butter, raw sesame butter, a vegetable protein drink and wheat, corn or oat bran daily. Yohimbe and Ephedra Daytime Combination is believed to be a natural type of "high" (Cocaine sensation).

SIGNS AND SYMPTOMS OF CRACK AND COCAINE USE

Smoked Crack reaches the brain within eight to ten seconds after the smoke is inhaled. Snorted cocaine reaches the brain within two to three minutes. Crack is similar to Ritalin. It stimulates the central nervous system, causing involuntary movements and possibly raises the body's temperature. The poisonous impact of the drug begins within two minutes of smoking, usually peaks in less than half an hour.

Central Nervous System

Stimulation of this system causes euphoria, talkativeness, hallucinations, irritability and suspicion. The user may hallucinate and feel as if there are bugs crawling under the skin.

Arteries

Blood pressure increases from ten to fifteen percent. This depraves the brain of air, increases waste in the blood, decreases circulation, dehydrates tissue, weakens digestion and the sex organs. Blood circulating through the vessels at a rapid speed may cause the brain hemorrhage.

Eyes
Pupils may dilate and become more sensitive to light. This can cause the appearance of "halos" surrounding objects. Users often call the halo effect "snowlights."

Heart
Heartbeat becomes more rapid, increasing by 30 to 50 percent, and may become irregular. This increases the aging of the body. This weakens the heart and in rare instances can cause a heart attack.

Lungs
Chronic crack smoking may lead to hoarseness and bronchitis, similar to effects of marijuana or tobacco smoking. Smoking decreases the oxygen supply to organs causing oxygen starvation.

Limbs
May spasm or convulse as muscle involuntary contract. This causes the muscles to become congested with waste.

Weight
Cocaine use can lead to quick or severe weight loss. Users tend to lose their appetite and skip meals.

COLDS/FLU

Colds are a social term given to mucous congestion of sinus and/or lungs. Colds are a bodily defense reaction to toxins or a polluted septic body system and/or imbalanced body chemistry (minerals, vitamins, etc.). The common accepted belief is that one can "catch a cold." A "cold" is developed, not caught. You cannot "catch healthy" by standing near a healthy person. You cannot catch a cold by contacting some strange bacteria or dead cell particle called a virus. A dis-eased (toxic) weakened body has little defense against a strange bacteria and is the perfect septic environment to multiply. The catarrh (mucous) discharge called a "cold" is the body's attempt to rid itself of waste (toxic impurities) that it could not pass out through the bowels (manure) or urine or perspiration. The cold is a cleansing process and not a disease. The mucous drains out of the body via the lungs and nasal passage and is ignorantly called a "cold." It is usually caused by constipation, overeating or a diet of partial foods (junk foods) that produces partial health known as a disease. The body is not "at-ease," it is in a state of "dis-ease" called a "cold."

Supplements	Suggested Dosage	Remarks
Vitamin C with Bioflavonoids	5,000 to 10,000 mg., taken hourly or 3 to 6 times a day.	Combats infection.
Vitamin B-Complex	50-100 mg., 3 times daily.	Increases healing energy.
Vitamin B_6	50 mg. daily.	Relieves stress. Found in cold-pressed soy, sesame, safflower and flaxseed oil.
Vitamin A	50,000 IU.	Helps heal tissue.
Vitamin E	200 IU. daily.	Destroys free radicals.
Calcium	2,000 mg.	Stabilizes tissue.
Zinc		Fights infection.
Bee Pollen		
Garlic	400 mg., three times daily.	Defends against infection.
Folic Acid	200 mcg.	Stimulates health.
Iodine	150 mcg.	Aids development of health.
Silicon	10-40 mcg.	Stimulates immunity.
Digestive Enzyme	As directed.	Helps break down waste.

GLANDULARS

Raw Spleen, Raw Thymus	As directed.	Fights infection, stimulates immunity.

AMINO ACIDS

Cysteine, Ornithine, Histidine, Tryptophan, Arginine	As directed.	Repairs damaged cells. Stimulates immunity.

HERBS

Chamomile, Chaparral, Chinchoma, Comfrey, Desert Tea, Echinacea, Fenugreek, Ginger, Goldenseal, Hibiscus, Lemon Grass, Peppermint, Rosehip, Sage, Slippery Elm, Watercress, White Willow Bark.

FOODS

Carrots, Broccoli, Brussels Sprouts, Cauliflower, Collards, Currants, Dandelion Greens, Elderberries, Garlic, Grapefruit, Guava, Horseradish, Kale, Lemons, Onions, Oranges, Parsley, Peppers, Spinach, Tomatoes, Turnip Greens, Watercress.

HOMEOPATHIC

Calc. Phos., Ferr. Phos.		Fights infection, stimulates healing.

Books such as *Never Catch Another Cold* by W. Dimiscio and *Chronic Bronchitis* by A. Moyle are resources for help.

COLITIS

Colitis is the inflammation of the skin of the large intestines (colon) that tries to evacuate and excrete waste. When these fail to eliminate, it uses inflammation of tissue. The tissue of the colon becomes congested with waste due to junk foods, meat, dairy, drugs, stress and/or allergies. A stiff and waste impacted colon causes more waste to collect within the colon.

An inflexible colon has limited muscular movement. Limited colon movement causes excessive food gases and acids, which can result in inflammation. High acidity in the colon inflames it. The inflamed mucous membranes (tissue) develop pocket-like sac areas (diverted outward). Food waste collects in the pockets and dehydrates. Dehydrated manure, mineral salt waste, carbon dioxide and monoxide and poisonous gases stiffen the colon and waste accumulates. The mineral salt waste causes an increase in electrical current, which produces heat and dries and stiffens (crystalizes) the colon. The symptoms of Colitis are mucous and pus in watery stools, diarrhea, tenderness, cramps and spasms in the abdominal area, a continuous need to have a bowel movement and fever. Colitis can be of mucous membrane (skin) and intestines, which is called Enteritis. Colitis can be in the lower ⅗ of the small intestines with symptoms similar to colitis plus constipation. The intestinal wall thickens and swells, which narrows the opening of the intestines and limits the passage of manure.

See Bronchitis (page 39), for Vitamins, Minerals, Amino Acids, etc. Also take MSM antiflammatory.

HERBS

Bilberry, Cat's Claw, Catnip, Chaparral, Cleaver, Coltsfoot, Dandelion Root, Elecampane, Eyebright, Feverfew, Garlic, Hyssop, Lobelia, Mullein, Peppermint, Plantains, Red Clover, Sage, St. John's Wort, White Oak Bark, Wormwood, Yarrow.

FOOD

Bananas, Cabbage, Carrots, Corn, Dates, Eggplant, Figs, Okra, Parsnips, Pears, Persimmons, Squash, Tapioca.

HOMEOPATHIC

Arsenicum Album, Baptisia, Belladonna, Bryonia, Gelsemium, Lachesis, Muriatic Acid, Rhus Tox.

TISSUE SALTS

Kali. Phos.	12x or 3-200x, three times daily.	Reduces fevers.
Nat. Mur.	12x or 3-200x, three times daily.	Regulates moisture.
Ferr. Phos.	3x or 3-200x, every hour.	Helps protect tissue.

COMPUTER RADIATION

The body is composed of minerals, electricity, magnetism, melanin and various biochemical substances. It has specific ratios of frequencies, electromagnetism, pressure, pH, and fluid volumes and temperatures it maintains in order to be healthy. When the body is subjected to harsh bombardments of cancer causing synthetic radiation from computers, x-rays, electric blankets, appliances, hair dryers, subway trains, radios, air planes, cell phones, satellite dishes, electronic games, smoke detectors, televisions, cars, loud music, printers, monitors, radar devices, building materials, medical radiation therapies, cooling fans, microwaves, grocery store price scanners, oil storage tanks, etc. Radiation can cause cancer, blood clots, stress, boredom, headaches, cataracts, fatigue, neck aches, repetitive strain injury (i.e. carpal tunnel), discharges, shoulder pain, skin rashes, eye blink rate alternation, electrical hypersensitivity, mood swings, sleep disturbance, obesity, irritability, eating disorders, rigidity in thought sequence, dizziness, nausea, etc.

The body's cells communicate with natural electrical and magnetic pulses. The synthetic radiation (electromagnetic) congests the cells and/or, overheat them causes crystallization and inflexibility, which decreases their life span and your quality of life. Excess synthetic electrical and/or magnetic energy overloads the wiring of the body (nerves) and interrupts communications between cells, tissues and organs. This can result in static cling of radiation. Africans, with their high level of melanin, absorb the highest amounts of toxic radiation plus they develop synthetic electromagnetic cling. The high amounts of radiation from machines alters the rythmaticity and cyclic nature of the body causing diseases of rythmaticity. Metals worn by melanin-dominate Africans can amplify and absorb the radiation and raise it to higher levels of danger. Metals, such as jewelry, watches, eyeglasses, false teeth, mercury fillings, beepers and zippers multiply the radiation levels in the body. Radiation, like all synthetics (nicotine, white sugar, alcohol, salt, etc.) is addicting. For example, a person asleep with the television on will awaken when it is turned off. Turning off the television takes away the radiation drug fix—radiation addiction. This causes electromagnetic disruptions in the sleep pattern. In the body, radiation can turn into an addicting chemical.

Synthetic radiation congests the cells, tissues, organs and nerves. It overrides the conscious filtering system of the brain and goes directly into the brain with undecoded information, thoughts and emotions. The nervous system's electromagnetic safety level is violated. Nerves overheat, which wears away the nerves insulation (myelinated covering) causing oversensitivity, numbing, tingling sensation and fraying of nerves. Electromagnetic charges get stored in the bones, which congests them. The overheating of nerves causes them and muscles around them to dehydrate. This results in the muscle getting pickled (excessive mineral salts, congestion) and they lose elasticity, plus they drain the body of energy and natural electromagnetism causing fatigue. Synthetic radiation can reduce the oxygen in the body and weaken immunity. The cells get congested with synthetic radiation and their moisture evaporates causing a build-up of carbon dioxide and a reduction in oxygen. The radiation increases the aging of the body and can cause genetic mutation. The best defense is constant nutritional defense by using the following supplements. See Cancer (page 47), for Vitamins, Minerals, Amino Acids, etc.

HERBS

Barberry, Burdock, Chaparral, Dandelion Root, Echinacea, Feverfew, Goldenseal, Milk Thistle, Oregon Grape, Pokeweed, Red Clover, Sassafras, Wormwood.

FOOD

Asparagus, Avocado, Barley, Beets, Broccoli, Cabbage, Collard Greens, Eggplant, Jackfruit, Kale, Mango, Mushrooms, Oranges, Papaya, Peaches, Peas, Raw Peanuts, Rice, Romaine Lettuce, Soybeans, Tomatoes, Turnip Greens, Yams.

HOMEOPATHIC

Liver Radiation
Arsenicum Album 7   2 gr., once daily. Alternate.   Stops cell degeneration
  and China 4   stabilizes tissue.

Radiation Waste in Tissue
Kali. Phosphoricum 7   2 gr., once daily.   Maintains structure of cells.

Agitation Reducer
Rus. Tox. 9   2 gr., once daily.

Stress Reducer
Nux. Vomica 8 and Aconile 7   2 gr., once daily. Alternate.

Eye Stress Reducer
Arsenicum Album 7
and Agarieus 7   2 gr., once daily. Alternate.

You can use a Diode and/or Polarizer to protect against radiation.

CONSTIPATION

Constipation is hard or loose (diarrhea) fecal (manure) matter. Several reasons for this are:

- Too little water (should be one fluid ounce for each two pounds of normal body weight)
- Non-fiber foods such as refined or processed foods (bleached white flour, white sugar)
- Preservatives (retard digestion)
- Too little exercise
- Eating too late (should have last meal four or five hours before going to sleep)
- Digestive organs' weakness, disease or stress (liver, stomach, pancreas, etc.)
- Improper food combining
- Junk foods
- Nutrient or emotional imbalances

It takes four hours for the stomach to empty. No meal or snacks should be eaten until the stomach is emptied or else constipation will result. Bad breath, and a coated tongue can indicate constipation.

Supplements	Suggested Dosage	Remarks
Vitamin A	10,000 IU.	
Vitamin C	5,000-20,000 mg.	Helps heal.
Vitamin B-Complex	50 mg., 3 times daily.	Improves digestion
Vitamin B_1	50 mg.	Enhances digestion.

Brewer's Yeast	As directed.	Aids metabolism.
Wheat Bran	3 to 4 tbsp.	Cleanses colon.
Rice Bran, Oat Bran, Corn Germ	As directed.	Cleansing fiber.
Magnesium	750-1,000 mg.	Helps transient food.
Calcium Lactate	1,500-2,000 mg.	Enhances colon muscles.

GLANDULARS

Raw Liver, Raw Thyroid, Raw Thymus.	Improves digestions.

AMINO ACIDS

Methionine, Phenylalanine.	500-1,000 mg.	Stimulates colon.

HERBS

Black Root, Buckthorn, Cascara Sagrada (Laxative), Dandelion, Flaxseed, Ginger, Licorice, Mandrake, Psyllium, Raspberry, Rhubarb (Laxative), Senna (Laxative) Slippery Elm.

FOODS

Apricots, Asparagus, Avocado, Barley, Beans, Beets, Blackberries, Black Radish, Black Walnuts, Blueberries, Broccoli, Brussels Sprouts, Cabbage, Cantaloupe, Carrots, Cauliflower, Celery, Chard, Cherimoya, Cherries, Coconut, Collard Greens, Corn, Cranberry, Currant, Dandelion Greens, Dates, Dulse, Eggplant, Elderberries, Endives, Figs, Garlic, Gooseberries, Grapes, Jackfruit, Jerusalem Artichoke, Kale, Lettuce, Millet, Mustard Greens, Oats, Olives, Onions, Peaches, Peanuts, Pears, Peas, Pecans, Peppers, Persimmons, Pineapple, Plum, Potatoes, Prunes, Pumpkin Seeds, Quince, Radish, Raisins, Raspberries, Rhubarb, Rutabagas, Sauerkraut Juice, Sesame Seeds, Soy Beans, Spinach, Squash (Summer), Strawberries, Tomatoes, Turnips, Walnuts, Water Chestnuts, Watercress.

HOMEOPATHIC

Laxative

Pangelox or Delpech	As directed.

Infrequent Bowel Movements

Nux. Vomica 8	2 gr., in the a.m.
Lycopodium 7	2 gr., at noon.

Absent Bowel Movement

Opium 7	2 gr., in the a.m.

TISSUE SALTS

Nat. Phos.	6x or 3-200x, every 30 minutes until bowels move.	Helps colon muscles move food.
Nat. Mur.	6x or 3-200x in the a.m. and p.m. until bowels move with difficulty and are dry.	Improves transient time.
Nat. Sulph.	6x or 3-200x in the a.m. and p.m.	Stimulates the colon.

Coated yellow tongue

Kali. Sulph.	6x or 3-200x in the a.m. and p.m.	Stimulates colon moisture.
Calc. Flour. and Silicea	6x or 3-200x, both in the a.m. and p.m.	

Difficulty evacuating

Kali. Mur.	6x or 3-200x in the a.m. and p.m.	Aids excretion of waste.

Coated white tongue
Kali. Phos. and Calc. Flour.   12x or 3-200x in the a.m. and p.m.

Feel like you are going to have a bowel movement
Ferr. Phos.   6x or 3-200x every 30 minutes   Pain or inflammation.

CROHN'S DISEASE

Crohn's disease is inflammation of the digestive tract that has been going on for a long period of time (from months to years). Basically, it is colitis of a long duration and a combination of ileitis (inflamed intestines). Long-term inflammation such as Crohn's will cook the intestinal flesh, then the inflammation stops for a period of time. The cooked skin heals and leaves a scar, which narrows the tube-like opening of intestines. The inflammation causes the skin of the digestive tract to become too thick to absorb nutrients (mal- absorption) and damages the muscles. The villi (small hairy-like drinking straws that are in the intestinal skin) cannot suck the food's nutrients into the bloodstream because inflammation damaged the skin and destroyed villi. This further decreases the ability to absorb nutrients and move food through the digestive tract.

Crohn's disease can begin around age twenty or older. The inflammatory attacks can be sporadic or long-term. The symptoms can include periodic cramping, pain in the lower area of the abdomen (so-called stomach), anemia, bleeding, diarrhea, fever, loss of weight and appetite and lack of energy. It can be misdiagnosed as appendicitis. The skin of the intestine can develop holes and undigested food and/or pus can leak into the abdomen's cavity. This can cause inflammation of the skin lining the abdomen. Undigested food particles can get into the blood and cause allergies. Crohn's can be caused by cellular mineral waste embedded in the skin of the intestines, junk foods, dairy, meat, synthetic chemicals, radiation, stress and drugs (legal and illegal). See Bronchitis (page 39), for Vitamins, Minerals, Amino Acids, etc.

FOOD
Inflammation
Cantaloupes, Cranberries, Garlic, Grapefruit, Kumquats, Mangos, Parsley, Tangerines.

HOMEOPATHIC
Arsenicum Album, Baptisia, Belladonna, Bryonia, Gelsemium, Lachesis, Muriatic Acid, Rhus Tox.

TISSUE SALTS
Kali. Phos.   12x or 3-200x, three times daily.   Stimulates release of mucus.
Nat. Mur.   12x or 3-200x, three times daily.   Helps heal tissue.
Ferr. Phos.   3x or 3-200x, every hour.   Reduces fever.

CROUP

Croup is an early childhood disease associated with junk food, meat and dairy diet. The typical fat bloated child on such a diet has pictures on cereal boxes, paper diaper boxes, body food labels and in all commercial advertisements. These children are overfed, overweight, overwasted, fat bloated, drools from the mouth and have stomach gas. They are promoted as being healthy and have the early symptoms of a variety of adult diseases. In croup, the skin of the larynx (vocal chords) and trachea (windpipe) swell with mucous waste and get inflamed. The larynx and trachea tissues get congested with mineral filled mucous waste, which causes electrical friction, resulting in excess heat called an inflammation. Croups gets its name from abnormal "croup" sounding noise that is made when air is breathed in over the inflamed vocal chords through the mucous constricted windpipe. A croup attack usually occurs at night when resistance and circulation is decreased. The child starts a dry, hoarse and constant barking cough with shrill wheezy sounds when they breathe in air. Croup is a self-limiting disease that can last up to three days. It does not require treatment with poisonous prescription drug concoctions. In the case of children, supplements are best in liquid spray, chewable or powder forms. Liquid herbal supplements should not contain alcohol or vinegar. Herbal extracts in a vegetable Glycerin base are best. See Bronchitis (page 39), for Vitamins, Minerals, Amino Acid, etc.

HERBS

Catnip, Chickweed, Comfrey, Echinacea, Goldenseal, Mullein, Peppermint, Red Raspberry.

FOOD

See "Colds," page 63.

HOMEOPATHIC

Hepar Sulphur 7	5 gr., immediately or as directed.	Fights infection.
Bromium 7	5 gr., quarter of an hour afterwards or as directed.	
Sambucus Nigra 4	5 gr., quarter of an hour afterwards or as directed.	Helps expectorate.
Spongia 4 and Sambucus 4	2 gr., every 30 minutes or as directed. Alternate.	Cleanses tissue of waste.

TISSUE SALTS

Ferr. Phos.	12x or 3-200x or as directed.	Excretes mucus.
Kali. Mur.	12x or 3-200x or as directed.	Reduces inflammation.

DIABETES

Diabetes a dis-ease of the pancreas. The Melanin centers of the pancreas (Islet of Langerhaus) are harmed or damaged. The condition exists when the body has sugar (natural fuel for the body) available, but fails to recognize it. This

causes excess sugar to accumulate, which the body gets rid of by excess urinating. The urine will become morbid and change in odor and color. Excessive
urinating causes thirst, dehydration, weight loss, loss of appetite, and an overworked kidney and pancreas. The pancreas secretes the hormone insulin,
which stimulates the use of sugar. Diseases, emotions and/or social stressors
can overstimulate the pituitary and/or adrenals, which overtaxes the pancreas
resulting in diabetes. Black folks can have misdiagnosed or subclinical diabetes because the Caucasian race's diabetes test's normal range is 80-120 glucose. Black folks can have diabetes with a 90 glucose, along with diabetes
related diseases of high blood pressure, hyperactivity, kidney failure, cataracts,
nerve damage, glaucoma, infertility, mood swings, hair loss, bone loss, etc.

Diabetes is usually caused by overeating and refined carbohydrates
(bleached white flour, white rice, white grits, cooked white potatoes, and
refined white sugar). Eating excessive amounts of animal flesh and cooked animal fats (fats and proteins change to sugar in the body) can cause diabetes.
Bleached white flour, white rice and cooked white potatoes turn into sugar rapidly, weaken the pancreas and kidneys and cause diabetes.

White sugar is the primary cause of sugar diabetes. Diabetes is an emotional illness that can be caused by the inability to love and/or receive love.
Sugar represents love and the dysfunctional love emotions are medicated by
eating sugar (sweets, candy, sodas, cake, chocolate, ice cream, corn starch,
etc.). A weak liver that is unable to metabolize fats causes the craving for carbohydrates (i.e., sugar). The liver is made weak by drugs, processed foods,
processed oils, radiation, etc. The blood sugar level falls just before menstruation and this can cause a sugar craving. Sugar craving is stimulated by eating salt. Consequently, salt is found in candy bars, sweets, sodas, etc. Since
sugar is associated with love and love is associated with sex, perfumes are
made to smell sweet. Consequently, a craving for sex causes a craving for
sugar. Sexual frustration can cause a sugar craving. Sugar addicts refer to
each other with the terms, "Hi Sugar," "Hello Sweetie," "Hi Honey," etc.
Sugar is associated with nice and good behavior. Therefore, sugar is used to
reward yourself or others for good behavior.

Sugar diabetes can be caused by the inability to change stored sugar
(glycogen) into useable sugar (glucose). This inability can cause the body to
use fats as a source of sugar (ketones). Processed sugar weakens the pancreas' ability to use sugar for energy, so the body switches to fats (oil) for
energy. Thus, people drink a coke (sugar) with oily salty French fries or potato
chips (oil). Salt is associated with frustration and anger.

It is important to be aware that all processed sugars (fructose, honey,
maple syrup, sucrose, etc.) can be damaging to the pancreas, liver and health.
High amounts of fructose in hybrid fruits are stressful and damaging to the pancreas and can lead to diabetes. Fructose is a sugar that does not require insulin.
Therefore, diabetics believe they can use it. However, it damages the liver. The
treatment of the Glucose Imbalance can strengthen the pancreas.

GLUCOSE FROM GLYCOGEN AND GLUCOSE FROM FAT (OILS) IMBALANCES . . .

Tend to be associated with. . .	Relate specifically to. . .
- Diabetes	- Deficient oxidation activity
- Respiratory Rate	- Abnormal carbon dioxide levels
- Pulse	- Abnormal pH of blood
- Saliva pH	
- Blood Pressure	
- Glucose	

Glucogenic

These supplements help convert glucose to useable energy: L-Carnitine, L-Tyrosine, L-Phehylalanine, L-Leucine, L-Isoleucine, L-Methionine, Ribonucleic Acid, Liver, Vitamin A (Palmitate), d-Alpha Tocopherol, Niacinimide.

Supplements	Suggested Dosage	Remarks
Vitamin A	25,000 IU.	Protects glands.
Vitamin C	2,000-10,000 mg.	Destroys free radicals.
Vitamin B-Complex	50 mg., 3 times daily.	Enhances metabolism.
Vitamin B_6	50 mg.	Helps utilize nutrients.
Vitamin D	400 IU.	Combats calcium loss.
Vitamin F	As directed.	Stabilizes sugar levels.
Niacin (Niacinamide)	50 mg.	Aids absorption.
Chromium	400-600 mcg.	Helps utilize insulin.
Potassium	100-500 mg.	Regulates levels.
Manganese	5-10 mg.	Helps heal the pancreas.
Vanadyl Sulfate	100-200 mg.	Heals pancreas.
Lipoic Acid	100-200 mg.	Stabilizes, repairs nerves.

GLANDULARS

Raw Liver		Enhances the release of stored sugar.

HERBS

Alfalfa, Bilberry (blueberry leaves), Bitter Melon, Cayenne, Cedar Berries, Centeurea, Comfrey, Dandelion Root, Goldenseal, Gymnema Sylvestre, Mullein, Periwinkle, Raspberry, Sinta.

The underlined herbs are the best for diabetes. For Food, see Hypoglycemia, (page 84). Also, one cup of Raw Stringbean Juice equals two units of Insulin.

ENEMA

An enema is the use of water (distilled, spring or boiled) or herbal teas injected in the rectum and colon. The purpose of the enema is to remove feces, worms, and impurities.

A high enema is performed with a colon tube (which is 24" to 32" in length) attached to the tube of the enema bag and inserted into the anus; the tube passes through the rectum and into the colon. This type of enema reaches high into the large intestines (colon). A colonic irrigation is an enema performed by using ten to thirty gallons of water—a proctor is used and has a water in-flow tube and a waste out-flow tube attached. If the colonic irrigation is not available, then take ten gallons of water per high enema for three days. In this way, the body will not be strained by the colonic irrigation and the process becomes more rhythmical and natural. The enema tube should be lightly oiled and the anus should be lightly oiled before inserting the tube. Warm or slightly warm water is used. The herb teas are usually strained and used at a warm temperature.

Enema bags usually have a fountain syringe and can be purchased from a drugstore. Sometimes, the colon tubes have to be purchased at a medical supply store. Enemas are usually classified by the use desired.

Anthelmintic Enemas (gets rid of worms)
Worms feed off fermented and/or putrefied manure that is in the colon due to constipation, wrong food combinations, meat, contaminated yogurt, milk, lunch meat, unclean produce, slow digestion, spastic colons, stress, under-active appendices, feces that pack and line around the colon, etc. Worms can be felt crawling around, seen in the bowel movements or around the anus. They tend to crawl out the rectum at night, due to the warmth of sleeping blankets. They can be seen crawling out the anus at night. They can cause scratching the anus during the day as well as night. Worms come in all shapes and sizes and many are transparent.

Salt water: dissolve one to two cups of salt in warm water. Add lime or lemon to warm water and inject into the rectum.

Herbs
Aloe, Cascara Sagrada, Horse Radish and Senna, are laxatives that remove worms. (See anthelmintic). Asafetida, Elecampane, Garlic, Quassia and Wormwood remove worms.

Antispasmodic Enemas
The colon sometime becomes too weak to have natural muscle actions (peristalsis). The weakness can be caused by packed feces around the colon lining, constipation, etc. Parasympathetic spasm causes the colon to stay open (diarrhea). Sympathetic spasm of the sphincter muscles cause constipation.

Herbs
Chamomile, Hops, Lobelia, Valerian, (See calminitive herbs).

Astringent Enemas
A bleeding (hemorrhages) colon can be caused by straining when having bowel movements. Straining is caused by constipation, weak muscles (prolapsed), poor diet, etc. Ice cold-water enemas are good (See astringent herbs).

Emollient Enemas
This type of enema softens hard caked feces.

Herbs
Barley, Linseed Oil, Prune Juice, Psyllium, Castor Oil, Olive Oil.

Nutritive Enemas
One to two cup molasses; add 2 cups Horse Radish and lemon juice (use 2 lemons) to 2 quarts of water.

Sedative Enemas
Use Cannabis Sativa Seeds as a tea, Valerian or Catnip (See sedatives).

Purgative Enemas
Add liquid soap to an herbal solution of Ginger and Horse Radish.

Coffee and Garlic Enemas
This type of enema is used to detoxify the body and is commonly used for severe dis-eases.
　　The garlic is an antibiotic and rids the body of harmful toxins while the caffeine in the coffee stimulates the muscles of the colon to push waste out. The solution travels up to the gall bladder and causes it to eliminate its contents.

Diarrhea Enemas
Enemas of catnip or valerian for severe diarrhea were often used in Egypt. Comfrey, Wild Alum Root, Lobelia, Mullein, Wild Rue. (eat Arrow Root Powder), White Oak Bark.

An enema is not to be relied upon for proper bowel movements. A raw food and natural foods diet helps to regulate the bowels. The transitional time of food can be checked by eating five to six tablespoons of charcoal powder or tablets. Then look for the charcoal in the bowels. When it appears, it will give you the time to take for food to leave the body. The food should spend four hours in the stomach and four hours in the intestines (colon). Transitional time should be no longer than sixteen hours. If longer, an enema may be needed along with a good diet.
　　A way to avoid enemas and keep the colon clean is to take two tablespoons of Flax Seed Meal, Slippery Elm Powder, Psyllium Husk or Seed (or powder), Fenugreek or Chia Seeds daily. This will create natural fiber and mucous and it is not a laxative (irritant to digestive tract) or habit-forming.

EYE PROBLEMS

The eyes are often abused. They require exercise and a diet of colors. Colors are obtained from sunlight. Sunlight has a rainbow (iris-means rainbow) of color, light rays and heat. These colors nourish and stimulate the pineal, pituitary gland and cascades the stimulation to other glands. The eyes are abused by artificial light, distorted light (eyeglasses do this) and radiation from cars, television/computer screens, light reflected off cars, glass and artificial surfaces and poor reading light.

European eye doctors abuse the eyes by over-prescribing. They never recommend eye exercise. Their branch of medical science was created from an eyeglass fad and ignorance. In this science, they demand that every individual have the same 20/20 vision acuity. This is a physiologically absurd demand. For example, a group of athletes at peak performance cannot all run a 100-yard dash in 9.4 seconds. It is an undisputed fact and accepted by athletes and even medical doctors. Vision depends upon the eye muscles' ability to stretch and contract the eye lens. The eyes (another muscular apparatus like the legs) are asked to perform a physical task with no regard to the physical limitations of the muscle groups. Moreover, this so-called profession forces people to wear eyeglasses (contacts), which degenerates the eyes' muscles. Consequently, if an individual does not abuse his or her eyes, then medical science will. Eyeglasses and surgery indicate a failure of medical science to solve a vision problem.

A raw food diet, proper eye exercise, health awareness and full spectrum light bulbs can avoid eye problems.

Supplements	Suggested Dosage	Remarks
Vitamin A	50,000 IU.	Helps vision and eye problems.
Vitamin B Complex	50-100 mg.	Enhances metabolism.
Vitamin C	3,000-10,000 mg.	Helps heal.
Vitamin D	400 IU.	Aids tissue stabilization.
Vitamin E	400-1,200 IU.	Use for eye disorders.
Zinc	45-80 mg.	Repairs damaged tissue.
Calcium	1,500 mg.	Helps protect eyes.
Lipoic Acid	100-200 mg.	Repairs nerve damage.

GLANDULARS

Raw Thyroid, Raw Liver, Raw Pineal	As directed.	Helps protect eyes.

AMINO ACIDS

Glutamine	As directed.	Repairs damaged nerves.
Tryptophan		Relaxes tissue of eyes.

HERBS

Cayenne, Bayberry, Eyebright, Goldenseal, Orchic, Raspberry Leaves.

FOODS

All fresh fruits and vegetables, Karambola, no junk foods.

HOMEOPATHIC

Nat. Phos., Kali. Mur.   As directed.   Stabilizes eye tissue.

Eye Drops can be made from goldenseal and eye bright tea and a drop of honey. Squeeze the juice from fresh grape leaves; put a drop in each eye.

Books such as Better Eyesight without Glasses by H. Benjamin and Vision Victory via Vitamins, Vital Foods and Visual Training by D. Deimel are beneficial reading.

GOUT

Gout is a dis-ease reaction. It is a form of arthritis, which can be caused by white sugar and when uric acid collects in the feet. The body attempts to get rid of these impurities and places them around the joint, bone lining and connective tissues. Besides this, the impurities may be caused by excessive fat in the diet or the body's inability to break down (metabolize) fat. Gout is treated similarly to arthritis and rheumatism because it is the same dis-ease reaction. Gout is the failure of the body to dissolve excess electrolytes and/or crystallized waste. It is characterized by the onset of pain in the big toe followed by swollen feet.

Supplements	Suggested Dosage	Remarks
Vitamin A	50,000 IU.	
Vitamin B Complex	100 mg.	Enhances digestion and enzymes.
Vitamin C	3,000-5,000 mg.	Decreases uric acid waste.
Vitamin D	400 IU.	Protects joints.
Vitamin E	400 IU.	Removes cellular waste.
Potassium Bicarbonate	99 mg.	Decreases tissue swelling.

GLANDULARS

Raw Adrenal, Raw Pancreas   As directed.   Enhances immunity.

AMINO ACIDS

Glutamine, Lysine, Methionine   As directed.   Repairs and defends tissue.

HERBS

Alfalfa, Aloe Vera, Birch Leaves, Black Cohosh, Burdock, Chaparral, Comfrey, Ginger, Juniper Berries, Parsley, Sarsaparilla, Yarrow, Yucca.

FOODS

All tropical fruits. Carrots, Cherries, Pineapple Juice, Red Juice, Strawberries.

HOMEOPATHIC

Nat. Sulph., Mag. Phos.	As directed.	Helps excrete tissue waste.

HAIR (LOSS OF)

The hair is nourished at the root by your diet. The scalp and flat muscles of the head are subject to all dis-eases (i.e., Arthritis, worms, clogged blood vessels, stress, etc.). Hair loss can be caused by diabetes, skin disease, vitamin deficiency, thyroid disease, excess estrogen, iron deficiency, poor circulation, weight loss and acute illness. It can be caused by legal (over-the-counter) drugs, radiation, surgery, inadequate nourishment before menopause or during pregnancy and chemotherapy. Diet with excessive sex hormones (i.e., non-organic beef, chicken, dairy, eggs, milk, fruits, vegetables) and/or overproduction of sex hormones. This can cause galea tissue on top of the scalp to thicken and decrease blood supply to the hair, which results in baldness. Stress can tense the flat muscles of the skull and block nutrients from getting to the hair.

Hair loss/baldness is referred to as alopecia. If the hair falls out in patches, it is referred to as alopecia areata.

Supplement	Suggested Dosage	Remarks
PABA (Para-Aminobenzoic Acid)	50 mg., twice daily.	Used for graying hair.
Silica	2 tablets, twice daily.	Keeps hair looking shiny and sleek.
Unsaturated Fatty Acids (Primrose Oil, Linseed Oil)	As directed.	Enhances hair texture. Prevents dry, brittle hair.
Vitamin B Complex		B Vitamins are important for growth of hair.
Pantothenic Acid (B_5)	100 mg., 3 times daily.	Helps maintain hair.
Vitamin B_6 (Pyridoxine)	50 mg., 3 times daily.	Enhances growth.
Inositol	100 mg., twice daily.	Stimulates growth.
Niacin (B_3)	50 mg., 3 times daily.	Helps hair absorb nutrients
Vitamin C	3,000 – 10,000 mg.	Increases scalp circulation.
Vitamin E	Start with 400 IU and slowly increase to 800 – 1,000 IU.	Increases circulation, hair growth and oxygen to cells.
Zinc	50 – 100 mg., daily.	Promotes hair growth by enhancing immune function.
Copper Chelate	3 mg., daily.	Works with Zinc to aid in hair growth.
Coenzyme Q_{10}	60 mg., daily.	Enhances scalp circulation. Increases tissue oxygenation.
Kelp	5 tablets daily.	Supplies minerals for hair growth.
GH (Growth Hormone)	As directed.	Stimulates growth.
Pregnenolone (Progesterone Hormone)	100-150 mg.	Stimulates cell growth.

GLANDULARS

Raw Pituitary	As directed.	Stimulates growth.
Raw Thymus	500 mg., daily.	Stimulates immune function and improves functioning capacity of glands.

AMINO ACIDS

L-Cysteine	500 mg., twice daily.	Improves hair growth and texture.
L-Methionine	Take on an empty stomach with vitamins B_6 andC for better assimilation.	Helps prevent hair from falling out.
Glutathione	1,000-2,000 mg.	Stimulates skin, glands and soft tissue.
Ornithine	1,000-2,000 mg.	Releases growth hormone.

HERBS

Alfalfa, Birch Leaves, Burdock, Calendula (Marigold), Chaparral, Comfrey, Dwarf Nettle, Horsetail, Maiden Hair, Nettle, Rosemary, Wormwood (if worms in scalp is a factor).

FOOD

Asparagus, Barley, Buckwheat, Cabbage, Figs, Kelp, Millet, Oats, Onions, Rice, Romaine Lettuce, Rye, Sesame Seeds, Spinach, Strawberries, Tomatoes.

HOMEOPATHIC

Aurum 7 and Lachesis 7	2 gr., alternate. Take in the a.m.	Stimulates growth.
Thallium Aceticum 7 and Kali Phosphoricum 7	2 gr., alternate. Take in the p.m.	Enhances nutrients to hair.

TISSUE SALTS

Silicea	Daily, as directed.	Cleanses skin (scalp)
Kali. Phos.	Daily, as directed.	Useful for skin problems (hair follicles, scalp).

HEART DIS-EASE

It is usually caused by a combination of non-wholistic practices such as poor nutrition, environmental pollution, destructive eating habits and deteriorating body health internal and external. Many other factors can cause this dis-ease reaction such as, high and low blood pressure, acid ash, fat deposits, thermal glandular fatigue, loss of vein and artery flexibility.

The current fad that heart attacks are caused by high cholesterol levels resulting in arteriosclerosis was started in 1913. It is founded upon giving high levels of cholesterol to rabbits (liver too small to break down fats). Further, the researcher never realized that the research was on dis-ease damage and never gave dis-ease damage any significance. (N. Anitschkow's article entitled "On Variations in the Rabbit Aorta" in experimental cholesterol feeding, *Beitr Path. Anat. v. Allgem Path.* 56:379, 1913). Ironically, since 1877, heart attacks have been scientifically proven (over and over again) to be related to thyroid malfunctions. (Wm. Ord "Transaction Med-Surg Society London" 60-61:57, 1877-78; *Diseases of the Endocrine Glands* by Zondek, 1944; L.M. Hurxthal's article "Blood Cholesterol and Thyroid Dis-ease" in *Archives Internal Medicine* 53:762, 1934. Also, at Harvard University, in 1925, heart attack was related to thyroid weakness.)

The thyroid reacts to the bodily ill health condition of the individual. Illness can be caused by poor diet, cooked food (plants and flesh), immuno-suppressive drugs, and synthetic chemicals. It is the systemic (general) health of a person that causes this dis-ease (and all others). Claude Bernard and Louis Pasteur, in the 19th century, indicated that an individual who makes his body dis-eased is more dangerous than any bacteria.

Supplements	Suggested Dosage	Remarks
Vitamin C	3,000-6,000 mg.	Helps thin the blood.
Vitamin B-Complex	100 mg.	Helps nerves.
Vitamin B$_6$	50 mg.	Combats nerve damage.
Vitamin E	200 IU.	Enhances heart circulation.
Niacin	50 mg.	Dialates heart's valves.
Calcium	1,500-2,000 mg.	Helps control heart muscles.
Magnesium	705-1,000 mg.	Increases nutrients to heart.
Phosphorus	500-700 mg.	Aids heart muscles.
Potassium	99 mg.	Stabilizes electrolytes.

HERBS

Black Cohosh, Cayenne, Cinchona (rhythm disorders), Cramp Bark (relaxes heart muscles), Hawthorn Berries (all types of heart problems), Horsetail, Lily of the Valley (natural digitalis), Melissa, Mistletoe, Motherwort, Rosemary.

HEMORRHOIDS

A hemorrhoid is an outgrowth of skin tissue (tumor). They are varicose veins in the anus, which is a balloon expansion outgrowth of blood vessels in the anal area. The blood vessel is expanded, weakened, and can bleed. Constipation is the leading cause.

Constipation is the leading cause of strained, ballooned, bursted, weakened blood vessels in the anal area. A constipating diet, inadequate fiber and water, weak hemorrhoidal veins caused by sugar and/or sugar leaching their fluid, stiff inflexible veins due to electrolyte stress, straining during bowel movements, clogged hemorrhoidal veins, rheumatism of muscles of anus, weak or collapsed valves in the veins and junk foods cause hemorrhoids.

A suppository made with cocoa butter (melted), crushed garlic (or garlic powder), arnica herb, tansy or bee pollen or garlic clove suppository can bring temporary relief, as well as a hot sitz bath with teas (astringent herbs such as Witch Hazel, Wild Alum Root, Shepherd's Purse, Tormentil, etc.

Supplements	Suggested Dosage	Remarks
Vitamin C with Bioflavonoids	3,000-5,000 mg.	Normalizes blood and heals.
Vitamin B-Complex	50-100 mg., 3 times daily.	Reduces stress on veins.
Vitamin B_6	50 mg., 3 times daily.	Reduces tension in veins.
Vitamin E	600 IU.	Enhances blood clotting.
Vitamin A	1,500 IU.	Heals vein tissue.
Vitamin K	50-80 mcg.	Clots blood and heals.

GLANDULARS

Raw Adrenal, Raw Kidney	As directed.	Enhances vessel cleansing.

AMINO ACIDS

Glutamine, Phenylalanine, Methionine	As directed.	Helps repair vessels. Aids flexibility of vessels.

HERBS

Collinsonia, Rosehip, White Oak Bark, Witch Hazel, Yarrow.

FOODS

Citrus Fruit, Kamamboa, Kiwi, Mango, Papaya, Pineapple.

HERBAL ABORTION

The termination of pregnancy before the fetus reaches the 20th to 28th week of gestation (growth) is an abortion. Abortion can be induced by the use of drugs or herbs. Abortifacient herbs prevent the continuation of pregnancy. Herbs can cause the ejection of the fetus from the womb. Natural abortions occur when the fetus (foetus) is not healthy, or the mother is not healthy or when the fetus is on a different frequency from the mother. Herbs help to alter the physical frequency (or chemistry, vibration, temper, rhythm, cycle) of the mother. Further, this alteration puts the mother on one frequency and the child on another. This is a biochemical conflict imbalance between mother and child. In this case, the fetus is rejected and an abortion can be achieved by extremely low blood sugar or the allopathic, homeopathic and/or naturopathic use of herbs. An abortion in progress is characterized by bleeding and painful spasms that increase. The cervix is usually dilated or spread apart. Abortion herbs can be drunk and/or used in a douche. The most effective method is the herbal douche. It should be a very strong solution of 2 to 3 tablespoons of herbs to a cup. The herbs should be combined (three or more) for the tea and douche. Usually, three glasses of herb teas drank four times a day is a suggested dose. A therapeutic (effective) level is not achieved by a stronger solution, but by the right quantity. Anything above the therapeutic level is rejected (urinated) out of the body.

Herbs

Angelica, Black Cohosh, Blue Cohosh, Celery, Cotton, Ergot, Hemlock Spruce, Horse Radish, Hyssop, Mistletoe, Pennyroyal, Ragwort, Shepherd's Purse, Tansy, Tormentil.

For inducing an abortion, the herb cotton was used during slavery. Tormentil is the strongest astringent. It is often used as a douche to cause the vagina to become tight (virgin-like). It also can cause scarring of the sensitive tissue in the reproductive organs. The spiritual, emotional, mental and physical consequences of inducing an abortion is an issue that women and men have to answer for in their consciousness and answer to the ancestors, God and the murdered child's spirit.

HYPERTENSION, HIGH BLOOD PRESSURE AND STRESS

High blood pressure, stress, and hypertension are usually caused by a lack of proper nutrition. Improper nutrition weakens the internal organs, immune system, and lowers the organs' abilities to utilize nutrients, which feed the body. The body begins to starve because of the loss of proper nutrients. This starvation creates a nutritional debt. The nutritionally starved body tries to get more nutrients to pay the debt. Consequently, the body demands more food (nutrients in the blood) by drawing on poor (below-nutrient-level) blood. In order to increase the nutrients the body needs, it must get nutrients from the blood, so it increases the quantity of blood by increasing the pressure. The increase in pressure is the body's attempt to feed itself. This increase in pressure is the body's last resort to defend itself against the bodily pollutions, gland disorders, free radicals, kidney weakness, hypertension, overweight, emotional stress, toxemia, deteriorating metabolism, etc., and a foodless food (junk food) diet.

An inflexible vascular system is unable to bring pressure down. The pressure gets high and cannot come down to normal. However, the increased blood pressure fails to nourish the body, because junk foods (fiber-less enzyme depleted) are depleted of nutrients. This results in hypertension and stress. The blood nutrients can only be supplied by a natural whole foods diet. Additionally, the blood can have an accumulation of waste floating in it. This waste gets into the veins and arteries causing them to lose flexibility. The more cellular and chemical waste there is in the blood, the less oxygen and nutrients. The pressure is elevated in order to get more nutrients delivered to starved tissue, but instead brings more waste and less air. This rise in blood pressure demands more nutrients to sustain the high blood pressure, in the blood—thick with waste—stresses the heart and causes a nutritional unpaid debt. This is a case of nutritional suicide as high blood pressure causes high pressure, which in turn causes an extreme nutrient loss called low blood pressure. Subsequently, high and low pressure is caused by dis-ease. The high blood pressure diminishes the ability of the kidneys to filter waste, regulate hormones, aide mineral absorption and cell formation. The kidneys require the temperature and pressure to be normal in order for them to function.

The stress reaction does not cause diseases such as heart dis-ease, arterial hypertension and nervous disorder. Stress reactions triggers the release of adrenaline. However, wild animals have larger adrenal glands than tamed (domesticated) animals. Consequently, wild animals produce more adrenaline and are under more stress. They do not have dis-eases associated with stress such as high blood pressure because their diet is raw whole foods, uncooked foods and no processed junk foods.

It is the junk food diet and immunosuppressive drugs and malnourishment that causes stress. If stress were the cause of dis-eases rather than nutrient poor diet then the Black chattel slaves would have died from stress and high blood pressure.

It is the nutrient poor health, which is caused by immunosuppressive-drugs (antibiotics, etc.), fiber-less food, cooked food and free radicals (waste) that causes the dis-ease reaction of hypertension, stress, etc.

Supplements	Suggested Dosage	Remarks
Vitamin C	3,000-6,000 mg.	Thins blood and relieves stress.
Vitamin B Complex	100 mg., twice daily.	Lowers pressure, helps circulation.
Vitamin B_6	50 mg., twice daily.	Reduces heart stress.
Vitamin E	100-400 IU.	Thins blood, helps heart.
Inositol	50 mg.	Aids circulation and heart function.
Choline	50 mg.	Improves circulation and heart function.
Coenzyme Q_{10}	100-300 mg.	Normalizes pressure.
Lipoic Acid	100-200 mg.	Relieves nerve stress.
Plant Sterolins	As directed.	Combats stress.

GLANDULARS
Raw Adrenal, Raw Orchid (for men only).

AMINO ACIDS

Tryptophane	As directed.	Relaxes tissue, heart and nerves.
Taurine	As directed.	Aids heart function.

HERBS
Catnip, Chamomile, Hops, Passion Flower, Valerian.

FOODS
Avocado, Almonds, Brewer's Yeast, Dates, Eggplant, Tomatoes.

HOMEOPATHIC

Kali. Phos., Sulph. Calc., Nat. Phos.	As directed.	Normalizes pressure.

HIGH BLOOD PRESSURE

Vitamin B-Complex	100 mg., twice daily.	Improves circulation.
Vitamin B_6	50 mg., twice daily.	Relieves nerve and heart stress.
Inositol	50 mg., twice daily.	Enhances circulation.
Pantothenic Acid	50 mg.	Relieves stress.
Vitamin C with Bioflavonoids	3,000-6,000 mg.	Helps thin blood-lowers pressure.
Vitamin E	200 IU.	Thins blood. Lowers pressure.
Coenzyme Q_{10}	100-200 mg.	Lowers pressure.

GLANDULARS

Raw Spleen, Raw Pancreas, Raw Kidney	As directed.	Helps to thin blood.

AMINO ACIDS

Methionine, Cysteine	As directed.	Aids normalization of pressure.

HERBS
Butcher's Broom, Cayenne, Garlic, Hawthorn Berry, Rosemary, Tumeric, Water Chestnut.

FOODS
Barley, Broccoli, Cantaloupe, Guavas, Jujube, Kumquats, Spinach, Turnip Greens.

HOMEOPATHIC

Calc. Flour.	As directed.	Helps relax heart muscles.

LOW BLOOD PRESSURE

Vitamin B-Complex	100 mg., twice daily.	Improves circulation.
Vitamin C	3,000-5,000 mg.	Increases circulation.
Vitamin E	100-400 IU.	Thins blood, improves circulation.
Vitamin K	50-80 mcg.	Strengthens vascular tissue.
Bee Pollen	As directed.	Increases energy.
Octocosanol	As directed.	Stimulates circulation.

GLANDULARS

Raw Adrenal, Raw Liver	As directed.	Stimulates circulation.

AMINO ACIDS

Phenylalanine	500-1,000 mg.	Increases circulation.

HERBS
Astralagus, Cayenne, Garlic, Ginger, Ginseng, Goldenseal, Parsley, Yohimbe.

FOODS
Black Walnut, Currants, Dates, Figs, Pignolia Nuts, Pumpkin.

HOMEOPATHIC

Calc. Flour.	As directed.	Enhances heart's energy.

STRESS

Vitamin B-Complex	100 mg., twice daily.	Relieves stress.
Pantothenic Acid	50 mg.	Helps regulate adrenal hormone.
Inositol	50 mg., twice daily.	Increases nutrients to cells.
Niacinamide	50 mg., twice daily.	Aids relaxation.
Calcium	1,500-2,000 mg.	Stabilizes energy.
Magnesium	250-1,000 mg.	Relaxes tissue.
Coenzyme $Q10$	100 mg.	Aids circulation, decreases tension.

GLANDULARS

Raw Adrenal, Raw Liver	As directed.	Combats stress.

AMINO ACIDS

Phenylalanine	500-1,000 mg.	Stimulates energy.

HERBS

Alfalfa, Cayenne, Fo-ti, Ginseng, Saffron, Teng, Valerian.

FOODS

Barley, Brewer's Yeast, Broccoli, Corn, Kale, Lecithin, Pecans, Tomatoes.

HOMEOPATHIC

Calc. Flour.	As directed.	Nourishes heart muscles.

HYPOGLYCEMIA

Hypoglycemia is a dis-ease symptom reaction. It occurs because the body is low (hypo) in blood sugar (glycemia). When the body gets large amounts of sugar, it receives a rush of energy, but it also requires large amounts of energy to burn the large amounts of sugar. The body becomes exhausted from burning great quantities of sugar. This exhaustion occurs because the body is low in blood sugar. All fats, proteins and starches are naturally changed to sugar within the body and thus create more blood sugar. This blood sugar is used up burning the large amounts of processed sugars. The processed sugars are usually taken in the form of refined concentrated sweeteners, white sugar and refined, bleached white flour (both are refined carbohydrates). In order for the body to burn sugar, the pancreas must make insulin. The excess insulin released to burn up the processed sugars also burns up the normal blood sugar, causing a drastic drop. The drop in blood sugar level has many symptoms (warnings of dis-ease) such as fatigue, depression, nervousness, irritability, memory failures and it damages the nerves.

The typical junk food diet is composed of between 75 to 150 pounds of white sugar per year. Aside from obvious sugars, there are sugars in milk, table salt, catsup, mustard, mouthwash, salted nuts, medicines, toothpaste, salted chips, pizzas, fruit juices, tabacco, etc.

Sugar is added to salted products to make the salt taste saltier. Sugar is added to foods to make them addicting (get you hooked on the product). It is used to hide the chemical taste and poor quality foods and the taste of spoiled foods. The majority of Black folks are sugar addicts. If they are not addicted to white sugar, then they are addicted to fast burning processed carbohydrates (white rice, bleached white flour, potato chips, French fries, etc.) that turn into sugar quickly in the body. Sugar is the first addiction of alcoholics, marijuana smokers, sex addicts, video game addicts, phone addicts, cigarette addicts and drug addicts (legal and/or illegal drugs).

A hypoglycemic person should avoid all white sugar (read labels), concentrated sweeteners, bleached white flour, and junk foods.

Supplements	Suggested Dosage	Remarks
Vitamin A	10,000-50,000 IU.	Heals urinary tract.
Vitamin B Complex	50-100 mg.	Enhances metabolism.
Vitamin B_6	50 mg., twice daily.	Stimulates enzymes.
Vitamin B_{12}	300 mcg., twice daily.	Helps nutrient absorption.
Vitamin C	3,000-5,000 mg.	Enhances energy release.
Vitamin E	400 IU.	Stabilizes energy.
Pantothenic Acid	5-50 mg.	Combats stress.
Zinc	50 mg.	Enhances insulin release.
Manganese	10-50 mg.	Stabilizes blood glucose.
Garlic Capsules	As directed.	Thins blood.
Magnesium Chloride	750-1,000 mg.	Helps utilize carbohydrates.
Potassium Chloride	99 mg.	Stabilizes energy release.
Chromium	300-600 mg.	Helps cells release blood sugar.
Lipoic Acid	100-200 mg.	Stabilizes blood sugar.

GLANDULARS

Raw Liver, Raw Brain, Raw Adrenal, Raw Pancreas	As directed.	Help increase energy.

AMINO ACIDS

Glutamine, Cysteine, Carnitine	As directed.	Improves absorption of nutrients.

HERBS

Bilberry, Dandelion, Horse Radish, Juniper Berries, Kelp, Kiwi, Licorice, Milk Thistle, Spirulina, Wild Yam.

FOODS

Whole-wheat nuts, grains, seeds. Apples, Jerusalem Artichoke, Avocados, Bananas, Broccoli, Brown Rice, Cantaloupes, Carrots, Grapefruit, Lentils, Lemons, Persimmons, Pomegranates, Potatoes, Raw Spinach, Squash, String Beans, Yams.

Nat. Phos.	As directed.	Emulsifies fats causing energy.

It is sometimes recommended to eat at least eight small meals a day and eat snacks in order to stabilize blood sugar.

Books such as *My Battle with Low Blood Sugar* by G. Thienell; *Syndrome X* by J. Challen; *Body, Mind and Sugar* by C. Abrahamson and A. Pezet are informative.

KIDNEY STONES

Stones are crystallized waste (can be in the form of minerals or fats). This waste has not been broken down (catabolized by the body and properly filtered by the kidney). The kidney is like a filter, which works by water pressure. If pressure is unstable due to high or low blood pressure or the diet is of junk foods, it affects the kidney. Both of these effects can cause kidney stones. The kidneys help to recycle minerals (i.e., iron) and electricity in the body. They concentrate and dilute mineral salts. Kidney stones can cause pain on the sides of the middle and lower back.

There are two kidneys, one on each side of the body. They are about the size of a drinking cup and each kidney has a tube that leads from it to the bladder. The bladder lies between the hipbones. The bladder stores liquid waste (urine) until it is ready for release. When waste collects in the body due to constipating foods and/or weak, improperly fed organs, stones result. Stones can cause the kidneys to slightly sag and to become misaligned due to the extra weight of the stones. The kidneys are related (organ compliment) to the testicles and ovaries and can indicate a dis-ease in the reproductive system. When the kidneys are inflamed, have stones or lose their ability to recycle minerals the testicles and ovaries accumulate more waste and decrease their functions.

Supplements	Suggested Dosage	Remarks
Vitamin A	25,000 IU.	Aids healing kidney and urinary tissue.
Vitamin B_6	50 mg.	Reduces stones.
Vitamin C with Bioflavonoids	3,000-6,000 mg.	Inhibits stone formation.
Vitamin B Complex	50 mg., twice daily.	Helps reduce stones.
Garlic Capsules	2 Capsules, 3 times daily.	Helps reduce stones.
Lecithin	1,200 mg., 3 times daily.	Dissolves stones.
Choline	50 mg., twice daily.	Helps dissolve stones.
Calcium	1,500 mg.	Aids mineral use.
Magnesium Oxide	750-1,000 mg.	Helps proper mineral use.
Digestive Enzyme	As directed.	Helps metabolize stones.
Zinc	50-80 mg.	Decreases stone formation.
Potassium	99 mg.	Helps dissolve stones.

GLANDULARS

Raw Kidney   As directed.   Helps cleanse kidney.

AMINO ACIDS

Phenylalanine, Arginine,   As directed.   Aids healing urinary tract.
Methionine

HERBS

Catnip, Gingko, Goldenseal, Horse Radish, Juniper Berries, Kelp, Kidney Bean Pod, Lobelia,
Marshmallow, Orris, Parsley, Spirea, Uva Ursi, Wild Yam.

FOODS

Alfalfa, Aloe Vera Juice, Apples, Apricots, Asparagus, Cantaloupe, Carrots, Cranberry Juice, Garlic,
Lemons, Limes, Melons, Pumpkin, Squash, Sweet Potatoes, Yams.

HOMEOPATHIC

Nat. Sulph., Kali. Mur.   As directed.   Excretes stones.

Books such as *Kidney Disorders* by H. Clements and *Health Secrets of a
Naturopathic Doctor* by N. Garten are useful.

LIVER DIS-EASE AND
GALL BLADDER DIS-EASE

The liver is the largest gland in the body. Glands are organs that are similar to sponges. They secrete and absorb fluid. The liver secretes digestive
fluids, which are stored in the gallbladder. They are used for breaking down
carbohydrates and protein. The liver stores at least a six-hour supply of
reserved natural sugar (glycogen), which can be used in emergencies.

Dis-eases of the liver usually cause digestive problems, sluggishness,
weakness, vomiting, headaches, fever, weight loss, nausea, mental disorders, hemorrhages, fatigue, and low energy levels. The most common dis-
ease of the liver is jaundice, which is characterized by yellowish eyes, fingernails, toenails and skin. The liver is secreting more yellow bile in order
to dissolve toxins (impurities) in the system. Jaundice is a reaction to dis-
ease. The dis-ease created the need for extra yellow bile. Drinking alcohol,
sodas or vinegar damages the liver and causes the liver to get hard (cirrhosis). All drugs, synthetic chemicals, hormones and toxins go to the liver.
Drugs, synthetic chemicals, chemicals made in the body by radiation (computers, television, etc.), chemicals in polluted air, water (public drinking
water), noise (makes chemicals) and synthetic hormones decreases the
liver's functions such as making blood thinners (heparin), blood clotting
(thickeners) constitutents, red blood cells for the fetus, body heat, cholesterol, buffers (ammonia) that neutralize acidic blood, storage of Vitamin B_{12}
and Vitamins A, D, E, and K and destroying the bacteria in the blood.

When the liver gets weak, enlarged, inflamed or hard (cirrhosis), the spleen and kidney become weak.

Meat eaters should never eat an animal's liver because it is the most toxic (polluted) organ in the animal's body.

Supplements	Suggested Dosage	Remarks
Vitamin A	25,000 IU.	Enhances healing of tissue.
Vitamin B Complex	50 mg., twice daily.	Nourishes tissue.
Vitamin B_6	100 mg.	Eliminates toxins.
Vitamin B_{12}	300 mcg.	Stimulates cellular repair.
Vitamin C	3,000-6,.000 mg.	Combats toxins.
Vitamin E	400 IU.	Helps rebuild liver.
Garlic Capsules	2 Capsules, 3 times daily.	Detoxifies liver.
Niacin	100-500 mg.	Enhances circulation.
Choline	50 mg., twice daily.	Stops fatty buildup.
Inositol	50 mg., 3 times daily.	Stimulates cleansing.
Lecithin	1,200 mg., 3 times daily.	Emulsifies impurities.
Manganese	10-50 mg.	Helps liver repair.
Magnesium	750-1,000 mg.	Reduces waste.
Zinc	50-80 mg.	Helps repair tissue.
Digestive Enzyme	As directed.	Enhances detoxification.

GLANDULARS

Raw Liver, Raw Thyroid.	As directed.	Cleanses and strengthens liver.

AMINO ACIDS

Threonine, Lysine, Glycine.	As directed.	Helps excrete toxins.

HERBS

Alfalfa, Balmony, Barberry Root, Bayberry, Birch Leaves, Black Horse Radish, Bolbo, Catnip, Cramp Bark, Centaury, Dandelion, Fennel, Ginger Root, Goldenseal, Horsetail, Liverwort, Lobelia, Oregon Grape, Parsley, Red Beet Root, St. John's Wort, Wahoo, Wild Yam, Yellow Dock.

FOODS

Apple, Artichoke, Beet, Black Radish, Cucumber, Garlic, Grapes, Kiwi, Lemon Juice, Papaya, Pear, Red Beet Juice Tops.

HOMEOPATHIC

Nat. Sulph.	As directed.	Eliminates impurities.

Books such as *Liver Ailments and Common Disorders* by S. Tobe and *Natural Treatment for Liver Troubles and Associated Ailments* by J. Sneddon are informative.

MARIJUANA
(CANNABIS SATIVA)

Marijuana is a plant in the grass family and is classified as a weed. It has some limited curative properties and as a curative, it must be drank as a tea, used as a poultice or eaten raw. Interesting to note, as a food, raw marijuana is difficult to digest because people are not natural grass eaters. Humans lack the large flat molar teeth and the three stomachs found in natural grass eaters. However, the plant mineral content is good for lung dis-eases. When marijuana is burnt and smoked, it is transformed into a processed toxic chemical with cancerous deadly oils. The synthetic chemical droplets in marijuana smoke are a depressant. They depress the bodily function and nerve activity, lessens heart action, dulls thinking, lessens muscle contraction, lessens frequency and depth of breathing, decreases gland secretions (prostate, thyroid, pituitary, etc.) and increases the aging process.

Tiny droplets of chemicals in the smoke of Marijuana directly weaken the liver, lungs, brain, eyes, and sex organs (produces low quality and quantity of sperm). It alters the breath and the rhythm of internal organs. Marijuana synthetic chemicals disorientate cellular control of the body. In *The Low Fat Way to Health and Longer Life* by L. Morrison and a pamphlet report *Marijuana, The Health Hazard* by Dale Dominy, M.D., this subject is scientifically reviewed.

The tiny droplets of chemicals, in Marijuana, smoke reduce the sperm count and damages the nerve receptor site. The tiny droplets of chemicals in smoke contain more cancer-causing chemicals than tobacco smoke. Emphysema, lung cancer, bronchitis and related diseases that once only affected tobacco smokers are common in marijuana smokers. The chemicals in Marijuana smoke can cause scarring of the lung tissue and the oily droplets of chemicals in the smoke clogs the lungs. This reduces oxygen to the cells, tissue and organs such as the liver. Reduced oxygen to the liver causes weak digestive enzyme fluid, reduces mineral absorption, disrupt hormone balance, weakens the pancreas and thyroid and decreases the nutrients to the brain. The bitter oils stimulate the appetite.

The new hi-tech plants contain 200% more tetrahydrocannabinol (THC). It is not the same marijuana of twenty or thirty years ago. It is a cloned and hybridized plant concoction. It is not natural. Those that grow their own plants do not research the origin of the cloned seeds. They grow them in synthetic fertilized soil or nutrient depleted soil. The private growers do not test the soil and ground water for contamination or toxic chemicals.

Marijuana is deliberately bred to be addictive and can result in mild, severe, or delayed withdrawal symptoms. Some of the symptoms of withdrawal are chills, anxiety, food craving (related to liver damage), headaches, temper tantrums, diarrhea, hot flashes, apathy, family and relationship problems, hypersensitivity, mood swings, tremors, excessive talking, sleeplessness and illusions about self worth.

TREATMENT

See Cocaine Addiction, on page 61, for vitamins, minerals, aminos, etc. A two-week raw juice fast and the elimination of all junk food, alcohol and drugs.

Substitute Herbs (which can be smoked):
Catnip, Mullein, Peppermint, Corn Silk, Rabbit Tobacco and Wild Lettuce.

ADDICTION

The effect that smoke from burnt Marijuana gives is a chemically addicting state. The synthetic chemicals in the smoke cause sickness and malnutrition of the body. Marijuana causes the body to malfunction and biochemistry to be sickly, blocks nerve receptor sites, decreases oxygen and increases waste in cells. The tiny poisonous oil droplets within the smoke gums the lymph fluid, hormones, red and white blood cells and corpuscles. This self-induced sickness is called "feeling good." This malnutrition or disease state (depression) is commonly called a "high." The synthetic chemicals in Marijuana smoke creates mental, emotional, behavioral and physical dependency. Dependency behavior can mean smoking once a day, once a week, once a month or once a year. The regularity of smoking the chemicals in Marijuana reflects the individuality of the addictive person. Synthetic chemicals made from Marijuana smoke is addicting and causes the Marijuana to freely control and alter the mind, mood and behavior of the addict.

MARIJUANA EFFECTS ON THE SPIRIT

Burnt (cooked) Marijuana is a chemical that alters the attachment of the spirit to the breath. It causes the spirit to lose its guiding effect on the mind, mood and body. It can alter or destroy levels of spirituality.

MENOPAUSE

A woman's sexuality has three phases: menstruation (hemorrhaging of uterus), birthing, and menopause. Menopause is the apex of the sexual cycle. In this phase, ovulation and menstruation cease and reproduction ends. While the body is making the transition from fertility to sterility, nutritional, spiritual, emotional and mental imbalances occur. These imbalances begin months or years before menopause. Menopause requires transitional supplements (Pregnenolone) and herbs. When the body does not have adequate reserve energy to help make the hormonal transition, a nutritional deficiency can occur. Nutritional and hormonal deficiencies cause mood sings, unexplained pain and feelings, bone loss, hot flashes, insomnia, irritability, sore breasts, night sweats, respiratory problems, heart problems, itching, depression, loss of interest in sex, fatigue, bladder problems, anxiety, aging of skin, dry skin, vaginal dryness and tantrums.

It is natural for the sex drive to change to another orgasmic level. Ignorance of this change and failure to make spiritual transition can cause a "lost sex drive." The common menopausal dis-ease symptoms are related to poor nutrition, excess estrogen and steroids from non-organic fruits, vegetables, eggs, milk and meat. There are no Menopausal dis-ease symptoms in many colored cultures on organic foods (Incan, Chinese, Aborigines, Eskimos, etc.). These women eat organic foods, have maintained good nutrition, have unpolluted air, water, soil, and have a cultural education to support their three phases of sexuality.

Each woman has a natural "baby space." Baby space is the uniquely individual time that a woman should have a baby. A space (time) for a woman to have a child is hormonally, spiritually and emotionally programmed into the biochemistry. This space is usually finely adjusted by her male partner's pheromone level. Because of oppression, the social conditions deny the space and Black males that have not had "rites of passage" for adulthood and marriage also participate in denying the woman fulfillment of the baby space. Added to this, females are denied their "rites of passage" education and the cultural atmosphere conducive for having children, adulthood, parenthood and menopause. White Supremacy has denied the "baby space," "rites of passage," and the culture (village) needed to make menopause symptomless.

Supplements	Suggested Dosage	Remarks
Vitamin A	25,000 IU.	Improves immunity.
Vitamin B Complex	50 mg.	Enhances circulation.
Vitamin B_1	50 mg., 3 times daily.	Aids absorption.
Vitamin B_6	50 mg., 3 times daily.	Helps nerve function.
Vitamin B_{12}	300 mcg.	Stimulates energy.
Vitamin C	3,000-6,000 mg.	Used for hot flashes.
Vitamin E	400 IU.	Decreases hot flashes.
Vitamin K	50-80 mcg.	Stabilizes bones.
Pantothenic Acid	5-50 mg.	Reduces stress.
Calcium	1,500-2,000 mg.	Helps decrease nervousness.
Zinc	50 mg.	Prevents bone loss.
Boron	1-9 mg.	Improves Calcium absorption.
Silica	As directed.	Strengthens tissue and Calcium.
Evening Primrose Oil	As directed.	Helps relaxation, hot flashes.
Black Currant Oil	As directed.	Aids calmness and decreases edema.
Magnesium	750-1,000 mg.	Protects bones.
PABA	50-100 mg.	Decreases irritability and nervousness.
Lecithin	1,200 mg.	Soothes nerves.

Brewer's Yeast	As directed.	Improves nerves' function and circulation.
Pregnenolone	100-150 mg.	Balances hormone levels.
Progesterone (Wild Yam) Crème/Lotion	As directed.	Balances hormones; stimulates libido.

GLANDULARS

| Raw Ovary | As directed. | Aids hormone balance. |

AMINO ACIDS

| Glutamine, Cysteine, Methionine,Phenylalanine, Lysine, Arginine. | As directed. | Relieves symptoms. |

HERBS

Anise, Black and Blue Cohosh, Chaste, Cramp Bark, Dong Quai, Elder, False Unicorn, Fennel, Ginseng, Licorice, Pennyroyal, Red Raspberry Leaves, Sarsaparilla, Saw Palmetto, St. John's Wort, Squawvine.

FOODS

All fresh fruits and vegetables, Amaranth, Mustard Greens, Watercress.

HOMEOPATHIC

| Ferr. Phos. | As directed. | Provides iron. Improves circulation. |

MUSCLE, MENSTRUAL CRAMPS

The muscles not getting the proper nutrients or not getting enough oxygen,causes a buildup of lactic acid waste and cramps. The nutritionally starved muscles cannot relax; this is called a cramp. In addition, the body may not be able to burn (metabolize) the nutrients if they are present. Muscles rely largely upon minerals—particularly magnesium, potassium calcium, and vitamins B_6 and D. Furthermore, an acid condition of the body can burn up the alkalis (minerals). *See* Acid/Alkaline.

Supplements	Suggested Dosage	Remarks
Vitamin B_6	50 mg.	Relieves stress, tension.
Vitamin D	400 IU.	Stabilizes muscles.
Vitamin E	400 IU.	Useful for PMS.
Pantothenic Acid	100 mg., 3 times daily.	Anti-stress.
Calcium	1,500-2,000 mg.	Prevents cramps.
Magnesium	750-1,000 mg.	Decreases irritability.
Potassium	50-80 mg.	Reduces nervousness.
Silica	2 tablets.	Strengthens tissue.
Chondroitin& Glucosamine	1,000-2,000 mg.	Relieves muscle pain.
GABA	50 mg., twice daily.	Helps control behavior.

GLANDULARS

Raw Adrenal, Raw Liver, Raw Prostate	As directed.	Relieves symptoms.

AMINO ACIDS

Tryptophan	As directed.	Relaxes and calms.
Glycine	As directed.	Anti-anxiety.

HERBS

Alfalfa, Belladonna, Blue Cohosh, Cayenne, Comfrey, Dandelion, Kelp, Licorice (female), Lobelia, Oatstraw, Orris, Saffron, Sarsaparilla (female) Shavegrass, Thyme.

FOODS

Beets, Carrots, Cucumber, Seawater, Sesame Seeds, Sweet Fruits and Juices, Whole Grains.

HOMEOPATHIC

Mag. Phos.	As directed.	Nourishes nerves and brain.

OVERWEIGHT/OBESITY

Overweigh/Obesity is usually caused by malfunctioning digestive organs and/or overeating. Overweight is weight of five to ten pounds above normal weight. Obesity is the accumulation of excess fat. A person can have obesity and not be overweight. A person can be overweight and obesity. A body builder with large muscles is considered overweight (i.e., Arnold Schwartzenagger). Fat accumulates around the gut because the liver is too stressed to break down fat, the pancreas is weak, excess protein is turned to fat, overeating and/or a diet of junk foods. However, the reason for overeating must be wholistically solved or else the overweight/obesity will continue. Excess weight (fat) is actually extra cells the body has to maintain. These cells are homes for toxic waste. Fat steals energies that could be used for immunity. The fat tries to insulate the weak organs by keeping their low energy production protected. The fat increases as the organs' functions decrease. Fat becomes a storage place for waste and the fat cells stop the body's abilities to cleanse and maintain health.

The appestat (appetite control mechanism) can be imbalanced by emotional stress, physical shocks (dis-eased organs) and spiritual causes. Cases of overwaste (overweight) due to glandular disorders are infrequent, whereas cases of overwaste obesity are caused by the malnutrition from eating the wrong foods and junk foods. Undernourishment causes deteriorated organs to accumulate waste, toxins and fat. This begins to choke the healthy cells, decrease cell life and alter the path of the nutrients in the blood supplies. The body allocates nutrients to the fat cells and decreases nutrients to the healthy cells. The fat of obesity is another symptom of nutrient starvation and dis-ease.

Supplements	Suggested Dosage	Remarks
Vitamin C	3,000-5,000	Helps regulate appetite.
Vitamin B Complex	100 mg.	Relieves depression.
Vitamin B_6	50 mg.	Reduces irritability.
Vitamin B_{12}	300 mcg.	Aids metabolism.
Vitamin E	400 -1,000 IU.	Relieves stress.
Vitamin A	50,000 IU.	Aids weightloss.
Vitamin D	400 IU.	Helps store energy.
Niacin	50 mg., e times daily.	Improves circulation.
Calcium	1,500-2,000 mg.	Improves metabolism of fate.
Choline	100 mg.	Aids fat metabolism.
Magnesium	750-1000 mg.	Soothes nerves.
Zinc	50-100 mg.	Reduces craving.
Inositol	100 mg.	Enhances energy.
Lecithin	200-500 mg.	Dissolves fat.
Garlic Capsules	As directed.	Cleanses tissue.
Brewer's Yeast	As directed.	Anti-stress.
Cravex	As directed.	Reduces craving for sugar, etc.

GLANDULARS

Raw Thymus	As directed.	Regulates energy levels.

AMINO ACIDS

Phenylalanine	As directed.	Appetite control.
Ornithine, Carnitine	As directed.	Dissolves fats.

HERBS

Black Chaparral, Chickweed, Echinacea, Fennel, Gotu Kola, Irish Moss, Licorice Root, Mandrake, Saffron.

FOODS

Cabbage bottoms, Celery, Cherry, Grapefruits, Karamboa, Lemon, Orange, Pomegranate. All fresh fruits and vegetables.

HOMEOPATHIC

Calc. Phos.

DIET FADS AND BOOKS

All rapid weight loss diets or programs may seem healthy, but the slim foods eaten and weight loss supplements will cause health hazards and temporary loss of weight (usually water and protein from the organs, bones and muscles).

Diet Fads

The Beverly Hills Diet
The Cottage Cheese Diet
The Egg Diet
The Grape Diet
The Grapefruit Diet

Diet Books

Amazing Hypno-Diet
Calories Don't Count
Diet and Blood Types
The Doctor's Quick Weight Loss Diet
The Drinking Man's Diet

The Ice Cream Diet	*Eat Fat and Grow Slim*
The Lollipop Diet	*How Sex Can Keep You Slim*
The New York Diet	*The No Will Power Diet*
The Rice Diet	*The Psychologist's Eat Anything Diet*
The Roman Orgy Diet	*Pray Your Weight Away*

The largest selling books are cookbooks and diet books. It is essentially the cookbooks that cause weight gain, which necessitates diet books. The books never treat the food addiction and snack food habit. Therefore, weight gain and diets to lose weight continues.

FAT FALLACIES

Weight Loss Phrases	**Considerations**
"Doctors agree"	What are the names of the doctors? Do they have a degree in nutrition or medicine?
"Authorities agree"	What type of authorities? Do they speak with authority or are they authorities of English?
A diet that eliminates one or more entire food groups (such as carbohydrates)	We need whole foods from all food groups for physical health.
A diet that says eat only rice or meat.	Vegetable protein can be substituted for meat. Meat can be eliminated.
When a weight loss diet says you can lose more than two pounds per week	Water weight can be lost rapidly. Rapid weight loss causes craving for food and weight increase. Protein and water is lost from muscles and organs. This is dangerous and unhealthy.
"Lose up to five pounds overnight."	This type of weight loss is caused by the diet inducing a disease state.
"No pills! No exercise! Eat your favorite foods! Lose weight while you sleep!"	This is stupidity disguised as knowledge.
"New fat-burning system slims down pounds in ten days."	Water and muscle weight loss takes place over a ten-day period, not fat. This may cause subclinical malnutrition.
"Rapid weight loss."	Rapid weight loss supplements usually have addicting epinephrine or a herbal speed, such as Guarana, Ephedra, Yerba Mate or caffeine. They speed up your system, which is believed to speed up the burning of fats.

TYPES OF FAT

Saturated
These are the visible fats, such as butter, lard, tallow, and blubber. Most saturated fats are found in animal flesh. All animal fats are unsafe and contain cholesterol. They are usually cooked and contain very high amounts of chemicals and waste. Coconut oil is a safe saturated fat. Processed and cooked saturated fats are used in the diet. They are dangerous. Raw saturated fats are good.

Unsaturated
Unsaturated fats are desirable. They may prevent eczema and help circulate and break down cholesterol. Cooked and/or processed unsaturated fats are harmful. Raw unsaturated fats (found in raw food) are good.

Mono-Saturated
A type of unsaturated fat. Reduces total cholesterol. Includes canola, olive and peanut oils, as well as avocados and natural raw peanut butter.

Polyunsaturated
A kind of unsaturated fat. Lowers total cholesterol. Includes sesame, safflower, sunflower, soybean, and corn oils.

Omega-3
A type of polyunsaturated oil that lowers total cholesterol. May help decrease deposits of cholesterol in the arteries. It is in tofu, salmon, trout, mackerel, flaxseeds, soybeans and tuna.

PREGNANCY AND CHILDBIRTH

Pregnancy is the period of childbearing. The nutritional balance of the mother before pregnancy is very important; natural whole foods should be maintained for at least one year before conception. The female and male parents must avoid alcohol, cigarettes, sodas, drugs, refined foods and other junk foods. The man fathering the child should maintain a natural food diet. A poor diet creates poor sperm and eggs. Unhealthy sperm and eggs produce unhealthy children. Pregnancy is wholistic and the mother's and father's spirits, emotions and thoughts have an impact on the unborn child. The unborn child's spirit and aura (electromagnetic force field) is connected to the father (an emotional umbilical cord). The man fathering the child, as well as the birth father, can make mental and spiritual impressions upon the unborn child.

The difficulties with pregnancy are caused by inadequate nutrition, poor posture, high heels, nylon panties, hormonal changes, a shift in gravity and weight distribution, pressure on the bladder (increases urination), pressure on the colon(may cause constipation), inadequate exercise, failure to take Red Raspberry leaf tea consistently, muscle-relaxing effect of progesterone, increase in estrogen (cause bleeding gums, fluid retention) drop in blood pressure (causes dizziness), morning sickness, digestion problems (gas), spasms of ligaments, insomnia, leg cramps, mood swings, and inadequate holistic support from the male fathering the child and/or birth father.

The woman's body is delicately balanced. This delicate state allows the woman to transmit and receive energies from the environment (physical and mental), from the child, from the father and from herself. She can also act as receiver of negative energies which can cause the pregnancy to be difficult and full of problems.

Supplements	Suggested Dosage	Remarks
Vitamin A	5,000 IU.	Aids eyes, skin, bones, antioxidant.
Vitamin B Complex	100 mg.	Maintains skin, nerves, muscle and brain function.
Vitamin B_6	50 mg.	Enhances mental and physical health.
Vitamin B_{15}	2,000 mcg.	Stimulates energy production.
Vitamin C	3,000-6,000 mg.	Enhances tissue growth and repair.
Vitamin D	400 mg.	Aids growth of bones, protects heart.
Vitamin E	400-1,000 IU.	Combats diseases, enhances, circulation.
Vitamin K	100 mcg.	Helps repair cells, stabilizes bones.
Calcium	1,500-2,000 mg.	Regulates cholesterol, growth and development.
Magnesium	750-1,000 mg.	Stabilizes nerves, reduces stress.
Manganese	10-50 mg.	Aids reproductive organs, nerves and growth.
Folic Acid	800-1,000 mcg.	Regulates fetal development.
Potassium	50-80 mg.	Enhances nutrient level, nervous system.
Zinc	50-80 mg.	Nourishes glands.
White Clay	1-2 tbsp. daily.	Cleanses colon.
Bee Pollen	As directed.	Provides, protein and energy.
Vegetarian Iron	18 mg.	Essential for blood.
Quercetin	As directed.	Aids digestive tract used for cancer.
Coenzyme Q_{10}	30-100 mg.	Enhances immunity, lungs, muscles and glands.
Beta Carotene	15,000 I.V.	Combats diseases.
Vegetable Protein (Soy Free)	As directed.	Needed for bodily functions.

Vegetarian Acidophilus	As directed.	Aids digestion.
Chromium	100-200 mcg.	Regulates glucose.

HERBS
Alfalfa, Blessed Thistle, Ginseng, Gotu Kola, Kola, Spikenard, Raspberry leaves, Uva Ursi.

Stretch Marks (Prevention)

Aloe Vera Oil, Glucosamine and Chondroitin Crème/Lotion, Shea Butter, Vitamin E Oil	Rub on abdomen, thighs and hips.

Milk Production
Alfalfa, Blessed Thistle, Borage, Caraway, Oat Straw, Fennel, Milkwort, Rosemary.

Enrich Milk
Alfalfa, Burdock Rood, Dandelion, Nettle.

Uterine Contractions
Cramp Bark, St. John's Wort, Shepherd's Purse.

Avoid During Pregnancy
Angelica, Barberry, Black Cohosh, Bloodroot, Cat's Claw, Celandine, Cottonwood Bark, Dong Quai, Feverfew, Goldenseal, Lobelia, Oregon Grape, Pennyroyal, Rue, Tansy.

FOODS
All fresh vegetables and fruits, Beans, Beets, Raw Nuts, Raw Seeds, Whole Grains, Flaxseed Meal.

PROSTATE PROBLEMS

The prostate is partly muscle and gland. It is about the size of a walnut with a donut shape. It is directly underneath the bladder and surrounds the tube (urethra) that allows urine to flow out the bladder and pass out through the penis. The prostate secretes a thin cloudy alkaline fluid that helps make up seminal fluid. The muscular contractions of the prostate squeeze the prostatic fluids and help mix it with semen and sperm. The muscles help to ejaculate. There are many types of prostate diseases and many factors that can cause prostate problems. Drugs (legal and illegal) harm it.

Prostatic Hypertropy is enlargement of the prostate. It can slow down, interrupt, block, or stop the flow of urine as well as cause urine to stay in the bladder too long, resulting in infections and/or inflammation. This can lead to kidney disease and destroy the kidney.

Prostatitis is the inflammation of the prostate. Diseases can directly and indirectly affect the prostate such as Sugar Diabetes, High Blood Pressure, Rheumatism, Arthritis, Varicose Veins, as and Hypoglycemia, which damages prostate nerves.

There are early warnings of prostate problems. Premature baldness and/or ejaculation can indicate weakness and/or deterioration of the prostate. Young boys dribble urine after it stops flowing and often leaves urine stains in their underwear. This may be indicating the beginning of prostate problems. Men that need to shake their penis several times because urine dribbles after urination stops may have the onset of problems. Usually, early warnings are ignored until the male reaches middle age and has an enlarged prostate, cancer of the prostate or infertility.

Infertility is rising, as twenty-five percent of married couples cannot have children. The sperm count was 120 million per milliliter in 1938 and dropped to 20 million per milliliter in 1991. It has been steadily decreasing each year. Imbalanced sex hormone levels (estrogen, progesterone and testosterone) can result in decreased sperm counts. Excess estrogens in non-organic foods lower the progesterone and a testosterone level, which lowers the sperm count and deteriorates the prostate.

There are estrogen and steroid-type chemicals in non-organic meats, milk (dairy), egg, fruit, and vegetables. Excess estrogen weakens the prostate, causes cancer of the prostate and breast cancer in men. Synthetic estrogen in foods given to childbearing women can cause undescended testicles. Women eating non-organic commercial foods with excess estrogen have more synthetic estrogen in their breast milk than is found in non-organic cow's milk. Therefore, the consumption of excess estrogen in breast and cow's milk starts the deterioration of the prostate.

Prostaglandin hormones, as well as Adrenalin hormones are released as a reaction to High Blood Pressure, Stress, Diabetes, Obesity, Drugs, Junk Food, Non-Organic Meat, Egg, and Dairy consumption. Prostgalandins cause prostate muscle contraction and are anti-inflammatory. They can be high in semen. An overly high prostaglandin level weakens the tissue of the prostate, the prostate reacts by getting thicker, developing scar tissue and becomes hypertrophied (enlarged).

The prostate is harmed by white sugar, alcohol, vinegar, salt, processed foods, the toxic synthetic chemicals in commercial deodorants, colognes, cough suppressants and allergy remedies. They enter the blood and prostate. They cause cellular waste to be suppressed (kept) in the prostate and alter normal function. It is best to use natural products purchased from health food stores. Sexual intercourse with ejaculation causes the same nutrients' energy loss as running 20 miles. A lifestyle with junk foods and excessive sex without nutritional supplementation and prostate herbs will eventually destroy the prostate.

SIGNS AND SYMPTOMS OF PROSTATE PROBLEMS

- Pain between the rectum and the scrotum
- Decreased force of urination
- Difficulty starting and stopping urination
- Frequent day and/or night urination
- Burning feeling when urinating
- Blood in urine (pink or reddish)

- Pus in urine
- Decreased amount of semen (less than the normal one-half teaspoon)
- Decreased force of ejaculation
- Lower back pain
- Series of kidney infections or Urinary Tract Infection
- Semen dripping from penis instead of being ejaculated
- Thin clear semen instead of opaque
- Premature ejaculation
- Inability to maintain or get an erection or to ejaculate.
- Smell of semen changes. Semen usually has a slightly sweet odor. A salty odor indicates kidney excretory and venereal disease or diseased bodily condition. Bittersweet odor indicates spleen and/or pancreas disease.
- A hard rubbery mass is felt between the anus and the scrotum sack with the testicles. It can be painful if touched.
- Too much sexual intercourse (can cause prostate problems) or sex while having an active urinary tract infection further weakens the prostate.
- Constant kidney and/or bladder infection caused by urine backing up when the enlarged prostate blocks flow.
- Difficulty starting and stopping urination.

Supplements	Suggested Dosage	Remarks
Vitamin A	50,000 IU.	Protects sex organs.
Vitamin B$_6$	50 mg.	Enhances healthy gland function.
Vitamin C	3,000-6,000 mg.	Aids repair of tissue.
Vitamin E	400-1,000 IU.	Increases circulation.
Lecithin	1,500 mg.	Dissolves cellular waste.
Calcium	1,500- 2,000 mg.	Aids development of good tissue.
Magnesium	750-1,000 mg.	Strengthens glands and muscles.
Manganese	10-100 mg.	Nourishes sex organs.
Zinc	50-100 mg.	Heals and protects glands.
Pumpkin Seed Oil Capsules	As directed.	Nourishes and heals glands.
Bee Pollen	As directed.	Provides nutrients to build tissue.
Niacinamide	50-100 mg.	Increases circulation to prostate.
Pregnenolone	100 mg.	Progesterone hormone balance.
MSM	1,000 mg.	Anti-inflammatory.
Plant Sterols	As directed.	Protects and heals.
Plant Sterolins	As directed.	Promotes repair.
DHEA	50 mg.	Hormonal balance.

AMINO ACIDS

Lysine, (Infection), Glutamine (Increase circulation), Glutathione (Cleanses prostrate).

HERBS

Maca, Muira Puama, Pygeum, Saw Palmetto, Yohimbe.	Increase blood to sex organs. Cleanses, strengthens all types of prostate disease.
Cat's Claw, Chickweed,	Stops inflammation.
Echinacea, Feverfew, Goldenseal,	Decreases enlargement.
Sarsaparilla, Witch Hazel	Hormone balance, shrinks.
Cranesbill, Horsetail	Shrinks, cleanses.
Shepherd's Purse	Shrinks prostate.
Buchu, Juniper Berry, Uva Ursi	Reduces discomfort of urination.
Gingko, Gotu Kola	Increases prostate circulation.

FOODS

No alcohol, coffee, salt, non-organic eggs, meat and milk, white sugar, fried food, white flour, white rice, caffeine, black pepper (use cayenne), fermented foods (vinegar, beer, wine, soy sauce, etc.). Eat raw almonds, fruit, pumpkin, sesame seeds, sunflower seeds, vegetables; cold pressed oils and whole grains. Drink ½ gallon or more of distilled water daily.

SICKLE CELL ANEMIA

This protective reaction of the body helps to fight off malaria. In Africa, while one was on a natural foods diet, sickle cell anemia did not present a problem. It is a dis-ease today because the diet is of processed foods, meats, dairy, drugs, white sugar, salt, etc. This dis-ease is caused by the blood cell taking on a sickle shape and blocking the circulation of blood, nutrients and air, which causes toxins to stay in the body. The blocked blood vessels cause weakness and pain in the muscles, deterioration and weakening of organs and systems, energy loss, depression, mood swings and can result in death.

The cells naturally sickle after exercise or stress with people without sickle cell disease. If the person is under-nourished, has weak immunity or diseased, suffers from chemical or emotional stressors, the sickle cell will not rebound (return) to their natural shape. This can be diagnosed as sickle cell. Thiocyanate protects people of African descent from sickle cell anemia. Thiocyanate is abundant in cassava and yams (Wild Yam Extract).

Supplements	Suggested Dosage	Remarks
Vitamin A	50,000 IU.	Protects blood cells.
Vitamin B_6	50 mg.	Enhances cell function.
Vitamin B_{12}	300-400 mcg.	Regulates blood cell formation.
Vitamin C with Bioflavonoids	3,000-6,000 mg.	Protects cell's structure.
Vitamin E	400-1,000 IU.	Improves circulation.

FOODS

Chickpeas, Lentils, Lima Beans, Millet, Flaxseed, Cabbage.

See Overweight (page 92) for additional supplements. Follow the remedies as listed for Liver dis-ease and Gall Bladder dis-ease and take iodine supplement.

SKIN ERUPTIONS

Skin eruptions can be in the form of bumps, rashes, acne, boils, black and whiteheads, pimples, herpes and pus-filled bumps. The pus is actually nature's liquid bandage, and is filled with curative nutrients.

The diet to assist skin cleansing should consist of raw fruits and vegetables, whole grains, beans, brown rice, sprouts, millet, raw nuts, raw seeds and other whole foods. Avoid processed foods, processed fat, fried foods and animal fats.

There are many drugs to avoid such as alcohol, cigarettes, white sugar, coffee, soft drinks, cocoa, commercial tea, synthetic deodorants (they keep in toxins) and commercial toothpaste. Junk foods cause the body to use the skin for a bowel movement.

TREATMENTS

Wash skin with a natural soap, black (herbal/mineral) soap and clay soap. Do not use commercial cosmetics, shampoos, lotions or creams.

Skin dis-ease (acne) is usually aggravated and worsened by emotional tension and stress. See Acne (page 4) for supplements.

These books can be useful: *Herbs for Clearing the Skin* by S. Beckett; *Self Treatment for Skin Troubles* by H. Clements; *Skin Troubles* by B. MacFadden; and *Diet to Help Acne* by A Moyle.

STOMACH ULCERS

These ulcers are open sores on the skin, which can be on the esophagus, duodenum or stomach. Sores can be caused by inadequate nutrition and junk foods. The Sympathetic Nervous System is used for a crisis, fight or flight response, anxiety, fear, hypertension, danger, disease, alcohol, drugs, excess estrogen, arguments, accidents, steroids, harmful chemicals, radiation, polluted air and water, hyperactivity, etc. When the system is active, it causes waste retention and decreased blood, oxygen and nutrients to mucous tissue and underlining muscles of the digestive system. This increases retention of waste, cellular waste and toxic mineral salts waste. Mineral salts and cellular waste impacted tissues becomes stiff and breaks open causing a sore (ulcer). The tissue surrounding the ulcer is usually inflamed, swollen and irritated.

There are two common types of ulcers, duodenal and gastric (stomach). Duodenal ulcers usually cause pain during mid-morning, one to three hours after meals, between 1:00 and 2:00 a.m., before meals or between meals. Pain is usually relieved by food. Gastric ulcers usually cause a mild or severe pain, usually one hour or less after eating, burning and/or aching sensation, and/or pain at night. The pain decreases or stops by eating food, drinking water or vomiting. Peptic (stomach) ulcers can cause headaches, itching, back pain, nausea, vomiting or a choking sensation. The stomach constantly secretes slime (mucous). This mucous lines the stomach and protects it from acids produced in the stomach. Junk foods can cause excess stomach acid. However, the natural usage of mucous during digestion causes the sores to be exposed to the strong stomach (gastric) acid, which causes pain. Strong digestive fluids leave the liver and go through a tube (duodenum) to the stomach to aid digestion. When the sores (ulcers) are exposed to the digestive fluids with insufficient mucous lining the stomach or duodenum, it causes pain. When the liver secretes this fluid, it irritates and pains the duodenum.

Supplements	Suggested Dosage	Remarks
Vitamin A	50,000 IU.	Helps heal gastrointestinal ulcers.
Vitamin B Complex	100 mg.	Maintains healthy skin in digestive tract.
Vitamin B$_6$	50 mg.	Anti-stress.
Vitamin B$_{12}$	300-400 mcg.	Promotes tissue growth.
Vitamin C	3,000-6,000 mg. growth.	Needed for tissue repair and growth. Vitamin E
400-1,000 IU. Strengthens skin.	Enhances tissue repair.	
Vitamin K	50-80 mcg.	Protects stomach lining.
Chlorophyll	As directed. cells.	Increases healing oxygen to
Bromelain	500 mg.	Aids digestion. Reduces inflammation.
Pycnogenol	As directed.	Increases healing.
Grape Seed Extract	As directed.	Prevents infection.
Zinc	50-100 mg.	Heals and protects skin.
Iron	18 mg.	Necessary for growth and blood.
Calcium	1,500-2,000 mg.	Maintains healthy skin.
MSM	500-1,000 mg.	Anti-inflammatory.
Phosphorus	500-700 mg.	Protects bones and skin.
Magnesium	750-1000 mg.	Skin problems and metabolism.
Garlic Capsules	1,500 mg. and sores.	Used for intestinal infections
Curcumin	As directed.	Stimulates healing.
Beta Carotene	15,000-20,000 IU.	Used for infections and skin problems.
Deglycyrrhizinated Licorice	As directed.	Used for ulcers and inflammation.

GLANDULARS

Raw Stomach	As directed.	Enhances healing.

AMINO ACIDS

Glucosamine and Chondroitin Sulfate	1,000-2,000 mg.	Heals tissue.

HERBS

Aloe Vera, Butcher's Broom, Canagra, Cat's Claw, Chamomile, Chaparral, Cinta Oregano, Cloves, Comfrey, Goldenseal, Licorice, Marshmallow Root, Myrrh, Slippery Elm, Tumeric, Violet Flowers.

Bleeding Ulcers
Cranesbill, Shepherd's Purse, Witch Hazel, Vitamin K.

FOODS

Raw Aloe Vera Juice, Avocados, Bananas, Broccoli, Raw Cabbage (contains Glutamine), Carrots, Kiwi, Potato Juice, Yams. Avoid sours and citrus fruits.

HOMEOPATHIC

Nat. Phos.	As directed.	Heals ulcerations.
Calc. Sulph.	As directed.	Used for ulcers.

TOOTH DECAY

A natural foods nutritional approach can protect teeth and prevent tooth decay (dental caries). Tooth decay is primarily caused by under-nutrition, an imbalanced diet, excess estrogen, sugar, salt, processed, chemicalized devitalized, genetically modified and demineralized foods.

Commercial tooth powders and toothpaste contain abrasives and detergents, which are harmful to teeth and gums. Brush teeth with a soft-bristled brush and use distilled or spring water. The gums should be massaged daily. Avoid sticky foods as they can lead to gum disease and cavities. Toothaches can be herbally treated with oil of Hops, Yarrow, Origanum and Clove. The oil is put on a piece of cotton, then in the cavity of the tooth. Yarrow leaf, Origanum, Clove and Ginger can be chewed to relieve the pain of toothache. White Willow and/or Boswella can be taken for pain. Feverfew can be used for nerve pain.

Tooth decay is related to an acidic diet and calcium imbalance. Calcium imbalance causes the gradual breakdown of the tooth support (gums and bone). This is seen in periodontal (around teeth) dis-ease. Periodontal dis-ease is the leading cause of tooth (bone) loss in adults. Bone loss is usually a gradual process that starts with the lungs, then sex organs, then the teeth and finally bones. Calcium is related to phosphorus. The body must have one part phosphorus for each part of calcium (1:1) ratio. If this ratio is not maintained, then bone loss results.

The phosphorus-calcium ratio of the average denatured junk food diet is 22:1 instead of the ideal 1:1 ratio. The problems with refined processed foods are that there is an imbalance of phosphorus. Eating animal flesh (meat) contributes to this ratio imbalance in that meat has twenty parts phosphorus to one part calcium. Refined cereals, bleached white flour and sugar products are about 6:1, and cooked potatoes 5:1. Soft drinks (soda) contain large amounts of phosphorus in the form of phosphoric acid. As a consequence of eating these denatured junk foods, people are losing bone (teeth, jawbone, skeletal bone) at early ages. This bone loss is caused by the body's attempts to get the proper amount of calcium to balance the phosphorus. Calcium is taken from the bones and this results in bone deterioration. Bone loss or weak bones of the jaw causes teeth to shift. The solution to this bone loss is braces for the teeth. In books such as, *Eating for Sound Teeth* by F. Miller and *Nutrition and Physical Degeneration* by N. Price, this is reviewed.

The problem of tooth (bone) loss can be solved with natural unprocessed whole foods. Natural foods contain a good phosphorus-calcium balance. Interesting to note, a person short of minerals such as phosphorus, potassium, magnesium or calcium is almost invariably short of other vital nutrients. Salt causes bone loss, as well as diseases. Tooth decay indicates undiagnosed disease in the entire body. In the book, *Nutrition Against Disease* by R. Williams, this is highlighted. Tooth decay has to be treated as part of a bodily disorder and not as an isolated dis-ease.

Tooth decay has a definite pattern. It usually affects the teeth one by one. For example, if a tooth in the lower left jaw is decaying, the corresponding tooth (the tooth on the direct opposite side) in the lower right jaw is usually decaying. The tooth directly above on the upper left jaw will probably be decaying. The thirty-two teeth are related to the thirty-two vertebrae of the spine, and consequently relate to all major bodily organs and glands. Tooth decay can indicate that the tooth corresponding to an organ or gland is also deteriorating. Some of the major tooth-organ relationships are: incisor teeth (front) are related to the respiratory and circulatory organs; canines are related to the stomach, liver, spleen, pancreas; pre-molars are related to the excretory system and intestinal region; molars (wisdom teeth) are related to the small and large intestines and reproductive organs. The tooth that has a cavity is indicating the internal organs are stressed, weak or diseased.

Ancient Africans chewed raw plants and the wooden parts of plants in order to cleanse the teeth. Raw fibrous plants were used to cleanse the teeth along with plant fiber tooth brushing devices and chew sticks. The Inca Indian civilization did not brush their teeth and they were 90% tooth cavity-free. Ironically, the Caucasian "civilized" society spends more time and monies on dental care items and 90% of the population has cavities. Ancient Africans were over 95% cavity free.

Supplements	Suggested Dosage	Remarks
Vitamin A	5,000-50,000 IU.	Essential for bone formation.
Vitamin B$_6$	50 mg.	Useful for nerve pain.
Vitamin B Complex	100 mg.	Aids absorption of nutrients.

Vitamin C with Bioflavonoids	3,000-6,000 mg.	Aids healing of bones and tissue.
Vitamin D	400 IU.	Helps build and maintain teeth.
Vitamin F	50 mcg.	Helps prevent bone loss.
Niacinamide	100-200 mg.	Aids bone formation.
Rutin	25 mg.	Increases cell health.
Hersperidin	100 mg.	Strengthens.
Iron	10 mg.	Necessary for blood to build bone.
Manganese	10-50 mg.	Enhances bone formation.
Calcium	1,500-2,000 mg.	Essential for bone development.
Phosphorus	500-700 mg.	Strengthens bones.

GLANDULARS

Raw Adrenal, Raw Pituitary	As directed.	Helps relieve symptoms.

AMINO ACIDS

Aspartic Acid	1,000-2,000 mg.	Used for nerve pain.

HERBS

Balm, Bistort, Brown Bugleweed, Comfrey, Goldenseal, Horsetail, Majoram, Mullein, Myrrh, Oat Straw, Pennyroyal, Pimpernel, Plantain, Savory, Tansy, White Oak Bark.

FOODS

Apricots, Asparagus, Beans, Beet Greens, Broccoli, Cabbage, Cantaloupe, Carrots, Corn, Dandelion Greens, Endives, Kale, Lettuce, Mustard Greens, Oranges, Papaya, parsley, Peaches, Peas, Pecans, Sweet Potatoes, Prunes, Spinach, Turnip Greens, Watercress.

HOMEOPATHIC

Kali. Mur.	As directed.	Infections.
Ferr. Phos.	As directed.	Used for inflammation.

VARICOSE VEINS

The arteries become hard or lose their flexibility due to dis-ease. Hardening is not the primary dis-ease, it is a secondary dis-ease reaction. Hardening can be caused by absence of liquid or fluid within the arteries. Salt, white sugar and animal flesh are substances, which cause the arteries to harden. The body reacts by secreting oil (cholesterol) to soften the arteries, which causes a high cholesterol level in the body. The excessive eating of refined, bleached white flour and white sugar will cause hardening of the arteries. Processed hydrogenated fats (cooked) and large amounts of saturated (animal) fats such as tallow (has a high accumulation of toxins) can cause the condition.

Supplements	Suggested Dosage	Remarks
Vitamin A	50,000 IU.	Maintains healthy veins.
Vitamin C	3,000-6,000 mg.	Strengthens veins.

Vitamin B Complex	100 mg.	Maintains healthy veins.
Vitamin F	50 mcg.	Cleanses veins.
(Found in cold-pressed soy, sesame, safflower and flaxseed oil.)		
Niacinamide	100-200 mg.	Helps dialate veins.
Dolamite	As directed.	Cleanses veins.
Zinc	50-80 mg.	Protects veins.
Primrose Oil	500 mg., 3 times daily.	Helps dialate veins.
Multiple Vitamin and Mineral	As directed.	Essential nutrients.

GLANDULARS

Raw Adrenal	As directed.	Helps dialate veins.

AMINO ACIDS

Lysine, Aspartic Acid	1,000-2,000 mg.	Cleanses veins.

HERBS

Cayenne, Comfrey, Garlic, Goldenseal, Hawthorn, Kelp, Marigold, Mistletoe, Rosehip, Witch Hazel, Yarrow.

FOODS

Brewer's Yeast, Grapefruit, Green Plants, Kiwi, Lecithin, Lemon, Mango, Pineapple, Star Fruit (also known as carambola).

HOMEOPATHIC

Calc. Flour.	As directed.	Strengthens blood vessel walls.

VITILIGO

Vitiligo (leukoderma) is a symptom of melanin insufficiency or deficiency. It is characterized by white spots or patches appearing on the skin. Vitiligo is a symptom of malnutrition as well as a gland and organ dysfunction. A stressed liver and/or pancreas can cause a deficiency of hydrochloric acid in the stomach resulting in Vitiligo. Melanin can be continuously drained due to stressors to the body, mind, emotions and spiritual situations, as well as oppression, radiation, synthetic chemicals, junk foods, drugs and environmental stress. Melanin is a free radical scavenger used to fight a polluted environment. Consequently, environmental factors can rob the skin of melanin. Artificial light, a polluted environment and radiation (i.e., computers, television, etc.) can cause insufficient skin melanin while an undernutritional diet can cause deficient skin melanin. A loss of skin melanin indicates a disease process. Synthetic chemicals in soaps, lotions, deodorants, hair concoctions and public water is harmful to skin melanin. Cold hands and feet, emotional instability, over waste (overweight), headaches, fatigue, brittle nails, thicken skin (chelated), arthritis and constipation can indicate low thyroid function (hypothyroidism), which can result in Vitiligo.

Supplement	Suggested Dosage	Remarks
Zinc	50-80 mg.	Protects and heals skin.
Pumpkin seed oil capsules	As directed.	Skin disease.
Manganese	10-50 mg.	Enhances healthy skin formation.
Vitamin B_6	50 mg. and skin disease.	Used for eczema, dermatitis
PABA	100 mg., and up, 3 times daily.	Helps to stop discoloration of hair and skin.
Pantothenic Acid (B_5)	300 mg., in daily divided dosage.	Vital in skin pigmentation.
Primrose Oil (Essential fatty acid)	500 mg., 3 times daily.	Enhances skin health.
Vitamin B Complex	100 mg.	Necessary for proper skin tone and texture.
Betaine Hydrochloride	As directed.	Alkalines chemistry and promotes healing.
Creatine	1,000-10,000 mg.	Promotes cell growth.
Glucosamine and Chondroitin Sulfates	1,000-2,000 mg.	Heals skin, stabilizes glucose. Heals tissue, strengthens heart.

GLANDULARS

Raw Thyroid, Raw Pituitary, Raw Liver	As directed.	Aids the healing and cleansing of skin.

AMINO ACIDS

Tyrosine	500-1,000 mg.	Helps stimulate color.

HERBS

Burdock, Calendula, Chickweed, Clove, Dandelion Root, Echinacea, Evening Primrose, Eyebright, Ginger, Goldenseal, Lavender, Red Clover, Sanicle, Thuja.

FOOD

Buckwheat, Cherry, Chestnuts, Hazelnuts, Lentils, Plums, Red Grapes, Rice, Rye, Sesame Seeds, Soybeans, Sunflower Seeds.

HOMEOPATHIC

BarytaCarbonica and Aurum Metallicum	As directed.	Used for gland skin problems.
Zincum Muriaticum	2 gr., once daily.	Used to heal and protect skin.

TISSUE SALTS

Kali. Sulph. and Nat. Mur.	3x or 3-200x.	Used for sores, dry skin and eruptions.
Nat. Phos.	As directed.	Skin sores and problems.

WATER RETENTION - EDEMA

Water retention occurs when excessive water is collected in an area of the body. A blow (trauma) to the head, arm, body or an organ can result in edema to that area or organ. A deficiency of minerals in the cells causes the cells to burn more carbon dioxide gas, which expands the cells resulting in water seeping into the cell (edema). The pressure of one water-filled cell against another water-filled cell causes the cells to spill water out—edema. Water goes out a cell that was built with inadequate nutrients (junk food diet, nutrient stress due to disease or emotions) causing edema. Weakly constructed cells die faster and shrink and throw out water—edema. Cells that generate excessive heat because they are filled with cellular mineral salt waste cause moisture to be lost—edema. Water is a solvent and primarily helps to dissolve waste by rusting it (ionization). Excessive fluid (edema) is not the disease, but a reaction to a disease. For example, excessive fluid retention in the left leg can be related to uterus and prostate problems. Swollen (edema) ankles and/or feet before or during menstruation can be related to a mineral deficiency (manganese, iron, calciums) excess estrogen and/or cellular waste congestion in the uterus.

Water retention (edema) is a dis-ease symptom that can be related to heart or kidney disorders. The heart must have the strength (nutritionally balanced chemistry) to pump, thick sludge waste in the blood and pump out the excess fluids that are in the extremities (feet, hands, etc.) or else fluid is retained. The kidneys can be stressed by cellular waste, uric acid (meat, dairy, etc.), high blood pressure, sugar, salt and excessive sex and fail to filter and release fluid from the blood. Do not use salt as salt retains fluid and is a poison classified as a drug. Edema can be a result of a mineral deficiency and/or an electrolyte (the body is an electrical magnet) imbalance. The body retains the fluids in order to retain the minerals in the fluid. Fluid may be retained around weak joints (mineral drained bones) and organs to dissolve waste.

Water is retained inside, and on the body due to weak tissue. For example, pus is fluid. It comes when tissue is traumatized (wounded). Swelling (watery blood) occurs when a joint is bruised, injured, weak or the skin is harmed by inflammations. Incidentally, tears (water) come when the emotions are weakened by sadness or pain. Water is a solvent used to break down bodily waste and serves as a liquid band-aid. Fluid retention is used to help the weakened (deteriorated) health of an individual.

Supplements	Suggested Dosage	Remarks
Vitamin A	10,000 IU.	Promotes drainage of fluids, sinus, lungs, etc.
Vitamin B Complex	100 mg.	Maintains fluid levels.
Vitamin B_6	50 mg.	Diuretic.
Vitamin C	3,000-6,000 mg.	Prevents accumulation of fluids.

Vitamin E	10,000 IU.	Improves circulation of fluids.
Magnesium Oxide	750-1,000 mg.	Helps fluid flow.
Calcium	1,500-2000 mg.	Stabilizes tissue causing fluid release.
Potassium	50-80 mg.	Enhances the flow of fluids.
Bromelain	500 mg., 3 times daily.	Reduces swelling.
Silica	As directed.	Helps prevent fluid retention.
Zinc	50-80 mg.	Helps excrete fluids.

HERBS

Black Cohosh, Buchu, Cornsilk, Cubeb, Ginger, Horsetail, Jewel Weed, Juniper Berry, Kidney Bean Pod, Lobelia, Marshmallow, Parsley, Uva Ursi.

FOODS

Cucumber, Green Leafy Vegetables, Karamboa, Melons, Pineapple, Whole Grains.

WOMEN'S SEX ORGAN RELATED DIS-EASES (HERPES, VD, ETC.)

There is no mystery to the increasing number of sex organ related dis-eases among women. The dis-eases are caused by biochemical imbalances, birth control pills, excess estrogen, dioxin bleach in sanitary napkins, stressors, synthetic chemicals, latex, and polyurethane condoms.

The destructiveness of these chemicals amounts to a chemical attack. Ironically, these chemicals are designed by men who will not suffer penis flesh scraping (dilation and curettage) or penis removal (total hysterectomy). These procedures are confined to women. It is a war against the womb.

Chemicals attack the woman's sex organs in various forms. The synthetic chemicals are alien to the body and cause the body to eject them. This ejection takes months or sometimes several years. Chemicals such as those found in synthetic condoms, birth control pills and gels, and douches contain substances that are not proven to be unharmful. If these chemicals were actually safe, then the douche solution could be drunk. If a solution is not safe enough for the stomach or eyes, then it cannot be safe for the sensitive uterus. The use of these synthetic chemicals or any synthetic chemical alters the natural body chemistry and vaginal flora (natural fungus, yeast, bacteria found in vagina and intestines). These chemicals can cause cancer and skin irritation. The skin reacts with cleansing actions, which are bumps, abscesses, cysts, tumors, herpes, sores and rashes. The synthetic chemicals in sanitary napkins and tampons, such as dioxin, are equally dangerous. Tampons cause the skin to reabsorb dead and diseased cells and dry the uterus. Birth control foams and gels, pills and intrauterine devices (IUD's) can cause inflammations and skin irritation. Hormonal and biochemical imbalances can weaken the uterus and destroy vaginal flora. Synthetics are released in the form of skin eruptions, cysts, tumors, bumps, catarrh and other dis-ease states. Toilet paper treated with synthetic perfumes, bleach, dyes and paper bonders and softeners cause skin eruptions. The use of synthetic cough suppressants, deodorants and antihist-amines dries up nasal mucous and vaginal mucousal fluid, causes uterus rheumatism, dehydrates the uterus, congests the uterus with waste, hardens the uterine arteries and veins, which contributes to fungus, yeast and bacterial dis-eases. Antibiotic usage kills natural uterus bacteria flora, resulting in yeast and fungus dis-ease.

Tight pants, nylon stockings and nylon (non-cotton) panties stop proper air ventilation of the vagina. This can cause vaginitis (inflammation), skin eruptions and create a moist environment for excessive fungus, yeast, and bacteria to grow. The introduction of feces on the penis from anal sex and alien bacteria through oral sex can contribute to altering the natural flora and cause dis-eases known as abscesses, cysts, sores, herpes, etc.

There is a basic question that has to be understood in the dis-ease process. How did the first person contact Venereal Disease (VD)? There must have been a first person to have VD in order to sexually transmit it to another person. A conscious analyst reveals that the body produced the dis-ease. The body will always produce herpes, VD and other symptoms whenever it is trying to cleanse itself from toxins, cellular waste and dis-ease. An unhealthy state is created by perversions of the natural laws. The law says a whole person must eat whole foods. Whole foods are made by nature, not by man. Man-made foods are partial foods. Partial foods pro-duce partial health, which results in dis-ease. The synthetic foods, chemi-cals, radiation and drugs make the body mildly or severely sick and even-tually collapse the immunity. This causes diseases.

VD and herpes can be triggered by foods. Allergic reactions to the syn-thetic chemicals, additives, dyes or preservatives in foods can cause the uterus to react. The skin reaction can result in eruptions, which try to eject the chem-icals. VD can be triggered by hormonal imbalances. Consequently, a woman with an excess estrogen hormone imbalance will get various types of VD before, during and after menstruation.

Treatment for types of VD varies and can be specific. Both hot and/or cold baths can be used. Baths aid in cleansing the body. Chaparral, Red Clover, White Oak Bark and herbs can be used in baths. Herbs are beneficial in douches.

Syphilis, like all dis-eases, affects the entire body. A cleansing diet of fruit or a high enema with herbs should be taken. No non-organic meats, dairy, eggs, processed foods or synthetic chemicals in foods should be eaten. There are many herbs that can be used such as Burdock, Chaparral, Goldenseal, Dandelion Root, Devil's Claw, Oregon Grape, Uva Ursi, Buckthorn, Spikenard and Yellow Dock.

Herbal treatments for venereal diseases of all types should be rigidly fol-lowed. Herbs can be used for douche solution, enemas and baths. In the case of baths, a shallow sponge bath is suitable.

Gonorrhea, like syphilis, is attributed to a germ. In Caucasian thought, they believe that either they are being attacked or that they must be attacking something or someone. They believe that if they are not preparing for war, engaged in war or someone's not trying to attack them, then they are weak. Their predatory militaristic logic causes them to believe that a germ has attacked them and caused the dis-ease. This thought process would lead to the conclusion that the body can attack itself and cause dis-ease. Caucasian science never states that healthy germs are attacking the body and giving health. Disease is erroneously blamed on the germs that are only reacting to a disease state. The germ population increases because they have bodily waste to eat. The waste causes the germs (effects). The germs do not cause the waste (i.e., disease). The effect cannot be the cause.

Imbalanced nutrition causes the internal and external skin to deteriorate, split and lacerate, producing sores. The sores associated with this dis-ease can be treated with the herbs such as Goldenseal, Comfrey, Aloe, Garlic, Thyme and Myrrh can be applied, combined with clay and charcoal.

Discharge disorders such as leukorrhea can be treated. Leukorrhea can be treated with astringent herbs such as White Oak Bark, Witch Hazel, Shepherd's Purse, Barberry, Tormentil (often used to make the vagina tight), Hemlock, Hickory and Queen of the Meadow. Of course, a strict diet and health program is always indicted in dis-eases such as leukorrhea.

Other vaginal problems can be treated naturally. A partial list of treatment is as follows:

Vaginitis
Cat's Claw, Feverfew, Gum Arabic, Marshmallow Root

Excessive Menstruation
Burnet, Cranesbill, Pilewort, Shepherd's Purse, Sorrel, Witch Hazel, Yarrow

Excessive Discharge
Alum Root, Bayberry, Beth Root, Plantain, Oregon Grape, Shepherd's Purse, Witch Hazel

Estrogen Imbalance
Black Cohosh, Chaste (Vitex), Damiana, Dong Quai, Licorice, Sarsaparilla, Squaw Vine

Progesterone Imbalance
Wild Yam

Cancer
Chaparral, Pau D'Arco, Red Clover

Prolapsed Uterus
Comfrey, Slippery Elm

Cramps
Blue Cohosh, Cramp Bark, Fennel, Pennyroyal, Rue, Wood Bethany

A preventive douche could consist of herbs such as Marshmallow, Fennel, Fenugreek, Bayberry Bark and Uva Ursi.

Prevention is the best method of avoiding dis-eases. A balanced whole foods natural foods diet, exercise, a healthy mental outlook and a healthy spirit are the foundation for prevention of all dis-eases.

Diseases of women's sex organs may seem to be local or confined to the uterus, fallopian tubes, ovaries and uterus. However, all dis-eases indicate a biochemical imbalance, weak immunity and degenerated health. Sexual intercourse should be limited or avoided while treatment is taking place. You would not use a car that has no brakes, oil or lights, so do not use your sex organs when they are ill.

WORMS

Worms are parasites that live off of waste in the gastrointestinal tract (stomach, intestines, rectum, etc.). They also live off of waste in the prostate and vagina. When food stays in the body too long and putrefies causing poisons such as ptomaines and leucomaines or ferments causing poisons such as carbon dioxide, ammonia, ascetic acid (vinegar) and alcohol. Improper food combining such as eating meat and starch together (i.e., hamburger, milk and cereal), sugar and starch (cake, cookies, pastries) or fruit and starch (i.e., pies, jelly sandwiches) causes worms. Eating late at night, which causes food to ferment and putrefy in the stomach can cause worms. Eating fried foods, unwashed vegetables and fruits, milk, cheese, ice cream, eggs and any type meat causes worms. Worms multiple and hatch eggs all over the body (muscles, blood, intestines, etc.) Worms can be found under the scalp and eat away the hair, resulting in baldness. They can be under facial skin and in facial bumps. Worm colonies result in decreased absorption of vitamins and minerals from the gastrointestinal tract. People with worms tend to be hungry because the worms are eating the food. Worms can cause diarrhea, rectal (anus), facial and scalp itching, muscle pain, loss of weight and appetite, digestive problems and a crawling feeling in the stomach and under the skin. Worms can invade the body from walking barefoot on soil contaminated by dog, cat, human and rodent manure, letting worm infested animals lick your face or touch your skin or walk in your home, eating uncooked or partially cooked meat that has worm eggs or larvae (USDA meats usually has worms) and kissing, having sex with or touching worm infested people can cause you to get worms. There are many types of worms such as threadworms, roundworms, tapeworms, pinworms and hooked worms. The most dangerous worms are in seafood. Worms have many shapes, colors and sizes and some are transparent. A child or adult may scratch their anus area while they are asleep because the warmth of the bed tends to make the worms crawl out the rectum. Nose itching or nose scratching can indicate pinworms or false teeth that vibrate. People who scratch excessively are usually scratching worms. Hair that has a dull sheen to it can indicate worms. Vaginal itching can be caused by worms. The feeling of worms crawling around in the prostate or sex organs can be misinterpreted as the feeling of sexual arousal. It is a worm sensation, not a sex sensation.

Supplement	Suggested Dosage	Remarks
Garlic capsules	2 capsules 3 times daily with meals.	Expels worms.
Pumpkin extract	As directed.	Aids in expelling the worms.

HERBS

Aloe, Areca (Betel) Nut, Black Walnut Hulls, Buckbean, Catnip, Elecampane, Larkspur, Life Everlasting, , Male Fern, Mugwort, Mulberry, Pinkroot, Quassia, Senna, Tansy, Tarragon, Thyme, White Oak, Wormseed, Wormwood.

For severe worm infestation, take an enema with any combination of the above herbs and also drink the herbs.

FOOD

Black Walnut, Carrot, Cayenne, Garlic, Endive, Fig, Leeks, Onions, Papaya, Plum, Pomegranate, Pumpkin, Raw Pumpkin Seeds, Radish, Raw Sesame Seeds, Tamarind.

HOMEOPATHIC

China (Cinchona)	As directed.	Treats worms, inflammation and infection.
Spigelia (Pinkroot)	2 gr. in the p.m.	Used for worms.
Hydrastis (Goldenseal)	1st x: 5 drops at noon.	Cleanses and expels worms.
Poconeol 82	5 drops before dinner.	Purifies and expels worms.

Note: Fresh Garlic (minced) or garlic powder in the shoes kills worms. Eat fresh Papaya Seeds to expel worms.

TISSUE SALTS

Nat. Mur. and Nat. Phos	3-200x 4 times daily. Alternate.	Expels worms.

Threadworms
Nat. Phos.	3x
Nat. Mur.	3x and 4 doses dissolved in a cup, then give an enema with the cup of liquid.

Various types of Worms
Nat. Mur.	12x or 3-200x 4 times daily.
Nat. Phos. and Silicea	12x or 3-200x 2 times daily.

YEAST INFECTION

A fungus-like yeast called candida albicans is called yeast infection. Yeast, fungus and bacteria (bacteria flora) are present at all times in a healthy person's lungs, mouth, intestinal tract, skin and vagina. The bacteria flora can get out of balance and yeast, fungus or bacteria can multiply whenever excessive food (waste) is provided for them. The acidity and sugar content of the vagina can become altered due to the eating of refined carbohydrates (white sugar, bleached white flour etc) and eating foods with yeast in them, fermented foods (vinegar, beer, wine etc). Synthetic drugs, antibiotics and oral contraceptives can cause yeast infection. Those that are borderline diabetic or diabetic tend to have many yeast infection. The symptoms of candida can be itching, cheesy discharge, burning sensation and slight inflammation of the vagina. It is the leading cause of vaginitis.

Supplement	Suggested Dosage	Remarks
Caprylic Acid	1st week; 1 tablet twice daily. 2nd week; 2 tablets twice daily. 3rd week; 3 tablets twice daily.	Destroys fungus.
Grape Seed Oil	As directed.	Combats infection.
Garlic capsules (Can be odorless)	2 capsules 3 times daily.	Inhibits the infecting organism. Garlic suppositories also effectively treat Candida vaginitis.
Multivitamin and mineral complex (zinc, iron, and yeast free) with	Daily as directed on label.	Vital nutrients for proper proper immune function.
Vitamin A and	25,000 IU.	Enhances protection.
Selenium	200 mcg.	Aids expelling worms.
Maxidophilus (Milk free) or Megadophilus	Use as directed on label.	
Omega Oils, Flaxseed Oil or Primrose Oil	1-3 grams.	Vital essential fatty acids.
Coenzyme Q_{10}	100 mg., daily.	Enhances tissue oxygenation.
Vitamin B Complex with extra biotin	100 mg., 3 times daily	Faulty absorption is common in candidiasis.
Vitamin B_{12} lozenges	1 lozenge (2,000 mcg) under the tongue 3 times daily, taken between meals.	Vital for digestion. Needed for metabolism of carbohydrates, fats, and proteins. Candida prevents the absorption of nutrients from the intestinal tract.
Germanium	100-200 mg., daily.	Enhances tissue oxygention.
Vegetable Protein	As directed.	Helps build healthy tissue and balances flora.

GLANDULARS

Raw Thymus	As directed.	Protects systems.
Raw Liver	As directed.	Stimulates detoxification.

AMINO ACIDS

L-Cysteine	500 mg., on an empty stomach. twice daily.	An antioxydant and free radical destroyer.

HERBS

Clove Tea, Grape Seed Oil, Pau D'Arco, Uva Ursi.

FOOD

Raw Cranberry Juice or Fresh Cranberries.

HOMEOPATHIC

Kreosotum 7	5 gr., once daily.	Soothes irritation, itching and swollen vagina.
Mercuris Cyanatus 7	2 gr., once daily.	Soothes burning sensation.
Canella 4	2 gr., 2 times a day.	Used for skin problems.
Borax 7	2 gr., once daily.	Inflammation, sores.

TISSUE SALTS

Kali Phos. and Nat. Sulph.	6x or 3-200x, 3 times daily.	Soothes irritation.
Nat. Phos.	6x or 3-200x, 3 times daily.	Heals sores.
Silicea	6x or 3-200x, 3 times daily.	Heals tissue.

MEDICINE

It's a Simple Case of "Black and White"

European Medicine is for People of European Decent.	African Medicine is for People of African Decent.

The Caucasian Junk Foods are destroying African Americans. At the current rate of

dying, African Americans could be near extinction in

100 years or less!

Section 2

Remedies

Herbs for Dis-eases
A to Z

Abscesses
Lobelia, Mugwort, Slippery Elm

Abrasion/Cuts
(Bruises Under the Skin)
Aloe Vera, Arnica, Bittersweet, Bugleweed, Chickweed, Comfrey, Hyssop, Lobelia, Mugwort, Pennyroyal, Primrose

Aches
Angelica, Boswella, Catnip, Hops, Peppermint, Skullcap, Valerian, White Willow

Anemia
Agrimony, Century, Comfrey, Dandelion, Fenugreek, Red Clover, Yellow Dock

Poor Appetite
(or lack of desire to eat)
Calamus, Chamomile, Gentian, Ginseng, Goldenseal, Marjoram, Organum, Woodsage

Appendicitis
Cayenne, Buckthorn, Vervain

Arthritis
Alfalfa, Black Cohosh, Buckthorn, Burdock, Cat's Claw, Chaparral, Comfrey, Devil's Claw, Parsley, Yucca

Asthma
Chickweed, Coltsfoot, Comfrey, Elecampane, Flaxseed, Horehound, Hyssop, Lobelia, Mullein, Pleurisy, Sage, Skunk Cabbage

Backache
Boswella, Nettle, Pennyroyal, Tansy, Uva Ursi, White Willow, Wood Betony

Bed Wetting
Buchu, Corn Silk, Fennel Seed, St. John's Wort, Plantain, Wood Betony

Bladder
Aloes, Broom, Goldenseal, Hemlock, Lily Pond, Nettles, Uva Ursi, Valerian, Vervain, Wintergreen, Yarrow

Bleeding
Alum Root, Mullein, Self Heal, Shepherd's Purse

Blood Circulation
(Increase)
Cayenne, Gentian, Goldenseal, Holy Thistle, Hyssop, Witch Hazel

Blood Cleaner	Bittersweet, Burdock, Chickweed, Dandelion, Echinacea, Hyssop, Nettle, Sassafras, Sorrel, Red Clover, Yellow Dock
Blood Impurities	Bayberry, bugleweed, Chaparral, Chickweed, Comfrey Root, Gentian, Goldenseal, Myrrh, Primrose, Red Clover, Yellow Dock
Bowel *(Digestive Problems, Constipation)*	Catnip, Comfrey, Dandelion, Fenugreek, Goldenseal, Magnolia, Marshmallow, Tansy, Witch Hazel
Breast *Inflamed, Sore, Swollen, etc.*	Black Cohosh, Comfrey, Ginger, Goldenseal, Myrrh
Sore Nipples	Parsley, Poke Root, St. John's Root, Slippery Elm
Bronchitis	Chickweed, Coltsfoot, Elecampane, Ginger, Goldenseal, Mullein, Pleurisy, Saw Palmetto, Skunk Cabbage, Slippery Elm
Burns	Aloe Vera, Bittersweet, Burdock, Calamus, Calendula, Comfrey, Onions, Primrose, Poplar
Cancer:	Blue Flag, Blue Violet, Chaparral, Dandelion, Goldenseal, Pau D'Arco, Sage, Sorrel, Yellow Dock
Childbirth	Plantain, Red Raspberry, Squaw Vine
Chills	Bayberry, Catnip, Cayenne, Colombo, Fleabane, Sage
Colds/Flu/Fever	Bayberry, Cat's Claw, Chickweed, Cloves, Elecampane, Horehound, Mullein, Pleurisy, White Pine Bark
Convulsions	Arnica, Black Cohosh, Catnip, Fennel, Hyssop, Mistletoe, Peppermint, Self-Heal, Skullcap, Valerian
Corns/Calluses	Bittersweet, Garlic Powder (Sprinkle in Socks). Horsetail Powder and Chamomile (Make into a poultice or ointment and apply)

Coughs Black Cohosh, Coltsfoot, Comfrey, Flaxseed, Ginseng, Goldenseal, Horehound, Hyssop, Lungwort, Myrrh, Origanum, Pleurisy, Red Sage

Cramps Bayberry, Blue Cohosh, Coral, Fennel, Masterwort, Motherwort, Pennyroyal, Squaw Vine, Thyme, Twin Leaf, Wood Betony

Dandruff Aloe, Burdock, Indian Hemp, Rosemary, Sage

Diabetes Bilberry, Blue Cohosh, Gymnema Sylvestre, Periwinkle, Poplar, Raspberry Leaves, Saw Palmetto

Dizziness Catnip, Peppermint, Rue, Wood Betony Burnet, Hops, Origanum, Pimpernel. Fenugreek, Garlic, Yellow Dock

Eczema Balomy, Bloodroot, Calendula, Chickweed, Dandelion, Goldenseal, Nettle, Plantain, Primrose, Yellow Dock

Epilepsy Black Cohosh, Elder, Lady's Slipper, Mistletoe, Skullcap, Valerian, Vervain

Eyes Bilberry, Chamomile, Chickweed, Eyebright, Goldenseal, Hyssop, Rosemary, Sassafras, Slippery Elm, Squaw Vine, Tansy

Fainting Cayenne, Lavender, Motherwort, Peppermint

Fever Angelica, Bitterroot, Borage, Buckbean, Calamus, Catnip, Cat's Claw, Cayenne, Cinchona, Cleavers, Dandelion, Echinacea, Feverfew, Hyssop, Indian Hemp, Lily of the Valley, Lobelia, Mandrake, Nettle, Parsley, Pleurisy, Poplar, Sage, Sarsaparilla, Shepherd's Purse, Sumac Berries, Tansy, Thyme, Valerian, Vervain, Wahoo, Willow, Wintergreen, Yarrow

Gallstones	Bitterroot, Cascara Sagrada, Chamomile, Cherry Bark, Hydrangea, Mandrake, Milkweed, Parsley, Rhubarb, Wood Betony
Gangrene	Chamomile, Comfrey, Echinacea, Hemlock, Myrrh, Poplar, Willow
Gargle	Bayberry, Bistort Root, Goldenseal, Hyssop, Myrrh, Pilewort, Sage
Gas *(Type of Constipation)*	Agrimony, Aloe Cape, Balmony, Bay Leaves, Bitterroot, Cascara Sagrada, Cayenne, Chamomile, Ginseng, Goldenseal, Hyssop, Red Sage, Senna
Genitals *Burning, Itching, Irritations*	Chickweed, Marshmallow, Peach Leaves, Pleurisy, Raspberry Leaves, Slippery Elm
Glandular Organs	Bittersweet, Echinacea, Mullein, Parsley, Poke Root, Sea Wrack, Stinging Nettle, Yellow Dock
Goiter	Bayberry Bark, Echinacea, Irish Moss, Poke Root, Sea Wrack, White Oak Bark
Gonorrhea	Bittersweet, Bistort Root, Black Willow, Blood Root, Cleavers, Goldenseal, Hops, Juniper Berries, Parsley, Poplar, Red Root, Rock Rose, Squaw Vine, Uva Ursi, Wintergreen
Hair	Burdock, Indian Hemp, Nettle, Rosemary, Sage
Halitosis *(Bad Breath)*	Cascara Sagrada, Echinacea, Goldenseal, Henna, Myrrh, Rosemary
Hay Fever	Black Cohosh, Coltsfoot, Mullein, Poplar, Skunk Cabbage
Heart	Angelica, Bloodroot, Borage, Cayenne, Cinchona, Goldenseal, Hawthorn Berry, Holy Thistle, Mistletoe, Motherwort, Peppermint, Skullcap, Sorrel, Tansy, Valerian, Vervain, Wood Betony

Heartburn	Anise, Catnip, Fennel, Ginger, Nutmeg, Peppermint, Sage, Sassafras, Thyme, Wood Betony, Yarrow
Hemorrhoids	Aloes, Bittersweet, Burdock, Goldenseal, Myrrh, Nettle, Shepherd's Purse, White Oak Bark, Uva Ursi
Headache	Blue Violet, Calamine, Chamomile, Coltsfoot, Elder, Feverfew, Holy Thistle, Marjoram, Pennyroyal, Rhubarb, Rosemary, Rue, Skullcap, Tansy, Vervain, Wood Betony, Yerba Santa
Hemorrhages	Alum Root, Bayberry Bark, Beth Root, Burnet, Comfrey, Fleabane, Goldenseal, Nettle, Pilewort, Plantain, Red Sage, Shepherd's Purse, Sorrel, Tormentil, Uva Ursi, Witch Hazel, Wood Betony, Yarrow
Hernia	Aloe Vera, Barberry, Comfrey, Plantain, Witch Hazel
Hiccoughs:	Blue Cohosh, Cinnamon, Dill, Hyssop
High or Low Blood Pressure	Aloes, Black Cohosh, Blue Cohosh, Broom, Cayenne, Garlic, Ginseng, Goldenseal, Hyssop, Myrrh, Parsley, Skullcap, Valerian, Vervain, Wild Cherry
Hips *(Painful)*	Strawberry Leaf, Thyme, White Willow
Hypnotics	Chloral Hydrate, Ephedra, Hops, Orange Blossom Oil, Yohimbe
Hysteria	Black Cohosh, Blue Cohosh, Catnip, Mistletoe, Pennyroyal, Peppermint, Rue, Saffron, Skunk Cabbage, Tansy, Valerian, Vervain
Influenza	Indian Hemp, Peppermint, Poplar, White Pine
Inflammation	Arnica, Cat's Claw, Cayenne, Chickweed, Fenugreek, Feverfew, Goldenseal, Hops, Hyssop, Lobelia, Marshmallow, Mugwort, Slippery Elm, Sorrel, Tansy, Witch Hazel

Insomnia   Catnip, Chamomile, Hops, Kava,
                                Skullcap, Valerian

Impotence   Damiana, Dopa Bean, Fo-ti, Gotu Kola,
                                Maca, Mucana Purine, Muira Puama, Saw
                                Palmetto, Siberian Ginseng, Tribulus, Wild
                                Oats, Yohimbe

Kidney Problems   Aloes, Balm, Beech, Beth Root,
                                Bitterroot, Broom, Cayenne, Celadine,
                                Chamomile, Chickweed, Cleavers,
                                Dandelion, Goldenseal, Hemlock,
                                Hyssop, Masterwort, Milkweed, Oregon
                                Grape, Parsley, Poplar, Poke Root,
                                Sage, Sanicle, Sea Wrack, Spearmint,
                                Tansy, White Oak Bark, White Pine

Laxative   Aloes, Cascara Sagrada, Chia Seeds,
                                Elder, Flaxseed, Goldenseal, Henna,
                                Horehound, Hyssop, Mullein, Rhubarb,
                                Sage, Senna, Wahoo

Leukorrhea   Slippery Elm, Squaw Vine, White Oak Bark
Vaginal Discharge   Bayberry Bark, Comfrey, Tormentil,
                                Wormwood

Douche   Alum Root, Bistort Root, Goldenseal,
                                Magnolia, Plantain, Ragwort

Liver Bile   Bitterroot, Cascara Sagrada, Celandine,
(Aids Digestion. Bile   Hops
Leaves Bitter Taste
in Mouth)

Liver Problems   Bayberry Bark, Bistort Root,
                                Bittersweet, Bloodroot, Borage, Broom,
                                Buckbean, Celandine, Chamomile,
                                Chicory, Cleavers, Dandelion Root,
                                Fennel, Gentian Root, Horehound,
                                Indian Hemp, Lungwort, Mandrake,
                                Milk Thistle, Origanum, Parsley, Peach
                                Leaves, Pennyroyal, Plantain, St. John's
                                Wort, Senna Leaves, Sorrel, Tansy,
                                Wormwood

Low Back Pain   Arnica, Black Cohosh, Boswella,
                                Queen of the Meadow, Shepherd's
                                Purse, Uva Ursi, Valerian, Vervain,
                                White Willow

Menstruation	Wild Alum Root, Tormentil, Bayberry Bark, Sage, Shepherd's Purse, Uva Ursi, Bistort Root, Burnet, Sorrel, Pilewort, Sanicle, Lungwort, Witch Hazel, Wood Betony, Arnica, Horsetail, Yarrow, Saffron, Raspberry Leaves, Cleavers, Pleurisy Root
Mental Illness	Arnica, Catnip, Holy Thistle, Peppermint, Rosemary, St. John's Wort, Skullcap, Vervain, Wood Betony
Mucus *(Phlegm)*	Borage, Coltsfoot, Hyssop, Nettle, Pennyroyal, Vervain, White Pine, Wild Cherry
Muscle Spasms	Blue Cohosh, Cayenne, Cedron, Clover, Fennel, Fit Root, Masterwort, Red Root, Rue, Sassafras, Skunk Cabbage, Spearmint, Twin leaf, Wild Yam
Nausea	Anise, Ginger, Goldenseal, Lavender, Mint, Origanum, Peach Leaves, Peppermint, Red Raspberry, Spearmint, Solomon's Seal, Sweet Balm, Wild Yam
Nose Bleed	Bayberry, Blood Root, Buckthorn, Wild Alum Root, White Oak Bark, Witch Hazel
Pancreas	Bilberry (Huckleberry Leaves), Bittersweet, Blueberry Leaves, Cayenne, Dandelion, Goldenseal, Uva Ursi, Wahoo
Paralysis	Black Cohosh, Cayenne, Cramp Bark, Ginger, Lady's Slipper, Skullcap, Valerian
Pneumonia	Black Cohosh, Bloodroot, Coltsfoot, Comfrey, Elecampane, Horehound, Marshmallow, Peruvian Bark, Red Sage, Skunk Cabbage, Spikenard, Vervain, Wild Cherry, Willow
Prostate	Dopa Bean, Goldenseal Root, Gravel Root, Horsetail, Juniper Berry, Maca, Marshmallow, Muira Puama, Nettle, Pygeum, Saw Palmetto, Yohimbe
Ruptures:	Arnica, Bistort Root, Comfrey, Solomon's Seal

Sexual Excess

Arnica, Black Willow, Lily Root, Mountain Grape Root, Plantain, Sage, Skullcap, Star Root

Skin Eruptions
(Sores/Bumps)

Beech, Birch, Bittersweet, Blue Flag, Blue Violet, Buckthorn, Burdock, Chickweed, Cleavers, Comfrey, Dandelion, Elder, Flaxseed, Goldenseal, Hyssop, Hops, Lobelia, Magnolia, Oregon Grape, Origanum, Pennyroyal, Plantain, Poke Root, Primrose, Prince Pine, Red Clover, Red Root, Rock Rose, Saffron, Sarsaparilla, Sassafras, Sorrel, Spikenard, Turkey Corn, Vervain, White Clover, Wintergreen, Wood Sage

Spleen Problems

Aloes, Angelica, Balm, Bittersweet, Broom, Cayenne, Gentian Root, Chicory, Dandelion, Fennel, Goldenseal, Hyssop, Marjoram, Parsley, Uva Ursi, Wahoo, White Oak Bark

Stomach
(Indigestion, Upset)

Aloes, Angelica, Anise, Balomy, Bay Leaves, Bayberry, Calamus, Caraway Seed, Catnip, Cayenne, Cedron, Chamomile, Chicory, Comfrey, Cubeb, Echinacea, Goldenseal, Hyssop, Marjoram, Milkweed, Mugwort, Pimpernel, Rue, Sage, Sassafras, Slippery Elm, Strawberry, Thyme, Valerian, Vervain, Willow, Witch Hazel

Swellings

Burdock, Chamomile, Comfrey, Dill, Elder, Fenugreek, Ginger Root, Hops, Indian Hemp, Mugwort, Origanum, Parsley, Tansy, White Lily, Yellow Dock

Syphilis

Barberry, Bittersweet, Bloodroot, Blue Violet, Buglewood, Chaparral, Echinacea, Elder, Goldenseal, Milkweed, Oregon Grape, Palmetto, Parsley, Plantain, Poplar, Prickly Ash, Red Clover, Sanicle, Yellow Dock

Throat
Irritated/Sore

Barberry, Bloodroot, Cayenne, Fenugreek, Ginger, Goldenseal, Hops,

	Horehound, Hyssop, Mullein, Sage, Saw Palmetto Berries, Vervain, White Pine, Wild Alum Root, Wood Sage, Wood Sanicle
Thyroid	Cayenne, Irish Moss, Kelp, Pau D'Arco, Parsley
Tonsillitis:	Cat's Claw, Echinacea, Goldenseal, Mullein, Red Root, Sage, Tansy, White Pine
Toothache	Arnica, Balm, Broom, Clove Oil, Cloves, Hops, Mullein, Origanum, Origanum Oil, Pimpernel, Plantain, Tansy, Yarrow Oil
Tumors	Burdock, Cat's Claw, Cranesbill, Sanicle, Shepherd's Purse, Thuja, Witch Hazel
Tuberculosis	Bayberry Bark, Burdock Root, Coltsfoot, Comfrey, Elecampane, Goldenseal, Myrrh, Sanicle, Skunk Cabbage, Wild Cherry Bark, Yellow Dock
Spleen Problems	Aloes, Angelica, Bittersweet, Balm, Broom, Cayenne, Chicory, Dandelion, Fennel, Gentian Root, Goldenseal, Hyssop, Marjoram, Parsley, Uva Ursi, Wahoo, White Oak Bark
Ulcers	Angelica, Ash, Beech, Bistort Root, Blue Violet, Borage, Bridgewood, Calamus, Cayenne, Celandine, Chickweed, Comfrey, Fenugreek, Gold Thread, Goldenseal, Hemlock, Mullein, Pilewort, Poplar, Prickly Ash, Psyllium, Rock Rose, Sage, Saint John's Wort, Sorrel, Twin Leaf, Wild Alum Root, Wood Sanicle, Yarrow
Urine	Buchu, Burdock Seed, Cloves, Cubeb, Peach Halves, Spearmint, White Poplar Bark
Varicose Veins	Bayberry Bark, Burnet, Horsetail, White Oak Bark, Wild Alum Root, Witch Hazel

HOMEOPATHIC QUICK REFERENCE

ALLERGY/HAY FEVER

Remedy	Dosage	Remarks
Apis (Made from Honeybee)	30c potency, to be taken every 30-60 minutes during an acute attack or twice per day during an ongoing allergy reaction. Stop the remedy once you notice signs of improvement.	Use for swelling, blotching of skin and edema.
Carbo Veg. Vegetable Charcoal)	30c potency, to be taken every 30-60 minutes during an acute attack or twice per day during an ongoing allergy reaction. Stop the remedy once you notice signs of improvement.	"Air hunger," wants to be fanned
Arsenicum	30c potency, to be taken every 30-60 minutes during an acute attack or twice per day during an ongoing allergy reaction. Stop the remedy once you notice signs of improvement.	Food allergy, vomiting and diarrhea, burning pains, desires sips of warm water.

BOILS/BUMPS

Remedy	Dosage	Remarks
Belladonna (Herb = Belladonna)	30c potency. Take the remedy 3-4 times per day until the pain and swelling resolve (early stages) or until the boil erupts and discharges (later stages).	First Stage: Swollen, painful and redness.
Hepar Sulph	30c potency. Take the remedy 3-4 times per day until the pain and swelling resolve (early stages)or until the boil erupts and discharges (later stages).	Second Stage: The boil starts to develop a pocket of pus. Hepar Sulph will cause skin eruption to discharge or resolve.
Silica	30c potency. Take the remedy 3-4 times per day until the pain and swelling resolve (early stages) or until the boil erupts and discharges (later stages).	Causes the boil to discharge pus. Silica enhances the healing of a boil.

BROKEN BONES

Remedy	Dosage	Remarks
Arnica (Herb = Arnica)	30c. Take one dose every 15-30 minutes as needed for the first 3-4 hours after injury, continue taking Arnica as needed for the first 36-48 hours after injury.	Severe pain, swelling, trauma to bone and soft tissues.
Eupatorium (Herb = Boneset)	30c. Take one dose every 15-30 minutes as needed for the first 3-4 hours after injury.	Bone pain. Start taking after severe swelling and trauma has passed.
Synphytum (Herb = Comfrey)	30c. Take one dose every 15-30 minutes as needed for the first 3-4 hours after injury.	Enhances bone healing.
Calcarea Phosphorica	30 c. Take one dose every 15-30 minutes as needed for the first 3-4 hours after injury.	Decreases bone pain. Calc. Phos. is available as a cell salt (6x potency).
Hypericum (Herb = St. John's Wort)	30c. Take one dose every 15-30 minutes as needed for the first 3-4 hours after injury.	For shooting, nerve-like pain.
Ruta (Rue)	30c. Take one dose every 15-30 minutes as needed for the first 3-4 hours after injury.	Enhances the healing of the periosteum (surface layer of the bone). Ruta stimulates the final stages of healing, e.g., resolve pain that persists after a cast is removed.

BRUISES

Remedy	Dosage	Remarks
Arnica	30c. Take every 30-60 minutes immediately following injury, then 2-3 times per day until improvement.	For injuries to the head. Taking Arnica immediately after an injury can stop bruising and swelling.
Hypericum	30c. Take every 30-60 minutes immediately following injury, then 2-3 times per day until improvement.	Injuries to highly enervated areas (e.g., eyeball, hands, feet, genitals) or in case of nerve damage or bruising.
Aconite	30c. Take every 30-60 minutes immediately following injury, then 2-3 times per day until improvement.	Hot, throbbing, no discoloration; patient is anxious.
Belladonna	30c. Take every 30-60 minutes immediately following injury, then 2-3 times per day until improvement.	Discolored, throbbing, hot.

BURNS

Remedy	Dosage	Remarks
First Degree Burn		Pain, inflammation, redness.
Cantharis	30c. Repeat one dose	Burning pain that improves with
(Insect = Spanish Fly)	(three pellets) of the remedy	cold applications. For second-
	every 2-3 hours until pain	degree burn with blister
	and inflammation diminishes,	formation.
	then stop the remedy.	
Hypericum	30c. Repeat one dose	For very tender, painful burns;
	(three pellets) of the remedy	shooting, nerve-like pain.
	every 2-3 hours until pain	
	and inflammation diminishes,	
	then stop the remedy.	
Apis	30c. Repeat one dose	For stinging, itching pain.
	(three pellets) of the remedy	
	every 2-3 hours until pain	
	and inflammation diminishes,	
	then stop the remedy.	
Second-degree Burn		Inflammation, redness and blistering of the skin.
Cantharis	30c. Repeat one dose	Burning pain that decreases
	(three pellets) of the remedy	with cold applications.
	every 2-3 hours until pain	
	and inflammation diminishes,	
	then stop the remedy.	
Third-degree Burn		Charring of the skin, tissue damage.
Cantharis	30c. Repeat one dose	Burning pain that improves
	(three pellets) of the remedy	with cold applications. Blister
	every 2-3 hours until pain	formation.
	and inflammation diminishes,	
	then stop the remedy.	
Causticum	30c. Repeat one dose	Severe burns and chemical
	(three pellets) of the remedy	burns.
	every 2-3 hours until pain	
	and inflammation diminishes,	
	then stop the remedy.	

COLDS

Remedy	Dosage	Remarks
Occiloccoccinum	30c. Take three pellets 2-3 times per day until improvement, then stop taking the remedy.	Use at the very first sign of a cold, right after the first sneeze. The remedy will not be effective after the first twenty-four hours. Take six of the small pellets every 3-4 hours.

Aconite	30c. Take three pellets 2-3 times per day until improvement, then stop taking the remedy. wind.	Take after the first sneeze, when feeling anxious or fretful; symptoms may have developed following exposure to a cold, dry
Allium Cepa (Red Onion)	30c. Take three pellets 2-3 times per day until improvement, then stop taking the remedy.	Mucous discharge, sore upper lip, excoriating discharge from the nose, bland discharge from eyes; feels worse in a warm room, better in fresh air.
Arsenicum	30c. Take three pellets 2-3 times per day until improvement, then stop taking the remedy.	Affected by changes in weather; thin painful, burning discharges.
Pulsatilla (Wind Flower)	30c. Take three pellets 2-3 times per day until improvement, then stop taking the remedy.	Thick, bland discharges, green or yellow discharge. Changing symptoms: pains move around and do not localize. May feel better outside, worse in stuffy room.
Gelsemium (Yellow Jasmine)	30c. Take three pellets 2-3 times per day until improvement, then stop taking the remedy.	Slow onset, for colds that begin in warm weather or during a mild winter. May feel achy, the limbs heavy. No thirst.
Byronia	30c. Take three pellets 2-3 times per day until improvement, then stop taking the remedy.	Feels worse with motion, better with pressure. Very hot, very dry, aches all over. Thirsty for cold drinks.
Nux Vomica (POison Nut)	30c. Take three pellets 2-3 times per day until improvement, then stop taking the remedy.	Very chilly, even while dressed very warmly. Worsens with slight coolness or the least movement. Feels chilled from drinking. Aching in limbs and back. Nose stuffed at night. Can have upset stomach or other digestive symptoms.

COLIC

Remedy	Dosage	Remarks
Magnesium Phosphorica	30c.	Cramping pain; improves with warm applications.
Chamomilla (Chamomile)	30c.	Child is extremely irritable, wants to be carried, then demands to be put down. Inconsolable. One cheek has redness, the other pale.
Cholocynthis (Bitter Apple)	30c.	Cramping, abdominal pain that is relieved by pressure and by drawing the knees toward the chest.
Bryonia (White Bryony)	30c	Feels worse following the slightest motion; generally irritable.

CONSTIPATION

Remedy	Dosage	Remarks
Nux Vomica	30c.	"Ineffectual urging to stool," never feel completely emptied. Overuse of laxatives. Chilly, irritable.
Sulphur	30c.	Frequent urge with incomplete evacuation. Hard, dry, black stools expelled with great effort, pain and burning, especially around the anus. Alternating constipation and diarrhea.
Bryonia	30c.	Dry mouth, dry lips, and dry tongue. Stools dry and hard. Thirst for large quantities of water.
Calc Carb	30c.	Feels better "if doesn't" have a bowel movement.

CUTS

Remedy	Dosage	Remarks
Arnica	30c. Take three pellets every 15-30 minutes for acute bleeding. Stop taking the remedy when the bleeding stops.	Helps stop bleeding and bleeding associated with soft-tissue injury.
Phosphorous	30c. Take three pellets every 15-30 minutes for acute bleeding. Stop taking the remedy when the bleeding stops.	For arterial bleeding (bright red blood).
Belladonna	30c. Take three pellets every 15-30 minutes for acute bleeding. Stop taking the remedy when the bleeding stops.	Helps infection, especially staph and strep.
Mag. Phos.	30c. Take three pellets every 15-30 minutes for acute bleeding. Stop taking the remedy when the bleeding stops.	Releases muscle tension associated with cuts and other physical trauma.
Ferrum Phos.	30c. Take three pellets every 15-30 minutes for acute bleeding. Stop taking the remedy when the bleeding stops.	Helps stop bleeding.

DIARRHEA

Remedy	Dosage	Remarks
Arsenicum	30c.	For explosive diarrhea with vomiting. Can feel exhausted,

restless, anxious; desires hot
drinks, in small sips.

Bryonia   30c.   Following exposure to cold, dry
wind, or after a fright.

EARACHE

Remedy	Dosage	Remarks
Aconite	30c.	Earache begins after exposure to cold, dry wind. Ear redness, high fever, sudden onset. Extremely sensitive to noise. Sharp pain. Anxious, restless. Thirst for cold drinks. Onset after shock.
Belladonna	30c.	Sudden, violent onset. Dilated pupils. Throbbing blood vessels in the neck. Pain causes delirium. Child may have nightmares and call out in sleep. Throbbing, shooting, sharp pains. Ear redness and throbbing. No thirst.
Chamomilla	30c.	Irritable; intense pain. Redness to one cheek, the other pale. The child wants to be held and carried, yet arches her back. Inconsolable. Earaches from teething. Grass green stool.
Ferrum Phos.	30c.	Use at the beginning of infection, before pus develops. Pulsating, throbbing pain. Flushed face. High fever with few symptoms. Use when Belladonna fails.
Hepar Sulph	30c.	Mucous, pus in ear. For later stage of infection, when pus has developed behind the eardrum. Sensitive to drafts, wants to cover ears or head. Chilly, oversensitive, sweats easily. Feels better with hot, damp weather.
Pulsatilla	30c.	For a "ripe" (second or third stage) cold and ear infection. Copious, thick, yellow-green discharge. Feels better in fresh, cold, open air; worse in warm, stuffy room. Feels worse in the evening. No thirst. Symptoms fluctuate.

EYE INJURIES

Remedy	Dosage	Remarks
Hypericum	30c.	Redness, burning pain; very sensitive or burn.
Ruta	30c.	For burns to the eyeball.
Apis	30c.	Swollen lids. Profuse, hot tears. Photophobia (aversion to bright light), can't tolerate covering eyes.
Silica	30c.	Pushes out foreign objects.

FEVER

Remedy	Dosage	Remarks
Aconite	30c. Take three pellets 2-3 times per day until improvement is noted, then stop taking the remedy.	Hot, dry, cranky. Fever that may develop after exposure to cold cold wind. Fearful, anxious.
Ferrum Phos.	30c. Take three pellets 2-3 times per day until improvement is noted, then stop taking the remedy.	Fever with no other specific symptoms.
Belladonna	30c. Take three pellets 2-3 times per day until improvement is noted, then stop taking the remedy.	Glassy-eyed, dilated pupils; hot, red, dry face; sweaty body; possibly delirium. Sudden onset. No thirst.

HEADACHE

Remedy	Dosage	Remarks
Belladonna	30c.	Intense, throbbing pain. Very sensitive to noise, light, touch, strong smells. Pain starts abruptly, usually in the frontal area. Pain may travel to the back of the head. Feels worse after jarring. Face may have redness and feel hot, extremities cold. Pupils may be dilated.
Bryonia	30c.	Increases with any motion, even slight movement of the head or eyes. Better with firm pressure to the painful area. Constant, aching pain may be intense over the left or over the forehead area. Irritable, wants to be left alone. Improves with warmth.

Nux Vomica	30c.	Headaches that follow excesses in eating or drinking; hangovers. Generally sick feeling, with possible digestive upset. Aversion to light and sound. Avoids company. Irritable.
Gelsemium	30c.	Heavy head. Dull headache. Sensation of having a band around the head. Joints are achy, heavy. Desires to be alone.

INDIGESTION

Remedy	Dosage	Remarks
Nux Vomica	30c.	Overeating and overdrinking. May be stressed, overworked and keep a demanding schedule, which irritates a weak digestive system. Tendency to have constipation.
Arsenicum	30c.	Burning pain in the stomach, wants to drink small sips of water, although water may cause vomiting. Food poising with both diarrhea and vomiting.

MENSTRUATION

Remedy	Dosage	Remarks
Belladonna	30c.	Heavy sensation in abdomen. Menses bright red, profuse. Restless. Head feels worse after jarring or touched or in a draft.
Borax	30c.	Fears downward motion. Membrane and tissue pass with menses. Early profuse bleeding, with colic and nausea. Feels better during cold weather.
Bryonia	30c. menses)," i.e., nosebleed	"Substitute (vicarious) and/or gum bleeding rather than menstrual flow. Inter-menses pains with pelvic and abdominal soreness. Avoids the least motion. Thirsty for large amounts of water.

Calc. Phos.	30c.	Extremely intense backache. Chilly. Menses is early, excessive, bright red; occurs every two weeks.
Chamomilla	30c.	Dark, clotted blood with labor-like pains. Mood swings, irritable, cross, quarrelsome. Thirsty. Feels worse at night.
Colocynthis	30c.	Bends over double in reaction to pain. Pain "bores into" ovary. Pain eases with pressure. Restless. Fluctuating severe gripping pain.
Pulsatilla	30c.	Sensation of band around throat just before menses. Clotted intermittent, changeable menses.

MOTION SICKNESS

Remedy	Dosage	Remarks
Borax	30c. Take the remedy one hour before travel, then every 15-30 minutes as needed once travel begins.	For motion sickness during air travel. Symptoms worsen with downward motion.
Rhus. Tox.	30c. Take the remedy one hour before travel, then every 15-30 minutes as needed once travel begins.	Nausea and vomiting with complete loss of appetite. Giddiness on attempting to rise. Severe frontal headache. Unquenchable thirst.
Cocculus (Herb = Cocculus)	30c. Take the remedy one hour before travel, then every 15-30 minutes as needed once travel begins.	Car sickness, morning sickness in pregnancy. Sensitivity to the sight or smell of food. Hollow, empty feeling.

PHYSICAL TRAUMA

Give homeopathic Arnica as soon as possible after the injury. Arnica is specific for trauma, bruising, head injury, and soft-tissue injury, and can also slow bleeding and treat shock. Often, someone needing Arnica will deny being injured.

Continue giving Arnica as needed for 3-4 days. Can repeat the remedy as often as every thirty minutes immediately after the injury. Homeopathic remedies act according to the frequency of dosage, not the amount.

Remedy	Dosage	Remarks
Ledum (Marsh Tea)	30c.	Bruised area that is cold and blue. Follows Arnica well, after three or four days.

Ruta	30c.	Injury to ligament or periosteal tissue (surface of the bone). Area is red; condition worsens with motion.
Rhus. Tox.	30c.	Sore, painful joints which improve with warmth and motion (painful when first moved, better with continued movement).
Hypericum	30c.	Injury to areas with nerve tissue (eyes, hands, genitals). Sharp, nerve-like pain.

SHOCK

Remedy	Dosage	Remarks
Aconite	30c. Give every 15-30 minutes until improvement is noted.	Fear, fright, anxiety. Sudden, violent onset. Numbness. Vomiting from fear. Face is pale when sitting up. Fear of death.
Carbo. Veg.	30c. Give every 15-30 minutes until improvement is noted.	Icy coldness. Stagnant blood. "Air hunger" (can't catch breath). Wants windows open; wants to be fanned; wants cold drinks during chills.
Gelsemium	30c. Give every 15-30 minutes until improvement is noted.	Dull, droopy, drowsy, dazed. Dilated pupils. Heat stroke. Heavy, drooping eyelids. No thirst.
Arnica	30c. Give every 15-30 minutes until improvement is noted.	After head injury. Denies need for help.

SUNBURN

Remedy	Dosage	Remarks
Hypericum	30c.	For first-degree sunburn (no blistering).
Cantharis	30c.	If blistering is present (second-degree).

TEETHING

Remedy	Dosage	Remarks
Calc. Carb.	30c.	Late dentition (teeth slow to grow). Fontanelles slow to close. Ear infections sometimes accompany teething.

Chamomilla	30c.	For teething, inconsolable children, or children who are extremely irritable and demand to be carried, yet arch their back away from whomever is carrying them. Redness to one cheek, the other pale. Stools may be grass green and runny.
Ignatia (St. Ignatius Bear)	30c.	Child is distressed, but not extremely irritable. The baby sobs, sighs and cries. The whole body or single body parts may tremble.

Section 3

Dis-ease,
Diagnosis,
Examination

Simple Diagnosis of Organs

The skin of the body can be used to diagnose dis-ease. The body consists of the upper, middle and lower section (see Organ Regions on the Body, p. 291).

The upper section contains essential organs such as the lungs, heart, liver (on right side near lower ribs), the heart (on the left mid-center side), stomach, pancreas and spleen on the left. The middle section contains the small intestines, large intestines, appendix, lower right side of the abdomen, two kidneys in the back near the last rib and two adrenal glands that rest on top of the kidneys.

The internal organs leave an imprint on the outer skin. The internal organs have nerve endings on the external skin. If the outer skin changes in complexion, texture, or a series of scratches, rashes and bumps appear, then the internal organ connected to that skin portion (meridian) is stressed or in a diseased condition. Accidents (there are no accidents in African medicine) will occur to the skin-related external organ. When in a dis-ease state, dis-eased organs call accidents such as burns, scratches and scars as a way of attracting needed energy. An individual who falls may strike a diseased organ's meridian area (or energy). There may be longer hair growth on a meridian of stressed or diseased organ (see hair chart). The longer hair growth is the body's attempt to protect a weak organ. Finger pressure (acupressure) upon the internal organ's outer skin energy field (meridian) can be used to diagnose. The finger pressure should be between two and four pounds. If the individual feels pain with two pounds (check finger pressure on a household scale) of pressure on the meridian, the organ is dis-eased (see Acupressure Meridians, p. 309).

The individual parts of the body can be divided into three sections for diagnosis (*see* organ regions chart). For example, the upper leg (thigh) sections are as follows: the part of the upper thigh closest to the hip is the lower section, the part closest to the knee is the upper section and the mid-part is the middle section. Try to divide the sections into three equal parts.

The parts of the lower leg (calves) are as follows: the part closest to the knee is the upper section, then the middle section and lower section is the part closest to the ankle.

The upper arm has three sections (see p. 291). The upper section is closest to the shoulder, then the middle section and then the lower section that is closes to the elbow.

The lower arm has three sections; the part closest to the elbow is the lower section then the middle section and the upper section that is the closest to the wrist. The feet and hands are divided into three sections (*see* foot chart). A reflexology chart can help to visualize the sections. The palm of the hand and sole of the foot's three sections are: the part closest to the knuckles is the upper section, then the middle section and the lower section that is closest to the heel of the hand or foot (see Hand Chart, p. 289).

Finger pressure and skin complexion (see Color Chart, p. 275) can indicate dis-eased organs.

The fetus position may help one to see the connection between parts. Assuming a fetal position will be helpful in understanding the section's relationship to internal systems and organs.

The eyes are divided into three sections (see Eye Chart, p. 285). The upper part of the eye's iris or whites (sclera) —visualize the eye as a clock—between 10 and 2 is the upper section. The middle section is between 10 and 7, and also between 2 and 4. The lower section is between 5 and 7. The eye whites should have no more than three or four red veins in them. Red veins in the sections indicate that the organs or body part in that section is stressed or dis-eased. The color of the whites (such as light yellow, blue green, etc.) indicates dis-ease (see Colors, p. 275).

The teeth can indicate dis-ease by their surface and color (see p. 291). The upper section is the front teeth, the middle section starts at the canine teeth, and lower section is at the molars. Tooth loss, cracked teeth, white or dark spots, and color deviation from normal (see Colors, p. 275) indicate stressed or dis-eased organs or systems.

Any part of the human body can communicate a dis-ease of the internal organs. The human body is wholistic and every part of the body is connected to each organ of the body. The tongue, ears, hair and odors can be an indication of dis-ease or stressors to organs and/or systems.

HOW FLUID SECRETIONS SHOW DIS-EASE

The fluid secretions of the body indicate health and dis-ease states. However, the fluid is also secreted to heal or cleanse the body and its organs.

Fluid can also correct a flora (friendly bacteria, fungus, yeast and virus) imbalance. A flora imbalance such as that found in the uterus can be caused by synthetic antihistamines (suppress nasal fluid), anti-sperm gels, latex or polyurethane condom as well as their talc, cough suppressants, deodorants, (dry up vaginal fluids) antibiotics that kill friendly bacteria in uterus and vagina and chemicals in tampons and toilet paper. Nylon, other synthetic underwear and tight pants can cause Venereal Dis-ease (V.D.). Fluid secreted is usually a defense reaction of the body to stop further deterioration. Fats and protein matter give off an offensive smell. This indicates the inner skin's fats and proteins are rotten and breaking down. The fluid from the vagina is usually clear, the uterine mucous is white, while the fallopian tube fluid is yellow. Any deviation from typical colors can appear in the mucous (fluid) discharge. This will indicate reproductive problems. For further color information, see Color Chart.

The fluid secretions of the body have been distorted by societal values. For example, the perspiration (sweat) of the forehead (brow) is considered respectable while the sweat of the feet is disrespectful. The saliva from the mouth is considered offensive while tears are considered acceptable fluid of emotional tenderness. The perspiration (head, feet) and tear fluids are chemically the same. Ironically, if an individual spits in a glass several times and then this same individual is asked to drink his own spit, the individual will not because one's spit outside of the mouth is considered offensive. Another fluid such as the connective tissue called blood is the least alive of the bodily fluids. Yet, blood is culturally valued as having a deep connection between relatives while actually its function is to carry oxygen and waste. Blood corpuscles, called Red Blood Cells and White Blood Cells reproduce themselves by dividing apart. They are corpuscles, not cells. Cells grow from a root (melanin template) then the body and organelles of cell grows from the root. The cell dies, then another template grows. Cells do not divide. They grow and have a nerve attached to them with a blood supply attached to the nerve. In any case, in Germany they tried to use blood transfusions to harmonize married couples with problems. This scientific experiment was a failure. Organs that secrete fluids are given non-scientific cultural values. The brain secretes biochemical thoughts; the heart pumps (secretes) blood mixed with oxygen and the liver secretes digestive fluids. Yet, the societal values for the brain's fluid are high. In the Caucasian past, the liver was given a high status because it was believed to secrete emotions. However, all fluids are regulated by the Pineal, are equal in value, and should be considered as instruments for reading the state of health in the body. The hierarchy of importance given to fluids is socially defined and not a biochemical hierarchy (classification).

MELANIN (PINEAL) NUTRITION

Melanin is the foundation for immunity. It is a free radical scavenger; aids digestion antioxidant, bones, nerves, cellular and hormone functions. The following are essential for Melanin production.

MELANIN HORMONES:	*Serotonin /*	*Melatonin*
NERVOUS SYSTEM STIMULATED:	*Sympathetic Stress*	*Parasympathetic Stress*

SUPPLEMENTS

Vitamin A	d-Alpha Tocopherol
B_6	B_1
B_{12}	B_2
Calcium	Magnesium
Chromium	Vanadium
Cobalamin	Coenzyme Q_{10}
Copper	Vitamin E
Vitamin C	Vitamin D, Iodine
Niacin	Niacinamide

Serotonin / Sympathetic Stress	Melatonin Parasympathetic Stress
Folic Acid	Folic Acid
Manganese	Manganese
Potassium	Panthothenic Acid
Riboflavin	Phosphorous
Silica	Pyridoxal 5 Phosphate
Selenium	Riboflavin
Bromelain	Choline
Zinc	Zinc
Chondroitin Sulfate	Glucosamine Sulfate
Tablets/Liquid Serotonin	Tablets/Liquid Melatonin

HERBS *Combine:*	*Combine:*
Gingko or Gotu Kola Damiana, Eyebright Echinacea	Gingko or Gotu Kola, Chamomile, Echinacea

AMINO ACIDS	
Ornithine, Arginine	Phenylalanine, Tyrosine
SULFUR AMINO ACIDS Methionine, Cysteine, Taurine	**ALKALINE AMINO ACIDS** Histidine, Lysine, Arginine, Glycine

ACID AMINO ACIDS	
Glumatic Acid, Aspartic	Glutamine

GLANDULARS	
Pancreas, Liver, Brain	Pancreas, Pituitary, Adrenal, Brain

FOODS

Apples, Apricots, Bananas, Blue Grapes, Blueberries, Broccoli, Cauliflower, Red Cherries, Collard Greens, Currants, Dandelion Greens, Dates, Figs, Guava, Lemons, Mangoes, Fresh Olives, Oranges, Papaya, Peaches, Raw Peanuts, Plantains, Soybeans, Spelt, Star Fruit, Strawberries, Turnips, Wild Rice, Yams

HERBAL FORMULA

Combine these herbs in equal amounts. Drink 1 cup daily. Alfalfa, Black Cohosh, Burdock, Dandelion Root, Eyebright, Fo-Ti, Gingko

FOOD CLASSIFICATION

- Carbohydrates increase Tryptophan = Calmness
- Protein increases Dopamine/Norepinephrine/Tyrosine = Alertness
- Fruits stimulate Melanin energy
- Vegetables stabilize Melanin energy

Section 4

Easy Remedies

Athlete's Foot Sprinkle Garlic Powder, Pau D'Arco Powder and Horseradish Powder on feet. Put Tea Tree Oil between toes and affected areas daily. Drink Pau D'Arco.

Bedbugs Put Wild Thyme in the bed and corners of the room. Make sure the room is closed and the temperature is warm.

Bedwetting Cinnamon tea. No fluids after 6:00 p.m. Drink diuretic (Uva Ursi, Juniper Berry) around noon time.

Bleeding Pour Aloe Vera Juice on area. Apply Clay, Goldenseal Powder and Spider Webs. Take as much Vitamin K as needed to stop bleeding.

Candles Last longer if refrigerated for one week before using.

Cataracts Put one drop of Castor Oil in each eye before sleep. Take Vitamin B_2 to help absorb oil into eye.

Chapped Lips Make lotion of Lavender, Aloe Vera and Witch Hazel. Add Vegetable Glycerin and a little bee's wax and apply to lips.

Cigarette Smoke Fill a small pot full of vinegar. Add baking soda and put in area.

Corns Soak feet in cabbage juice, lemon juice, ginger root and turpentine.

Dandruff Use 2 ounces Nettle, 2 ounces Aloe, 2 ounces Rosemary. Steep in 1 pint of boiling water.
Herbs to drink: Anise, Rosemary.
Vitamins: A, E, F, B_6, B Complex, Zinc, and Selenium.
Glandulars: Adrenal, Liver.
Amino Acids: Lysine, Cysteine, and Alanine.
Homeopathic: Nat. Mur., Kali. Sulph.

Deodorant Clay mixed with Witch Hazel, a drop of Peppermint, Tea Tree Oil and/or Orange Extract.

Disinfectant   Basil, Myrrh and Frankincense in Vinegar and sprinkle in room.

Dizziness   Catnip tea.

Dog Bite   Make a strong tea of Sea Salt, Gentian and Myrrh and apply. Mix crushed Garlic and Tobacco; put on area and cover with ace bandage.

Eye Drops   2 tsp. each of Goldenseal, Eyebright and Aloe tea. Strain and add a drop of honey. Use eye drop bottle or eyecup.

Falling Hair   Boil Wild Cherry Bark for 10 minutes. Remove
(Baldness)   from heat, add Nettle and Horsetail and drink.
Herbs to drink: Dried Dates, Nettle, Shave grass, Horsetail.
Food: Brewer's Yeast, Lecithin.
Vitamins: B_6, B Complex, C, E, F, Biotin, Inositol, Niacin, Choline, Growth Hormones, Progesterone, PABA, Iron, Silicon, Sulfur.
Amino Acid: Cysteine.
Homeopathic: Silicea.

Flea Repellent   Equal parts of Cedar Wood Shavings (Thuja), Pennyroyal, Chamomile; put into a small (cat or dog,) size pillow.

Foot Cooler   Rub a little Peppermint, Spearmint, or Lemon
for Summer   Grass Oil on the feet, especially between the toes.

Foot Warmer   A little Cayenne powder sprinkled in the socks.
for Winter

Gas   Psyllium, Bay Leaves, Calamus, Peppermint, Slippery Elm, Papaya Juice, Garlic.
Food: Bee Pollen, Sprouts, Charcoal, Yogurt, Digestive Enzyme, HCL.
Vitamins: C, B, Calcium.
Glandulars: Pancreas.
Amino Acids: Glutamine.
Homeopathic: Mag. Phos.

Gout   Pure Cherry juice and 6 to 9 Raw Almonds or a tablespoon of raw almond butter.

Gray Hair	Boil 8 tbsp. Henna and 1 ounce of Sage in 1 quart of water. Let cool and rinse hair. Apply 1 ounce of Sage oil mixed with 2 pint of Almond Oil. *Food:* Brewer's Yeast, Wheat Germ. *Vitamins:* B Complex, Pantothenic Acid, PABA, Silicon, Folic Acid, Zinc, Calcium, Magnesium, Selenium. *Glandulars:* Adrenal, Pancreas, Spleen. *Amino Acids:* Cysteine. *Homeopathic:* Silicea.
Hair Rinse	4 tablespoons of Nettle, Sage, Rosemary and Hyssop. Make into a tea, add to rinse water.
Hair Oil	Crush Pine Needles (leaves), put in 2 pints of Olive Oil. Let soak 1 week, then strain and use.
	1 ounce Sage oil, 2 ounces Aloe Oil, 1 pint of Sesame, Sunflower, Almond or a light oil. Add Lavender or Jasmine, etc. for fragrance.
Hay Fever	Bee Pollen capsules or tablets, Jimson Weed, Black Cohosh.
Insect Repellent	Mix equal parts of Pennyroyal, Bay Leaves, Cloves, Tansy, Lavender, Cayenne and Spearmint. Sprinkle Tea Tree Oil and Citronella Oil on herbs, then put into cloth bags and put around clothing. Spread powder herbs in area where insects crawl.
Itchy Skin	Arnica, Chickweed, Violet, Yarrow, Marjoram. *Food* (externally): Apple Cider Vinegar. *Vitamins:* A, C, E, F, B Complex, Ferrous Sulfate. MSM (Methysulfonylmethane) Lotion. *Glandulars:* Adrenal, Thyroid. *Amino Acids:* Tryptophane. *Homeopathic:* Mag. Phos, Kali, Mur.
Mildew	Soak mildewed clothes in sea salt and vinegar solution, then dry.
Mildew Stains	Remove by using Raw Potato, Raw Tomato, Sea Salt and Vinegar.

Natural Contraceptives Acacia and Stone Seed. Apply to sponge tampon, corn stalk pulp or douche.
Food: Kelp, Brewer's Yeast.
Vitamins: B, B$_6$, C, Folic Acid, Iodine.
Glandulars: Thyroid.
Amino Acids: Triptophan.
Homeopathic: Calc. Sulph., Nat. Sulph., Calc. Phos. Also the rhythm method and a daytime cyclical method.

Natural Hair Relaxer *(Straightener)* Simmer Henna neutral, 2 pints of Sesame Oil, 10 ounces Sage Oil and add 2 ounces Beeswax. Add ¼ ounce Tincture Benzoin, 4 drops Citronella Oil and Bergamot Oil. Remove from heat. Pour into glass container and use or call 1-800-324-7136 for Herbal Tame.

No Taste or Smell Zinc tablets (60 mg.)

Rats Mix cement, powdered glass and dry corn meal. Put in a dish.

Red Eyes Vitamin E drops in eye and a drop of fresh raw lemon juice. Orally, Vitamin A, Vitamin B$_2$ and Nutritional Brewer's Yeast.

Refrigerator Freshener Put lemon and orange peels into an open container with apple halves and sprinkle with charcoal powder.

Ringworm Combine poultice of Gunpowder, Vinegar, Pau D'Arco and Charcoal Powder and apply to area. Drink Pau D'Arco and Wormwood Tea. Prepare an infusion of Burdock, Thyme, Gentian Root and mix with equal parts of Apple Cider Vinegar and apply to area.

Rinse Water Add a little vinegar and Epsom Salt to rinse water after washing clothes.

Skin Oil ¾ pint olive oil, 2 tbsp. Lecithin Oil, a little Wheat Germ Oil.

Split Fingernails Put your finger into half a slice of lemon or white potato for 10 minutes daily. Also soak fingernails in olive oil.

Swollen and Baggy Eyes

Apply cloth tea bags to eyes while lying down for about 15 minutes.
Use herbs such as Agrimony, Alum, Cranesbill, Hemlock, Kola, Pilewort, Tormentil, Uva Ursi, Wild Indigo.

Tension and Anxiety

Nutritional Brewer's Yeast, Arnica, Chamomile, Hops, Catnip.
Vitamins: B_6, B Complex, Pantothenic Acid, Phosphorus, Calcium, Potassium.
Glandulars: Adrenal, Liver.
Amino Acids: Tryptophan, Tyrosine, Alanine.
Homeopathic: Calc. Sulph., Silicea.

Tired Feet

Soak feet in Arnica, Yarrow, Ginger and Lavender.

Warts

Rub with combined Plantain Juice, Marigold Juice and Turpentine. Drink Thuja and/or Sanicle.
Externally: Digestive Enzyme, Green Papaya Juice.
Food: Fig Juice, Papaya Juice.
Vitamins: A, E, Calcium Lactate.
Glandulars: Thymus.
Amino Acids: Lysine, Alanine.
Homeopathic: Silicea, Kali. Mur.

Whiten Teeth

Brush with Charcoal and mashed fresh Strawberries.

Worms

Pure Turpentine (Pine Oil), Wormwood, Elecampane and Honey. Use fi to 1 teaspoon.

Wrinkles

Mix Tormentil (herb) and Aloe Vera Gel and apply. Massage Aloe Vera oil into area. Apply L-Lysine Cream, Pau D'Arco or Primrose Oil is effective for all types of skin problems.

Lotion

For chapped hands or dry skin. Shake well and apply.

½ ounce Glycerin (vegetable)
½ ounce Sage (darkens gray hair)
½ ounce Aloe Oil
¼ ounce scented oil (i.e., Lavender)

Lips
Aloe Oil and Honey. Mix together and apply. Rub Shea Butter on lips.

Facial Mask
Mix equal parts Wheat Germ Flour, Honey and Clay; apply to face thoroughly.

Dry Skin Cleanser
Mix 1 ounce Aloe Oil with 2 ounces Almond Meal and Honey. Leave on for about 15 minutes then rinse off with warm water.

Facial Vegetable Pack
Blend Cucumber, 2 tablespoons of Kelp and mash 2 medium sized tomatoes to a pulp and apply to skin; leave on for 20 minutes then rinse with water.

Section 5

Vitamin Guide

Vitamins

Vitamins are given the name of vitamins because they are considered "vital minerals" = vita-mins.

Vitamins energize the body while minerals stabilize. Each vitamin has a complex (a family such as C Complex: C_1, C_2, C_3, C_4). All vitamins are hormones, all hormones are enzymes and all enzymes are vitamins. Vitamins are either water-soluble (dissolve in water) or oil soluble (dissolve in oil). Oil soluble vitamins can be dangerous at a high dose because they are stored in bodily fat, remain in the body too long and cause toxins (poison to the body). They can cause hypervitaminosis (vitamin overload).

There is a small degree of separation between one vitamin and another. In fact, all vitamins and minerals are composed of the same ingredients just in different proportions (ratios).

The science of alchemy teaches that the human body has a vital force (i.e., aura, electromagnetic cloud, and energy to mutate, resistive and transmutative strain) that allows the body to change one type vitamin into anther type vitamin and/or one type mineral into another type vitamin. This wholistic, alchemic bodily property allows humans to survive severe nutritional crisis.

Buy vitamin and mineral tablets that are made from plants. Do not buy synthetic vitamins and minerals. They are made from harmful chemicals (coal tar), have additives and addicting (caffeine, white sugar, etc.) substances in them.

The label's indication of milligrams, grams and/or micrograms in a vitamin and mineral is somewhat questionable. For instance, the total amount of Vitamin C in a bottle is 50,000 milligrams and it costs $5.00 (approximations). The label will indicate Vitamin C (Ascorbic Acid). Ascorbic Acid is a fragment of Vitamin C. It is not the vitamin. Ascorbic Acid is synthetic. A rubber tire (Ascorbic Acid) is not a car (Vitamin C). The label has dysinformation—it lies. While one orange contains 300 milligrams of Vitamin C and costs 25 cents, 50,000 milligrams of Vitamin C in fresh oranges would cost $250. A total Vitamin C would include the fragment Ascorbic Acid so it would be expensive. Besides, it is obvious that the Vitamin C milligrams in a live orange is natural. Vitamin C is high in Rosehip and Ascerola. Therefore, they are used in concentrated form for their Vitamin content. Rosehip and/or Ascerola is sprayed on synthetic ascorbic acid. This is the devious way in which vitamin companies charge Rosehip/Ascerola prices for Ascorbic Acid. The use of synthetics causes the price to be low. Manufacturers use very small amounts of Rosehip/Ascerola and call the combination of Ascorbic Acid with Rosehip and/or Ascerola Vitamin C or natural Vitamin C. Furthermore, it has been proven that colored women on a natural food diet can make Vitamin C in their bodies. This was verified in the book *Biological Transmutations* by Kervan.

Vitamins, made from plants and/or medicinal herbals are more active than dead processed synthetic vitamins. Synthetic vitamins and minerals eventually drain the body of nutrients, alter pH and body chemistry, and have a negative effect on health as well as immunity.

The recommended dosage on the label is for stopping starvation. Since vitamins, minerals and supplements are classified as foods, the products must indicate a serving/dosage. A serving/dosage is not a therapeutic dosage. It is not the amount you need to be healthy or fight diseases. When you are dis-eased, you need a higher dosage because the body still needs its normal amount plus the additional dosages to fight dis-ease.

It is suggested that the dosage be doubled or tripled for water-soluble (Vitamins B and C, etc.). Oil soluble vitamins (A, D, E, K) can be doubled. The minerals can be doubled with the exception of Iron. It is suggested that Vitamin C can be taken in the highest amount (example: 5,000 to 10,000 mg. for adults and 500 to 1,000 mg. for children under 9 years of age, while 300 mg. for children under 4 years of age). The dosage is dependent upon the age, race, weight, sex and state of wellness or disease. For example, a male, aged 20 with digestive disorders and weak muscles due to lack of exercise would take a different dosage than an 80-year-old woman in excellent physical health. There are vitamin precursors (Beta Carotene), water dispersible, oil soluble vitamins, chelated nutrients, sustained release, acid-free Vitamin C, soft capsules, free form, crystal forms, capsules, liquid and tablet forms of supplements which have to be considered. The choice of type is based upon preference, age and disease state. Further, oil soluble vitamins and some minerals have toxic levels and ratios to be considered. Supplements can inhibit, compliment and excite each other; i.e., Vitamin C has to be increased if taking Cysteine. Phenylalanine can increase high blood pressure; Glycine neutralizes the acid effect of other amino acids; RNA requires alkaline fluids and water to neutralize its acidity; Calcium requires acid to be metabolized, etc. There are many more precautions that must be considered and are listed on labels.

Vitamin A

Maintains health of tissue, hair; builds resistance, helps eyes, nasal passage, lungs, stress, etc.

Deficiency	Herbs with Vitamin	Foods
Eye inflammation, weak vision, respiratory problems, skin diseases (boils, acne, pimples, dry skin, etc.), poor sense of taste and smell, get infections easily, teeth and gum problems.	Alfalfa, Burdock, Comfrey, Dandelion, Eyebright, Okra Pods, Paprika, Parsley, Rosehip, Watercress.	Carrots, Green Leafy Vegetables, Melons, Tomatoes, Yams, Fruits.

Vitamin B₁ (Thiamine)

A nutrient for the nerves and brain. Increases the use of body proteins, aids digestion, helps the red blood cell count, enhances circulation, brain function and carbohydrate metabolism. Helps prevent fluid retention (edema).

Deficiency	Herbs with Vitamin	Foods
Weight loss, Beriberi, edema, fatigue, forgetfulness, numbness, digestive problems, loss of appetite, constipation, muscle weakness, agitation, nervous exhaustion and mental depression.	Alfalfa, Brewer's Yeast, Burdock Root, Catnip, Cayenne, Chamomile, Chickweed, Dandelion, Eyebright, Fennel, Fenugreek, Garlic, Hops, Nettle, Oat Straw, Peppermint, Red Clover, Red Raspberry Leaves, Sage, Spirulina, Yarrow, Yellowdock.	Asparagus, Brown Rice, Broccoli, Brussels Sprouts, Parsley, Peanuts, Peas, Plums, Raisins, Rice Bran, Watercress, Whole Grains.

Vitamin B₂ (Riboflavin)

Vital for blood formation, growth, metabolism.

Deficiency	Herbs with Vitamin	Foods
Eye problems, inflammations, sores, skin problems, cracks at corners of the mouth.	Alfalfa, Burdock, Chickweed, Garlic, Kelp, Parsley.	Almonds, Asparagus, Avocados, Brewer's Yeast, Broccoli, Brussels Sprouts, Currants, Green Leafy Vegetables, Mushrooms, Nuts, Sunflower Seeds, Wheat Germ, Whole Grains.

Vitamin B₃ (Niacin)

Aids metabolism of carbohydrates (starches), fats and protein. Useful for the nervous system, skin, circulation, cold feet and hands, digestion, sex hormones, mental illness, memory and lowers cholesterol.

Deficiency	Herbs with Vitamin	Foods
Nervousness, coated tongue, anemia, insomnia, forgetfulness, headaches, mental problems, diarrhea, headaches, dizziness, low blood sugar, loss of appetite, sores.	Alfalfa, Burdock, Catnip, Cayenne, Chickweed, Garlic, Fenugreek, Mullein, Nettle, Parsley, Peppermint, Red Raspberry Leaves, Red Clover, Rosehips, Yellowdock.	Broccoli, Carrots, Green Leafy Vegetables, Nuts, Peanuts, Potatoes, Rice Bran, Sunflower Seeds, Tomatoes, Whole Wheat.

Vitamin B₄

Classified as a protein (amino acid).

Vitamin B$_5$ (Pantothenic Acid)

It is useful for stress, adrenal glands and adrenal hormones, toxins, growth, skin, nervous system, cortisone production, anxiety.

Deficiency	Herbs with Vitamin	Foods
Allergies, asthma, hair loss, fatigue, mental problems, skin dis-ease, burning feet, insomnia, headaches, nausea, tingling in hands, dizziness, low blood sugar (hypoglycemia), constipation, low blood pressure.	Alfalfa, Dandelion, Parsley, Wheat Grass, Yellowdock.	Bran, Beans, Green Leafy Vegetables, Mushrooms, Nuts, Peas, Wheat Germ, Whole Wheat and Grains.

Vitamin B$_6$ (Pyridoxine)

Aids metabolism (utilization) of proteins and fats. It is useful for the nervous system, mental problems, skin dis-ease, arteriosclerosis, PMS, Carpal tunnel, teeth, fluid retention before menstruation, balancing minerals, enzymes and pregnancy.

Deficiency	Herbs with Vitamin	Foods
Skin problems, edema, anemia, mental problems, migraine, nervousness, insomnia, tooth decay, bad breath (halitosis), convulsions, arthritis, irritability, sores on the mouth, hair loss, numbness, oily skin, tingling.	Alfalfa, Catnip, Oat Straw.	Avocados, Bananas, Nutritional Brewer's Yeast, Broccoli, Cabbage, Cantaloupe, Corn, Green Leafy Vegetables, Pecans, Plantain, Potatoes Rice Bran, Soy Beans, Sunflower Seeds, Walnuts, Wheat Germ.

Vitamin B$_{12}$ (Cyanocobalamin, Cobalt)

It is useful for red blood cell growth and production, anemia. metabolism and enzyme action.

Deficiency	Herbs with Vitamin	Foods
Poor appetite, fatigue, poor mental energy, feeling of stiffness and/or numbness, pernicious anemia, constipation, depression, digestive problems, labored breathing, moodiness, headache, liver problems, ringing in ears, palpitations.	Alfalfa, Bladderwrack, Catnip, Comfrey, Dong Quai, Dulse, Hops, Kelp.	Bananas, Brewer's Yeast, Bee Pollen, Concord Seeds, Soybeans, Wheat Germ.

Vitamin B$_{13}$ (Orotic Acid)

Good for reproduction of cells.

Deficiency	Herbs with Vitamin	Foods
Cell growth problem, liver troubles.	Fermented (rotten) Foods, Herbs. They naturally rot in the intestines.	Fermented foods.

Vitamin B$_{13}$ (Pangamic Acid)

Helps body use oxygen, regulates fat metabolism. Good for nervous system, regulating cholesterol, circulation.

Deficiency	Herbs with Vitamin	Foods
Hypoxia (reduced levels of oxygen to cells and tissues), heart disease, nervous problems.	*See* B$_{12}$	Nuts, seeds, whole grains, brown rice.

Folic Acid
(Inositol and Vitamin B)

Good for building red blood cells, growth of cells, healing, skin, hair (gray hair).

Deficiency	Herbs with Vitamin	Foods
Skin dis-eases, baldness, discoloration, mental problems, impotency, poor circulation.	Alfalfa, Kelp, Dandelion, Parsley, Garlic.	Lima beans, mushrooms, wheat germ, nuts, peanuts, broccoli, Irish potatoes, asparagus.

Biotin (Vitamin H)

Vital nutrient for hair, skin, metabolism of fats, carbohydrates and protein, muscle pain, sweat glands, nerve tissue.

Deficiency		
	Alfalfa, Kelp, Wheat Grass, Parsley, Dandelion.	Mushrooms, Spinach, Whole Grains.
Infertility, reproductive dis-ease, fatigue, anemia, eczema.		
Herbs with Vitamin	**Foods**	

PABA (Para-Amino-Benzoic Acid)

A nutrient for skin, hair, growth and production of cells.

Choline

Assists in the production of cells, metabolism of fat (cellulite), regulates liver, gallbladder, and blood pressure (good for high blood pressure). A preventive for hardening of arteries and kidney, Aids nerves, memory and brain function. Useful for Parkinson's and Tardive Dyskinesia.

Deficiency	Herbs with Vitamin	Foods
Hardening of arteries, high blood pressure, liver dis-ease, heart problems, kidney and liver problems.	Alfalfa, Dandelion, Kelp, Parsley, Wheat Grass.	Brewer's Yeast, Green Leafy Vegetables, Lecithin, Legumes, Soybeans, Wheat Grains.

Inositol

Vital nutrient for blood cholesterol, overweight, mental problems, hair and heart, metabolism of fats.

Deficiency	Herbs and Foods
High blood cholesterol, constipation, eczema, hair loss, eye problems, irritability, mood swings, arteriosclerosis, constipation.	See Choline.

Vitamin C (Ascorbic Acid is a fragment of Vitamin C)

Increases the health of glands, organs, teeth, protection against all diseases, infections, stomach disorders, toxins, skin, gums and an antibiotic.

Deficiency	Herbs	
Slow healing wounds (sores), varicose veins, tooth decay, gum dis-eases, anemia, "pinpoint" hemorrhages under skin, recurring colds and infections, edema, bleeding gums, lack of energy, tooth loss.	Alfalfa, Boneset, Burdock Root, Catnip, Cayenne, Chickweed, Coltsfoot, Dandelion, Elderberries, Eyebright, Fennel, Fenugreek, Hawthorn, Hibiscus, Hops, Horseradish, Horsetail, Lobelia, Marigold, Mullein, Nettle, Oak Straw, Oregano, Paprika, Parsley, Peppermint, Pokeweed, Red Clover, Red Raspberry Leaves, Rosehips, Shepherd's Purse, Yarrow, Yellowdock, Watercress.	Ascerola Cherries, Asparagus, Avocados, Beet Greens, Citrus Fruit, Grapefruit, Green Peas, Guavas, Kiwi, Lemons, Limes, Mangos, Mustard Greens, Onions, Oranges, Papaya, Persimmons, Rosehips, Star Fruit, Strawberries, Turnip Greens.

Foods

Vitamin D (Ergosterol)

A nutrient for glands; absorption and utilization of minerals, bones, and teeth. Vital for growth, muscles, heart, thyroid, normal blood clotting.

Deficiency	Herbs with Vitamin	Foods
Tooth decay, softening of bones, lack of energy, in children slow growth and poor bone structure, loss of appetite, diarrhea, insomnia, weight loss, eye problems.	Alfalfa, Horsetail, Nettle, Parsley.	Dandelion Greens, Lettuce, Oatmeal, Sweet Potatoes, Watercress.

Vitamin E

A nutrient for tissues, sores; stabilizes energy and reduces need for oxygen, improves circulation, reduces blood pressure. Vital for lungs, PMS, skin, blood, heart, veins, arteries, sterility, impotency, menopause and all infections and dis-eases. Improves stamina, relaxes muscles, reduces keloids and scarring from wounds.

Deficiency	Herbs	Foods
Lung problems, strokes, heart dis-ease, cell, muscle and skin disorders, infertility, menstrual problems, miscarriages.	Alfalfa, Dandelion, Dong Quai, Flaxseed, Kelp, Oat Straw, Red Raspberry Leaves, Rosehip, Spirulina, Watercress.	Green Leafy Vegetables, Nuts, Soy Beans, Sprouted Seeds, Sweet Potatoes, Wheat Germ, Whole Grains.

Bioflavonoids (Vitamin P):

Assists the building and strengthening of tissue and cells. Helps prevent hemorrhaging. Vital for all injuries, infections, skin, and liver diseases. Aids circulation, lowers cholesterol, reduces herpes.

Deficiency	Herbs	Foods
Dark blue spots on skin, eczema, hemorrhoids, varicose veins, infections, hypertension.	Chervil, Elderberries, Hawthorn Berry, Horsetail, Rosehips, Shepherd's Purse.	All fresh fruits and vegetables. Emphasize Apricots, Black Currants, Buckwheat, Cherries, Citrus Fruit, Green Peppers, Prunes, Strawberries.

Vitamin F (fatty acid):

Essential for heart, adrenal glands, skin, growth, cholesterol, and all mucous membranes.

Deficiency	Herbs with Vitamin	Foods
Falling hair, reproductive problems (menstruation and prostate), skin diseases, kidney and liver disorders.	Burdock, Orris, Uva Ursi, Flaxseed, Kelp, Echinacea, Dandelion.	Corn, sunflower seeds, soybeans. Also unrefined and unprocessed oil made from above foods.

Vitamin K

Vital for blood clotting, liver, bone formation, bone loss, nervous system and energy.

Deficiency	Herbs	Foods
Nosebleeds, bleeding ulcers, hemorrhaging, low energy.	Alfalfa, Kelp, Nettle, Oatstraw, Plantain, Shepherd's Purse.	Asparagus, Broccoli, Brussels Sprouts, Cabbage, Cauliflower, Green Plants, Oatmeal, Rye, Soybeans, Wheat.

Vitamin T

Essential for blood, cell production.

Deficiency	Herbs	Foods
Memory problems, bleed easily.	Plantain.	Sesame seeds, vegetable oils, Brewer's yeast.

Vitamin U

Assists the healing of wounds.

Deficiency	Herbs	Foods
Ulcers (peptic, duodenal).	Alfalfa.	Cabbage, White Potatoes.

Vitamin G

A nutrient for nervous system.

Herbs
Alfalfa, Dandelion, Kelp, Capsicum, Gotu Kola, Watercress.

Vitamin L

A nutrient for cell production, breast-feeding.

Herbs

Foods

Alfalfa, Rosemary

Wheat Germ, Brewer's Yeast.

Vitamin P (Rutin)

A vital nutrient for stomach, liver, hemorrhoids.

Herbs

Foods

Rosehip, Rue, Paprika

Lemon, Buckwheat

Section 6

Mineral Guide

Minerals

Purchase minerals (chelated) from a health food store or a natural food store. Do not buy synthetic minerals. Synthetic minerals are made from harmful chemicals. Natural minerals are made from plants and other natural sources.

When using minerals to treat a dis-ease remember that the listed dosage is what the body requires when it is healthy. However, a dis-ease requires a higher dosage of minerals because the body has to use its normal amount and an additional amount to fight the dis-ease.

It is suggested that for a dis-ease two or three times the normal dosage serving (listed on label) be taken.

Iron

Vital for the making of blood.

Deficiency	Herbs	Foods
Mental problems, nervous disorders. Anemia, tired, fatigue, poor resistance to disease, pale complexion, headache.	Burdock Root, Catnip, Cayenne, Chamomile, Chickweed, Devil's Claw, Dong Quai, Eyebright, Fennel, Fenugreek, Horsetail, Kelp, Parsley, Plantain, Peppermint, Sarsaparilla, Shepherd's Purse, Strawberry Leaves, Uva Ursi, Yellow Dock	Almonds, Apricots, Avocados, Bananas, Beans, Beets, Lentils, Millet, Peaches, Pears, Prunes, Pumpkins, Raisins, Rice, Rye, Sesame Seeds, Spinach, Some Mineral Springs, Sunflower Seeds, Turnip Greens, Walnuts, Watercress, Whole Grains.

Calcium

Essential for bones, teeth, muscle action, clotting of blood, and vital activities of the body.

Deficiency	Herbs	Foods
Soft bones, decay, nervousness, mental problems, muscle spasms, cramps, high blood pressure, brittle nails, eczema, high cholesterol, numbness, arthritis and heart problems.	Aloe Root, Bittersweet Root, Burdock Root, Cayenne, Chamomile, Chickweed, Chives, Fennel, Flaxseed, Fenugreek, Hops, Horsetail, Mistletoe, Peppermint, Red Clover, Red Raspberry Leaves, Rosehip, Shepherd's Purse, Sorrel, Toad Flax Chives, Yarrow.	Almonds, Walnuts, Raw Vegetables, Beans, Millet, Broccoli, Brussels Sprouts, Oats, All Leafy Greens

Phosphorus

A nutrient for bones and teeth, mentality, nerves, heart and kidney function.

Deficiency	Herbs	Foods
Skin problems, nerve and mental problems, anxiety, numbness, trembling, respiratory problems, weakness, soft bones, poor sexual activity.	Alfalfa, Caraway, Dulse, Kelp, Licorice, Marigold, Rosehips, Rosemary, Sorrel, Watercress	Asparagus, Bran, Corn, Fruits, Garlic, Legumes, Nuts, Seeds, Whole Grains

Potassium

Vital for muscles, heart, digestion, allergies, prevents strokes, stabilizes blood pressure, depression, constipation, diarrhea, mental problems.

Deficiency	Herbs	Foods
Edema, heart problems, high blood pressure, nervous disorders, fatigue, dry skin, chills, thirst, high cholesterol, headaches, respiratory problems, depression, constipation, diarrhea, mental problems	Calamus, Catnip, Dandelion, Dulse, Eyebright, Fennel, Hops, Horsetail, Mullein, Nettle, Parsley, Peppermint, Plantain, Red Clover, Rosemary, Sage, Skullcap, Watercress	Apricots, Avocados, Bananas, Brown Rice, Carrots, Dates, Figs, Garlic, Nuts, Oranges, Papayas, Plantains, Potatoes, Raisins, Squash, Sunflower Seeds, Green Leafy Vegetables, Whole Grains, Yams

Choline

Essential for digestion, liver

Deficiency	Herbs	Foods
Poor digestion, imbalanced body fluid	Alfalfa, Betony, Burdock, Chickweed, Dandelion, Kelp, Myrrh, Nettle, Spirulina	Asparagus, Avocados, Cabbage, Celery, Cucumber, Endive, Kale, Oats, Pineapple, Tomatoes, Turnips

Sulphur

A nutrient for skin, nails, hair, disinfects blood, helps resist bacteria

Deficiency	Herbs	Foods
Skin problems, blemishes, rashes, split ends, brittle nails.	Asafetida, Broom, Eyebright, Horseradish, Horsetail, Irish Moss, Pimpernel	Brussels Sprouts, Cabbage, Celery, Kale, Onions, Plantain, Soybeans, String Beans, Turnips, Wheat Germ

Iodine

Essential for regulation of mental and physical activity, healthy skin and thyroid, metabolizes fat.

Deficiency	Herbs	Foods
Goiter, fatigue, anemia, obesity, breast cancer, low blood pressure, loss of sexual activity	Black Walnut Hulls, Iceland Moss, Jojoba, Kelp, Sarsaparilla, Watercress.	Asparagus, Garlic, Lima Beans, Mushrooms, Sesame Seeds, Soybeans, Spinach, Squash, Turnip Greens.

Manganese

Vital for digestion nerves, brain, regulates blood sugar, bone growth, metabolism, reproduction and muscles.

Deficiency	Herbs	Foods
Digestion problems, asthma, female and male sex activity, poor bone growth, confusion, eye problems, atherosclerosis, heart problems, memory loss, tremors, tooth grinding, hypertension, convulsions	Alfalfa, Burdock Root, Broom, Chickweed, Dandelion, Eyebright, Fennel, Fenugreek, Hops, Horsetail, Mullein, Parsley, Primrose, Wintergreen, Yarrow, Yellow Dock	Apricots, Avocados, Beets, Blueberries, Brussels Sprouts, Garlic, Grapefruit, Nuts, Oranges, Peas, Pineapples, Spinach, all Green Leafy Vegetables

Zinc

A vital nutrient for cell and tissue growth, prostate, healing wounds and burns, helps taste and smell, vital for enzymes

Deficiency	Herbs	Foods
Impaired sexual functions, acne, hair loss, high cholesterol, recurrent colds, white spots on toe and/or fingernails, poor sense of taste and smell, hair problems, slow healing, poor resistance to dis-ease, impotence, fatigue, memory problems	Cayenne, Chickweed, Dandelion Root, Eyebright, Hops, Milk Thistle, Mullein, Nettle, Parsley, Rose Hips, Sage, Sarsaparilla, Skullcap	Kelp, Nuts, Pumpkin, Spirulina, Sunflower Seeds, Green Leafy Vegetables, Wheat Germ

Chromium

An essential nutrient. Regulates levels of Manganese. Vital for digestion of protein and glucose. Stabilizes blood sugar.

Deficiency	Herbs	Foods
Diabetes, low blood sugar, heart dis-ease, hardening of arteries, anxiety, fatigue	Alfalfa, Catnip, Horsetail, Kelp, Licorice, Nettle, Oatstraw, Red Clover, Sarsaparilla, Spirulina, Yarrow	Beans, Brown Rice, Corn, Mushrooms, Potatoes, Whole Grains

Selenium

Essential for improving liver function, reducing energy loss, protecting body from toxins, aids the prostate, is an antioxidant.

Deficiency	Herbs	Foods
Liver damage, digestive problems, muscle weakness, cancer, fatigue, infections, high cholesterol	Alfalfa, Burdock Root, Catnip, Cayenne, Chamomile, Chickweed, Fennel, Fenugreek, Ginseng, Hawthorn Berry, Hops, Horsetail, Kelp, Lemon Grass, Milk Thistle, Nettle, Parsley, Sarsaparilla, Yellow Dock	Brazil Nuts, Broccoli, Brown Rice, Garlic, Mushrooms, Onions, Spirulina, Vegetables, Whole Grains

Lithium

Vital for nerves, brain.

Deficiency	Herbs	Foods
Mental problems, nervous disorders.	Kelp.	Seawater, Some Natural Mineral Springs.

Vanadium

Vital for sugar and insulin production, metabolism, bones and teeth.

Deficiency	Herbs	Foods
Heart and kidney disease, diabetes.	Dill.	Olives, Radishes, Snap Beans, Whole Grains.

Magnesium

Promotes mineral absorption, digestive enzyme activity; helps bone formation; helps metabolize carbohydrates, helps dissolve kidney stones.

Deficiency	Herbs	Foods
Nervousness, irritability, rapid heartbeat, insomnia, tantrums, asthma, fatigue, pain, depression, seizures, bone loss.	Alfalfa, Dandelion Root, Lemon Grass, Mullein, Nettle, Oat Straw, Parsley, Peppermint, Red Clover, Sage, Shepherd's Purse, Yarrow, Yellow Dock.	Apples, Apricots, Avocados, Bananas, Brown Rice, Cantaloupe, Figs, Garlic, Grapefruit, Lemons, Lima Beans, Millet, Nuts, Black-eyed Peas, Sesame Seeds, Soybeans, Whole Grains, and Green Leafy Vegetables.

Section 7

Flushes
(Cleansers)

Liver Flush Drink

½ Cup Fresh Lemon Juice
¼ Cup Lecithin Granules
1 tsp. Horseradish Root Powder
1 Garlic Clove or 2 tbsp. Garlic Powder
1/8 tsp. Cayenne (a pinch)

Kidney Flush Drink

½ Cup Fresh Lemon Juice
½ Cup Fresh Grapefruit
1 Garlic Glove or
1 tsp. Garlic Powder
1 tsp. Ginger Root Powder
⅛ tsp. Cayenne

Stomach Flush Drink

1 Cup or more of distilled water
1 Cup Cabbage Juice
½ Cup Raw White Potato Juice
½ tsp. Cascara Sagrada Powder
1 tsp. Comfrey Powder
1 tsp. Horseradish Root Powder
⅛ tsp. Cayenne (a pinch)

Spleen Flush Drink

1 Cup Carrot Juice
1 Cup Celery Juice
¼ Cup Parsley Juice
1 tsp. Lecithin
1 tsp. Sunflower Oil

tsp. = teaspoon
tbsp. = tablespoon

Section 8

Herb Classifications

ALTERATIVES

Alterative herbs are used to slow down the action of an herb used as a curative. In many dis-ease states an abrupt cure would shock the body and cause a secondary illness. Dis-eases are often developed slowly and consequently require a slow exit from the body. In some cases a dis-ease can require emergency action, such as herbal allopathic remedies.

Alteratives are usually combined with bitter tonics, astringents, aromatics, demulcents, expectorants and stimulants.

Spikenard Root, Sarsaparilla Root, Bittersweet Twigs, Black Cohosh Root, Burdock Root, Chaparral, Echinacea Root, Red Clover Flower, Yellow Dock Root, Stillingea Root, Nettle Root, Garlic, Anise, Allspice, Caraway, Catnip, Celery Seed, Cinnamon, Cloves, Cumin Seed, Eucalyptus, Ginger, Valerian, Fennel, Nutmeg, Peppermint.

ANTHELMINTICS (WORMS)

Anthelmintics or vermifuges remove intestinal worms that inhabit the body.

Areca Nuts, Elecampane, Pomegranate, Pumpkin Seed, Uva Ursi, Senna (Bark, Seeds Or Juice), Balomy Leaves, Male Fern, Wormwood, Garlic, Horseradish, Wild Violet.

ANTIPERIODICS

Herbs that reduce seizures caused by fevers or nervous disorders (example: epilepsy).

Vervain, Arnica, Cinchona Bark, Red Raspberry, Skullcap, Eucalyptus, Senna, Rue, Peruvian Bark, St. John's Wort, Feverfew.

ANTI-INFLAMMATORY

Herbs used in reducing or stopping inflammatory dis-ease states. They are usually never used on partially damaged tissue.

Arnica, Blue Cohosh, Cayenne, Lobelia, Wormwood, Hops, Burdock, Chaparral, Garlic, Slippery Elm, Feverfew, Cat's Claw.

ANTIPYRETICS

These herbs are used to reduce body temperature (example: fever). They work by slowing down blood circulation and opening the pores in tissue and skin, which allows heat to escape. This also causes water and toxic waste to escape in the form of perspiration.

These herbs can be used in baths (hot or cold), wet packs (saturate flannel cloth with herbs and cover cloth with plastic and place on body) or they can be drunk as teas.

Eucalyptus, Wild Indigo, Indian Hemp, Feverfew.

ANTISEPTICS / DISINFECTANTS

Herbs that kill or retard the growth of germs or bacteria, which can rot internal flesh.

A disinfectant herb is prepared stronger (approximately 2 tablespoons to a cup of water) than an antiseptic (approximately 1 teaspoon to a cup). All dis-infectants kill germs.

Anise, Myrrh, Wormwood, Cassia, Thyme, Peppermint, Clove, Garlic, Cayenne, Comfrey, Eucalyptus, Witch Hazel.

ASTRINGENTS

These herbs cause internal and external skin to tighten (contract). They can cause tissue to become firm and can close the pores of mucous membranes found in nasal passages, mouth, uterus, stomach, intestines, etc. They allow heat and nutrients to stay within the body.

These herbs temporarily reduce excessive fluid secretions and can be used in baths, douches, washes, mouthwashes, drinks, gargles or skin lotions.

Alum root, Barberry, Black Alder, Congo root, Kola nuts, Pilewort, Shepherd's Purse, Sumac, Tormentil, Wild Indigo, Witch Hazel.

BITTER TONICS

These herbs are primarily used to aid digestion and for temporary loss of appetite. They increase the flow of saliva and digestive fluids, and can increase the fluid secretion of mucous membranes.

Balomy, Chamomile, Hops, Dandelion, Wormwood, Yellow Root, Barberry, Gentian, Blessed Thistle, Bayberry, Goldenseal, Black Haw.

CALMATIVES

These herbs are used to excite and stimulate the body through the organs of smell and taste. The fragrance of the herbs creates a feeling of warmth and alerts the senses. They stimulate the stomach and transmit a feeling of relaxation to the body.

Valerian, Hops, Chamomile, Catnip, Skullcap, Nerve Root, Kava, Passion Flower.

CATHARTICS
(Laxatives and Purgatives)

These herbs are used for constipation. Constipation causes the bowel movements to be irregular. Further, the feces of the body are either hard or loose (example: diarrhea).

Cathartics either create mucous or irritate the internal skin to increase mucous and digestive system muscle action. The effect of the herbs is the removal of human waste (usually ¾ % dead body cells) from the large intestines.

Cathartics are considered strong laxatives or purgatives and should be used with discretion, especially if symptoms of appendicitis are present and if pregnant. They should never be used consistently as they weaken digestive muscles, inflame tissue and may cause dependency.

Cascara Sagrada, Rhubarb, Senna, Aloes, Butternut, Buckthorn, Elder, Balomy.

DEMULCENTS

Demulcents are slimy (mucilaginous) and bland in nature. Internal organs are soothed and protected by the slime, which provides a mucous coating. They are good for irritated stomachs, constipation, common colds, irritated throat and vaginal problems.

Licorice, Agar, Coltsfoot, Flaxseed, Solomon Seal, Sassafras, Marshmallow, Oatmeal, Irish Moss, Psyllium, Comfrey, Okra Pods.

DIAPHORETICS

These herbs open the pores and increase bodily perspiration, which helps to rid the body of impurities. They also help to lower fevers and speed up cleansing of the body of dis-ease.

Ague Weed, Ginger, Hyssop, Angelica, Blessed Thistle, Pleurisy, Pennyroyal, Indian Hemp, Serpenturia, Lobelia, Sage, Yarrow

DIURETICS

These herbs increase urination. They act faster on an empty stomach and are often taken for kidney and bladder problems. Also, they help speed up the flushing out of toxins in the body. However, they can cause weak kidneys to be strained. These herbs are usually combined with a demulcent herb in order to soothe their reactions in the body.

Buchu, Burdock, Cleavers, Corn Silk, Cubeb Berries, Juniper Berry, Kava, Parsley, White Birch

EMOLLIENTS

Emollients are herbs of an oily or slimy nature. They are used topically (externally) for their soothing and softening properties and internally for digestive problems and for skin irritation in the uterus, vagina, throat or digestive tract.

Quince, Marshmallow, Oatmeal, Comfrey, Slippery Elm, Flaxseed.

These herbs are usually mixed with meal (corn meal, oatmeal, wheat flour, clay), wrapped in cloth and placed on the skin. A little oil should be rubbed on the skin before applying the cloth (can be muslin, flannel, cheesecloth).

EXPECTORANTS

Expectorants cause one to spit out phlegm (mucous) from the lungs and nasal passages. Subsequently, they are good for bronchitis, stuffy nose. chest colds and irritated lungs. Further, lungs become irritated by polluted air (marijuana and tobacco smoke, automotive exhaust, toxic chemicals). These herbs speed up the cleansing of excess toxins from the nasal passages and lungs and are usually combined with demulcents.

Elecampane, Pleurisy, Chickweed, Coltsfoot, Horehound, Mullein, Comfrey, Lobelia, Skunk Cabbage, Asafetida, Marshmallow, Echinacea.

NERVINES
(Relaxants)

These herbs act upon the nervous system and are good for fatigue, exhaustion, nervous irritation (stress), strain, and relaxation.

Nerve root, Valerian, Hops, Passion Flower, Yarrow Leaf, Catnip, Betony, Chamomile, Skullcap.

STIMULANTS
(Nerve)

These herbs increase nerve reactions (speed up). They are allopathic.

Yohimbe, Cocoa Bean, Coffee Bean, Guarana, Yerba Mate.

REFRIGERANTS
These herbs cool the body.

Mints, Lemon Grass, Sorrel, Melissa, Borage, Burnet, Pimpernel, Eucalyptus, Tamarind, Licorice.

SEDATIVES

These herbs soothe and calm pain. They are allopathic and can tend to hide the cause of pain. Pain is an alarm which signals that the disease is well developed, and accordingly, requires a nutritional balancing. These herbs are often used for female menstruation pains. They should not be used for delayed menstruation.

Squaw Wine, Catnip, Yarrow, Cramp Bark, Chamomile, Black Haw, Black Cohosh, Motherwort.

STIMULANTS

These herbs excite and increase the action of organs and bodily systems. Individuals who tend to have mucous overloads in the intestinal tract (colds and bronchitis) tend to react to stimulants rapidly. While, individuals with blood, liver or circulatory disorders require less as it is bounded in the blood longer. Subsequently, stimulants are required in smaller amounts in order to reach a therapeutic level (effective action).

Mustard, Cayenne, Yellow Root, Pennyroyal, Cinnamon, Damiana Blood Root, Angosturn Bark, Black Pepper, Cloves, Sarsaparilla, Prickly Ash, Camphor, Yarrow, Bayberry Leaves, Nutmeg, Fo-Ti, Sumac, Schizandra, Ginseng, Yohimbe.

VULNERARY
These herbs are applied to open wounds (example: cuts, bruises, scratches, burns) and all types of skin diseases. They cause the body to rush healing nutrients to the wound and lessen the degree of scarring. Additionally, they are used for ulcers, respiratory and digestive disorders.

Aloe Vera (the juice can be used also), All Heal, Calendula, Centauria, Horsetail, Comfrey, Marshmallow, Plantain, Clown's Woundwort, Live Forever, Blood Root, Goldenseal.

WHITE JUNK FOODS
ARE KILLING BLACK AMERICA

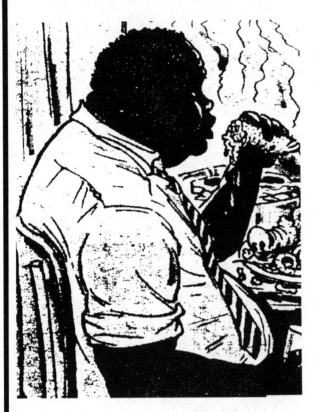

White Sugar

White Flour
(Bleached)

White Rice
(Polished)

White Salt

White Cow's Milk

*If It's White
Don't Trust It!*

Section 9

Food

Food is composed of nutrients (vitamins and minerals), carbohydrates (starches), fats and proteins, which provide energy. Carbohydrates are quick energy foods. They are usually classified as starches, sugars, cellulose (fiber-nondigestible food stuff), gums (not chewing gum) and storage food energy called glycogen. The pancreas secretes the hormone insulin, which stimulates enzymes to break down the carbohydrates.

Fats are the slowest burning energy source. They are composed of smaller substances called fatty acids. Some fatty acids can build themselves into larger groups of fatty acids. These types of fatty acids are called poly (many)-saturated. Other fatty acids will not build larger fatty acids and they are called saturated fatty acids. This type of fat is usually in a solid form. Polyunsaturated fats are found in vegetable oils, soybeans, corn, etc. Saturated fatty acids are usually found in animal fats, cow's milk, beef, pork, etc. The fat intake in the diet of people in Caucasian countries is over 40% of the calories (a unit of measuring heat). The traditional African type diet is usually composed of 10% or fewer units of fat energy.

Proteins (vegetable and animal flesh) are composed of smaller substances called amino acids. The body does not store excess protein. Excess protein is changed into fat and absorbed in organs (heart, kidney, etc.) or in muscle tissue or as stored cellulite. It is dangerous to eat too much protein, especially from animal sources.

Protein consumption has become an ignorance in Caucasian science. It is commonly felt that in order to build human muscle (and proteins) one must eat lean animal flesh muscle (protein). This is clearly not the case. The protein requirement was established by evaluating an upper middle class group of Caucasians that ate a junk food diet. However, normal protein levels in other diets are different. The vegetarian, lacto-ova vegetarian, vegan and fruitarian have protein levels which are optimum at low levels. Vegetarians eat high amounts of raw chlorophyll. Chlorophyll stabilizes protein; thus, vegetarians require less protein. Carbohydrates build protein and can also reduce protein requirements. Eating meat increases cellular destruction, raises the blood acid level, and therefore increases protein requirements.

A combination of various nuts, seeds, whole grains (wheat) and beans is a good protein balance. Animal flesh is not composed of all the amino acids and meat is not a balanced protein. The nutrients in fresh fruits and vegetables have amino acids, as well as chlorophyll that stabilize amino acids and this reduces the protein requirement for vegetarians. Vegeterians use amino acids to make protein.

The protein standards of the Hunza people have proven to be adequate. They live on an almost all fruits, nuts, and seeds diet with animal flesh eaten twice a year for religious reasons. An article in the American Heart Journal 1964 by E. Toomey and P. White validated that the Hunza diet of beans and nut proteins is healthy. An article in the *Journal of American*

Dieters Association, 1969, by N. Scrimshaw also validated that protein requirements are met by a vegetarian diet. Cattle get their protein from plants. Plants are the source of amino acids, which are used to make proteins. Meat eaters wait for the animal to eat the plant protein and then they eat the animal. Meat is second hand protein. The food animals merely act as a middle passage for protein. Vegetable proteins such as corn, millet, legumes, nuts and seeds (these are fruits) are sources of protein in Africa and this diet produced high fertility rates until the Caucasian junk foods and synthetic medicines were forced on African society. The Unites States Public Health Service publication No. 822 in1968 had an article by D. Jeliffe, titled *Child Nutrition in Developing Countries,* which further validates vegetables as *a good* protein source.

The high meat protein diet of Caucasians was started by the meat industry and is related to the high profit margin of the animal flesh industry. An article by J. Store and G. Thorn in the *American Journal of Public Health* in 1943 titled "Some Medical Aspects of Protein Food" validates that a variety of vegetables supply a complete protein balance. Again, a proper combination of beans, raw nuts, raw seeds and whole grains does provide complete protein balance. Eating the sex hormone and adrenalin saturated, antibiotic steroid, growth hormone, pesticide and chemicalized animal corpses does not provide complete proteins. It does increase the acid content of the blood; degenerates the health, causes cancer, fibroid tumors, arthritis, bone loss, diabetes, prostate disease, sex addiction, allergies and is highly constipating. Meat does harm the health.

FOOD COMBINING

Food requires acid and alkaline digestive fluids and enzymes for digestion. Digestion is a complex process. However, food combining is a simple way to understand digestion.

Digestion starts with smell. Smell stimulates the digestive organs to get ready for food. Once the food enters the mouth, it should be chewed until it is a liquid so that acidic salivary digestive enzymes such as ptyalin (breaks down starches) can be mixed into it. The liquid food then enters the stomach, which secretes hydrochloric acid that further breaks down starches and acidic gastric enzymes that break down proteins and emulsifies fats. The liquid food leaves the stomach and enters the duodenum. The duodenum triggers the stomach's peristaltic activities and triggers the liver and pancreas to secrete digestive enzymes. The main activity of digestion occurs in the duodenum. The alkaline digestive fluids of the pancreas neutralize the acidified food that leaves the stomach. The alkaline pancreas enzymes saturate the food while it is in the duodenum. The liver secretes Bile, alkaline digestive fluids that break down fats. The digestion enzymatic sequence actually wraps (saturates) foods with a mucous code. The code puts the food on a waiting list for digestion and dictates the proper strength of enzymes needed to break down a particular kind of food.

Digestion is a sequence or chain reaction of enzymes that require specific strengths of alkaline and/or acid enzymes. Wrong food combining interrupts, blocks and stops the sequence. This results in putrefaction and fermentation of foods. Wrong food combinations end the building of cells and immunity and start the destruction of cells and immunity. Wrong food combination causes colds, allergies, skin eruptions, clogged veins and arteries, constipation, diarrhea, bad breath, plaque on teeth, coated tongue, diseases, stomach gas, addiction, mood swings and irritability. Wrong food combinations make chemicals such as vinegar, alcohol and salts. Consequently, the person becomes addicted to the chemicals they make inside their body, crave them and use them to season foods (i.e., vinegar, salt, wine, etc.).

Animal flesh requires an acid fluid for digestion. These acid fluids are destroyed by carbohydrates and fruits. Animal protein or vegetable protein should not be combined with carbohydrates. When they are eaten at the same time, the animal flesh is not properly digested and the carbohydrates (starches) are not properly digested. Protein (vegetable, animal flesh) can be combined with vegetables. Ideally, meat should not be combined with any vegetable, fruit or starch. Meat should be eaten alone and after eating meat, at least one hour should pass before eating another type food. In other words, a hamburger and bread sandwich is not proper food combining. It is harmful to health. *Never mix starches with meat.*

Never mix sugars (honey, maple syrup, molasses, etc.) with starches. The sugar burns quicker than the starches. The heat the sugars generate causes the starches to ferment (rot) before they can be properly digested. Sugar does not combine with fruits, starches or protein. When sugar is combined, it weakens the digestive fluids and creates toxins.

Never mix oil with starches (example: fried potatoes or meats). The digestive system only receives one signal at a time. For example, one hears in one ear at a time and sees out of one eye at a time. The signal's message to the brain is switched rapidly between both of the ears or eyes that the mind makes it appear as though it is one signal and one message. Once a fried food enters the stomach, the brain receives the signal to digest oil. The oil around the starches or meat causes the body to secrete strong fluids in order to metabolize the oil. These strong digestive fluids emulsify fats and cannot metabolize starch or meat. After the breakdown of the oil, the digestive fluids must switch to the alkaline or acid fluids needed to break down the starch or meat, which the oil saturated. While the oil was broken down, the starch or meat became rotten and created toxins that destroy health.

Never mix sweet fruits with green fruits (cucumbers, squash, okra). This causes both fruits not to be digested properly. They begin to ferment and rot. This causes the body to deteriorate. Mixing sweet fruits with grains causes the spoilage of the grains and fermentation and stops digestion. The grains (wheat, rice, corn, rye, barley, millet) cause the sweet fruits to burn (metabolize) too slowly. This mixture of fruits causes constipation. Cow's milk mixed with grains or sugars works against digestion. Cow's milk cannot be combined with any food. Milk must be drank by itself, then after drinking the milk, wait an hour before eating another type of food. Milk requires lactose to be digested. Lactose enzymes are only needed until the child is five-years-old. Then, the child no longer makes lactose enzymes (lactose intolerance). Adults usually cannot digest cow's milk, colostrum milk or breast milk.

The end result of wrong combining is dis-ease. Food is forced to be utilized without proper digestive juices and it becomes rancid (rotten) before it is absorbed. An acid-alkaline imbalance occurs, cellular waste congests the tissues and toxins pollute the blood, nerves, bones, tissues and brain. Whatever is fed to the body is fed to the brain. Wrong combining decreases the nutritive level of the body and decreases the brain's ability to function. The culminating effect of wrong food combination is constipation, weak immunity, mood swings, irritability, diseases, a short life span and nutritional death.

Another simple food combining method is the "doctrine of signatures." Foods that grow in the ground combine together harmoniously. Green fruits combine with each other, leaves combine with leaves, sweet fruits with edible skin combine with each other, sweet fruits with the skins that are peeled combine with each other, sour fruits combine, citrus fruits only combine with citrus, sweet fruits that change skin color (melons) combine with each other, green fruits that change skin colors (squashes) combine with each other and the grains (seeds) of grasses (wheat, rice, etc.) combine with each other. Food combining works on the principle that everything can be married (combined). It is safer to combine within the families (sweet fruits, squash, beans, grasses) than outside the plant family. The method used to combine vegetables outside of a plant family requires herbs. Herbs can help marriages between different families to be harmonious.

These herbal medicaments (medicinal herbs, erroneously called spices) were used in Africa. The Caucasian invaders of Africa misinterpreted food-combining herbs and labeled them as spices. These spices (medicaments) put both plants (families) in harmony. For example, garlic can neutralize the disharmony between acid and alkaline plants and unite mismatched combinations. There are many such herbs. Usually, they do not have the taste of either plant to be combined or they have a dominating flavor. These herbs are used to make a marriage (mediate) between plants of different tribes (families). Incidentally, spice originally meant a small portion. A small portion of herbs was used in foods. Therefore, the ancient Caucasians called the herbs "spices." The herbs can have a cold taste (peppermint) or a hot taste (black pepper). Consequently, the ancient Caucasians believed the herbs had powers to change the seasons (weather) in the body from winter (coldness) to summer (hotness). Therefore, they called the herbs "seasons or seasonings."

WHITE SUGAR IS . . .

White sugar is sweet, delicious, good tasting and a dangerous concentrated sweetner. White sugar is a refined carbohydrate and is technically classified as a *drug*. It takes four pancreases to process white sugar. Humans have one pancreas. White sugar stresses the pancreas, kidneys, liver, starves the brain of oxygen, causes adrenal weakness, baldness, attention deficits, blindness, tooth decay, high blood pressure, allergies, bone loss, infertility, cataracts, glaucoma, nerve damage (i.e., Multiple Sclerosis), brain damage (Alzheimers), senility, kidney failure, diabetes, mood swings, hypoglycemia, hyperactivity and arthritis. It causes cellular waste to congest the soft tissue and bones, requires large amounts of water to flush it out the system and it is one of the most addicting and harmful drug used.

A Black man named Norbert Rillieux invented the refining process used to make white sugar. He invented the process to help produce better minerals and metals. However, his good invention was turned into a weapon against Blacks. His refinement process when used for sugar became a health destroyer and weapon of enslavement.

White sugar was a weapon for the enslavement of Blacks. Historically, slaves were used to plant and harvest sugar cane and refine the sugar. Then the sugar was sold to buy slaves. The slaves were in turn sold by the pound, as individual livestock or as a group (by the dozen) to buy rum made from the molasses (white sugar). Then the rum was sold to buy slaves. This resulted in the sugar and slave and rum triangle trade. Blacks have been the victims of white sugar and other Caucasian inventions. This victimization of Blacks by a harmless invention (refining) is nothing new. For instance, the Chinese gunpowder toy called the firecracker (small explosive) was used in the European inventions called the cannon, dynamite and bullet. Bullets, guns and cannons were in turn used to invade Africa for dry goods, natural and human (slave) resources, medicinal herbs and plants. In fact, Blacks still do not associate chattel slavery or colonialism with sugar.

Sugar enslaves the internal organs of the body. Sugar is a form of synthetic dirt and it contains no vitamins, minerals or fibers. Sugar causes addiction. Sugar causes a biochemical craving for sugar and this results in psychological and physiological slavery to sugar. White sugar robs the body of minerals and vitamins, especially Vitamin E. This robbery results in drowsiness, temper outbursts hyperactivity, mood swings, tantrums, mischievousness, delinquency, laziness, and violence. Sugar indirectly causes poor digestion of starches. Sugar causes the tissue to starve for nutrients; the body compensates for sugars nutrient drain by taking vitamins and minerals from the liver, eyes, kidneys, heart and nervous system. White sugar causes children to have memory lapses, hypertension, allergies, kidney weakness, obesity, bone loss, cavities, absent-mindedness, laziness, mental fatigue and causes unacceptable behavior.

Tooth decay is an obvious result of white sugar consumption. Anything strong enough to destroy hard teeth must be strong enough to destroy or damage the soft tissues of the heart, sex organs, eyes, kidney and liver.

Combining white sugar with other foods is dangerous. White sugar (or concentrated sweetners—honey) combined with meat causes the rapid spoilage of meat, creates toxic chemicals, gases and acid in the stomach. The toxins are absorbed, causing cellular aging and degeneration. Meat does not combine sugar, milk (cheese) or other carbohydrates (bread). Sugar combined with carbohydrates (i.e., bread, grains, rice, cereal) causes rapid spoilage of the grain, poisons and constipation. Meat and carbohydrates creates toxic mucous causing catarrh (colds, sinus congestion, asthma, running nose).

Sugar is synthetic dirt, white manure, a white turd and technically classified as a drug. The factory's processing machines imitate the digestive system, the machines chew the food, use chemicals similar to that of the liver and pancreas and the dehydrating effect of the colon is imitated. The end result of eating (processing) food is a bowel movement. The factory processes the sugar cane and has a bowel movement (white manure) = white sugar. The sugar cane or sugar beets vitamins, minerals, enzymes and fiber are destroyed by the factory. The sugar cane or beets are reduced to an addicting dehydrated empty calorie starvation drug. White sugar destroys the melanin centers of the pancreas (Islets of Langerhans). Destroyed Melanin centers cause diabetes.

The modern diet consists of over 150 pounds of sugar a year. There is no physiological requirement for this amount of sugar. The commonly accepted religious belief that white sugar calories are needed is the propaganda of the sugar industries. White sugar damages the pancreas, kidney, eyes and the immune system. White sugar requires taking whole calories (vitamins and minerals) from the body's energy reserves. It is quick because it raises the sugar level in the blood—this causes an energy drain called low blood sugar (hypoglycemia) and high blood sugar (diabetes). Refined sugar rusts or breaks down (oxidizes) the organs, nerves, bones, muscles, arteries and veins and causes obesity. Sugar is believed to be a pure food. It is a pure synthetic chemical—a non-food. Brown sugar and raw sugar is white sugar with brown caramel dye on it. Concentrated sweetners are drugs and addicting. The other names for processed sugars are honey, maple syrup, barley or rice syrup, molasses, corn syrup, sucrose, concentrated fruit juice, pasteurized (cooked orange juice), dextrin, dextrose, maltose, dry cane juice, Succanat, sorbitol, fructose and mannitol.

Avoid processed sugar; it is unhealthy. Sugar is hidden in many foods such as mustard, salt, tobacco, catsup, beans, milk, soups, chili, pizza, popcorn, salted nuts, aspirin, seltzers, baby foods, meat dishes, mouthwash, toothpaste, etc. The only official sugar is sucrose. Therefore, a product can have another form of white sugar and be labeled sugar free.

White Sugar and Murder

> If one family (Caucasian) using five pounds of sugar a week would abstain from it for 21 months, one Negro would be spared enslavement and murder.
> *—William Fox, 1792*

Black folks have always been victims of white sugar. Today, their health is victimized by it and countries are colonized by it. Its color (white) more than anything else reveals more about it. It creates good (sweet taste) only to produce evil (disease). The Caucasians create evil (crime, wars, slavery, etc.) to create good (wealth). They create good only to control evil. Good is not defined by Maat, but by power (economic, military, psychological).White sugar is a symbol of Caucasian power and slavery.

The Two Types of Sugars

Glucose
- Found in complex carbohydrates
- Found in grains and vegetables

When added to foods, causes diabetes, blindness, high blood pressure, nerve damage, Alzheimers, Parkinsons, senility, fatigue, heart disease, kidney failure, arthritis, cataracts, glaucoma, hyperactivity, mood swings, addiction, etc.

Processed Fructose
- Free radical oxidation (destroys tissue, cells, organs, etc.)
- Causes aging, weak immunity and ten times more diseases than glucose
- Excessive amounts are in hybrid commercial fruits; makes them dangerous
- Damages the liver, kidneys, nerves, blood vessels, eyes, etc.

Sucrose, which is glucose plus fructose
- Humans lack sucrase enzyme for digesting sucrose
- Causes same diseases as glucose, damages pancreas and liver, reduces fluid in bones, nerves, muscles, veins and arteries

Lactose milk sugar, which is glucose plus galactose
- When cooked, it turns into processed sugar with the same dangers as white sugar
- Adults lose ability to digest milk sugar (i.e., breast milk)

OILS (FAT)

The two types of dangerous processed fats, which are synthetics and used in sugary foods (snack food) are:

Saturated
   • When cooked, causes clogged and blocked veins and arteries, resulting into many diseases

Polyunsaturated
   • Cooked, processed and/or rancid is the primary cause of every disease

HIGH SUGAR AND FAT DIET

Step One
• High processed sugar and high fat diet (cooked, processed and/or rancid fats/oils)

Step Two
• Insulin Resistance
   - Losing ability to use natural bodily made sugars (glucose)
   - High Serum Insulin (Stresses system, organs, nerves, arteries; causes vision and reproductive problems)

Step Three
• High serum triglycerides (Causes hardening of arteries, strokes, heart attacks)
• Increased size of abdominal fat cells (Clogs veins and arteries, makes blood into thick sludge, stresses heart, increases cellular waste, decreases oxygen to cells, etc.)

Step Four
• High blood pressure
• Thick blood that can cause strokes, kidney disease, heart attacks
• Serum cholesterol. Normal to somewhat elevated, but usually not as high as triglycerides

Step Five
• Obesity
• Loses ability to digest fats and craves carbohydrates, which stress pancreas causing loss of ability to digest carbohydrates
• Emotionally and chemically addicted to sugar

Step Six
• Type II Diabetes Mellitus

The substitution of white sugar with artificial sweeteners is dangerous. The bodily damage done by artificial sweeteners such as Sweet 'n Low™ and Nutrisweet™ (Aspartame) are dangerous. It is safe to say that white sugar is less damaging than artificial sweeteners (Aspartame, Sweet 'n Low).

Professional athletes have found that sugar taken after a workout causes muscle soreness. Sugar taken before exercise causes weakness and interferes with sweating.

Mental patients and criminals have been found to have low blood sugar caused by white sugar.

An alternative to sugars can be the herb, Stevia or date sugar or dried fruit. White sugar is an enslaver (nutrition destroyer) and a Slave Master (addictor).

WHITE SUGAR
(Brown Sugar, Turbinato Sugar, Molasses, Raw Sugar, Honey)

Causes ...

Diabetes	Blindness	Arthritis
Hyperactivity	Mood Swings	Glaucoma
Cataracts	High Blood Pressure	Addiction
Hardening of Arteries, Nerves and Veins	Low Blood Sugar	Bone Loss
Tooth Decay	Hair Loss	Skin Diseases
Dehydration	Fatigue	Nerve and Kidney Damage
Respiratory Problems	Headaches	Diarrhea
Hives	Shock	Eye Problems

ASPARTAME
(Nutra-Sweet™, Equal™, Spoonful™, etc.)
Contains wood alcohol, Aspartic Acid, etc. (Changes into formaldehyde – embalming fluid)

Causes ...

Metabolic Acidosis [rusts (degenerates) cells]
Diabetic's sugar levels to fluctuate (memory loss, coma)

Methanol Toxicity (poisons cells)	Mental Confusion	Violence
Mood and Thought Disorders	Menstruation Problems	Rage
Headaches (Brain Aches)	Nerve Damage	Panic Attacks
Multiple Sclerosis	Leg Cramps	Systemic Lupus
Manic Depression	Blindness	Cancer
Alzheimer's to worsen	Birth Defects	Genetic Mutations
Alteration in Brain Chemistry	Nerve Damage	

The Food and Drug Administration (formerly called the Bureau of Chemistry) only classifies sucrose (white sugar) as sugar. All other sugars are not called sugar (i.e., sugarless). Therefore, something sweetened without sucrose (white sugar) is technically classified as "sugar free." The other sugars are just as dangerous and sugary as sucrose. Suggested reading: *Excitotoxins: The Taste that Kills,* by Dr. Blaylock and *Defense Against Alzheimer's* by H.J. Roberts and *Syndrome X* by Jack Challen.

Sᴡᴇᴇᴛ 'N Lᴏᴡ™ Iɴɢʀᴇᴅɪᴇɴᴛs

Dextrose (Glucose, Corn Syrup)

Causes: Diabetes, Cancer, Reproduction problems, Digestion problems, Genetic alterations, Mutations, Hardening of arteries, Decreased oxygen to brain and blood circulation

Calcium Saccharin (made from Coal Tar)

Causes: Cancer, Digestive disorders, Skin diseases, Blood clotting and collagen formation problems

Calcium Silicate

Causes: Headaches, Diarrhea, Hives, Shock, Eye problems, Respiratory problems

Used to make: Cement and glass, Aspirin, Food dyes, Cosmetics, Anti-caking agent

Cream of Tartar

Causes: Skin Problems, Edema, Mineral imbalances,

Can contain: Salt, Dyes, Emulsifiers, Non-food dirt (waste), etc.

FOODS TO AVOID AND THEIR SUBSTITUTES

Avoid	Substitutes
For Baking, fl cup Sugar	2 cups apple juice or ½ cup fruit juice concentrate, ½ cup maple syrup or 1½ cup brown rice syrup
Black pepper	Cayenne, cumin, marjoram, oregano, thyme
Butter, margarine	Soy or safflower margarine, raw tahini (sesame butter), raw almond, raw sunflower, raw sesame, raw cashew or raw peanut butter milk
Candy Bars	Carob bars, fruit bars, honey bars
Cheese	Soybean cheese, rice cheese
Cinnamon	Almond extract, coriander, orange rinds
Cocoa (1 cup)	1 cup carob powder
Cooking Wine	Vegetable broth or tomato puree with lime and lemon juice
Drugs	Herb teas
Flour	Pureed oatmeal
Gelatin (1 tbsp)	1 tbsp granulated agar-agar or 1 tbsp flaked agar-agar + 3½ cups liquid
Ice Cream	Soybean ice cream, rice cream, tofu ice cream
All Meats	Beans, nuts, meat substitutes, nuts, textured vegetable protein, vegetables (fresh), vegetable protein (soy free powder)
Muffins or Quick Breads	Use three ripe, well-mashed bananas instead of ½ Cup butter or oil
Pie Crust	Use only ½ cup margarine for every 2 cups of whole grain flour
Prepared Mustard (1 tbsp)	1 teaspoon dry mustard
Pastries	Fruit
Peanut Butter, Nut Butter	Raw nut or seed butter (non-hydrogenated)
Popsicles	Slice and freeze watermelon, honeydew melon, cantaloupe. Peel grapes and freeze, etc.
Salt (made from rocks) (Sea Salt)	Dulse, Kelp, Soy Sauce and Tamari cause the same diseases as Salt. Potassium Chloride has somewhat salty taste and causes diseases. Use Celery or Bragg's

	Amino Acid
Shortening (1 Cup)	½ - ¾ Cup oil, olive canola or sesame
Sodas	Concentrated or unsweetened juices (apple, orange, pineapple, grape, pear, apricot). Add carbonated water
Sugar, Maple Syrup, Honey, Molasses, Stevia, date sugar	Grain Syrups
Syrup	1 tbsp Honey and Fresh Fruit (i.e., cherries) or use concentrated juices
Thickeners	Arrowroot, kudzu, agar-agar
Sautéed Vegetables, Soups	Use water or low-sodium vegetable broth, stews, sauces
Vinegar	Raw lime and/or lemon juice
Fruit Flavored Yogurt	Plain soy yogurt. Add fruit or concentrated fruit juice
White Bread	Sprouted grains or whole wheat bread
White Flour	Whole grain flours (wheat, soy, rice, spelt, amaranth, kamut, etc.)
White Grits	Soy grits, yellow grits, couscous
White Sugar, Brown Sugar, Confectioner's Sugar	Less dangerous is honey, date sugar, maple syrup and grain (i.e., rice, barley) sugars. Stevia is the safest.

VEGETABLES AND FRUITS

The difference between a vegetable and a fruit is sometimes unclear. Every plant that vegetates on the earth is a vegetable. "Vegetation" eaten from a "table" is called a "veg-table."

A fruit is a part of the plant. It is the part that contains a seed (exposed or covered with flesh) or some other reproductive device of the plant (flower). The roots, leaves, stems and branches are classified as the plant vegetable and the remaining part is classified as fruit. For example, the corn plant has parts that do not have seeds such as the leaves, stalk, roots and the remaining part is the seed. Corn is the fruit of the corn plant.

Some fruits of vegetables are: asparagus tips, okra, broccoli (flower tops), peppers, cauliflower (tops), squashes, cucumber, tomatoes, avocado, beans (navy, soya, etc.), corn, peas, eggplant, stringbeans, berries, wheat germ, oats, lima beans, nuts and seeds.

Excluded on this partial list are the sweet fruits such as apples, melons, oranges, strawberries, pears, as these are quite obvious and classified correctly.

TYPES OF DIETS

The cooked food diet is the single most destructive diet. It can consist of totally or partially cooked food. Cooking processes the food. Processing destroys fiber and enzymes. Cooked food has no live digestive enzymes needed to break down the food. This is its most dangerous factor. Lightly steamed vegetables are safer because the fiber and enzymes are not destroyed. Unfortunately, beans and grains may require cooking because they are sold unripe. Ripe beans and grains are partially green. Ideally, the beans and grains should be sprouted and then eaten.

The danger of cooked food to African people has been untold. Holistic Africans were forced to abandon a raw food diet and accept the European enslaver's cooked food. European-cooked, fried, salty, sugary, slimy, pasty, constipating concoctions have caused mucous congestion, thermal fatigue and changes in the functions of glands. For example, the liver and pancreas have become more involved in digestion and have abandoned their other emotional, spiritual and mental functions. Cooked foods have caused vegetarian animals (this includes man) to lose the digestive functions of the cecum and appendix (former stomachs). They have atrophied (shrank) to their present size.

Harvard Medical School researchers Drs. N.B. Marshall, S. B. Andrus and J. Mayer found that the brain gets smaller and the internal organs such as the kidney, liver, pancreas and heart get bigger on refined processed foods (junk food). The endocrine glands such as the pancreas, pituitary and thyroid get larger from eating refined, processed and cooked food.

Charles Darwin verified that the brains of enslaved (domesticated) rabbits are smaller in size than those of wild (unhumanized) rabbit. Other European scientists, such as Donaldson, further noted that the wild guinea pig, rabbit, rat, fox and lion have larger brains than enslaved (zoos) and circus domesticated (tamed) ones. Interesting to note that the fossil skulls of the Neanderthal man (approximately 100,000 years old) indicated that they had larger brains and the brain was heavier than that of so-called modern man (*The Rat,* by Dr. H. Donaldson).

Cooked food causes a rise in organ temperature. The constant demand on digestive organs to try to metabolize cooked foods and neutralize the harmful chemicals made by cooked foods causes thermal fatigue. The United Nations World Health Organization data indicates that 97 percent of primary cancers start at heat exhausted (thermal fatigue) organs such as the prostate.

The toxic chemical and digestive stressors of cooked foods cause the glands and organs to age and get larger. This is the same thing that happens to a deteriorated thyroid or prostate (hypertrophy = enlarges). The glands and arteries get weaker as they get larger. Minerals are too hard to be broken down, vitamins and enzymes are dead. The endocrine interrelated chain of glands become over stimulated, which results in an increase in body weight (suggested source is "Comparative Experiments with Canned, Home Cooked and Raw Food Diets" by Kohman, Eddy, White and Sanborn in the *Journal of Nutrition* 14:9-19 [1937]). Cooked plant or animal foods cause health quality to deteriorate (*The Status of Food Enzymes in Digestion and Metabolism* by Dr. Howell, 1946).

Enzymes are alive in raw food and help to digest (break down) and metabolize the raw food. In ancient Africa, enzymes were utilized to improve food metabolism. For example, grains were allowed to partially germinate (sprout) before they were eaten; this caused an increase in the plant's enzyme. The Caucasian junk food industry has eliminated the germination phase. Processed grains (seeds and fruits of plants), do not have enzymes. Africans utilize enzymes in their animal flesh diets. For example, the Pygmies of equatorial Africa eat the flesh of elephants after they have been dead several days. Allowing the elephants' flesh to partially rot combats ptomaine poison because the natural enzymatic ratio is in balance. Other colored cultures, such as the Eskimo, utilize enzymes in eating raw flesh. They, like the *Pygmies, allow* the intact carcass to putrefy (rot) a few days before devouring it (*The Eskimo* by K. Birket-Smith).

The cooked food diet shortens the life span. It causes weak organs, thermal fatigue, increases bodily toxins and weakens immunity. Cooking food is based upon Caucasian mythology and superstitions, not facts. For example, an ancient Caucasians belief is that there is one stomach and it digests proteins. Humans have two stomachs (lower and upper portiandas well as proteins when the food rises up to the top of the stomach and touches the skin of the stomach (digestion takes place) and then slides down into the intestines (*Journal of Laboratory and Clinical Medicine* and the "*American Journal of Physiology,* 1941). Enzymes are holistic and get tired, have life spans, react to environment and have spiritual and mental functions. ("Enzyme Intelligence, Illustrating That Enzymes and Ferments are the Ultimate, Indestructible and Invisible Units of Life and are Conscious and Intelligent" by Nels Quelui).

The local environment, culture and lifestyle of a people determine their diets. The culture teaches a person what foods to like and dislike. For instance, the so-called Eskimos live in the cold Arctic region of the earth. Their environment has scarce vegetation and in many cases, none. Consequently, they eat a totally animal flesh diet. The medicines they use are made from the flesh (glandulars) and bones (minerals) of animals.

When people live near the sea or bodies of water and near vegetation, their diets consist primarily of sea animal flesh and vegetation. When people live in an environment of vegetation and animals, they eat animal flesh and vegetables and use animal flesh and bones coupled with vegetation (herbs) as medicine. However, the biochemistry and anatomical structure of humans indicates a vegetarian, fruitarian, liquidtarian and breathtarian diet. Humans adapting to a food supply or environment does not indicate evolution or that ideal diet. Adaptation is not evolution.

A vegetarian diet, for humans, is based upon their biochemistry and anatomy. Animal flesh eaters have a short digestive tract (approximately 2/3 the length of their bodies) while vegetarians have a longer digestive tract (humans 30 to 35 feet long). The total surface area of the digestive intestinal tract is equal to the size of a football field and the number of microbes (animals) and flora (plants) living within the intestines totals more than the number of cells in the body. These microbes have various tribes, territories (hills and valleys) and personalities in the body. Humans have an intestine that resembles that of vegetarian animals. Humans do not have strong digestive enzymes or fluids and cannot digest raw animal flesh, hair, feathers or scales. Humans do not have the ability to perspire (sweat) through the mouth like flesh eaters. Humans lack the strength and speed and claws for killing animals and canine (hollow) teeth for cutting into raw animal flesh. The human jaw moves in a circular motion (like vegetarian cattle), while raw flesh eater's jaws move up and down only. All natural meat eaters eat animal flesh raw. All fetus-eaters (bird eggs) eat the fetus raw and can eat the animal that laid the egg raw. Humans cannot physically chase, attack, fight and kill their prey. Humans lack the biochemistry for eating the worm-infested and poisoned meat of dead animals (i.e., buzzards, and hogs can eat it).

The life span of animal flesh eaters is short. The age span of an animal increases as the quantity of animal flesh diet decreases. Vegetable consumption increases the age span and this increase is according to diet as follows: breathtarians live the longest, then liquidarians, fruitarians and vegetarians.

Fruitarians eat the fruit of plants (sweet fruit, non-sweet fruits). The fruitarian eats the highest concentration (largest amount) of nutrition that the plant produces, which is its fruit. This diet has the highest nutrient content because the plant seeds store high amounts of vital nutrients for its offspring in its fruit. Seeds and nuts are classified as fruits. Fruit flesh (meat) contains distilled water. The body distills water (i.e., lungs, intestine, kidney) before it is digested. The fruitarian has a high content of liquid and a very low content of earth minerals. Vegetarian (fruitarian, vegan) diet does not require the killing of the plants and fruits. The food can be eaten raw. No natural vegetarian, animal flesh eater or fruitarian animals eat cooked food, fried foods, sweeten or season foods or mixes many different type of foods together.

The liquidtarian lives basically on a diet of spring or sweet creek water. Some liquidtarians live on a diet of organic raw vegetable or fruit juices and water. The breathtarian lives on a diet of unpolluted air. This diet is the highest on the scale and has the longest life span. They seem to use electromagnetic energy and are biochemically capable of organizing the ions in air in such a way as to produce a energy-food. They use their breath as the breath of life. It is a spirito-physical life.

The diet should be determined by the diseased or wellness state, type of work (laborer, desk job), social and economic condition (jail, poverty), environment (polluted air, computer, radiation), emotional and social stressors. A diet change requires learning different types of foods, seasonings, recipes, cooking methods and in some cases, changing friends and social lifestyles, losing friends to socialize with, elimination of alcohol and marijuana. It is usually the loneliness, caused by eating health food, junk food addiction, eating disorders, peer pressure and cultural homelessness that keeps Black people on bad diets.

ACIDS AND ALKALINES

Diet Guide
Human nutrition is often measured and regulated by acids and alkalis. Acid foods usually have a sour after-taste. They cause deterioration or are cor-

rosive by nature. Alkaline foods are non-acid and make an acid solution weak. They usually taste bitter and feel slippery in the mouth. The acid-alkaline balance of the body is usually measured by pH. The pH scale measures from 0 to 14; from 1 to 7 is acid,7 is neutral, and 7 to 14 is alkaline. Everything has its own pH, such as the vagina, stomach, skin, head, feet, and mouth, Anger is acid, happiness is alkaline, tears of sadness are acid, tears of joy are alkaline; stress is acid, relaxation is alkaline, exercise is acid, rest is alkaline, etc. The pH is also a measure of the speed of digestion or biochemical activity. An acid pH means fast activity while an alkaline pH means slow chemical activity.

Foods are oxidized (burned) in the body. Digested (burned) foods leave a waste matter called ash. The ash can be neutral (7.0), acid (1 to 6.9) or alkaline (7 to 14). The objective of nutrition is to keep the acids and alkalis in balance (proper ratio) and to avoid acid ash.

The normal ratio for acid-alkaline varies with type of diet. The junk food, animal flesh eater's diet is the highest acid diet. It is the most corrosive and destructive diet and creates numerous dis-eases.

A diet that consists of animal flesh and cooked vegetables is the second highest acidic diet. The vegetarian that includes raw and cooked foods has the lowest acid levels. The healthiest alkaline-acid ratio is a diet with a 4:1 or 80% alkaline and 20% acid. This ratio gives optimum health and the highest protection against dis-ease.

Acid foods have a high content of phosphorus, sulfur and chlorine. All animal flesh, poultry, seafood, chicken fetuses (eggs), most nuts, legumes, alcohol, nicotine and all synthetic foods are acid.

Alkaline foods have a high content of magnesium, sodium, calcium and potassium. Most fresh fruits and vegetables are alkaline. Without large amounts of alkaline mineral elements in the diet, the body becomes diseased. The body robs the tissue and bones for the alkaline elements to balance a high acid diet. This causes a nutritional debt (deficit). The nutritional debt is paid by the organs, nerves, bones and connecting tissues. The drain of minerals (alkaline) nutrients from the lungs, reproductive organs, jaw, teeth, then the bones results in dis-ease (colds, flu, reproductive problems, jaw deterioration, rotten teeth, etc.).

The alkaline drain causes holes in the connective tissues (joints) and bones, which results in fluid filling up the holes. This causes inflammation of joints and soft bones (deterioration of skeletal structure), and reverse osmosis, which causes disease by draining fluid from bursae, muscles, connective tissue, arteries, nerve mylein, etc.

The eating of large amounts of animal flesh adds large amounts of protein to the diet. Consumption of large amounts of protein (even vegetable protein) is a nutritional drain. Excess protein is converted to fat and stored by the body. The burning of protein causes the accumulation of toxic acid ash in the body. It requires more air and water consumption to cleanse (flush out) acid ash and impurities. The body cannot meet the extra cleansing demands and loses reserve energy. This extra cleansing demand and reserve energy loss is usually the reason why a high protein diet causes rapid weight loss. The tissue is robbed of its fluids and alkalinity in order to flush out acid ash. Chemically, the cells that lose alkaline become acid while the system maintains alkalinity. High acid diets can cause the alkaline minerals to be lost in each urination. An obvious mineral drain, malnutrition and disease state is the end result of this diet.

All refined, processed, denatured man-made foods are acid. All animal flesh is acid; all cereals and grains (grasses) are acid. Animal by-products (egg, milk, cheese) are acid. Acid nuts are walnuts, cashews and peanuts; all other nuts are alkaline. Acid vegetables are lentils, rhubarb, artichokes, beans (kidney, navy, white beans) and brussels sprouts. All other vegetables and beans are alkaline.

All fresh fruits and all vegetables (except those mentioned) are alkaline. Citric and malic acids found in fruits are alkaline. In balancing the diet, keep the acid (20%) and alkaline (80%) ratio as a standard.

ALKALINE AND ACID FOODS

ALKALINE-ASH FOODS		ACID – ASH FOODS	
Apples	Lemons	Bacon	Oatmeal
Apricots	Limes	Barley, pearled	Oysters
Avocado	Mushrooms	Beef	Peanuts
Bananas	Muskmelon	Brown Rice	Pork Chops
Beets	Onions	Butter	Roasted Peanut Butter
Blackberries	Oranges	Cheese	Salmon
Blueberries	Parsnips	Chicken	Sardines
Broccoli	Peaches	Chocolate Cake	Sausage
Brussels Sprouts	Pears	Codfish	Scallops
Cabbage	Pineapple	Corned Beef	Shrimp
Cantaloupe	Prunes	Dried Lentils	Soda Crackers
Carrots	Radishes	Eggs	Veal
Cauliflower	Raisins	Fresh Corn	Wheat Bran
Celery	Raspberries	Honey	Wheat Germ
Chard Leaves	Rhubarb	Ice Cream	White Bread
Cherries, Sour	Rutabagas	Lamb/Turkey	White Flour
Cucumbers	Sauerkraut	Macaroni/Spaghetti	Whole Wheat Bread
Dried Dates (Sun)	Spinach (Raw)	Milk (Cow, Goat)	Whole Wheat Flour
Dried Figs (Sun)	Strawberries		Yogurt
Grapefruit	Sweet Potatoes		
Grapes	Tangerines		
Green Beans	Tomatoes, Ripe		
Green Limas	Watercress		
Green Peas	Watermelon		
Green Soy Beans	White Potatoes		
Honeydew Melon	Lettuce		

For Food Effects on the Body's Acid/Alkaline Balance, see page 531.

WHAT'S EATING YOU?
(Consumer and Food)

The commercial fast foods are non-organic processed, genetic altered and chemicalized dirt and are synthetic food look-alikes. In fact, there is no commercial food safe to eat. Commercial foods have an overabundance of toxic, poisonous, synthetic chemicals, hormones, antibiotics, steroids, terminator codes (block nutrient absorption) additives, preservatives and coloring which destroy and deteriorate the human body and are addicting. They use synthetic chemicals to purposely make junk foods (synthetic food contraband) addicting. This makes the consumer a junk food addict that constantly spends money on food so that the junk food industry can constantly make money (profit). The snack food addict goes from one fast food store to another store and is constantly eating snacks, sodas, burgers, candy, sweets, pizzas, chewing gum, cookies, coffee, chips, etc. They have a chemical craving for junk food and a mental illness called an Eating Disorder/Food Addiction. Instead of the consumer eating the foods, the foods are eating the consumer's health.

The trillion dollar chemical food industry makes look-alike foods, which are tasteless, odorless, flavorless and use chemicals flavor enhancers to hide chemicals used in processing. White sugar and salt are sued to hide the bad taste of chemicalized food. These chemical companies have decided to use the consumer as a synthetic chemical garbage can. (*Handbook of Consumer Motivation, The Psychology of the World of Objects* by B. Dichter).

Synthetic chemical foods devour the body and destroy its life and health sustaining ability. The Pharmacological and Toxicological Division of the FDA has admitted that their analysis of synthetic chemicals in foods is inadequate for measuring the amount of chemicals or the danger of chemicals (*Chemicals in Food and in Farm Produce: Their Harmful Effects* by F. Bicknael). Synthetic chemicals in water, soil, highly processed food animals, seeds and plants, combined with those chemicals used to process foods can boost each other's strength and combine to form new chemicals with lethal reactions. These chemicals interfere with the body's ability to function, use enzymes, amino acids, minerals, fats and vitamins. Synthetic chemicals age and deteriorate the health. Synthetic chemicals have slow and delayed effects that do not appear for weeks or months after they are consumed. When the effects of the chemicals appear, they are misdiagnosed as flu, infection, V.D., heart attack, AIDS, allergies, headaches, tension, stress, depression, fatigue, tingling toes or fingers, constipation, etc. The chemicals slowly eat away the body, putting it on a downward progression, which affects the body in 5, 10, and 15 to 50 years. The effects can be a small malfunction or an increase in the size of the liver, spleen or kidney. The body can become weak in cyclic stages of every two weeks or once a month and this can be labeled a chronic disease. These chemicals are slowly eating the body. Every time the consumer has dinner—he is the dinner. *(The Poison in Your Food* by W. Longwood).

The consumer is merely a food-eating garbage disposal puppet of the food chemical industry. They are walking hospital out-patients that must take aspirin, laxatives, Viagra, cold medicine, etc. Ironically, the FDA "decertifies" and "delists" chemicals for use in foods because of health danger. However, they do not forbid the "decertified" and "delisted" chemicals from being used by the food industry. The FDA does not stop the delisted chemicals from being used. They put the dangerous chemical on a decertified status and the industry continues to feed the dangerous chemicals to the public. Further, the GRAS (Generally Recognized as Safe) chemicals are a title given to dangerous chemicals by food manufacturers who economically feel that they are safe. Moreover, the USDA withholds reports on the dangerous chemicals used in food from the public (*History of Crime Against the Food Law* by H. Wiley, M.D.). They continue to allow poisonous chemicals to be used in food by adjusting the level of safe use for the poisonous quantity. This is similar to correctly doing something wrong. The FDA sets standards for correctly doing something wrong. The synthetic chemicals (poisons) cause an emotional and mental illness called an Eating Disorder/Food Addiction. Food Addiction guarantees profits for the Food Industry and diseases for the Disease Industry (hospitals, doctors, etc.) The majority (95%) of the Addicts do not realize they have a problem because all their friends, peers, movie stars, athletes, ministers, heroes, idols and role models are food junkies. The poisons (synthetic chemicals) are approved by the FDA, which makes the food junkies feel safe. Aside from this, all diseases are blamed on bacteria, not the synthetic chemicals in foods. The use of poisons in foods is wrong and no level of safe poison eating is acceptable. In other words, eating a little arsenic is safe because it does not immediately kill you or harm you while eating a log of arsenic is unsafe because it will kill you. However, the constant eating of a little arsenic (safe level) has accumulation effects and causes minor diseases aside from being in your system and combining with other synthetic chemicals to cause minor diseases.

The following are charts that can help you recognize a Food Addiction/Eating Disorder and some addicting foods.

Signs and Symptoms of Food Addiction and Eating Disorders

Junk foods are chemically made addicting. The indications of addiction are:

- Compulsive overeating
- Constantly eats snack foods, sodas, candy, chewing gum

- Eats when excited or happy
- Obesity
- Constantly talks or thinks about food (food obsession)
- Eats to relieve stress
- Eats to exert control
- Eats excessively when depressed and/or around Menstruation cycle
- Hyperphagia (eats when not hungry)
- Unable to stop eating
- History of unsuccessful dieting
- Abnormal body image pathology
- Eats to relieve painful emotional problems
- Are in denial about addiction
- Socializes with other food addicts

ICE CREAM—YOU BETTER SCREAM

Ice cream is totally unsafe. It is made from cheese by-products, butter, butter oil, evaporated milk, condensed milk, all types of buttermilk, all types of skim milk, milk treated with sodium hydroxide and disodium phosphate, plastic cream, dried cream, cheap poisonous thinners, propylene (paint remover, antifreeze), imitation flavors (used as flea killers, embalming fluid, leather tanners), extra strength synthetic deodorant industrial flavor chemicals (have caution and innocuous poison on labels), polyoxyethylenes (cancerous), sodium carboxymethylcellulose (cancer inciter), refiners syrup (cheap by-product with salty taste and off-flavor), white sugar, pork and beef gelatin (increases germ growth), antioxidants, buffers, synthetic perfumes (cancerous) neutralizers, stabilizers and other countless dangerous chemicals which have been approved by the FDA. The chemical content of ice cream does not have to be listed on the label as it has been exempted by the FDA. The FDA and USDA serve as a consumer delivery system for the junk food chemical companies. They give foods the cosmetic label of being safe. They can make you scream "No ice cream!"

CHEESE

Processed cheeses are made by heating cheeses and pumping the slimy mass with air. This cheese is a mixture of low quality green (uncured) and cured cheese, moles, yeast, bacteria-infested and recycled cheese of whatever cheeses are around at processing time. These cheeses are ground up, mixed with poisonous emulsifiers and other chemicals. Furthermore, they contain the combined contaminants of the milk, treated water, the cattle forage and feed, plus the processed chemicals. In the strict sense, it is neither a cheese nor a food.

Cottage cheese contains sodium hydrochlorite (speeds up the process), white sugar, diacetyls (butter flavor), hydrogen peroxide (bleach), cochineal or annatto (toxic dyes), salt (indigestible), plaster of Paris cast (plastic hardener), poisonous mold retarders plus the chemicals found in milk, water and cattle grass and feed. The FDA recognizes the poisons used but fails to do anything about these poisons. A Consumer Union study in 1964 revealed, dirt, rancid oil, over-acidic oil, mold, bacteria and yeast contamination and poor flavors in cottage cheese. Storage of cottage cheese in stores promotes bacterial infestation and spoilage, which goes undetected by the consumer because of the deodorizers used in the cheese. The cheese has the same chemicals found in extra strength synthetic deodorants plus synthetic perfumes.

Commercial cheeses are made by bleaching the cheese. Thus, destroying oil soluble vitamins. The bleach is not rinsed out. It is eaten.

Dyes, sorbic acid (mold inhibitor) and acidic synthetic vitamins are usually added, plus the toxic chemicals found in the milk, such as pesticides, steroids, sex hormones, growth hormones, antibiotics and penicillin in addition to the poisons used in the cattle forage. The synthetic vitamins in the cheese demineralize the bones—bone loss (*The Cheese Book* by V. Marquis and P. Haskell).

CREAM AND BUTTER

Cream and butter are usually made from stale cream and/or recycled milk. It is very acidic, and an acid neutralizer calcium carbonate or hydroxide is added. This stops the ability to use minerals. Then a bleach such as hydrogen peroxide is used, coupled with an antioxidant to retard spoilage. This causes a horrible smell and an awful taste, which is removed by adding a starter culture—then cancer-causing coal tar dyes are added. Contaminants found in milk are present in butter. Butter or oils that turn rancid (spoil) are injected with diacetyl, which hides foul odors and rancid taste. These rancid foods destroy nutrients in the digestive tract. The FDA does not require the presence of many chemicals on the label. High amounts of salt are added to salted butter because salt retards molds and yeast growth. Salt causes the body to rust, dehydrate, harden, break down and stop digestion. Saltiness is disguised by adding a neutralizing toxic alkaline salt. The combined effect of the dangerous drugs (chemicals) is not only an obvious health hazard, but immoral.

PEANUT BUTTER CRIMES

Peanuts or Niger Nuts (as they are called in Europe) are beans by definition and in a raw state are a good protein. However, the commercial peanut butter has been totally turned into a colorful brown liquid— synthetic chemical slime. Sweeteners (white sugar, corn syrup, dextrose) are added to peanut butter to hide moldy, inferior and rancid peanuts. The peanut is degermed (taking out its heart) before processing to increase shelf life in the stores—this lowers its protein value. Further, hydrogenated oil (or beef or pig lard) is added up to a level of 60% oil and 40% peanuts. Emulsifiers are added to keep the oil mixed with the small quantity of peanuts. Then additives plus texturizers are mixed in the brown slime. Aside from this, bleached peanuts are used. Bleaching denatures the peanut and destroys nutrients. Moreover, artificial flavors are added. All the combined ingredients are synthetic toxic poisons, which has the words "caution," "poison," "innocuous" on the industrial labels. The Food and Drug Administration's September 2000 Total Diet Study stated that non-organic peanut butter has over 259 disease and cancer-causing chemicals such as hexachlorobenzene (brain damage, tumors, bone-marrow poison, cancer), benzene hexachloride (skin irritant, leukemia, poison, cancer), dieldrin (causes diseases), methyl-parathion (poison, cancer), etc.

The sum total of commercial processing of the peanut renders it a non-food. This amounts to a nutritional robbery of the peanuts and a crime against the peanut and the peanut butter consumer.

TABLE SALT
(Sodium Chloride)

Sodium Chloride is a poison. It is a mineral salt commonly called Salt. There are many mineral salts (Magnesium Chloride, etc.). The mineral salts, already present, in the foods (except sea weeds) are not harmful. Salt was used to preserve meat. The eating of vegetables cooked with salted meat conditioned people to wanting to add salt to foods that were not salty. Salt is used in candy, baked goods, mouthwashes, eye drops, cereals, milk, cheese, prescription drugs, catsup, mayonnaise, mustard, yogurt, etc. It causes many health problems.

INGREDIENTS	REACTION
Alumino-Calcium Silicate	Irritates lungs and skin, Diarrhea, Nausea, Vomiting, Clogs glands, Bleeding. Used to make cement and glass.
Sodium Alumino Silicate	Skin irritant, Vomiting, Diarrhea. Used in detergents and preserves eggs.
Ferrocyanide	Poison, Stops perspiration, Constipation, Itching, Convulsions, Stops Enzymes.
Sodium Carbonate	Skin rash, Diarrhea, Vomiting, Digestion problems. Decreases circulation.
Yellow Prussiate of Soda	Poison, Addiction.
White Sugar	Addiction, Many diseases.
Chloride	Anemia, Diabetes, Eclampsia, Pneumonia, Kidney inflammation, Fevers, Liver problems. More dangerous than Sodium.

DISEASES SALT CAUSES

Addiction (Craving)	High Blood Pressure	Obesity
Heart Disease	Tooth Decay	Arteriosclerosis
Rheumatism	Tension	Insomnia
Hair Loss	Edema	White Spots (Bleaches)
Kidney Problems	Skin Rashes	Bone Loss
Root Canal Disease (irritates roots of teeth)		

Suggested reading: *A Consumer's Dictionary of Cosmetic Ingredients,* Ruth Winter; *Consumer Beware,* Beatrice Hunter; *Webster's Dictionary.*

Salt Facts

The body processes 5 grams of salt in twenty-four hours. Eating more than 5 grams causes the salt to get into the nerves, brain, muscles, bones, cells, glands, blood and organs. It then retards irritates, dehydrates and oxidizes (rusts tissues).

- Junk food diet has 20 to 30 grams of salt.
- You require 0.2 to 0.6 grams of salt daily.
- Salt consumed above 0.6 grams is stored in the body as a toxic poison.
- Do not add table salt, sea salt or salty seaweeds (kelp) to food. Salty rocks are washed into the ocean, causing seaweeds to be salty. Do not eat rocks.
- The mineral salt (baking soda) is not a deodorant or toothpaste.
- The salt is a natural part of foods. Do not add salt.
- Salt is addicting.
- Sweating gets rid of toxic mineral salts through the tissue. Sweating does not get rid of essential mineral salts. If your sweat tastes like salt, then the body is degenerating (oxidizing). The skin should not be used for a bowel movement to eliminate salts. The skin's primary function is to regulate temperature, protect and metabolize the sun (make Vitamin D).

SULPHUR AND DRIED FRUITS

Sulphur dioxide is a synthetic chemical that is toxic and poisonous. It alters the nutrient patterns and destroys vitamins and minerals. It especially destroys the B complex vitamins. It causes a calcium deficiency. The government has not set a limit on the amount that can be used in food. The Federal Food, Drug and Cosmetic Act has given the food industry the privilege of free use of this drug, despite the fact that it causes brittle teeth in animals (demineralizer).

Dried fruit is usually dried on trays that have been treated with pesticides. These pesticides soak into the fruit. One of the toxic chemicals used to dry fruit is fumigate methyl bromide. This poison is also used in chocolate, dairy products, beans, macaroni, nutmeats, flour, dried vegetables, spices, feeds, chestnuts, etc. The FDA still allows its use despite the fact that it causes temporary insanity and has poisoned industrial workers. According to its manufacturers, it is dangerous to all forms of animal and plant life.

SKIM MILK

Skim milk is a by-product once solely fed to hogs. It is stripped of enzymes, vitamins D, E, K and denatured. Cooked and acidic rancid fish oil is used for the Vitamin A added to milk.

Dry milk is usually dried at high temperatures. This destroys the vitamins, makes the fatty acids a type of transoil plastic and makes the minerals too coarse to be digested. It is contaminated by salmonella. and synthetic vitamins or cooked fish oil (Vitamin D) is added, making it difficult to digest. It is a non-food.

Canned evaporated milk contains roach killer, white sugar, salt, preservatives, synthetic vitamins, calcium chloride, disodium phosphate, and sodium citrate. All of these are dangerous to health.

Imitation milk has indigestible artery-clogging saturated hydrogenated coconut oil, excess estrogen, steroids, growth hormones, sodium caseinate from milk or soybeans, corn syrup (white sugar product), salt, emulsifiers, dyes, potassium phosphate, artificial flavors and acidic synthetic vitamins and minerals. These chemicals transform raw milk into liquid plastic white pus. Polluted milk is not equal in nutritional value to raw fig juice or human milk. Skim, dry, evaporated and imitation milk are unsafe for children, pregnant women and breastfeeding women, the poor and the elderly. It causes uterine fibroid tumors, prostate disease and breast cancer in men and women. In the strict sense, cow's milk is cattle food. This commercial milk contains toxic, cancerous detergents, genetic modifiers, pesticides, radioactive isotopes, hormones, bacteria, cooked pus, dirt (legally approved nonspecified impurities), cancer causing adrenalin, antibiotics; penicillin and chloromycetin are used to curb inflammation of the cow's breast. These chemicals get into the milk along with the other chemicals. These contaminants have been found in milk by the FDA. Pasteurization does not destroy antibiotics and it causes bacteria to multiply rapidly and allows milk to be recycled. Hormones in milk have caused cysts, tumors, cancer, early menstruation in girls, gender confusion and feminization of males in studies. Petroleum wax in milk (and other waxed containers) has cancer-causing hydrocarbons in them. The FDA acknowledges this but allows their use. Milk should only be consumed at the temperature of the mother's body (cow's body). It should be drank directly from the nipple and never exposed to light or air. Otherwise, the milk is dangerous as food.

Ironically, in Ancient Africa, raw fig juice was used as a substitute for human milk. Figs are similar in chemical composition to human milk. It can double the size of an infant in six months. Figs combined with dates were used to sustain the life of many desert African tribes. The Romans later used dates as food for training warriors and building muscles.

MARGARINE

Margarine is a combination of water and oil combined by a chemical emulsion similar to soap. It is hydrogenated and contains animal as well as vegetable products. There are high amounts of animal fats (lard) used to make it. Known poisons such as the benegoates and emulsifiers (sodium stearates, polysorbates, sterols, sulfated alcohols) are used. The corn oil in margarine is hydrogenated with poisonous barium peroxide and phosphoric acid and the added cottonseed oil (a non-food due to chemical contamination), soy oil and other oils are hydrogenated. Corn oil has to be hydrogenated in order to become solid at room temperature. Hydrogenated oils have germand enzyme killers, become rancid (spoiled), cause arterial deterioration (hardening of the arteries), build-up of fat around the heart and clogs and/or blocks arteries and veins. This leads to heart attacks, strokes and bypass surgery.

OIL

Oil is processed, cooked, filtered and refined. Nutrients destroyed, oil becomes a synthetic transoil to retard spoilage and prolong its shelf life. The vital vitamins and minerals and fiber is dissolved with toxic chemicals and filtered out of the oil. In the refinement process, a gasoline solvent is used to dissolve the oil after extraction. Then it is treated with toxic poisonous lye, alkalis and caustic soda. Next, it is bleached to make it nice and clear. These refinement chemicals and bleach leave a horrible odor and taste; so, the oil is then chemically deodorized and perfumed and poisonous antioxidants added. Residual amounts of the chemicals stay in the oil, which cause it to be unsafe for human consumption. Some refiners add trace amounts of white sugar to make the oil addicting. Processed oils are a highly concentrated synthetic chemical that are harmful. Polyunsaturated, saturated and hydrogenated oils that are processed are equally health destructive. However, the consumer watchdogs, USDA and FDA, approve this and law does not require the listing of all the chemicals in the oil. The final oil product has been heated several times and further reheating by the consumer causes it to be even more dangerous.

Cold pressed oils are the safest. They are concentrated and weaken the digestive system and thicken the blood making it into sludge (sewage). Processed or cooked oils cause unidentified diseases.

Polyunsaturated Fatty Acids (PUFA)
and Hydrogenated Oils
Oils that are isolated, processed and heated become drugs.

Processed Oils
- Increase the incidence and severity of cancer
- Contribute to inflammation of joints
- Weaken immunity
- Increase fluid retention (edema)
- Decrease and interrupt mitochondria function
- Increase cell death
- Slow down cell growth and development
- Heated, causes cancer
- Decrease the cells of the brain, liver, skin, etc.
- Mutate cells
- Decrease energy
- Impair, fetal and infant brain development
- Cause fats to become transoils and rancid (rotten
- Decrease communication between cells

Suggested reading: *British Medical Journal,* October 18, 1997; *The Journal of Bone and Mineral Research;* Oregon Institute of Science and Medicine, 1994 study; *Journal of the American Medical Association,* December 24, 1997.

CHEWING GUM

Chewing gum contains over 30 ingredients, which are not listed on the label. FDA does not require a list of ingredients. Many shipments of the chewing gum industry's gum bases have been seized because they had high dirt levels, which include rat manure and insects. Chewing gum is 60% white sugar with two teaspoons of sugar per stick.

Chewing gum reduces the acid in the stomach and hampers digestion. It raises the sugar content of saliva and causes a negative chain reaction in the gastrointestinal tract, as the stomach gets ready for food that never comes. It is categorized as a food probably because most of it is accidentally swallowed.

CHEWING GUM
(SAME INGREDIENTS USED IN COMMERCIAL TOOTHPASTE)

Ingredient	Harmful Effect
BHA (Butylated Hydroxyanisole)	Cancer
BHT (Butylated Hydroxyl toluene)	Cancer
Plasticizers	Solvent (dissolves skin), Digestive problems
Aspartame	Nerve damage, Cancer, Cysts, Tumors
Polysobutylene (lighter fluid)	Solvent, Skin irritant, Suffocation
Polyterpene (turpentine)	Respiratory failure (death), Skin irritant
Aluminum	Brain damage, Clogs glands
Propyl Gallate	Skin irritant
Polyvinyl Acetate	Damages lungs and kidney, Tumors
Coal Tar	Cancer, Degenerative diseases

Wood Tar	Cancer, Insanity
Petroleum Tar	Cancer, Degenerative disease
Paraffin	Cancer, Degenerative disease
Approved non-food dirt	Unknown
(Dead insects, rat manure, filth)	
Unspecified ingredients (Over 20 not listed)	Unknown
White sugar (Corn syrup, maltose	Kidney failure, Diabetes, Blindness,
dextrose, dextrin, etc.)	Addiction, Cancer
Dyes	Cancer

Suggested Reading: *Consumer Bulletin*, August 1961; *A Consumer's Dictionary of Cosmetic Ingredients* by Ruth Winter (Food and Drug Administration says ingredients do not have to be listed on package).

SYRUP AND HONEY

Syrups such as maple syrup can contain only 2% maple syrup and are labeled pure maple syrup. This syrup usually has white sugar, corn syrup, sodium citrate, sodium benzoate, salt, imitation maple flavor, dyes and citric acid. The maple syrup production of the trees is increased by using a toxic poisonous paraformaldehyde pellet. These pellets are put in trees to increase the tree's syrup production.

The filtration of honey filters out nutrients and the heating of it destroys nutrients. The commercial honey industry uses toxic poisons of benzaldehyde, carbolic acid, propionic anhydride, nitrous oxide, sulfa drugs, antibiotics, and mothballs, all of which leaves toxic residues in honey. Mothballs are used to fumigate combs; also, hydrocyanic gas (used in gas chambers) is used to destroy diseased bees. This gas also gets into the honey.

Honey contains 70% fruit sugar (fructose) and 30% sucrose sugar (white sugar). It causes:

Kidney fatigue and disease; nerve and blood vessel damage; hardening of the arteries; gouty arthritis; heart attacks; strokes; periodontal disease (teeth and gums); contributes to uterine fibroids, endometriosis, cystic mastitis, breast cancer; stomach ulcers; liver and adrenal glands get larger and damaged; pancreas shrinks and deteriorates; increases blood fats; increases uric acid, cholesterol, triglycerides, cortisone, blood levels of insulin; mood and thought disorders; hyperactivity.

DRINKING WATER

Nature's safe drinking water is found in springs, wells, and freshwater creeks. Water is the handmaiden of nutrition. It is a mixture of air, minerals, trace minerals and vitamins. There is always foreign matter floating in water, which is essential to its proper digestion. This matter is usually filtered out by public water purifying works.

Water is the main carrier of blood; it helps regulate body temperature and maintains the mineral salt balance of the blood.

Nature's best drinking water is filtered over stones, sand and plants as it flows in a stream. It is exposed to the sun and wind. The color light rays of the sun and electrical forces of the wind create an atmospheric mixture. This mixture is healthier for the body than man-made public water, which is heavily polluted by our poisoned environment. Public water is chemicalized synthetic water, which contains bacteria that does not need air to grow. Some of the chemicals are aluminum, ammonia, fluoride and bleach (chloride) is added. Aluminum Sulfate, which is a poison that irritates the skin, stops digestion, causes constipation and allergies. It gives water a fresh clean taste. Fluoride (acid salt) is similar to lye. It is made by dissolving tin in hydrofluoric acid. It brittles bones, causes cavities, irritates the skin, eyes and digestive organs. Ammonia is toxic, causes skin irritation, blisters and burns and harms the eyes, breaks hair and causes indigestion. Taking baths and/or showers with this water contributes to skin cancer. The unsafe public water has adjustable levels of acceptable pollution, which is set and reset by the Board of Health. The United Nations World Health Organization has classified public drinking water in all major American cities as polluted. The public drinking water is usually obtained from polluted lakes and streams. The lakes and streams meet substandard levels of safety. The water has active viruses, bacteria and chemicals, which cause kidney stones, arteriosclerosis, emphysema, constipation, gallstones, arthritis and inflamed gastro-intestinal tracts. It is estimated that over 40% of the population is drinking public water that has been used by animals, industry, and used five or more times by other people. The water does not meet low government standards and purification levels are usually raised to include more impurities. The chemicals from factories, hospitals, agriculture, along with atomic waste results in over two million new chemicals, which eventually get in public drinking water. Public drinking water is deodorized recycled toilet water. *(The Shocking Truth about Water* by P.C. Bragg, *The Coming Water Famine* by J. Wright).

Whenever spring water cannot be drunk, distilled water distilled spring water is the best substitute. If distilled water is not available, then boiled public water is the last alternative.

America has an overabundance of underground (aquavaults) clean spring water. The multinational companies control them in order to create water scarcity and economic profit.

The previously mentioned processed, synthetic, chemicalized, dangerous water, fertilized soil, meats, milk and eggs kill the body. They eat away the vital force of the body causing death. What this amounts to is that the water you are drinking and the food you are eating is eating you (*Chemical Carcinogensis and Cancers* by W. Huepser and W. D. Conway).

There is no safe level of poisons. This has been revealed time and again by the United States Department of Agriculture and by history. For example, Paracelsus used a safe level of mercury to cure syphilis. The safe level caused diseases, side effects and the poisons had delayed disease-causing reactions. Safe levels of poison medicines (allopathic) used by M.D. medicine cause heart attacks, diseases, birth defects, AIDS, locomotors ataxia and poresis. Historically, poisons were used as medicine by Ehrlich (1911), who used a poisonous arsenic compound "salvarsan" to cure syphilis without success. Poisonous Arsenic and Mercury were used in a Syphilis experiment on Tuskegee, Alabama Negroes. It was a behavioral modification experiment mislabeled Syphilis and a biochemical Caucasian terrorist attack. These toxic medicinal drugs were not safe nor is the public water or the so-called food industry's modern drugs safe as they quietly eat away the life of the human body by poisoning it. *(100,000,000 Guinea Pigs. Dangers in Everyday Foods, Drugs, and Cosmetics* by A. Kallet and F. J. Schlink *Drugs, Doctors and Disease* by B. Inglis).*

THE QUESTION IS . . .MEAT?

Meat consumption or the eating of dead animal corpses is sometimes overlooked and unquestioned. Eating meat is more of a religious belief than a nutritional belief. Meat is not a complete protein. Beans, nuts and seeds combinations provide complete protein. Mass media has focused upon meat's protein value. However, there are some other dimensions to it.

Historically, the eating of dead animal corpses in African cultures was a part of rituals and ceremonies or a substitute in cases where no other primary protein food supply existed. On the other hand, in Caucasian culture, animal flesh eating became a part of their diet due to the Ice Age (the absence of abundant vegetation), cannibalism, food shortages and cultural preferences.

It is believed to be safer to eat animals that eat vegetables, rather than to eat animals that eat animals. Biological magnification or the increased accumulation of toxins, chemicals and diseases occurs when one animal eats another animal. Subsequently, animals such as fish, scavengers such as crabs, snails and lobsters and especially the hog (also referred to as swine, pig and pork) are labeled as highly unsafe and unclean to eat.

The buzzard and hog are physically structured to eat rotten flesh, animal manure and decayed filth. Hogs are fed the rotten corpses of dead chickens in their diets. Non-organic chickens and cattle are fed meat protein, which can include chicken and cattle meat. This causes them to be contaminated by bacteria and worms that live in the rotten flesh of the corpse of the dead.

All animal corpses are contaminated and bacteria infested. It is the putrefaction of all animal flesh (chicken, cattle, lamb and fish), which causes it to be tender. Cooking flesh speeds up the putrefaction process and dehydrates the meat. It is the putrefied, decayed flesh, blood, waste and pus that give meat its delicious taste. The cooked blood and pus actually gives meat its flavor. Fat helps you taste the pus and blood. Food experts generally agree that putrefaction has set in when bacteria reach ten million per gram. Researchers have found that over 40% of all purchased packaged meats are spoiled (putrefied). Exposure to this spoiled flesh and radiation is harmful. Added to this, the meat is irradiated with nuclear waste. This causes cancer in humans. The U.S. Bureau of Labor lists exposure to slaughterhouse work as the third most hazardous occupation. This is due to the harmful bacteria, worms, chemicals, hormones and dis-eases that are carried by dead animal contaminated corpses of the food animals (i.e., chicken, cattle, pigs, etc.) Exposure to radiation in the meat compounds the hazard to a new level of danger.

Slaughtered animals are usually dis-eased with tuberculosis, parasites, worms, tumors, and cancer. Large cancer sores, tumors and diseased parts are usually cut out and the corpse is then allowed to pass U.S. inspection. There is a relationship between a dis-eased corpse and the increased cancer rate amongst humans. Aside from this, human anatomical factors are involved.

Natural meat eaters eat flesh raw. Accordingly, natural meat eaters have claws, sharp teeth, sweat through the mouth, have a short intestine which is two-thirds the length of their bodies (humans are thirty feet long), their jaws move up and down only and the stomach can digest hair. Humans lack all of these natural meat-eating traits. The human intestinal tract causes meat to stay in the body for up to three days. This causes toxins to be absorbed in the body creating diseases, while the natural meat eaters raw flesh diet allows meat to leave quickly (one day or less).

Flesh eating increases the workload of the kidneys and liver. It is usually cooked, which dehydrates the meat and dehydrates the consumer of meat. Consequently, this decreases immunity and degenerates the body. Aside from this, the animals secrete adrenaline into their bodies as a reaction to the fear caused by the slaughterhouse. This adrenaline poisons the flesh, creates toxins and becomes a chemical stress when eaten. It causes disease.

Many types of diseases are transmitted by dead animals. The disease of Salmonella poisoning causes symptoms which resemble "colds," "flus," and "viruses." These symptoms are misdiagnosed and treated with "cold" medicines. Botulism or food poisoning cannot be stopped by refrigeration or by cooking. Actually, the meat is poison and not a food. It cannot be a food and a poison. In other words, the phrase "food poison" is a lie. It is not food. It is poison. Cooking does not kill many strains of heat resistant parasites and worms. Meat is one of the most highly processed foods. It is processed with steroids, hormones, antibiotics and chemicals. When meat is cooked, some chemicals in it change to new harmful chemicals, which are dangerous. The fats in the meat become synthetic poisons.

Worms found in hogs are difficult to destroy. The worms get into the blood, muscles and nerves of humans. The worm eggs hatch and cause muscle pain, inflammation of the nerves and muscles. These worms hatch thousands of eggs into the entire body. The worms have toxic bowel movements. The worms dig into the intestines, which result in an upset stomach; get into glands such as prostrate, as well as uterus, vagina and rectum; causes breathing difficulties; vision problems; and sexual arousal and problems. The microscopic examination of slaughtered animals for parasites and worms is too expensive and has been abandoned by the health department. Many of these parasites live on and in farm animals and household pets (a dog, licking a person's face spreads worms), so, it is difficult to protect oneself in the presence of animals. There is no safe way to kill many types of worms and parasites. The reason for this is that anything that can kill these types of worms can also kill the person. Packaged fish and canned flesh are carriers of worms and they are putrefied and filthy. Because the U.S. Department of Agriculture has established "dirt" levels for meat and dry foods. Dirt is non-food items such as rat hairs, feces, worms and actual dirt.

Antibiotics and other chemicals cannot protect meat. The U.S. Meat Inspection Service recognizes over 42 diseases in animals. This makes flesh eating dangerous and antibiotics useless. There are over 80 diseases that can be transmitted from dead animals to man. The continued eating of antibiotics in animal corpses causes human resistance to antibiotics and immunity to penicillin. Antibiotics in food animals helps people to develop resistance to drug therapy. Chemicals added to meat to retard spoilage cause cancer. They also retard digestion and immunity. The chemicals give meat a nice red color and deodorize the rotten smell. The deodorizers do not stop the meat from having a bad taste nor do they kill the animals' diseases.

Animal flesh eating was never restricted to the muscles of cattle, fish, fowl, pigs and herbivores. Caucasians eat muscle because they believe to make human muscle you have to eat animal muscle. Carbohydrates build amino acids and amino acids build muscle. When you eat animal, protein in the body has to break it down to amino acids then build protein. Your body works twice as hard to use meat while vegetables are metabolized as amino acids then built into protein. Amongst the ancient African, Greek and Roman civilizations, the eating of insect's flesh and flesh eating plants were included in the flesh eater's diet. In these ancient civilizations, the flesh eaters would eat the organs of the animals and the entire insect. Eating organs gave rise to the internal organ medical system called glandular therapy. The book, *Glandular Extracts,* by Dr. Donsbach, is suggested. Don and Patricia Brothwell also review this concept in the book, *Food and Antiquity.*

Ancient African flesh consumption indicates a broad food nutritional base. For example, caterpillars and termites were food crops; termites were toasted or eaten raw by the Pygmies. The Bantu ate caterpillars as a source of B vitamins, minerals and proteins.

ANIMAL PROTEIN AND
VEGETABLE PROTEIN EQUIVALENTS

ANIMAL PROTEINS	ALTERNATIVE VEGETABLE AND GRAIN PROTEINS
Eggs	Navy and Black Beans
Fish	Millet, Lentils
Beef	Wheat, Barley
Cheese	Soybeans, Corn (Rice Cheese, Soy Cheese)
Poultry	Garbanzo Beans, Raw Peanuts, Sunflower Seeds, Green Peas

COMPLETE PROTEIN COMBINATIONS

- Beans and Brown Rice, (Wild, Basmati, etc.)
- Corn and Green Beans
- Corn and Lima Beans
- Millet and Green Beans
- Garbanzo Beans and Seeds
- Tofu and Rice (Brown, Wild, Basmati, etc.)
- Whole Grain Pasta (Wheat, Brown Rice, etc.), Sesame Seeds and Corn
- Bulgur Wheat and Dried Beans

HOT DOGS AND HAMBURGER:
A MOUTH FULL OF DEATH

Hamburger meat and other processed animal flesh have sodium nicotinate (a poison) to preserve color, and beef blood is used to add color. Fat levels ideally should be 20%. However, the federal and state governments have set a fat level of 30% to 50%. Aside from this, meat-wrapping paper has toxic preservatives in it and poisonous cancerous agents and the antibiotic chlortetracycline.

The hot dog was formerly called frankfurters. However, the German name was dropped after the Euro-American tribal war with Hitler's Germany. The USDA has no fat limit for hot dogs and the water content can be as high as 63%. Sodium sulfite or a similar chemical is used to hide the foul smell of rotten hot dogs, hamburgers and other meats. This chemical causes gastrointestinal diseases. The meats are usually contaminated and dis-eased before they are slaughtered. An "all meat" hot dog or processed meat includes steroids, excess estrogen, preservatives, deodorizers, dirt (unspecified matter), cereals, pork, cancerous coal tar, insect scales and dyes. If the label reads "all beef", it can have 70-80% beef mixed with chicken, pork, lamb and meat by-products. If it says pure beef, it merely means the beef in it is "beef," and the other meats are not beef. The mixture is beef = "pure beef."

MEAT INSPECTION

Federal meat inspection is largely a well-manipulated tool of the meat industry. The meat industry is basically the lord of the meat colonies (farmers). Federal inspection is totally inadequate and poor, yet the animal corpse peddlers avoid it by selling meat locally- within the state. Meat that crosses state lines must be federally inspected, not meat bought and sold within a state. Individual state inspection is much, much lower than the poor standards of federal inspection. The United Nation's Food and Agricultural Organization concluded that in the meat industry, diseases are more serious today than ever before. No current method of U.S. meat (includes seafood and poultry) inspection can assure non-contaminated and disease-free meat.

Meat Grading is confused with inspection for safety. Grading is merely the ratio of fat to meat and does not indicate that the meat is disease free. In fact, grading is a voluntary choice of the meat industries. The standards for grading are manipulated by the meat industry.

Pork
It is illegal to feed raw garbage to hogs. However, processed (cooked) garbage is legal. This cooked garbage is so-called animal feed food and causes anemia, ulcers and systemic disorders (dis-ease in the entire pig). Antibiotics, such as copper sulfate (a poison), are fed to hogs to increase their growth. Copper sulfate causes nerve and brain damage, senility and decreases the life span. The same cancer-causing chemicals that are in the animal are eaten by the consumer of the animal flesh. Giving animals inoculations makes the consumer believe that the cancerous and dis-eased hogs are safe. Pork has never been graded. The ratio of fat to meat (grading) is solely controlled by the pig industry, not the federal government. Fat is the storage place for high concentrations of estrogen, steroids, chemicals, preservatives and other non-specified chemicals. Pigs are being cloned and genetically modified, causing them to have new strains of diseases that cannot be killed or treated. The pig eaters eat new diseases.

Ham is injected with synthetic pickling fluid (smoked flavor) and phosphates. Phosphates allow ham to hold water. The poisonous chemicals used in pickling (smoked) ham are never listed. The USDA has approved these chemicals. The use of phosphates allows water to be sold at ham prices. Some hams have more than 10% water in them. The meat industry, wanting to avoid this federal health and safety standards and regulations buys pigs in the same state that they were sold. States not wanting to lose tax dollars or hurt the local farm, grain, drug, machine, labor and secondary supporting industries manipulate and lower health and safety meat standards and alter inspection procedures so that the state can keep revenues high.

Chicken

Chicken feed has poisonous arsenic (to speed growth), antibiotics, growth hormones, steroids, tranquilizers, anti-infective agents, aspirin, stilbestrol (causes birth defects) and pesticides. These chemical poisonous drugs get into the chicken flesh and are eaten by the consumer. The FDA approves these chemicals and more. USDA does not detect all contamination and diseases of fowls. In fact, they found one out of five birds are unfit for human consumption and yet they pass state inspections. Chickens are filthy garbage eating birds. They are pigs with feathers.

Synthetic urea (a chemical found in urine) is used as a protein substitute because it is cheap and partially eliminates the need for expensive soybeans. In others, they feed the animals unsterilized urine. Meat packers use meat tenderizers so that the tough, stringy flesh of old bulls, cows, pigs, lambs and chickens can be sold as high quality meat.

Synthetic cancerous pesticides are fed to animals in order to keep the manure free of flies. Pesticides are internally injected to kill worms that are in the animal. Once eaten, they interfere with digestion. DDT-like chemicals are used and it has been proven by the Texas Research Foundation in 1950 that meat is contaminated and rendered unsafe due to pesticides such as DDT and chemicals of similar molecular structure.

Cancer-causing drugs are put in animal feed to increase the animal's size. The Food and Drug Administration approved the use of stilbestrol in 1955. It was scientifically proven to cause cancer by the International Union Against Cancer in 1956. Additionally, antibiotics are given to food animals. This causes bacteria to develop a resistance to drugs in man and makes the prescribing of medications for infections a questionable therapeutic value. The Food and Drug Law Institute meeting in 1966 proved this to be true. Tranquilizers are given to animals to increase growth and it is given to cows to increase milk production. They also increase the effect of stilbestrol and antibiotics aside from being harmful to man. Notwithstanding, the FDA approved their use and has allowed doubling of the use of many of them. Ironically, stilbestrol (a hormone) is used to cause sterile cows to produce milk and to sterilize bulls. People who eat this hormone will develop reproductive problems and have children with birth defects. The effect of this hormone, combined with other chemicals has dangerous repercussions.

The FDA has approved the use of cancer-causing chemicals such as sodium nitrite, sodium nitrate, sodium ascorbate and a complete list of these would fill an entire book. Bulletin No. 4 of the federal government proves that these chemicals are cancerous. Many cancerous and AIDS causing chemicals are used just to give a good red color to meat and hide the spoiled smell and taste. Boston's Children's Cancer Foundation has scientifically proven that the meat industries' chemicals cause degenerative disease, cancer, AIDS and produce abnormal growths. Yet, the use of these synthetic chemicals continues with the federal government's approval.

Fish and seafood get the same chemicals in them via fish feed and seafood feed used by the fishery farms and the chemicalized ice that they are packed in for shipment. Many chemicals are used at the fisheries (seafood farms) and they use chemically polluted water.

The eating of the dead corpses of animals is an ethical, religious, moral, ecological, humanitarian and economical issue. However, the question of "Should you eat meat?" or "Should you not eat meat?" has to be answered by each individual.

FAST FOODS, EXERCISE OR DIE

Fast foods clog the veins and arteries, thicken the blood, cause heart attacks, strokes, diabetes, obesity, dehydration, degenerative diseases, constipation, aging, electrolyte stress (rust the tissue-oxidize), mood swings, food addiction and death. The calories, from eating them, must be immediately burnt off or else diseases will start. However, exercising to burn off calories speeds up the damaging effect while not exercising lets the damage happen slower. It is not a matter of if you will get sick—it is when you will get sick. The sickness actually begins when you eat the junk. Your nose running is your body getting rid of the junk. Cancer and AIDS means your body failed to get rid of the junk.

Cheeseburger
It has the same amount of fats as two cups of ice cream and over 300 calories. Burn the calories: Lift weights for almost two hours.

Soda
It is liquid chemicals with sugar, dye, artificial flavor and carbonated water that dehydrates you. A 64-ounce soda has 800 calories, 90 grams of sugar, and 3 grams of salt. Drinking sodas does not reduce your craving for food. You drink them and are still hungry. Sugar causes thirst.

Sodas have indigestible salts (i.e., synthetic electrolytes = mineral salts). This causes electrolyte stress, which oxidizes (makes rusts that breaks down tissue) the muscles, nerves and bones, resulting in bone loss, pancreas and kidney damage, heart stress, loss of oxygen to the brain, hardening of veins and arteries, mood swings, tension, eye problems, hair loss, sex organ problems, etc.

For each bottle (24 ounces, etc.) of soda, mix it with two bottles (48 ounces, etc.) of water, then drink. This will help avoid electrolyte stress and slow down the immediate damaging disease process.

Burn the calories: Ride a stationary bike for 120 minutes, jump rope for one hour or play basketball for two hours.

Sports Drinks

Sports drinks are non-carbonated sodas with extra indigestible electrolytes (mineral salts). They cause the same damage as sodas and dehydrate the body.

For each bottle of the drink, mix three bottles of water with it before you drink it. This will postpone the immediate damage of the electrolyte stress.

Burn the calories: Jump rope for two hours, ride a stationary bike for three hours or play soccer for two hours. Then ride a bike or walk to cemeteries and funeral homes to pick out your last resting place.

French Fries (Dies)

They are cancer causing cooked trans-fatty acid. It is grease disguised as a potato. Fifty grams or more of fat (depends on size) and greasy indigestible potatoes.

Burn Calories: Skate or swim for one hour or run at least seven miles per hour for one hour.

Potato Chips

They are greasy thin toilet tissue thin-sized slices of potatoes in the shape of chips.

Contains 80 grams of fat, 25 grams of salt, 2 grams of sugar, 75 grams of carbohydrates and 330 calories.

Burn calories: Play basketball for two hours or rock climb for thirty minutes.

Pork Skins

They can cause a pig to have bypass surgery, aside from giving it high blood pressure, a stroke and heart attack.

Contains 195 grams of fat, 60 grams of salt, 300 grams of carbohydrates, over 240 calories.

Burn calories: Ride a bike, jump rope for one hour or chase a pig for thirty minutes.

Glazed Donut

No fiber, no nutrients plus grease and white sugar.

Contains 30 grams of carbohydrates, 1 gram of protein, 9 grams of fat and 200 calories.

Burn calories: Jump rope for fifteen minutes, bike ride for twenty minutes or lift weights for twenty-five minutes.

Salad with Diced Meat, Cheese, Crouton (Bread Cubes)

Contains 65 grams of fat, 25 grams of carbohydrates, 43 grams of protein, 815 calories.

Burn calories: Go hiking with a 10 to 20 pound backpack for one hour and forty-five minutes.

Suggested source for information: www.mensfitness.com.

SHOULD WE EAT GRASS?

The African domestication of plants brought new vegetable foods to the diet. The breeding (domestication) of hybrids (special) in the grass family created a new diet. The plants in the grass family are wheat, rice, millet, oat, barley, rye, etc. These are the fruit part of the grass. They are technically fruits. The leaves are not fruit and difficult to eat. Ancient Africans use the leaves for paper (papyrus, etc.)

The grass family was part of the agricultural wealth of Africa. These grasses were used to create monies and the mercantile system. In ancient history, Greeks and Romans used Africa as a colony for food grass (granary) farming.

Cultivation of large portions of land for plant domesticated grass farming required the exploitation and deterioration of the soil. This caused ecological imbalances and interruption of the wild plants as well as soil cycle. It created disharmony in the ecology and altered the ecological balance of plants, insects, air, soil, water, animals and people. Cultivation farming was a large part of African agriculture.

Non-cultivation plant farming, which does not require stripping the land of minerals, clearing the land of plants and tilling of the soil was also performed. It was (and is) called non-cultivation plant farming. In this type of farming, the trees, plants, waters, animals and land resources were left as they were. Holes were dug and seeds planted according to the moon and astrology. This did not disturb the wild plants' ecological system.

Non-cultivation farming allowed the plants to live free and wild. These non-cultivated crops were not domesticated. The non-cultivation plants were of higher nutritional food value. This non-cultivation farming did not have a higher crop production, but it did require the humans to be in tune with the rhythm and cycles of the earth and planets (i.e., moon). Wild or free-living plants such as rye, millet, barley, and wheat are smaller, and higher in nutritional value. They excite the body's nutritive powers to a greater degree. The leaves of wild grass is too tough to eat raw which limits the humans to eating the fruit of the wild grass such as ripe wheat berries, rice, rye, corn, oat and barley. The fruits of the grasses are slightly green when eaten. Unripe rice is not partially green. Grains ripen early while sweet fruits ripen later in their growing season.

The eating of the wild grass stem and leaf in its natural state requires the human to get down on their hands and knees. Natural grass eaters' mouths are not high from the grass, just as a giraffe's mouth is not far from the leaves and fruits of trees. Natural grass eaters have more than one stomach, and a longer transit time (time it takes food to get from the mouth to the bowels and out the body). People cannot chew or digest wheat grass.

The grass-eating animals (cattle, sheep, goats) have flat teeth. They grind the grass with a circular motion of the jaw. Humans grind food up and down, segmentedly and circularly. Grass eating animals eat their grass raw and when it is in cycle. When the summer grass is out of cycle, they switch to the much tougher and shorter winter grass.

The grinding (chewing) and complete digestion of raw grass requires a very strong stomach acid. Humans cannot produce this type of stomach acid. If humans are natural grass eaters, then they are totally, anatomically ill-prepared for eating grass and would die from this diet. The fruit of grass can be eaten, such as wheat berries, oat seeds (oat meal), Rye, Buckwheat, Kamut, Spelt, Rice, Corn, etc. People cannot eat the leaves as only a grass eater can chew the leaves.

ARE YOU EATING FOOD OR DRUGS?

The herbal drugs in ancient African and European histories were simply labeled drugs. A drug is any substance that has been isolated, concentrated, or taken out of its natural state. Drugs can be made from (synthesized) organic matter, nonorganic matter, living things, or non-living things. Drugs are synthetic chemicals and synthetic dirt. Drugs cause the biochemistry to slow down, speed up, genetically altering and/or exhausting the body's melanin. Melanin malfunctions or is depleted in its response to a drug. Melanin has a malfunction reaction because drugs are synthetic dirt and dirt has no action. Drugs do not have actions or side effects – the body has them. A drug is an isolated concentrated substance and, the food industry has confused the public on the definition of a drug for capital gain. A drug, no matter how natural the food or herb may be, is still a drug. An isolated concentrated substance causes chemical imbalances when eaten and can cause a nutritional drain in the body. Consequently, all health practitioners use drug concentrates (i.e., vitamins, minerals, amino acids, glandulars) for the treatment of dis-eases. Herbs are heated (simmered, boiled) and heat brings out the curative properties of the herb. Heat also concentrates nutrients, which means they are put in a drug-like form. Heat simplifies (concentrates) the nutrients. Herbs were called simples.

Drugs can be used allopathically, that is they can be used to create a second illness in the body. The allopathic principle is based on introducing a dis-ease into the body. The prescriptions drug (a poisonous chemical) is a dis-eased substance. The body is biochemically altered and reacts by getting rid of the secondary dis-ease, which altered the body's chemistry and causes an immunity reaction. In this process, the primary dis-ease is supposedly cured by a rise in the body's immune defenses to get rid of the drug. In allopathic medicine, the patient can die from the cure.

Drugs can also be used homeopathically. In homeopathic drug medicine the dis-ease is excited. In other words, a drug is given that will produce (excite, stimulate) the same dis-ease in a healthy person. For example, a person with a venereal dis-ease would be given a homeopathic
remedy that causes venereal diseases. In this system, the patient can die
from the cause of dis-ease.

In naturopathic medicine, herbs are used as food medicine or heated to
concentrate them. This makes them drug-like, but not toxic. In naturopathic medicine, the patient is given a fresh, dried or heated herb that will
help the body defend itself. The herbs nourish and strengthen the immunity. Naturopathic medicine generally follows the defense reactions of the
body. For example, if a patient has mucous flow from the nose, then this
could indicate that the body is putting waste in the mucous and the waste-
filled mucous is being discharged out the nose. The mucous in the nasal cavities reduces the oxygen. This makes the body acid. Acidity helps break
down waste. The body is maintaining its healthy tissue and reducing the
waste from diseased tissue. The naturopathy modality would increase the
nutrients to the body's tissues. This can be done with herbs such as goldenseal, barberry, or boneset, etc. In naturopathic medicine, the patient dies
from natural causes, not from disease.

The treatments in all of the above systems are based on drugs. Sugar
removed from its natural plant state is a drug (honey, beet or cane sugar,
maple syrup). Honey was used as a medicine in ancient Africa and later
became a common food condiment. It is a concentrated sugar extract
(processed) from a flower by a bee. It is a drug obtained from flowers. In
this instance, the bee is turned into a drug pusher. The sugar, within the stalk
of sugar cane, sugar in the flower, barley, rice, malt and/or maple sap is safe.
In other words, you would have to eat a sugar cane stalk, a flower, barley,
rice or drink maple sap to have a safe sugar. Eating isolated concentrated
sugars are harmful. They weaken and/or destroy the pancreas, liver, kidneys and degenerate the health. They are sweet drugs.

Oil is another drug that was used by ancient African physicians. Olive
oil was used as an emollient, laxative aid, a solvent of cholesterol and
demulcent; stimulate peristaltic contractions and stimulated production of
chyle and liver bile. In later centuries, oil became a condiment. Any oil
taken out of its natural state causes a nutritional imbalance when eaten.
Oils were meant to be eaten in their natural nutritional tribes of vitamins,
minerals, fiber and water. Corn oil, safflower oil, peanut oil, all vegetable
oils should be eaten while within the plant, and not separated (extracted)
from the plant and then eaten. One teaspoon of corn oil would approximately take over 24 ears of corn to produce. Nature limits the amount of
oil that can be safely eaten without causing damage to the biochemical
balance and nutritional homeostasis. Oil drugs are processed, cooked and
refined and the nutrients are filtered out. Filtering out nutrients makes the
oil clear. The non-cold pressed oils usually use industrial solvents (lye,

acid) to dissolve the nutrients and process the oil. The oils usually have traces of toxic poisonous chemicals in them. Heating the oil turns it into a trans-oil, which is a plastic liquid that causes cancer. Processed oils are addicting. The temperature has to be at least 200 degrees Fahrenheit to digest (breakdown) oil. Oil clogs blood cells, causes waste to accumulate, decreases oxygen, and stresses the liver and heart. Medically, cold pressed oils (2 to 3 tablespoons) are used to stimulate the liver to secrete bile, which breaks down fats and helps digestion and oil is used to help constipation.

Oil and other drugs such as sugars, salt, bleached flour, etc. are partial foods. The body tries to make the partial food into a whole food. This is accomplished by taking the necessary nutrients from the eyes, immune system, brain, nerves, sex organs, heart, kidneys, liver, bones, muscles and other body parts. The body's nutritional Maat wisdom dictates that all partial foods (isolated and concentrated) must be restored to their original nutritional value and made into whole foods. Consequently, the whole body is traumatized and nutritionally shocked by a drug and robs itself of water, minerals and vitamins (commits nutritional suicide) and then sends its defenses to rid body of the drug. The high feeling that drugs such as sugar or alcohol give is the defensive reaction of the body. In due course, the body nutritionally loses this fight and submits to the alcohol dis-ease of intoxification or sugar drug dis-ease of hyper or hypoglycemia (diabetes) or submits to the oil drug triglyceride dis-ease of high triglycerides, loss of ability to metabolize oil, cellulite, obesity or hardening of the arteries and veins.

The average daily junk food diet consists of one to four cups of oil. There are hidden oils in pastries, ice cream, salad dressing, breads, catsup, cake, juices, mayonnaise, mustards, soups, gum, fried foods, candy, toothpaste, prescribed medicines, etc. Oil (butter, margarine) is used to enhance the flavor of food.

Bleached white flour and polished white rice are drugs. The roughage and more than thirty-two nutrients are milled and isolated from the white flour and rice. Bleached white flour and polished white rice are isolated concentrated starches. Again, a drug is any isolated, concentrated substance. Calling a drug a food, spice or condiment does not change its effect upon the body. The liver does not know the difference between a prescription drug, illegal drug or a food drug. A drug is a drug to the liver. Your mind may play tricks about what is a drug, but the liver does not. Drugs cause nutritional imbalances, addiction and a melanin drain.

A drug eater either dies from lack of knowledge of the drug or lack of knowledge of the dis-ease the drug produces. The ancient African healers believed that herbs should do no harm and food is the true medicine. The practitioners were trained in the proper preparation and use of herbal teas, extracts and concentrated herbs (drugs) to excite the body towards health. The consumer is being drugged by commercial food drug business. The drug foods are synthetic bowel movements. The whole foods are sent to a factory where machines similar to the teeth, liver, pancreas and intestines strip away fiber, nutrients and water, leaving a fully processed food = bowel movement = food drug.

An herb in its natural state is raw and fresh. Once the herb is cooked (as in tea) it becomes a drug. Heat causes the nutritional tribe of vitamins and minerals to segregate and concentrate. This isolation of the nutrients creates a drug reaction in the plant. The liquids (teas) made from herbs are firstly a food and secondly a drug. All heated herbs are drugs. Technically, all cooked or fired (heated by fire) foods are drugs. In this respect, most of the addicting substances are cooked, such as tobacco, cocaine, marijuana, coffee, sugar, heroin, cola drinks, sweet pastries, and alcohol.

The socially approved drug addicts are addicted to white sugar and they out number the alcoholics, heroin, cocaine and prescribed allopathic medicine addicts. The Caucasians take a predatory military approach to herbs and concentrated herbs called vitamins (vegetarian supplement). In ancient times, they would attack their enemy, kill them and cut the enemy's heart out and eat it. Today, they attack the herbs and vegetarian (concentrated herbs) supplement, kill them (processing) and take the vital nutrients out. This creates a drug. African Maat healers respect the herb and use it as a whole food in liquid or concentrated form; thus do not harm the ill person.

The Caucasians changed the use and purpose of herbs in order to gain profit and control the plants. They changed the definition to simple spices, condiments, and seasonings. It is the preparation of a drug (leaving it as whole as possible = African) or fragmenting it (Caucasian) that can excite the body to health or disease. African civilizations holistically perfected a harmless herbal drug system beyond the scope of contemporary Caucasian's knowledge. The ancient African healers used Maat and believed the body to be a holy temple and herbs were a way of worshipping the temple. The Caucasians believed the body to be a machine. Diseases attack the body so they attack diseases by attacking the body. Diseases are believed to poison so they use a bigger poison such as a drug or radiation to kill the attacker.

Today, the drug trade continues. Chemical behavior modifiers were synthesized in Germany during the Hitler regime. The modern name for Hitler's original drug company is Merck, Glaxo and Smith. The synthetic drugs created during Hitler's era were released and duplicated on the world trade market. The scientists had to make synthetic copies of herbs (heroin's synthetic equal is Methadone) because they could not obtain the herbs. Consequently, they synthetically made many drugs. Many of these synthetic drugs (behavior modifiers) became knows as preservatives and additives. The formulas for making these drugs were part of the Nuremberg trial papers and were not disclosed to the general public. They are exclusive property of multinationals, secret societies and clans that control Caucasian governments. The junk food companies and pharmaceutical cartel put synthetic chemicals in cosmetics, deodorants, toothpastes, skin creams, hair preparations, eyewashes, deodorized sanitary pads, toilet paper, mineral oil, hair sprays, soaps, detergents, mouthwashes, colognes, non-organic meat, eggs and dairy, baby foods, etc. The same chemicals used for bio-chemical warfare is in their products. It is biochemical war against the consumer. All drugs are addicting and alter the behavior and biochemistry of the consumer. The victim of the drug trade is the consumer.

MICRO-GRAVE / MICROWAVE
(Instant Cooking – Instant Disease)

The microwave oven is a dangerous machine that causes mental and phys-ical diseases. The initial German experiments were done at Humboldt Universitat at Berlin (1942-3). Further information on its dangers was reported in *The Journal of Natural Science* (April-June 1998) by Dr. Hans V. Hertel of the World Foundation for Natural Science in Switzerland. The former Soviet Union's report on microwaves caused them to ban them from use in 1976. William Kopp's paper in *The Journal of Natural Science* further verified the health hazards of microwaves. Microwaves kill, mutate and deteriorate all types of human cells. Melanin dominant Africans absorb the highest level of toxic radiation from the microwaves. The machines are not safe and are extremely dangerous for pregnant women, children, sperm and ovaries.

Biological Effects of Exposure
- Being around microwaves for long periods of time causes the loss of vital energies within humans, animals, plants and all liv-ing things. If you are within a 500-mile radius of the opera-tional equipment, it is considered dangerous.
- Causes imbalances, insufficiency and malfunctioning of hor-mones in males and females.
- The nervous system and lymphatic systems can get negative side effects resulting in emotional, mental, physical and immune deterioration.
- Brainwave disturbance in the alpha, theta and delta wave signal patterns.
- Destroys the bioelectric, biomagnetic and biochemical life energy field.
- Negative psychological effects (produced as a result of the brain wave pattern changes) that included: decreases memory, decreases the ability to concentrate, changes in intellect and emotional responses and sleep disturbances.
- Interrupts, alters, breakdowns and deteriorates nerve messages in the brain.
- Causes imbalances and deterioration of cells inside the body.

- Decreases the nutritional value of foods especially minerals and Vitamins B, C and E.

Cancer Causing Effects
- Eating food heated in microwaves causes a higher percentage of cancer cells within the blood.
- Can cause stomach and intestinal cancerous growth and the deterioration of the function of the excretory and digestive systems.
- It creates cancer causing agents in milk and cereal grains.
- Cooking or heating meat in them creates the cancer causing agent D-nitrosodiethanoloamine.
- Food becomes biochemically cloned and when eaten can result in bodily malfunctioning, which decreases the body's ability to stop some types of cancerous growth.
- Thawing frozen foods with microwave radiation biologically alters frozen foods.
- Biological alteration of foods occurs when they are briefly exposed to microwaves.
- Microwaves' electromagnetically alter foods and people, resulting in genetic caused diseases.

DYING TO LOOK GOOD
(The Eating of Harmful Cosmetic Ingredients)

Cosmetics and personal care products are usually made with harmful synthetic chemicals. The chemicals are absorbed into the skin and get into the blood. What you put on your skin you are eating. You eat your cosmetics. The following list is just a few of the many dangerous actions of chemicals used to improve skin beauty.

AHA's (Alpha Hydroxy Acids, i.e., Lactic and Others)
Removing the outer layer of the skin, IT exposes to environmental toxic agents. AHA's make you age faster. AHA is an acid produced by anaerobic respiration. Skin care products with AHA exfoliate by destroying live and dead skin cells and the skin's protective barrier. AHA causes long-term skin damage. AHA burns away your top skin layer and can cause keloids. It gives a temporary youthful appearance to the skin. However, later in life the skin appears older. AHA gets into the blood and exfoliates the tissue of organs.

Albumin
Formulas usually contain non-purified cow's bovine serum albumin. It dries the skin and forms a film over wrinkles. This film causes the skin to suffocate and hold more waste. The film temporarily covers wrinkles. It

does not remove wrinkles. Film causes the fingers to slip over wrinkles, the slippery feeling results in a smooth skin feeling.

Aluminum
A metallic element used to make pots, pans, cans, motors, aircraft components, prosthetic devices, etc. It is an ingredient in antiperspirants, antacids, and antiseptics. Aluminum clogs the pores of the skin, blocks blood flow and drains electrical energy from the body and brain. It can contribute to nerves overheating resulting in irritability and pain. It can cause Alzheimer's because it can cause the brain's blood vessels to get clogged, varicose, metallic, overheated and damaged.

Animal Fat (Tallow)
Oily solids or semisolids that are water insoluble esters of glycerol with fatty acids. The oil causes the skin to feel slippery and smooth. It does not make the skin smooth or soft. It can breed bacteria.

Bentonite
This natural mineral is used in facial masks. It is not a true clay. It is mixed with liquid and forms a gel, the clay particles have sharp edges that scratch the skin. Bentonites dry the skin.

Bentonite traps waste and carbon dioxide. It stops the skin from getting oxygen, which results in aging of the skin.

Boitin (Vitamin H)
The molecular size of Biotin is too large to penetrate the skin. The skin does not absorb it. A deficiency of Biotin is very, very rare in humans. A deficiency in fur-bearing animals (i.e. rats) causes them to get bald and have greasy scalps. Biotin stopping baldness in animals is the reason for its use despite the fact that human hair and animal fur are different in nutrient requirements.

Collagen
The collagen molecule cannot penetrate the skin because it is too large to be absorbed by the epidermis (skin). It provides a slippery coating on the skin and suffocates it. It does not nourish the skin or add to human collagen.

Coal Tar (D&C, FD&C)
Cancer causing, color pigments which cause skin sensitivity, irritation, depletion of oxygen in the body and death. The colors are used in foods, drugs, and cosmetics.

Diethanolamine (DEA)
A colorless liquid or crystalline alcohol that causes kidney and liver cancers and irritates the skin and mucous membrane. It is used as a solvent, emulsi-

fier, and detergent (wetting agent). DEA works as an emollient in skin soft-ening lotions or as humectants in other personal care products. Other poisonous ethanolamines are MEA (monoethanolamine), TEA (triethanolamine). DEA & MEA are listed on the ingredient label with the compound being neutralized. (Cocamide DEA or MEA, Lauramide DEA, etc.) These are hormone-disrupting chemicals and are known to form cancer causing nitrates and nitrosamines. These are in personal care products that foam, including bubble baths, body washes, shampoos, soaps and facial cleansers.

Elastin (Not cross-linked Elastin)
It cannot be absorbed by the epidermis (skin). It cannot restore tone to skin. It forms a film over the skin, which holds in waste, carbon dioxide and moisture.

Fluorocarbons
A colorless, nonflammable gas or liquid that causes mild upper respiratory tract irritation. They are used as a propellant in hairspray.

Fragrance (i.e., Perfume, Cologne)
A combination of up to 4,000 ingredients found in fragrances. It is used in most deodorants, shampoos, sunscreens, skin care, body care and baby products. Many compounds in fragrance are carcinogenic or otherwise toxic. Fragrances can cause headaches, dizziness, rashes, skin discoloration, coughing and vomiting, and allergic skin irritation, depression, hyperactivity, irritability, inability to cope, and other behavioral changes.

Glycerin
A liquid made by chemically combining water and fat. The water splits the fat into smaller components glycerol and fatty acids. It enhances the spreading qualities of creams and lotions and prevents them from losing water through evaporation. It is a solvent, humectants, and emollient that absorbs moisture from the air and therefore helps keep moisture in creams and other products. Unless the humidity of the air is over 65% Glycerin will dehydrate the skin by pulling the moisture out of the skin. Thus drying you from the inside out, while making your skin dry. It makes dry skin dryer.

Humectants
Moisturizers contain humectants that act as water attractors. They pull moisture out of your skin. The problem with humectants, including propylene glycol and glycerin is that they are only effective when you are in areas with high humidity, if you are going to be in an extremely low humidity atmosphere, such as in an airplane, school, office building, at home, stores, or even a dry room, they take moisture from your skin.

Hyaluronic Acid
It has a high molecular weight (up to 15 million) and cannot penetrate the skin. It forms a film over the skin and suffocates it.

Hypoallergenic
Hypoallergenic means "less than." The word hypoallergenic indicates that the manufacturer believes the product has fewer allergenics than other products. "Hypoallergenic" has little scientific meaning.

Imidazolidinyl Urea
Slows down the skins ability to absorb nutrients and oxygen while slowing the skin's release of carbon dioxide. It helps poisonous formaldehyde to be absorbed.

Isoprophyl Alcohol
It is in hair color rinses, body rubs, hand lotions, aftershave lotions, fragrances etc. It is made from petroleum and is a solvent used in shellac and antifreeze. Inhalation is dangerous and ingestion (one ounce) is fatal.

Kaolin
A natural clay originally from Mt. Kaolin in China, hence the name. It is drying and dehydrating to the skin. It can be contaminated with impurities. It is used in formulations and masks and forms films that stop the skin from breathing. It traps waste, toxins and carbon dioxide in the skin and suffocates the skin by blocking the vitally needed oxygen.

Lauramide Dea
It is used to make lather and thicken cosmetics. It is used in dishwashing detergents to cut grease. It causes the scalp and skin to itch and dries the hair.

Lipsomes
Lipsomes is believed to join with aging skin cells and restore youth to them. However the cell membrane of a young and old person are not alike. Consequently, the lipsomes probably would make young cells older. Thus, its antiaging effect is nullified. They merely coat the skin cells and suffocate them. Coating makes the skin feel smooth and youthful.

Mineral Oil
It is a mixture of liquid hydrocarbons and causes petrochemical hypersensitivity, which causes arthritis, migraine, cancer, hyperkinesis, epilepsy, and diabetes. Taken internally, Mineral Oil binds the fat-soluble Vitamins A, D, E, K and carries them unabsorbed out of the body. Mineral oil does not penetrate the skin and can produce symptoms the same as dry skin by stopping the natural moisturizing factor of the skin. Petrolatum, Paraffin or

Paraffin oil and Propylene Glycol are other common toxic cosmetic forms of Mineral Oil. Mineral Oil can dissolve the skin's own natural oil and increase dehydration of the skin. Mineral oils are probably the greatest cause of bumps, rashes and skin problems. Cancer causing carcinogens are commonly found in Mineral Oil. Baby oil is 100% mineral oil, which coats the skin like liquid plastic. The skin's immune barrier is disrupted as this plastic inhibits its ability to breathe. The oil slows down the skin's functions and normal cell development causing the skin to prematurely age resulting in skin disorders (i.e. acne). It is a petroleum waste product that suffocates the skin and waste accumulates. It was originally sold as a cure for cancer.

Natural Cosmetics
There is no legal definition for "natural." Most cosmetics called "natural" still contain preservatives, coloring agents, and other toxic chemicals.

pH
The term pH stands for the power of the hydrogen atom. Skin and hair do not have a pH. A scale from 0 to 14 is used to measure acidity and alkalinity of solutions, and pH 7.0 is neutral. Acidity is a low pH number (0 to 6.9). And alkalinity is a high pH number (7-14). The pH of cosmetics will not change the pH of the hair or skin because the hair and skin contain keratin, fatty acids, and other substances that adjust the pH. As long as a pH is not unusually high or low there is no pH problem. The high pH of cold wave solutions and hair straighteners damage the hair and skin. There is no such thing as a "pH balanced" product because a product's pH will change while it is on the shelf in the store and change when applied to the hair and skin.

Placental Extract
Extracts cannot nourish the skin and make it youthful. It provides nourishment for a fetus and embryo only. It can be from a human aborted fetus or animal fetus and is usually not sanitized.

Propylene Glycol (PG)
Called a moisturizer or humectant in cosmetics but is actually "industrial antifreeze" It is causes brain, liver and kidney damage and is the major ingredient in brake and hydraulic fluid.

It is used in industry to break down protein and cellular structure (what the skin is made of). It is in make-up, hair products, lotions, after-shave, deodorants, mouthwashes, toothpaste and used in food processing. The EPA requires workers to wear protective gloves, clothing and goggles when working with this toxic substance. The Material Safety Data Sheets (MSDS) warns against skin contact. There is no warning on the labels of products such as stick deodorants, where the concentration is greater than that in most industrial applications.

Polyethylene Glycol (PEG)
Used to dissolve oil and grease as well as thicken products. It is used in caustic spray-on oven cleaners. Polyethylene glycol's contribute to stripping the skin's Natural Moisture Factor. They are carcinogenic and weaken the immunity.

Royal Bee Jelly
It is worthless for skin care. If fresh in a container or stored for over two weeks, royal jelly loses its ability to nourish queen bees. The sugar in it is absorbed into the skin. Sugar has never been proven to improve skin.

Seaweed
This plant has gelatinous properties. Seaweed is used in clear facemask creams and lotions where it gives body and substance to the products, not to the skin. It makes a gelatin liquid. The gelatin liquid coats the skin, which keeps in moisture, waste and carbon dioxide. It blocks the skins ability to get oxygen.

Sodium Chloride (Salt-NaCI)
Sodium chloride is used to make cosmetics thick. It can cause eye and skin irritation if used in high concentrations. It dries the skin, which causes the need to buy more skin products.

Sodium Lauryl Sulfate (SLS)
It is a detergent, which is used in soaps and shampoos. It irritates the eyes, brain, heart, liver, etc. SLS and related substances get into the eyes and other tissues. This is dangerous to infants because they have a greater uptake absorption in the tissues of the eyes. SLS changes the amounts of some proteins in cells that form eye tissues. Tissues of young children's eyes may be more susceptible to alternation by SLS (Green). SLS forms cancer-causing nitrates. These nitrates are in shampoo, bubble bath, and shower gels and facial cleansers and get into the blood. SLS are used for their detergent and foam-building properties. They cause skin rashes, hair loss, scalp scurf similar to dandruff, and allergic reactions. They are in cosmetics with the parenthetic explanation "comes from coconut." SLS are used in garage floor cleaners, engine degreasers, and car wash soaps. It can retard healing, cause cataracts in adults, and can keep children's eyes from developing properly. SLS and SLES may cause carcinogenic nitrates and dioxins to form in shampoos and cleansers by reacting with ingredients. SLES is the alcohol form (ethoxylated) of SLS. Both SLS and SLES enter the blood stream.

Sodium Laureth Ether Sulfate (SLES)
An ether chain is added to SLS. It thickens when salt is added in the formula and produces high levels of foam to give the illusion it is thick, rich, and expensive. It is used as a wetting agent in the textile industry. SLES is

irritating to scalp can cause hair loss and gets into the blood causing an array of problems.

Talc
A soft gray-green mineral. It causes cancer, cysts and tumors. If inhaled, it causes respiratory problems.

Section 10

Vitamins
and Minerals

Do it Yourself
Multi-Vitamin and Mineral

Measure one cup of water for each teaspoon of herb; add two glasses for the pot. Let water come to a boil, then turn down heat to a low simmer. Simmer roots, barks and seeds. Let simmer 30 minutes or more, and then remove from heat. Next, put in herbs that are leaves and/or flowers. Let stand for 30 minutes or more. Strain while still warm and put in glass (preferably dark brown) container; keep in refrigerator. If you use a clear glass container, put the bottle in a paper bag or cover with paper so that the refrigerator light won't weaken the solution.

For larger amounts double or triple quantity or add extras according to needs. If you desire to increase strength, then, let herbs simmer and/or steep for a longer period of time. The herbal solution can be preserved by adding vegetable glycerin. Add 1 tablespoon for every 4 or 5 cups of liquid.

Honey can also be used as a preservative. Add 1 tablespoon of honey for every 4 cups of the herbal solution.

Suggested quantity ratio of 1 teaspoon per cup of water or 1 ounce of herb to 20 ounces of water. This herbal vitamin and mineral formula can be adjusted to treat a specific disease by adding the herbs needed for that dis-ease. However, it is suggested that the medicinal dis-ease herbs should be taken separately. Herbs can be substituted if they are in the same family and/or have similar nutritional content.

Herbs
Alfalfa, Shavegrass, Licorice, Peppermint, Blue Cohosh (or Black Haw), Red Raspberry Leaves, Mullein, Plantain, Burdock, Marshmallow, Moss (or Kelp), Lobelia, Dandelion Root, Yellow Dock, Cayenne, Garlic.

Caution
Lobelia should be used at 1 teaspoon to 4 cups of water. Use very small amount of Cayenne and Garlic (1/8 teaspoon to 4 cups of water).

EARTH MINERS AND
HUMAN MINERALS IN AFRICAN SCIENCE

Earth minerals, plant minerals and human minerals are different. The minerals are viewed as "the same" because they are in the same mineral tribe (family). The plant minerals are unique to plants and human minerals are unique to humans. To test this, pre-weigh four to six pounds of dried soil.

Put the soil in a closed flowerpot (one without an opening on the bottom). Then plant a seed (of your choice) in the filled pot. Let this seed grow to a reasonable size plant.

After the plant grows to the desired height, take the plant out of the pot, spread plastic on a table and shake the earth from the roots. Empty the remainder of the soil out of the pot onto a plastic sheet. Let the soil dry and then weigh the soil. You will find that soil weighs the same weight as it did before you planted the seed. This test demonstrates that plants do not eat soil or earth (soil) minerals. The earth soil minerals excite the plant's own unique minerals.

When you eat vegetables, their minerals are absorbed into your body. These minerals should be flushed from the body with raw fruits. Once the earth minerals have excited the body's minerals their job (function) is over and they should be cleansed (flushed) from the body. It is the eating of high amounts of earth minerals without flushing them out, which causes them to accumulate in the body and calcify the body. This accumulation is quite visible in the elderly. Years of accumulated earth mineral deposits cause their body motion to be slow, and rigid and inhibit the body from utilizing its own minerals, resulting in bone loss. This high mineral content causes a nutritional debt, which is paid for by death.

Earth minerals have a rotation cycle just as planets have a rotation cycle. These cycles (natural rhythms) excite and react to human and plant cycles. This causes a harmony between all things on the planet earth and in the galaxy. The Caucasian scientists assume that all minerals are the same. In African sciences, the Mineral Kingdom is given a status equal to the plant, insect, animal, human, ancestral and spirit (angels) kingdoms.

Section 11

Doctrine
of Signature

Natural Herb Guide

The doctrine of signatures is an African science concept. In this concept, the specific signature or medical purpose of an herb is written on it by its shape, color, texture, taste and/or odor. The color, shape, texture, taste and odor of a plant's leaves, stem, flower, fruit or roots identify the medicinal usage. The original herbalist did not have a textbook with pictures and definitions of herb use. They relied upon the signature, divining, astrology the herb's chemical analysis and the herb's anatomy to define the herb's usage.

ENVIRONMENTS

Herbs that grow in specific areas usually have adjusted to that area or environment. These herbs are generally good for dis-eases of that specific environmental area. Herbs that grow on mountains are good for the lungs, bruises, stabilization of temperature, resistance to cold (snow-capped mountains) and blood pressure regulation. Herbs that grow in water have medicinal properties, which help to control fluid absorption. These herbs carry electrical currents easier, aid in resistance to circulatory illness, aid the internal nerves and blood system of organs, are vital for the treatment of edema and have diuretic properties. Ninety percent of the herbs that grow in water are edible. Herbs that grow in the desert or desert-like areas aid electrolyte balance, regulate water in the body, hold moisture in the skin, stabilize the temperature, help heal burns and can protect you from ultraviolet rays. Herbs that grow near water are usually good for the hair, skin, lung dis-eases, dissolve waste and aid in the retention of oils in the body.

LEAF

Herb leaves that are wrinkled or well-convoluted are usually good for the skin. Smooth leaves are usually good for visceral (smooth) organs. Leaves that feel smooth to the touch are usually edible, while leaves that have irritating fine hair on them are not. A leaf with many veins is good for circulation. Leaves with straight veins or have no vein branches attached to the main vein's trunk are good for muscles. Veins in the leaf are similar to a tree; some veins have a vein trunk with a few vein branches. Other veins have a crooked trunk and many vein branches attached to each branch. The more complex the vein tree is the simpler its functions are in the body. Complex vein formations are good for nerve and circulatory diseases. Simple vein formations are good for muscles, digestive tissues and bones. Leaves that appear to shine generally have a high content of oil. While leaves that have a dull shine have a low oil content. Leaves that have the shape of a particular organ have an affect on that organ. For example, a leaf shaped like the lungs usually is healing for the lungs; good for colds and cause the lungs to speed up or slow down their action. Lung shape leaves are usually good for the lungs' complementary organ, which is the large intestine. Round-shaped leaves are healing for smooth tissues as well as the skin. Leaves that have dark, light or color areas that look like an organ usually treat that organ.

See Color Chart and various vein shapes in the Eye Chart. The vein shapes identify the disease or organ that the herb with similar veins can treat.

TASTE

Leaves that have a bitter taste indicate that the leaf liquid can close the pores. This leaf would be classified as astringent and may be alkaline. Leaves that have a sweet taste indicate that it has a liquid content and is high in minerals. A herb with this taste can open the pores. It is a diaphoretic.

COLORS

Leaves that have one color or uniformed coloring usually have one function in the body. This leaf would primarily act on one type of organ or one dis-ease symptom. Leaves with two or more color variations are usually good for many dis-eases. (See Color Chart).

GROWTH

Herbs that grow close to the ground or are short in height have a high mineral content. These herbs would generally be good for the bones, nerves and blood. Herbs that grow high in areas or are tall in height are generally good for the respiratory system and circulation. Vine type herbs are good for the nervous system, arteries, veins, blood and eyes. The flowers of herbs are generally good for the skin, reproductive system, digestion, lymphatics and brain. The short herbs that grow around trees or wrap themselves around trees are usually good for treating the spirit, circulation, arthritis and rheumatism.

SMELL
(Odor, Fragrance)

The medicinal usage of herbs can be defined by its primary smell or combinations of smells. A fragrance can be detected from the plant flower, fruit, leaf, stem or roots. The smell may need to be released by partially breaking the leaf open or by cutting an incision in the plant's flesh (root) or steeping the herb in hot water. (See Oil Chart). Herb smells are associated with the organs as follows: sour smell is related to the liver/gall bladder; bitter smell, heart/small intestines; sweet smell, spleen/pancreas/stomach; pungent smell, lungs/large intestines and salty smell are related to the kidney and bladder.

In many cases, the dis-eased organ can indicate the herb of choice. For example, the liver may give a smell to the urine or taste (you taste the vapors of an odor) in the mouth. A liver smell may have a predominantly sweet smell and a lesser sour smell or a pungent sour smell. This may indicate that there is too little sour in the liver or that the liver's enzymes are weak. The liver may give off a sour, salty or sour-pungent smell in response to a disease. This may indicate that the liver is stressing the kidneys by demanding too much support from the kidney (salty smell) or lungs (pungent). This may indicate that the primary treatment should focus upon the kidneys and lungs to the first degree and secondarily focus upon the liver to the second degree.

FRUIT

The fruit of herbs are flowers or seeds. The seeds can be covered with fruit flesh (i.e., apple) or exposed (sunflower seeds). Herbs that have thorns on the stem or branches generally have edible fruits. Usually, if you can eat the fruit, then, the roots are safe to use for their medicinal properties.

The skin of the fruit can be eaten if it changes color (e.g. apple, pear, orange). If the skin of a sweet fruit does not change colors, then, it cannot be eaten. The roots of sweet fruits or bushes are usually good for internal use.

Fruit skin that can be peeled generally has a high mineral content. Fruits from a vine herb, such as melons, have edible seeds. Green fruits such as the pumpkin or tomato usually have a change in skin color or two or more varieties of colors. These fruits have edible skins. If the sweet fruit's skin stays the same color, it usually is not edible.

The color of the skin or flesh of fruit indicates what organs it can treat. The color of a flower indicates what organs the herb (leaves, root, bark, fruit, etc.) can treat (See Color Chart).

STEMS

Herb stems, branches and trunks are used for medicine. They usually are prepared by boiling (simmering one hour or more). The stems can be ground into a powder and put in capsules or mix into juice and/or water and drank.

Within the stem are veins and arteries that transport nutrients and air. Stems tend to help the body transport its energy and aid circulation and help increase vascular flexibility and strength. They can assist in breaking down impurities in the body or building defenses for the body.

There are usually two types of flesh on the stems. The skin's outer flesh can be used to flush impurities out the body, and stabilize and protect vitality, nutrients and immunity. The inner flesh of the stem transports the root and fruit nutrients. The stem's muscular structure or flesh can help maintain the health of your muscles, regulate heat and aid circulation.

ROOTS

Roots are usually those parts of the herb that are beneath the soil. They have a high earth mineral content, assist the plant's respiration, stabilize nutrients, protect plant immunity and maintain a water and mineral balance. Roots can flush toxic minerals out of the body. Roots help to balance your electrolytes. All the cells in the body use electricity. The organs operate on an electro-chemical principle such as the heart, brain, muscles, eyes, ears, kidneys and liver.

The medicinal roots usage is sometimes based upon shape. Roots shaped like an organ or that have the colors associated with an organ are good for that organ. An herb such as ginseng is shaped like the human body and is good for the entire body. Roots that have bulbous portions such as beets, potatoes or turnips are good for the blood. Their use can be based on shape and/or color. White bulbous root portions such as potatoes are good for the under layer of skin, joints and the bones (white), stomach (it has white-like mucous) and nerve covering (mylinated). Roots have various lengths. Usually, long roots such as alfalfa are good for the upper portion of the body. Long roots reach more trace minerals. The medium length roots are good for the mid-organs. Short roots are good for the lower organs. Roots stabilize electrolytes and are in harmony with the mineral cycle.

ROOTS AND COLORS

The medicinal usage of a root can be indicated by the color of its fruit's flesh, skin and flower. The following is an example of treatment use.

- Red fruit roots are good for blood dis-ease, circulatory system.
- Yellow fruit roots are good for bowel dis-ease, diabetes.
- Brown root with inner yellow flesh is good for intestinal dis-ease.
- Brown root with soft inner flesh and white color is good for hollow organs (e.g., intestine, stomach, bladder).
- Brown root with hard inner white flesh is good for solid organs, e.g., kidney, heart, liver. (See Color Chart)

POISON

Herbs that cause the skin to itch, have fine thorns on the leaf, offensive odor, grow in stagnant water, or irritate your skin, are usually poisonous in some way (clinically or sub-clinically) inside the human body. Many poisonous herbs have antidotes. An antidote can be another herb that reacts chemically with the poison, making the poison harmless. The antidote can also block the absorption of the poison with charcoal or produce the opposite effect such as a sedative (Valerian) given to combat a stimulant (Guarana, Ephedra, Yohimbe) or combination of antidotes such as charcoal, tannic acid (goldenseal) and oil.

There are many theories for detecting poisonous herbs. Some theories advise you to eat only what birds eat. However, some birds and rodents (rabbits, squirrels) eat plants that are safe for them but poisonous to humans. Other theories say eat only what gorillas eat (this is the safest guide). However, gorillas eat some plants that are poisonous to man.

The overall diet of the animal used for poisonous and non-poisonous standards should be judged. Some animals include antidotes in their diet or their foods create antidotes. Subsequently, when setting a standard for poisonous herbs, it is wise to (1) examine the overall diet of the animal which is being used for a standard of poison, (2) assess any adaptational adjustments the animal has made to survive, and (3) measure the impact of the Caucasians on the animal's society and food source. Ironically, many of the animals and plants have had to adopt growth patterns that are not wholistic because the Caucasians have interrupted the plant lifestyles, ecology of their habitat and/or altered their natural food supply causing them to switch to plants that biochemically destabilize them.

These lifestyles are considered normal by unwholistic investigators. For example, today it is considered normal to live in soil, waste, air and radiation polluted and people congested city, use computers, play sex and violent computer games, eat junk foods, be watched by cameras, charge food with credit cards, buy air and water, etc. The behavior of humans under such conditions is viewed as normal. The constant massive people impact on people is abnormal. A wholistic diet and community is the only standard for normal. This same principle has to be applied to animals and plants. Many of the plants have been forced by multinational farms to live together in agriculture plantations while many of the animals have been forced to live together because the Caucasians have altered or destroyed the ecological system. Poisonous plants have developed a way of defending themselves against destruction. When you judge a poisonous plant, see what it is poisonous to, what plants live around it, how it defends itself from insects and/or animals and what animals do not eat it. Poisonous plants, combined with their antidote, can be used as a medicine if the healer is skilled in the science of using them. Gorillas, elephants, some monkeys, cattle, reindeer, hippopotamuses, fruitarian and other vegetarian animals are usually good indicators of which plants are poisonous. Birds usually eat animal flesh such as worms. The offensive irritating textures of plants (hairy leaves), position (place where it grows), color, odor (non-pleasing) smell or if it has an offensive taste it can indicate whether the plant is edible and to some degree, whether it is harmful or poisonous.

No herb is poisonous if it is combined properly with an antidote. In this way, the curative nutrients of the poisonous herb can be used for a treatment. A list of poisonous herbs can be found in the book, *Herbally Yours,* by P.C. Royal.

Section 12

Herbs

Herb Usage Guide

Herbal medicine is most effective when herbs are used fresh, live and picked the same day. Dried herbs are lesser in strength and in special cases more ineffective than fresh herbs.

In herbal medicine not all parts of the plant are used for treatment. Herbs may have a specific part that is used medicinally, such as the flower, seed, leaves (LF), root (RT), and branches.

Herbs can be annual plants that grow to full size, flower and die the same year. Herbs can be biennial plants that do not flower the first year, but produces only leaves. The second year of the plant's growth, it will flower and die. The leaves of the plant should be picked when they are in a flowering stage. If dried they should not be allowed to get moist while drying. Leaves that do not maintain their shape while drying should not be used. Herbs can be perennial plants. These herbs live for more than two years before they die. No herb dies completely (except from traumas). The upper portion dies while the root remains inactive until its next growing cycle.

Flowering herbs are called female and the same herb in a non-flowering state is called a male. Male plants are usually smaller and have more color, while female herbs are less colorful and larger in size.

Herbs belong to a family. Peppermint is in the mint family. Mints cause the body to feel cool. Generally, 99% of the mint family (tribe) is safe for humans. Some herb companies exploit the public by selling a herb's cousin or less potent next-of-kin (relative) instead of the authentic curative variety. The cousin or relative of an herb is in the same family (tribe) and resemble the authentic herb. It is best to purchase from a reputable herb dealer, health food store or buy a standard brand.

The overall effect of herbs is antidoted, lessened or not felt in the body whenever individuals take synthetic drugs, junk foods or alcohol. If junk foods, drugs or alcohol is consumed, then the medicinal herbs try to purify the body of the junk food, drug or alcohol and then act on the dis-ease. This may cause junk food eaters (synthetic, chemicalized individuals) to say that herbs do not work.

How to Prepare Herbs

Beverages and Teas

Use one teaspoon for each cup of water. The roots and barks are (boiled) simmered in water for twenty to thirty minutes or more. The longer they are simmered, the stronger they get in effectiveness. The leaves and flowers are added after the gas (heat) is turned off. Then the leaves and flowers should stay in the water (steep) for ten to thirty minutes. "Sun tea" is made by putting herbs in water, then placing them in the sun (cover pot) for several hours. The sun steeps the herb. Strain herbs while warm and drink three or more cups daily. Herbs can be combined.

Poultice
Mix herbs with water. Spread on white cloth or flannel cloth and apply to skin area. Put oil on area to be treated and cover the poultice with plastic (keeps in nutrients) and tape to skin.

Extract or Tincture
Put desired herbs in a jar filled with alcohol (pure grain, preferably corn liquor). Let herbs stay in the jar for two weeks. Shake daily. Strain and put in brown glass jar for storage.

Salves
Sixteen ounces of herbs desired (can combine those desired). Add 4 ounces of beeswax to 2 pound of natural oil. If you desire a smaller amount, reduce the quantities. Put in a pot and cover this oil and herb solution with water. Place in oven. Let simmer on medium temperature for three to four hours, then strain and put in glass container.

Syrups
Use honey, grain syrup (rice, barley, malt, etc.) or molasses; add herbs desired. Let simmer at low heat until thick. A ratio of ¾ honey to ¼ water can be used. Strain (with metal strainer or double cheesecloth) then put in glass container and store in refrigerator or cool place.

Liniment
Make with desired herbs (for pain, skin, boils, acne, pimples, arthritis, bruises, etc.). Combine 32 ounces of herbs. For example, 2 ounces of Goldenseal, 1 ounce of Arnica, 2 ounces of Comfrey, 2 ounces of Witch Hazel; add to 1 quart of rubbing alcohol. Put herbs in alcohol; let stand for 1 week; shake daily. Strain and put in glass bottle.

Seasoning
Seasonings were originally called medicaments and used for health reasons. For example, Turmeric for blood thinning, Oregano for infections, Juniper Berries for edema, Arrow Root for diarrhea, Slippery Elm Powder for constipation, etc.

Section 13

Sample Menu
and Recipes

Menu

Menu and diet are similar terms. A diet for African folks should consist of plants from the equator region. The equator area of the earth passes through many countries around the world. These countries where the equator region passes have similar plant growth similar to Africa. In the Americas, such states as Georgia, Florida, countries such as Panama, Cuba, the northern and mid-parts of South America and the islands of the West Indies, Barbados, Hawaii, Jamaica, Haiti, etc., are in equatorial regions.

Black African peoples and other colored races that lived in the equatorial area were raised for centuries on raw tropical plants. Black Africans' diets consisted of tropical vegetation for 100,000 to 200,000 years before Caucasian invaders destroyed plants and forced their cooked diet upon Africans. Biologically, the stomach flora (friendly germs, bacteria, fungus, yeast) has not changed in Black folks' stomachs. It will take over 2,000 years for the flora in Black folks' stomach to make a slight change. Black folks' specific flora makes digesting tropical plants easier, resulting in a proper metabolic balance. Raw fruits, vegetables (can be lightly steamed), whole grains and tropical plants are the best stabilizers of an African health. Herbs are the ideal medicine for Africans. Many of the African plants are grown in many countries because Caucasian exploiters (invaders) and merchants sold tropical plants to many countries.

Black Africans brought plants to many countries during their rule of the sea and earth. This African rule of the earth is sometimes estimated at 100,000 to 600,000 years prior to the Egyptian Dynastic Era. Black African slaves brought plants to many countries. The female slaves would cornrow seeds in their hair, thereby transporting plants to many places. Missionaries, invaders and slavers stopped cornrow hairstyles because it created a cultural connection to Africa. African slaves and tropical plants were taken to many countries. Places where Africans were taken as slaves, the plants of African can be found. Herbal folklores and remedies were brought to the Americas by African herbalists, agricultural scientists, doctors, midwives and African merchants (pre-slavery) and slaves. Black female herbalists were murdered as witches during the European 1600 witch-hunts. Fruits react quicker in the system and stabilize the health of Africans better than non-equatorial vegetables and fruits.

The Sahara desert is a climatic and vegetation shift. The Sahara Lake dried up and became a desert. Vegetation around the Sahara Lake were used as the food of Africans that lived around the lake. The dietary knowledge from that span of time was partially transmitted to Ethiopia, Egypt, etc. The present ecological plant life in northern Africa is recent and not a true herbal and dietary reflection of ancient African diets.

TROPICAL FRUITS

These fruits are typical of tropical lands and equatorial land regions. They are highly digestible and can be used in dried form or as a snack or fresh in a fruit salad.

Ascerola cherry, apricot, avocado, banana, breadfruit, kiwi, carambola, cantaloupe, cassava melon, cherimoya, coconut, dates, figs, crandilla fruit, guava, jackfruit, jujube, kumquat, loquat, mamey, mango, papaw, papaya, pineapple, pitanga, plantain, pomegranate, plum, quince, sapote, soursop, tamarind.

SAMPLE MENU

Breakfast
Upon waking drink one glass of water. This clears the digestive system of toxins and the nightly mucous build-up. Wait at least 30 to 40 minutes before you eat breakfast. Rolled oats can be eaten for breakfast (add a vegetable or fruit juice instead of water). Flax seeds or flax seed meal slightly heated in oatmeal milk, are also good for breakfast.

Drink one glass of fruit juice.

Lunch
Between 10:00 a.m. and 2:00 p.m. is the best time to eat a meal; especially one high in fats or protein. Make lunch your heaviest meal of the day.

Dinner
Brown rice and cauliflower. Sprinkle with Brewer's yeast and peanut flour (may also use peanut butter. Add water so it will pour easily).

Snacks
Dried fruit or fresh fruit.

RECIPES

The recipes that follow are meant to help you acquire a taste for health foods and crossover to a raw food diet; they have incorrect food combinations. Use glass and/or stainless steel pots and pans.

Salad of the Garden

1 cup of shredded beets	1 tbsp. caraway seeds
1 cup of shredded red cabbage	½ tsp. celery seeds
¼ cup raisins	½ tsp. mustard powder
½ tsp. horseradish powder	1 tbsp. honey

½ tsp. cayenne or desired amount   *¼ cup sunflower seed butter*
¼ cup sesame seed

Mix with ½ cups water, 2 tbsp. lemon juice. Pour into salad and mix.
Sprinkle salad with dill seed and ½ cup grated carrots.

Okra Stew

Cook one pot of Black eye peas and pour off water into a container for later use.

1 tbsp. peanut oil   *1 tbsp. sea salt*
1 tbsp. lecithin   *1 tsp. parsley*
1 tbsp. sesame oil   *¼ tsp. kelp*
2 onions, chopped (steamed)   *¼ tsp. cayenne*
4 tomatoes, chopped   *¼ tsp. ginger*
1 tsp. dill   *1 pound Okra (steamed)*
1 quart fluid (use water from Black eye peas)

Sprinkle with Almond meal. Wait 40 minutes, and then drink one glass of water.

Summer Salad

1 head lettuce   *1 garlic clove or 22 tbsp. garlic*
1 bunch spinach   *powder*
1 yellow squash, sliced   *2 carrots, cut into strips*
1 cup cauliflower   *6 tomatoes, cut into wedges*
  (cut in small flowers)   *1 bell pepper, sliced*
2 stalks celery, chopped   *(include seeds)*
1 green onion   *1 cup bean sprouts*
1 cup alfalfa sprouts

Sprinkle with Kelp, Dill and Lemon Juice.

Sweet Potato Mash

1 sweet potato or yam per person.   *½ tbsp. Almond meal*
  Boil potato (peel after boiling)   *½ cup lecithin*

Mix with wooden spoon until smooth (metal utensils decrease the electrical
charge of foods). Sprinkle with coconut (desiccated), cinnamon and nutmeg.
Mash can also be made with plantain, carob, green bananas, cornmeal.

Papaya Salad

Papaya, peeled and sliced   *Melon*
Grapefruit sections   *(honey dew, cantaloupe, etc.)*

Sprinkle with coconut (grated) and Sesame or Sunflower or Almond meal.
Sprinkle with Date Sugar.

Avocado Salad

1 ripe avocado, sliced   *1 tomato, sliced*

Put on lettuce leaves and spinach. Sprinkle with Lemon or Lime Juice, Kelp and grated coconut.

Almond and Corn Meal Fu-Fu

2 Cups stone ground Corn Meal   *2 tbsp. Lime Juice*
½ cup Almond Meal   *¼ tsp. Kelp*
1 tbsp. Sage   *½ tsp. Sea Salt*
½ tsp. Dill   *3 tbsp. Sunflower Oil*
1 tbsp. Poultry Seasoning   *1 Onion, chopped*
½ tsp. Parsley   *1 Bell Pepper (with seeds)*
1 tbsp. Origanum   *1 Celery stalk, sliced*
1 tbsp. Marjoram

Bake in pan for 20 minutes or until medium dry. This Fu-Fu can be stuffed in a hollow Bell Pepper.

Fudge Carob (Protein Balanced)

¼ Cups soy margarine   *¾ Cup soy isolate milk powder*
Combine / Cup lecithin granules   *Use enough milk to get mixture*
   (blend until creamy)   *slightly sticky*
½ cup raw honey   *¼ Cup sunflower seed meal*
½ cup carob powder   *¼ Cup almond meal coconut*
                            granules almond meal

Add to above ingredients and blend until creamy. Shape into balls and roll in this combined mixture. Refrigerate or freeze for firmness.

Millet Sandwich Patties

1 cup cooked millet   *2 cups of water*
2 tbsp. soy sauce.

Cook millet approximately 45 minutes.

1 cup chopped onion   *2 tbsp. soy oil*
¼ tsp. chives   *1 tsp. lecithin granules*
1 tsp. dill   *(sprinkle in mixture)*
¼ tsp. kelp   *¼ cup tomato sauce*
½ cup chopped celery   *½ tsp. sea salt*
1 tbsp. parsley flakes   *½ tsp. liquid chlorophyll*
¼ tsp. cayenne

Combine ingredients with cooked millet and soy sauce mixture. Then shape into patties and brown on both sides.

Almond Icing

¼ tsp. sea salt   1 cup water
¼ cup millet

Cook, combining approximately 40-60 minutes

½ cup coconut   ¼ cup honey
(Grind or grate finely)   ½ tsp. vanilla
¼ tsp. almond extract

Put combined ingredients in blender with hot millet. Water can be added. Chill.

Banana Milk

½ Cup coconut   ½ Cup cooked millet
¾ -1 Cup warm water   2 - 4 bananas

Pinch of salt and vanilla. Blend until smooth. Add an additional 1-2 cups of water.

Oatmeal Casserole (Protein Balanced)

3 Cups stone cut oats   4 cups of hot water
1 tsp. sea salt   ¼ cup almond meal
½ cup coconut   ½ cup raisins
¼ cup of sunflower seeds

Combine ingredients and stir. Pour in a casserole dish. Bake at 370° for approximately 35 minutes.

Corn Soup
(Protein Balanced)

1 onion,   2 cups cooked corn
   add 2 - 3 tbsp. of water and blend   1 cup diced cooked potatoes
2½ cups nut milk   (Combine and mix with onion)
   (almond, sesame, peanut or cashew)

Combine and mix with above.

1 tsp. salt   2 tbsp. parsley

Combine ingredients and bring to a boil. Garnish with parsley or chives.

Crispy Corn

1 cup yellow organic cornmeal   fi cup pecan pieces
¼ cup coconut   1 tsp. sea salt

Combine ingredients. Add 2 cups of boiling water and stir well. Then spoon onto a flour dusted and oiled cookie sheet. Bake at 400º for approximately 30 minutes or until crispy. Serve with soups or as a bread.

Corn Pudding

½ cup soaked raw soybeans
½ cup of water
1 tsp. sea salt or onion salt
¼ tsp. dill.
  (Stir into the combined mixture)

1½ cups raw corn
  (Puree in blender)
¼ tsp. of sage or basil
1 cup whole kernel corn
2 tsp. chopped parsley

Pour into 9"x 9" oiled baking dish, 9" or 10" pie plate. Bake at 450º for 10 minutes, and then reduce the heat to 350º for approximately 60 minutes.

Cake

1 pkg. yeast
¼ cup honey

1 cup warm water

To activate yeast, add the following combination of ingredients:

1 cup whole wheat flour
½ cup wheat germ
2 tbsp. almond butter
3 tbsp. water

½ cup unbleached white flour
½ tsp. sea salt
1 tbsp. sesame butter
¼ cup honey

Combine ingredients and mix with honey and water then dissolve yeast in ingredients. Pour combined liquid into dry ingredients immediately and lightly mix. Pour into a greased and floured cake pan. Let stand in warm place for approximately 20 minutes. Bake at 400º for 10 minutes, then 350º for 15-20 minutes.

Granola Peanut Butter

6 cups oats, coconut, flour, nuts seeds
⅓ Cup honey
⅓ Cup spring water
¼ cup peanut butter

1 tsp. vanilla
1 tsp. sea salt
¼ cup almond butter

Combine and blend liquids in blender. Mix with dry ingredients. Bake at 275º for 2 hours; stir occasionally to assist it being evenly toasted.

Granola Apple Sauce Mix

½ cup coconut
2 tsp. sea salt
4 diced apples
2½ cups applesauce
  (or 4 apples blended)

12 cups rolled oats
1 diced pear
½ cup chopped nuts
½ cup pineapple juice

Mix and bake at 300º for 2-3 hours.

Smoothy
(Protein Balanced)

¼ cup sesame butter
¼ cup almond butter
1 cup white whole wheat flour
1 tsp. lemon juice
2 – 2½ cups water

1 cup rolled oats
½ cup coconut
2 cups pineapple juice
1 pinch of sea salt
2 tsp. vanilla (or 4 tsp. almond extract, optional)

Fruit Tart Filling

Dried pineapple, soaked in spring water, purified or distilled and drain (save the juice). Frozen strawberries, thawed and drained (save the juice).

Combine all the juices and thicken with arrowroot, agar agar, cornstarch or tapioca. May add pear or apple juice concentrate, or date sugar and blend for sweetening. Add a pinch of sea salt and 2 tsp. vanilla.

French Toast
(Protein Balanced)

Use Blender to get smoothness

1 banana
½ cup cashew butter
7 dates
½ cup orange juice concentrate

1½ cups water
½ cup almond butter
⅓ Tsp. sea salt
2 tsp. flour

Dip each slice in batter and bake at 350º for approximately 2 hours.

Pizza

Pie Shell (3-4 Pans)

Combine and stir and let stand until bubbly

3 cups warm water
3 tbsp. yeast

3 tbsp. honey

Stir in bowl.

2 cups whole wheat flour
¼ tsp. kelp
3 tsp. sea salt

3 cups barley flour
3 cups unbalanced white flour

Should be mixed with ingredients until like sand. Add yeast and knead (press and squeeze) mixture. Let rise until double in size. Roll out. Bake.

Pizza Sauce

½ can (#10) tomato paste   ½ can crushed tomatoes
1½ cups sautéed onions   1½ tsp. sweet basil
1 tbsp. garlic powder   **Optional**: salt, thyme, marjoram,
                              honey

Combine and simmer on low heat. Spread on baked crust. Pour cashew pimento cheese on top. Decorate with sautéed red and green pepper rings, diced pimento, diced eggplant, diced onions and/or olive rings, etc.

Alternative Sauce

Sauté:
6 cups onions, finely chopped   1 cup water
½ cup oil (optional)   ¼ tsp. cayenne
/ cup honey   Then add ¼ cup sweet basil
¾ tsp. marjoram   ¼ tbsp. sage
1½ garlic powder   ¼ tbsp. chives
1½ cans tomatoes (crushed)

Blend juice and all ingredients. Let simmer approximately 1 hour.

Rice/Soy (Vegetable) Milk

1 cup rice,soy, oat, millet   ½ cup very warm water
  or other vegetable   1 tsp. honey
2 tsp. oil

Blend until very smooth and creamy. Next, add 1 Cup of water. Pour over breakfast cereals.

How to Make Soy-Rice Milk Base

Bring to a boil.
5 cups water   1 cup organic brown rice
1 tsp. sea salt

Then stir with a fork. Add 2 Cups soy flour. Simmer. Cook for approximately 14 hours.

Pancakes
(Protein Balanced)

Use blender for smoothness
¼ cup almond butter   ½ cup rolled oats
1 cup whole wheat flour   ¼ cup sesame butter
½ cup unbalanced organic white flour   ½ tsp. sea salt
1 tsp. per natural vanilla   5 cups spring or distilled water

Pour a thin layer of batter on a preheated pan. Set at 370⁰ (Use a Teflon, Silver Stone or lightly oiled glass stainless steel pan).

Cornbread
(Protein Balanced)
Mix

4 cups warm water	*3 tbsp. dry yeast*
¼ cup honey	*¼ cup lecithin granules*

In a large bowl, mix:

¼ cup sesame butter	*4 cups cornmeal*
½ cup whole wheat flour	*3 cups unbleached flour*
1 cup yellow grits	*¼ cup molasses*
¼ cup oil	*¼ cup almond butter*
½ cup honey	*1 tbsp. sea salt*

Mix any ingredients with hands. Pour yeast mixture over flour mixture immediately. Mix enough to combine. Oil pans. Dust with warm flour. Preheat oven to 375⁰; turn to 350⁰ and bake 40-45 minutes.

Oat Pie Shell Mix

2 cup rolled oats	*¼ cup apples*
¼ cup pineapple	*¼ cup papaya*
¼ cup peaches	*¼ tsp. sea salt*

Combine and mix completely and press into pie pan, smoothing with a spoon. Pie pan should be pre-oiled lightly. Bake at 350⁰ for approximately 30 minutes or until it becomes brown. Pour filling into shell and cool.

Apple Pie
Bring to boil and constantly stir for thickness:

2 cups pineapple juice	*4 tbsp. tapioca*

Partially let cool and then add: *2 cups shredded green or red apples.* Pour into pie shells, chill in refrigerator, then cut, and serve.

Chicken Seasoning

2 tbsp. brewer's yeast	*3 tsp. onion powder*
2½ tsp. garlic powder	*3½ tsp. sea salt*
¼ tsp. kelp	*2½ tsp. celery seed*
2½ tsp. thyme	*2½ tsp. sage*
1½ tsp. marjoram	*1¼ tsp. rosemary*
1¼ tsp. dill	

Seasoning ingredients for Italian dressing.

Soy Mayonnaise
(Protein Balanced)

2½ cups water

¼ cup almond butter

1 tsp. sea salt

¼ tsp. garlic powder

¼ cup lemon juice

1 cup soy isolate

¼ cup sesame butter

2 tsp. dill weed

¼ tsp. chives

Oat Sesame Coconut Waffles
(Protein Balanced)

1 cup raw sesame seeds

½ cup almond butter

½ cup fine coconut

3½ - 4 cups of water

1 cup quick oats

1 cup cornmeal

1 tsp. sea salt

Liquefy seeds in blender with part of water. Blend until smooth consistency. Next, mix remaining ingredients and water to a batter. Bake in hot waffle iron until done, approximately 6-10 minutes, or until it reaches golden brown.

Fruit Spreads

Fruit juices

4 Cups juice and 2 Cups tapioca
("minute")

Juice and fruit combined

4 cups juice fruit and 2 to 3
tbsp. tapioca

Combine fruit and juice with tapioca and let stand for 5 minutes. Next bring to a boil, stirring constantly until tapioca becomes clear. Let cool it, refrigerator.

Potato Soup

Per Person being served; bring to a boil:

1¼ cup spring or distilled water

½ cup potatoes (diced or sliced)

¼ – ⅓ Cup celery (diced)

¼ – ⅓ Cup onion (chopped)

1 tsp. chives

1 tsp. parsley

1 tsp. dill

Bring to a boil again and steep, turn burner down, and cook for approximately 20 minutes. Add cashew cream (2 tbsp. cashews and 3 tbsp. vegetable broth) (may need a little more broth to make a smooth cream). Add small amount of chopped parsley, stir until blended and serve with whole wheat, rye, zwieback, or crackers.

Sunflower Mayonnaise

¾ *cup sunflower seeds (raw)*
1½ *cup water*
⅔ *Cup soy milk or*
   1 cup blended puree brown rice
½ *cup lemon juice*

1½ *tsp. sea salt*
½ *tsp. garlic powder*
¼ *tsp. chives*
2 *tsp. onion powder*
¼ *tsp. kelp*

Blend sunflower seeds with water; add remaining dry ingredients. Add lemon juice.

Salad Sunrise Dressing

1 cup cashews
3 cups water
2-3 avocados
½ *tsp. chives*
3 tbsp. lemon juice

¾ *tsp. garlic powder*
1 tbsp. onion powder
1½ *tsp. sea salt*
½ *tsp. kelp*

Blend water with cashews until smooth. Then add remaining ingredients and mix.

Scalloped Potatoes
(Protein Balanced)

Blend together:
4 cups water
¼ *cup sesame butter*
¼ *cup almond butter*
½ *tsp. dill*

½ *cup raw peanuts*
2 *tsp. basil*
1½ *tsp. sea salt*

Pour over combined layers of sliced potatoes and onions. Bake at 400⁰ for approximately 1½ to 2 hours.

Pea Soup

1 Cup peas
1 Cup brown rice
3 fi cups water
fi tsp. dill

1 tsp. sea salt
fi tsp. chives
/ cup chopped onions
/ tsp. kelp

Combine ingredients in large pot and bring to a boil. Simmer on lowest heat for approximately 2 hours.

Caution: do not lift pot lid or stir until after 2 hours. Stir before serving.

Eggplant Sandwich Pattie

¼ *cup diced green onion*
½ *cup diced celery*
Combine and stir fry with
1 large eggplant, sliced and pared

2 minced garlic cloves
¼ *cup green bell pepper*
2 *tbsp. of oil*
¼ *tsp. parsley*

1 cup cooked white potato
  (cook with skin then dice
   after cooking)
¼ tsp. kelp

¼ tsp. dill
1 tsp. sage
1 tsp. sea salt

Steam eggplant. Combine with ingredients then add above ingredients. Shape into patties and coat patties with whole-wheat flour. Then, fry in lightly oiled pan until brown.

Vegetable Sandwich Burger

5 grated medium-size carrots
2 medium white potatoes
2 small diced onions
1 medium green pepper
1 tsp. dill
¼ tsp. kelp
¼ tsp. chives
2 diced celery stalks

1 tsp. garlic powder
1 tsp. cumin powder
½ cup quick oatmeal
1 tsp. sea salt
½ cup whole wheat flour
1 cup cold-pressed oil
½ cup lecithin oil (heat before
  adding to mixture)

Mix ingredients with whole-wheat flour. Flour should be used in order to produce paste consistency and to help shape into patties. Fry patties until brown on both sides.

Nut Loaf
(Protein Balanced)

¼ cup almond meal
¼ cup sesame meal
½ cup wheat germ or bread crumbs
1 cup walnuts
2 cup grated raw potatoes
⅔ Cup soy milk
1 tsp. lecithin oil

⅓ Cup oatmeal milk
1 tsp. sea salt
1 tsp. chives
½ tsp. dill
2 tbsp. grated onion
1 tsp. cold-pressed oil

Let stand 2 hour in a covered pan. Bake for 1 hour at 350°.

Date Muffins
(Protein Balanced)

¾ cup distilled or spring water
1 tsp. raw honey
1 package brewer's yeast
  (Combine and let stand
   approximately 10 minutes)
1 cup oats
¼ tsp. sea salt

¼ cup sesame meal
1 cup hot water
1 cup whole wheat flour
¾ cup almond meal
¾ cup chopped dates
¼ cup lecithin oil

Combine ingredients in the order written and mix until it reaches a smooth consistency. Pour in oiled muffin pan. Only half fill each pan cup. Bake for approximately 20 minutes at 350⁰.

Millet Fruity Cereal

2½ cups water
½ cup millet
½ tsp. sea salt
  Combine and cook for
  approximately 15 minutes

¼ cup raisins
¼ cup dried papaya
¼ cup dried pineapples
¼ cup chopped pecans
¼ cup chopped walnuts

Add to millet and cook for 15 minutes. Can serve with soymilk.

Bean Loaf
(Protein Balanced)

1 cup soy beans (or any type of bean)
1 tsp. garlic
¼ tsp. garlic
¼ tsp. chives
1 tsp. sage
½ tsp. dill
¼ tsp. cayenne

fi cup whole wheat bread
  crumbs
¼ cup almond meal
¼ cup sesame meal
¼ cup wheat germ
½ cup soy milk
½ cup tomato juice

Combine ingredients, bake in loaf Pan in the oven at 350⁰ for approximately 30 minutes.

Whole Wheat Bread

1 cup warm distilled
  or spring water
1 tbsp. honey
2 packages brewer's yeast
  (Combine and let stand in a bowl
  for approximately 10 minutes 3
  cups hot water)

⅓ Cup raw honey
3 tbsp. cold-pressed oil
2 tbsp. lecithin oil
1 tbsp. sea salt
4 cups whole wheat flour

Combine and blend in the sequence written. Let mixture cool before adding above yeast mixture. Then, blend and let rise in a large bowl for approximately 15 minutes.

5 cups whole-wheat flour (warm in oven at 250⁰)

Add warm flour to ingredients and knead for 5 minutes. This will make a soft dough that must be thrown with force upon table or board several times. Then shape into loaves and place in oiled bread pans. Let stand in pans for 12 minutes. Bake bread for 15 minutes at 250⁰ for approximately 45 minutes.

Mayonnaise

10 ounces firm tofu, drained   *3 tbsp. Vegetable oil*
1 tbsp fresh lemon juice   *½ tsp sea salt or salt free herb*
                                        seasoning

Blend mixture.

Herb Dressing

½ Cup olive oil   *½ Cup tofu mayonnaise*
⅓ Cup fresh lemon juice   *2 cloves garlic, minced*
1 tbsp dry mustard   *1 pinch salt or salt free herb*
                                        seasoning

Healthy Salad Dressing

2 tbsp olive oil   *4 tbsp. Tahini/Sesame Butter*
½ Cup water (spring or distilled)   *3 tbsp. minced red onion*
2 tbsp. Tamari

Blend together until smooth. Use on salads and vegetables.

Fruit Juice Dressing

1 Cup banana, apple, or any fruit   *4 tbsp. fresh lemon juice*
1 tbsp malt, barley or brown rice syrup *2 tsp herb mix salt substitute*
One pinch of cayenne or black pepper

Section 14

Chart Guide

Background of Charts

The charts are based upon the fact that the internal problems and diseases appear externally with various signs and symptoms. A physical (looking and touching) is far superior to a chemical examination (i.e., blood chemistry analysis). In doing a physical examination, it is best to use at least two methods (Eye and hand Charts, hair and Acupuncture Chart, etc.) before drawing a conclusion. And, use at least two methods of treatment (herbs and music, etc.) Use the art (Female Principle) of medicine by following your intuition, feelings and divining ability along with the science (charts). The charts reflect the Maat cultural foundation of medicine and the holistic nature of African civilization.

The foundation of the civilization is holistic. Holistic means that the spirit, mind and body are one. The past, present and future are one "now." Space, time and distance are one. Art and science are one. They function to serve God and God serves them. They function holistically. All art and artifacts have a function or effect upon the spirit, mind and body (*Esoteric Anatomy* by D. Baker, *Occult Principles of Health and Healing* by M. Heindel). The healing art and science practitioners included massage, herbalism, music, dance, psychology, spirituality, surgery, chemistry, biology, acupressure and chiropractic as remedies. The African healer sees the individual as a whole person (spirit, mind and body) and treated the whole person.

In African holistics, the spirit, mind and body are an indivisible = individual. A whole person is a verse of God. The Spirit is a verse (division, part of) of God, the mind is a verse and the body is a verse. They are one "united verse" = a universe. The spirit, mind and body are "members" of the whole person; they are united = "re-membered" as one.

The harmonic colors, music, dance and electromagnetic forces are wholistically generated by the body. Books such as *The Gurdjeff Work* by K. Speech explains the holistic scientific approach to dance. African Yoka, as practiced by civilization around the Pacific basin (Orient) demonstrates that specific Yoga body movements affect the mind and health. African dancers had specific healing gems or crystals that were worn to amplify the physical, mental and spiritual healing properties of the geometric shapes created during dancing. The book, *Crystal Power* by L. Arklinski, explores this and *Earth Energy* by J. Bigelow explains the vast array of holistic disease treatments that were created in Africa. The therapeutic affects of colors can be found in books such as *Color Therapy* by L. Clark.

The holistic healing usage of colors, fragrance, oil and incense, music, metals and crystals therapies were derived from nature. The ancient Africans used the Scientific Method or the structuring of phenomena based upon the holistic observation of facts. It was established before the Greeks stole and claimed the scientific method as their discovery. In the book, *Alchemists Through The Ages* by A. Waite, the origin of this truth is verified as African. Holistic Caucasians used the word "holistic" because they do not want to say "African." Instead of saying the African health system, the Caucasian say Holistic Health System.

The holistic healing usage of art, clothing, house decorations, music, colors and science has an African origin. The *Canon of Medicine* by O. Gruner explains the application of holistic colors in science. All civilizations that had social intercourse with Africa copied, stole and claimed the holistic (African) cultural practices and sciences as their own. In the book, *From Ancient Africa to Greece*, by Henry Olela, the Caucasian gravediggers and cemetery bandits (archaeologists) and their cultural cannibals (anthropologists) verified that holistic science is African.

Coprolith (fossil food and fecal remains) discovered in the tombs and pyramids confirm that a natural foods diet and a complex and yet simple food combining science is African. The usage of colors, oils, incense, metals, crystals and music are documented by pictures and words and fossil remains. In the book, *Supersensonics* by C. Hills, has explanations and examples of how to use ancient Black African Egyptian instruments of technology is validated. The Africans used the human body as the source of architecture, radionics, radio waves modified and converted the powers of crystals, colors, music, metals, oils, magnetism, electricity and radiation.

The interwoven, intermixed, interrelationship of one living universe, one God and the indivisible (individual/re-membered) is the foundation of holistic healing. Taste is part of all biochemical and organ functions. It is interwoven and a universe *(How to See Your Health Book: Oriental Diagnosis* by K. Michio). For example, the taste is connected to the organs and organ systems in the body. The tastes are as follows:

ORGANS	TASTE
Liver/Gall Bladder	Sour
Heart/Small Intestines	Bitter
Spleen/Pancreas/Stomach	Sweet
Lungs/Large Intestines	Pungent
Kidney/Bladder	Salty

An individual with a craving for sweets is having pancreas problems. The pancreas produces a sweet taste. For example, an alcoholic detoxing off alcohol has a craving for alcohol because this taste is produced in the body, and the body (specifically the liver) is trying to rid itself of the toxins from alcohol poisoning. An individual with a taste for sweets may be having problems with the emotion of love. The pancreas can be treated with the colors yellow, green and with the metal copper, the musical notes E and A, with the incense sandalwood, the oil patchouli and the medicinal herbs of juniper berry, thyme, sage and the plants celery and fruits such as olives, tangerines, soybeans and strawberries. The crystal Emerald can be useful. Mentally, they may be having problems with the Corpus Colostrum (Middle Thinking) or segregating thoughts. The above is a brief example of holistic treatments of a pancreas disease from an African holistic perspective. The charts on music, metals, oils, colors, crystals and should be used creatively and combined to use in various ways for treatments or used separately.

An African with impure blood due to infection or accumulation of toxins due to eating processed, preserved food, white sugar, bleached white flour and fried foods could be treated as follows:

IMPURE BLOOD TREATMENT

Music Note	E, G, C
(to be emphasized in songs)	
Colors	Red, Yellow, Green
(to be worn, painted on face	
or put in the home or around	
environment of ill person)	
Gems or Crystal	Amethyst, Coral, Garnet
(to be worn as jewelry)	
Metals	Gold, Mercury, Lead
Oil and Incense	Lavender, Styrax
(rubbed on body or burnt)	
Herbs	Chaparral, Red Clover, Yucca
Food	Sesame Seeds, Raisins, Cayenne, Guava, Garlic, Horseradish
Spirit	Needs to improve the ability to move the spirit
Mind	Needs to improve synthesizing reality and use sequential logic
Element Air	Needs respiratory herbs for blood and respiratory systems
Taste	Dis-ease can be indicated by sour, salty taste cravings

The chart usage can be simplistic or complex. Complex treatments do not indicate severity of dis-ease. Complex treatments may mean that the holistic health practitioners (healers) have a talent with complex modes. Healers can use one mode of treatment such as metal to get a cure while other healers need more healing modes. Complex mode usage is based on the healer's individual talent and not dis-ease complexity.

The objective of holistic science and healing is to allow everyone (no matter the talent) to have a tool to cure a dis-ease. The tool is based on the talent of the healer, availability, preference or patient. The tool serves as a medium to transport the energy of the whole (cosmic force and God) and serves only as a vehicle for treatment. God or cosmic forces cures disease, herbs merely serve to transmit the healing energy.

The African holistic approaches can be found in a denatured form in books such as *The Occult Causes of Dis-ease* by E. Densmore; *How Nature Cures* by E. Densmore; *New Concepts in Diagnosis and Treatment* by A. Abrams, M.D. These books reveal the negative impact of any dis-ease. Holistic concepts are a form of African communal science. African communal science focuses upon the relationship of families of energy. One family (spirit) of energy is not divided or separated from another family (mind or body) of energy. Each energy family shares and depends upon one another for survival. African healers possessed the scientific knowledge such as calculus, chemistry, physics, metaphysics and biology. The holistic (communal) approach followed the laws of Maat. The Caucasian science theme (method) is to divide and conquer. The African theme (method) is the direct opposite—united and heal. Holistically, a rainbow is a united family of colors, music is a united family of sounds, and when one member of the family (village) is ill, the entire family (village) is ill. The Caucasians laugh at this Maat communal concept. For example, when the White slave master was sick, the African slave would say "massa we sick." This indicated that on higher spiritual energy levels if one member of the racial family (White, Red, Black, Yellow, Brown) is sick, then the races on this planet share that sickness. White Supremacy psychosis of Caucasians has terrorized, destroyed and exploited all races and made them dysfunctional (sick). Consequently, one sick White race has made all races sick. The African slave and African peoples understand that the spirit and intelligence of this planet is ill because of White Supremacy Psychosis.

Holistic science balances all the energy to perfect a cure because all the energies (spirit, mind and body) are ill *(Yellow Emperor's Classic of Internal Medicine* by V. Ilza). Holistic approach to art and science is the foundation that built the African family and civilization and structured the world's knowledge.

A holistic approach takes into perspective the female, male and child energy force. It takes the equal energy of the female and male as a unit to define and use communal science properly. Caucasian holistic science is chauvinistic and the classification of colors, sounds (music), oils, crystals, and metals is unbalanced and causes an illness on other levels. African holism has been contaminated by Caucasian science and must use the Female Principle as defined by the female scientist before it can move to newer levels of Africanity. In Caucasian and oriental diets the foods are prepared, seasoned and cooked to please the biochemistry of the male. Notwithstanding, it is a male controlled science. Books such as *Diet and Nutrition* by Ballantine and *Origin of African Plant Domestication* by J. Horlan point to the total enslavement of females via the male scientist's unholistic domination of herbal and food science.

The charts are tools for self diagnosing.

Section 15

Charts

Colors

The holistic use of colors is very unique in African clothing, art, house decorations and science. Colors have a functional use.

Colors have a holistic effect upon the society, health, the mind, moods and impact growth. The Food, Drug and Disease industries use colors to sell products, to stimulate a child's growth, reinforce the symbolism of religion and government, and manipulate the mind, emotions and spirit.

Colors are combined in nature and naturally complement each other. Similarly, the colors of birds, matrix of flowers, rainbows, changing colors of plants and animals due to growth and seasons contributes to the African color science.

Colors have a holistic healing effect on the body and its organs. The color variations of the eyes, fingernails, and skin can indicate dis-eases as follows:

Kidneys/Bladder	=	black
Lungs/Large Intestines	=	pale
Spleen/Pancreas/Stomach	=	milky white
Heart/Small Intestines	=	red
Liver/Gall Bladder:	=	blue, gray

Plants that have colors that are the same as the color produced by an organ are good for treating a disease of that organ. Colors can be used to stimulate organs. For example, lemons (yellow) stimulate and cleanse the liver, the liver makes a yellow color (i.e., yellow jaundice).

Colors were extracted from medicinal plants and metals. Rituals and ceremonies were used to program the colors. These rituals and ceremonies were misinterpreted by Caucasians as superstitions, ignorance, paganism and exorcism of demons. The African Maat rituals and ceremonies reinforced the holistic intelligence, healing power and spirit that a color possessed.

The colors used in The Great Pyramids were scientifically combined. Incidentally, the color royal blue in the pyramids has only been duplicated by George Washington Carver. This feat established him as a modern day alchemist.

What colors mean and where they come from is distorted. The black color of African people is falsely attributed to the sun and heat of Africa. The black color comes from the Melanin and the pineal gland secretes Melanin. Melanin is a gift of God. Black people are not Black because they lived in Africa. Environment has an effect on people, environment does not create people. God created people. Colors come from the pineal gland's Melanin. The ancients call the location of this gland, in the center of the brain, the cradle of God. Colors have days that they radiate highest (energy level is high) and they have beneficial effects on organs.

Optimum Days

Sunday	orange	*Thursday*	purple
Monday	blue	*Friday*	green
Tuesday	red	*Saturday*	indigo
Wednesday	yellow		

Effects

Orange	lungs, pancreas	*Purple*	nerves, circulation
Blue	glands, kidney	*Green*	liver, heart
Red	blood cleanser	*Indigo*	bones, skin
Yellow	digestion, purification		

Colors can be rubbed on the chakras (Melanin clusters) and acupuncture meridians (Melanin pathways—highways) of the face to excite healing of dis-ease. This use of colors under and over the eye was called eye make-up by the Europeans. Colors applied to this area treat the kidneys. Colors were functional in ancient Africa. Retrospectively, Caucasian women color their eyelids and under the eye to indicate that they are fertile and to add color (Africanness) to their pale pink skin.

Many of the chambers in the Great Pyramid reflect this color science. The complementary combinations of colors speak to the organs, spirit and intelligence. They give a color story of Africa. The slower moving colors such as violet and blue relate to spirituality and the Female Principle. Fire colors move fast and relate to the mentality, Male Principle and heat.

ORGAN CLOCK AND CYCLES

Each organ and organ system within the body has a specific clock-like functional rhythm. The organ clock allows organs to singularly function at their best. However, if an organ fails to function at its best at a designated time, the individual will feel poorly at that hour. Each organ has an organ complement and if there is poor functioning of one, the complementary organ is affected.

Optimum Time	Part Affected	Optimum Time	Part Affected
1:00 am	Liver	1:00 pm	Small intestines
3:00 am	Lungs	3:00 pm	Bladder
5:00 am	Large intestine	5:00 pm	Kidneys
7:00 am	Stomach	7:00 pm	Internal system regulator
9:00 am	Spleen	9:00 pm	Energy regulator
11:00 am	Heart	11:00 pm	Gall bladder

COMPLEMENTARY ORGANS

Lungs ....Large intestines
Heart ....Small intestines
Kidneys ....Bladder (and sex organs)
Spleen............Stomach
Liver ....Gall bladder

BODY CYCLE

Sunday, Tuesday, Thursday   Physical Days
Saturday, Monday, Wednesday, Friday   Mental Days

The body cyclically fluctuates. On Sunday, Tuesday, and Thursday, it is external (physical, muscle organs, left-minded, acid, Male Principle, expansive), while on Monday, Wednesday and Friday it is internal (spiritual, visceral organs, right-minded, alkaline, Female Principle, expansive). Saturday, it is in the middle brain and balanced between the Male and Female Principle and worldly (external) and heavenly (internal). Exercise is best performed on physical days, light exercise can be performed on internal days.

WAIST AND POSITION CYCLE

- Above waist energy focus in the A.M.
- Below waist energy focus in the P.M.
- Vertical position energy in the A.M.
- Horizontal position energy in the P.M.

An understanding of human, planetary, celestial and ecology cycles reinforced Maat and African culture. Cycles were indicative of African peoples' culture and the calendar is a clocking of bodily and celestial cycles. The oldest calendar was developed by Black Africans in Egypt and is dated 4239-4235 B.C. The ancient clocks that used wheels and pendulums to keep time imitated the internal organs (cycles) rhythm.

OILS AND INCENSE
(Aromatherapy)

Oils and incense act upon the sense of smell. This sense is active (gives energy) and passive (receives energy). The oil can be applied and absorbed by the skin and blood or the healing aroma of the oil can be released when an oil saturated incense stick is burnt. The oil from medicinal plants and medicinal wood from herbs has the same curative properties of the plant.

The oils and incense have dominant aromas. These aromas have trace (smaller) aromas that cause the proper ingestion into the body. Aromas have an affect on spirit, mind and body.

Smell is related to the digestive system. Oil droplets (vapors) are tasted and digested as well as absorbed by the lungs. They enter the blood. The cell uses the oil and turns the oil into cellular waste (earth). All the senses operate chemically. The ears have water and hair inside them. The hair is stimulated by sound and the hair electrically triggers a chemical reaction. You hear chemically. Vision is a chemical process. The light strikes the retina inside the eye. This electrically triggers a chemical reaction that your brain interprets as vision. Taste and touch have sensors that electrically trigger a chemical reaction that your brain interprets. In any case, the final result of smelling produces earth (cellular waste). Smell is operated by the earth's element.

Ancient Africans used oils and incense smoke for healing therapeutic reasons. For example, Myrrh oil was used for antiseptic energies, Quassia for tonic effect, Gum Arabic for birth control and Sandalwood for spiritual effect, etc. The oils were functional and not a cosmetic perfume in African civilization.

The medicinal oils were used in lotions, body oils, hair oils and for waterproofing bandages.

The Effect of Oil and Incense

Myrrh	Used for nasal congestion, and as an antiseptic
Oilbanum/Frankincense	Vital for nervous system, vasoconstrictor, aids birth muscles.
Jasmine/Calamus Root	Good for kidney, blood purifier, mineral stabilizer
Pine/Burn Pine Cones	Good for respiratory, digestive organ cleanser, energy regulator, rejuvenator.
Lavender/Styrax	Use as cleanser of glands, pores and skin; mental tranquility.
Oak Moss/Cedar	Aids digestion, nerves, and blood purifier.
Rose/Sandalwood	Used for nerves, a cleanser, spiritual protector, pituitary gland, emotions

These oils/incense can be substituted (interchanged) for another member in its plant family.

Oils/Incense for the Weekday

Oils/incense are a cyclical and they have optimum days. The predominate days that they should be worn and burned are:

Sunday	Oilbanum/Frankincense
Monday	Jasmine/Calamus Root, Jasmine
Tuesday	Pine/Pine Cones
Wednesday	Lavender/Styrax
Thursday	Oak Moss/Cedar
Friday	Rose/Sandalwood
Saturday	Myrrh

Force of Oils/Incense

Oils/Incense have a downward circulatory (spiral) energy force and an upward circulatory (spiral) energy force. The downward spiral is related to the Male Principle, destruction of impurities, negative thoughts and behaviors, left mind thoughts, contraction (concentration), acid, action, etc. The upward spiral is related to the Female Principle, growth and development (building), right minded thoughts, expansion, alkaline, relaxation, etc. Therefore, to accentuate a particular characteristic or aid cleansing (destruction) or healing (building), choose the oil/aroma accordingly.

OIL/INCENSE

Upward Force	Oilbanum/Frankincense, Pine/Pine Cone, Lavender/Styrax
Downward Force	Jasmine/Calamus, Oak Moss/Cedar, Rose/Sandalwood

METALS

Metals are part of the Mineral Kingdom. This kingdom is composed of living substances. Minerals in the metals respond to music, drugs, electricity, magnetism, light, heat, color, crystals, and transmit and receive energy. Metals have a cycle, which is indicated in the charts by the days of the week. On specific days, metals have energy peaks and lows. Metals are active, give energy (Male Principle), neutral (conduct) and passive and receive energy (Female Principle). The body has many minerals in trace (very small) amounts. Metals are related to the generative system and function under the Fire Element of energy.

Metals have spiritual energy, intelligence and physical curative functions. Metals were worn on the fingers, hair, wrist, neck, ankles, toes and waist; woven into fabric; and used in make-up for the treatment of diseases and spiritual and/or mental problems. Malachite, a copper eye paint, was used by men and women around 4000 B.C., in Egypt.

Metals had a functional use for art, artifacts and the décor of the home. They were used to purify the home, spiritually protect the home and keep mental and emotional harmony in the home. Today, the African metal usage is not holistic and relegated to being nonfunctional decorations or art.

Metals and/or crystals were put in the ear to stimulate energy. The ear has points on it related to the internal organs and brain. See the Ear Acupuncture Chart. The book *Acupuncture for Americans* by L. Wensel has information on the subject of meridians. The ear is holistic and directly related to all parts of the body. Metal was placed in the ear as a healing therapy and for cultural reasons. However, the puncturing of holes in the nose and ear is self-mutilation and unholistic. The circumcised penis and clitoris and/or wearing rings in the penis and vagina and other body parts is mutilation and unholistic. The metals used to make or decorate musical instruments have holistic function. There are many combinations of ancient African so-called art, which had a holistic functional usage too broad in scope for this writing. The use of metals from holistic perspectives are revealed in *Esoteric Healing* by A. Bailey, *Healing with Radonics* by Baerlein and Dower. Besides this a few examples of the positive healing and negative usage of metal are in *It's Your Body* by M. Laversen, M.D. and S. Whitney.

The Effects of Metals
Metals have a holistic curative effect upon the body. In the body some organs have a higher content of one metal (mineral) than another metal (metal ratios). Therefore, a specific metal can biologically magnify and electrically stimulate a bodily process, organ and an organ system (i.e., circulatory system). The prostate is high in the metal zinc and selenium. The uterus is high in manganese; thyroid - iodine; bones - calcium; pancreas - vanadyl sulfate; heart - arsenic; eyes - zinc; vagus nerve (neck) - potassium, etc.

Metal	Remarks
Gold	For metabolic disorders diabetes, intestines, bowels, purification
Silver	Restores electrical current, adrenals, intestines, spleen, thyroid, brain
Mercury	Stabilizer of energy, purification lower digestive system
Tin	Anemia, nerves, and brain circulatory system
Copper	Blood, liver, pancreas, eye, ear, and emotions
Lead	Energy, counters destruction of cells, blood cleaner, blood pressure

Metals for the Weekdays
Metals have a cycle with a specific day for functioning at their optimum level as follows:

Sunday	Gold	*Thursday*	Tin
Monday	Silver	*Friday*	Copper
Tuesday	Iron	*Saturday*	Lead
Wednesday	Mercury		

Vibrations

Metals carry sound wave vibrations that reverberate in the body. The metals' vibrations enhance the energy force field (life force).

Metal vibrations are specific and related to musical notes (sounds) as follows:

METAL	MUSICAL NOTE
GOLD	D
SILVER	G
IRON	C
MERCURY	F
TIN	B
COPPER	A
LEAD	A

AFRICAN WHOLISTIC (ORGANIC) CHART

The body has a very fine sublime (Female Principle) inter-relationship between the spirit and mind. No primitive Caucasian theory about laws (i.e., two things cannot occupy the same space at the same time) can be applied to the body, because it is three things (spirit, mind, body) in one space at the same time.

Each organ, nerve, muscle and part of the body is related. Internal organs have nerve endings and energy imprints (acupuncture meridians) on each section of the body. The spirit has imprints (spiritual meridians) on the organs, the mind and body sections. The brain has intelligence imprints (meridians) on each organ and each section of the body. Elements have an influence on each section of the body. The organic (wholistic) inter-relationship began its existence in the human embryonic (egg or fetal) stage and it has continued to exist in the adult state.

This chart can be used by locating the problem organ or sense organ (sight, hearing or smell). For example, lung problems would mean balancing the upper thinking; spirit-soul and the element-air respiratory system and fire-generative system. The sex organs would be treated by balancing lower thinking; treating physical-spirit and form spirit and the elements of water (circulatory system) and earth (digestive system). The lung problem probably developed in the third trimester of the mother's pregnancy. This is when the lungs completed a growth phase.

This chart is prepared to increase the awareness of the psychic being, physical being and spiritual being...the sum total is the human being.

BODY SECTION	MIND	SPIRIT	ELEMENTS
Upper Organs	**Upper Thinking**	**Soul**	**Fire**
Lungs, Thyroid, Bronchi, Heart, Stomach	Abstract Thoughts, Universal Reality, Pineal	Directing the Spirit according to Ma'at, Pure Energy	Head, Sight Generative System
Middle Organs	**Middle Thinking**	**Life**	**Air**
Kidney, Pancreas, Spleen, Liver	Segregation of Thoughts, Synthesis	Moving the spirit of Humans, Animals *Contact: Kidneys*	Respiratory System, Hearing Thorax
Lower Organs	**Lower Thinking**	**Form**	**Water**
Bladder, Sex Organs, Small and Large Intestine, Rectum, Appendix	Congregation of Thought, Primitive Sense of Sex, Hunger, Thirst, Shelter	Creating your best spiritual nature. *Contacts: Heart, Lungs*	Abdomen, Circulatory System, Taste
Contacts the Physical Mind and Earth Spirit	*Contacts the Physical Mind and Earth Spirit*	**Physical**	**Earth**
		Spirit genetic code-- Purpose. *Contact: Pituitary*	Digestive System, Pelvis, Smell

FACE CHART

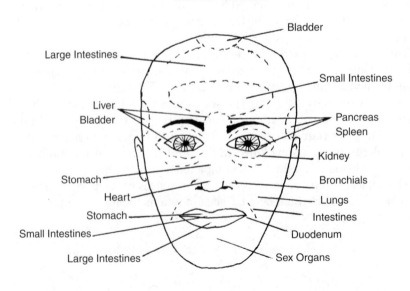

The face reflects good health as well as dis-eases. The skin color and texture should be consistent. A rash, dry, light or blotched area, variation in color, bumps (acne, pimples, blackheads, etc.), roughness, dry or oily texture indicates disease, stressors or a malfunction of the organ related to that specific area.

In African medicine, all scratches, bruises, and other so-called accidental marks that occur to the face are caused by a malfunction of the organs related to that specific area. The weak organ meridian on the face attracts a negative or positive energy causing a skin trauma, which is erroneously called an accident. Weak organs vibrate at an unstable, low or weak frequency, which is not in harmony, and this causes the organ meridian to attract negative or positive energy in order to re-establish harmony. The energy created by an accident is the weak or diseased organ's method of getting help or your attention to correct the dis-ease. In wholistic African sciences, there is no such thing as an accident. Accidents are controlled by the laws of accident. A lack of understanding of Maat causes the label of accident to be used.

THE FACE AND ZODIAC SIGNS

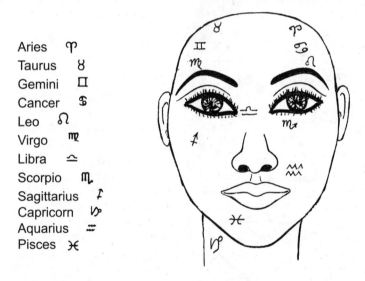

Aries	♈
Taurus	♉
Gemini	♊
Cancer	♋
Leo	♌
Virgo	♍
Libra	♎
Scorpio	♏
Sagittarius	♐
Capricorn	♑
Aquarius	♒
Pisces	♓

♈   Head, face, cerebrum, eyes, nose, pituitary
♉   Neck, throat, cerebellum, mouth, tonsils, vocal cords, thyroid
♊   Arms, shoulders, lungs, fallopian tubes
♋   Stomach, breasts, arteries, diaphragm, uterus, veins
♌   Cardiac region, spleen, heart
♍   Small intestine, pancreas, lower abdomen
♎   Small of back, adrenal, kidneys, bladder
♏   Pelvis, reproductive organs, gonads, colon, rectum

♐ Thighs, hips, buttocks, liver, sciatic nerve
♑ Knees, bones, gall bladder, teeth, cartilage
♒ Calves, ankles, bladder, retina of eyes, parathyroid
♓ Feet, circulation, pineal, lymphatic system

The face has areas that correspond to zodiac signs. Each side of the forehead has different signs while each side of the cheeks, chin, as well as the
neck have the same sign. A change in color (darkness, lightness), blotchiness, rash, oiliness, dryness, slight temperature variation (cold or warm
areas) and/or skin eruptions in a sign indicates stressors, problems, weakness or a disease with the body part that the sign represents.

THE FACE, PLANETS AND DISEASE

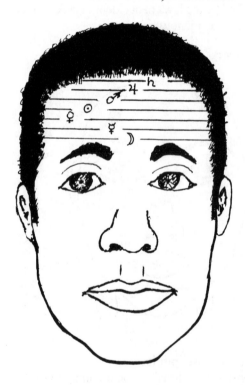

Sun   ☉
Moon   ☽
Mercury ☿
Venus   ♀
Mars   ♂
Jupiter ♃
Saturn   ♄
Uranus   ♅
Neptune ♆
Pluto   ♇, ♇

SYMPTOMS AND PLANETS

☉ Heart disease, artery and vein weakness
☽ Inflammation of mucous membranes, edema, dehydration,
   digestive problems, electrolyte stress
☿ Neuritis, respiratory diseases

♀ Throat infections, thyroid imbalance, kidney problems

♂ Swelling and inflammation, fevers, infections, accidents, hemorrhage and blood diseases

♃ Liver diseases (hepatitis), pancreatic diseases (hypoglycemia, diabetes), obesity, tumors, cysts, warts

♄ Arthritis, rheumatism, fractures, spinal ailments, dental problems, skin diseases, gall stones

♅ Cramps, spasm, shocks, paralysis, epilepsy, muscle problems, radiation toxicity

♆ Hallucinations, alcoholism, addictions, toxic conditions, schizophrenia, undiagnosed diseases, reactions to synthetic chemicals and hormones

♀ Diseases of the reproductive organs, degenerative diseases, weak tissue

The forehead has areas that correspond to planets. A change in color (darkness, lightness), blotchiness, rash, oily, dryness, skin eruptions, broken or uneven or deep furrows (wrinkles) in a planet's area indicate stress, problems, weakness or a disease with the body part the planet represents.

EYE CHART
(Sclera = Whites)

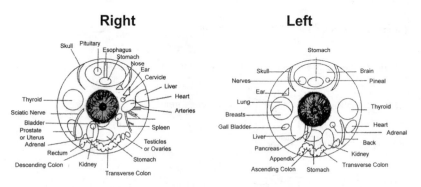

For enlarged chart, see page 523.

The eyes mirror the health of the body and internal organs as well as types of dis-eases. The colors of the whites (sclera) can show dis-ease (See Color Chart). The veins can point to the organ being stressed or diseased. Veins in the sclera have different shapes. Each shape indicates a problem. Whites of the eye normally should have no pronounced veins. Veins that are the closest to the iris indicate severe problem. Generally, in a healthy person three veins may appear in the whites of each eye. The iris of the eye can reflect the same illness by showing distinct color alterations.

VEIN SHAPES IN WHITES OF EYES

Vein shapes indicate illnesses such as:

Accident	Pregnancy	
Anemia	Pending Heart Attack	
Bladder Problems	Relaxing Stress	
Blood Clot	Rheumatism	
High or Low Blood Pressure		
Concussion/Congestion	Scar Tissue	
Congested Veins	Severe	
Infection	Stress	
Kidney Disease	Surgery	
Liver, Gall Bladder Problems	Traveling Line	
Low Grade Fever	Varicose Veins	
Narrowed Arteries		
	Poor Tissue Integrity	
Nerve Stress		
	Whiplash	
Poor Circulation		

EAR (AURICULAR) ACUPUNCTURE POINTS

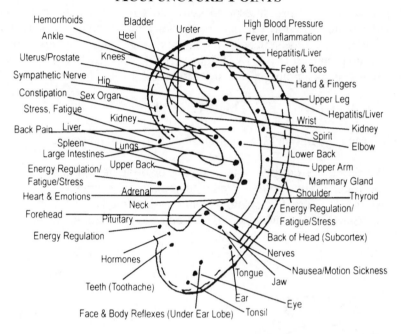

For enlarged chart, see page 525.

MELANIN CLUSTERS

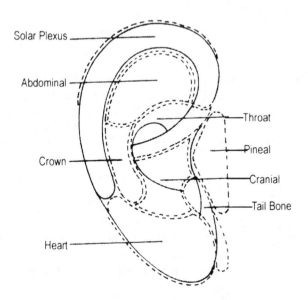

These points were used for metal and/or crystals called earrings or color or oil therapy called makeup or perfume. These parts of the body can be treated with finger pressure or an item that will not penetrate the skin (wooden match stick). If you put pressure on a point and it feels sore, tender or painful or if the skin color or texture changes at a point, apply pressure or rub points for two to five minutes. If a bump, rash, dryness, oiliness or soreness is on a point, it indicates a stressor, disease or malfunction.

HAIR CHART

Hair Area: Internal Organs represented by hair and scalp.

B Front   Excretory system, kidney, bladder, sex organs
L Side   Lungs, large intestines, respiratory system
A Top   Blood, circulatory system, small intestines, heart
C Back   Digestive system, stomach, side pancreas, spleen
K Back   Liver, gall bladder

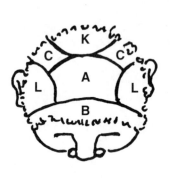
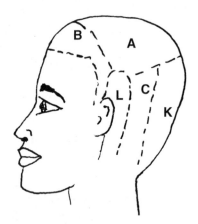

The hair color, split ends, length of hair, texture and falling out of hair, along with the condition of the scalp; oiliness and dryness of the hair and how slowly or quickly the hair grows in areas indicates deterioration of health or dis-ease of specific organs. Hair represents all the body and all the body represents hair.

Fibrin appears on the scalp and is called dandruff. Fibrin is a type of cell that is used to build fibers, tissue, muscles and ligaments. However, without enough potassium chloride in the blood, the fibrin will become loose (unattached) and is ejected as mucous, phlegm and catarrh. Most dandruff, fibroids, cyst, colds, adhesions, lung and sinus mucous are caused by unattached fibrin. An acid bodily state caused by synthetic foods, drugs, and cooked foods cause an excess of hydrogen, which causes acid, excess estrogen, lack of growth hormones, stressors that cause spasms of the head's flat muscles (stops hair growth), clogged scalp veins and arteries decreases nourishment to the hair and a mineral deficiency can cause changes in hair color, texture and baldness.

HAND CHART

The nervous system has nerve endings and acupuncture points in the hand, which are connected to the internal organs.

If you apply two pounds of pressure (females) or three pounds of pressure (males) to a nerve ending or organ region in the hand and feel pain, soreness or sensitiveness, the organ related to that region is malfunctioning and diseased. If the skin color (See Color Chart) is light, dark, blotched or altered in that organ region then the organ is stressed or dis-eased.

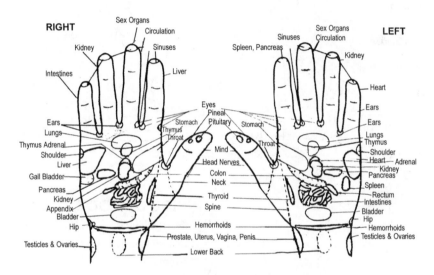

For enlarged chart, see page 524.

FOOT CHART

The feet have acupuncture points and nerve endings and areas, which are directly connected to every internal organ. Basically, the foot and hand charts are the same.

The Great Toe (big toe) and Great Finger (thumb) are related to the brain and contain the pineal and pituitary glands. The other toes and/or fingers contain the sinus.

The organ regions on the feet indicate the condition of the corresponding organ. If pain, tenderness or soreness is felt when two pounds of pressure (women) or three pounds of pressure (men) is applied, then the organ related to the area is dis-eased or stressed.The color of the skin can indicate problems or dis-ease. Extra pressure or a wooden match may be needed for tough skin. Calluses are often caused because a dis-eased organ will deposit acid waste in the feet; the acid will cause the skin to soften. The soft skin will rub against shoes and form calluses. Therefore, calluses, if not caused by physical traumas (improper shoe styles and high heels), are indications of dis-ease.

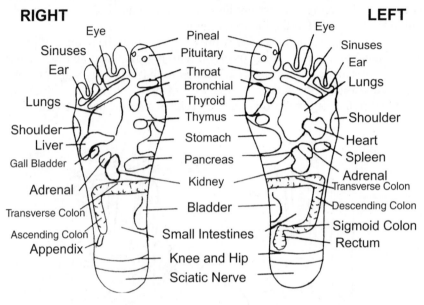

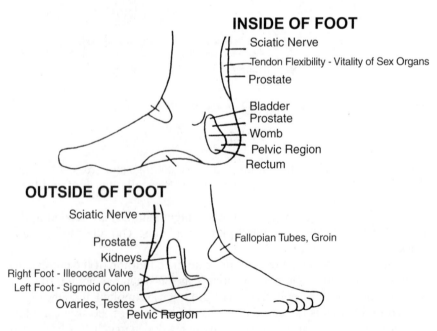

ORGAN REGIONS OF THE BODY

The body was once an undifferentiated mass (an egg). All parts of the body were related to each other and specialization of parts of the egg produce organs and limbs. When parts of the egg began to separate and form organs and parts, the nerves related to those specific organs remained attached and grew longer. The nerves never lost their connection to the nucleus and/or central nervous system.

The three major divisions of the body are A = Upper Region, B = Middle region, and C = Lower Region. Spiritual regions are C = Creating your Spirit, B = Spiritual Interactions and A = Willing (moving) Spirit. Holistic regions are C = Physical, B = Mental and C = Spirit. Gestation regions are C = First Trimester, B = Second Trimester and A = Third Trimester. See Wholistic Chart for organs in each region.

Any color inconsistency, skin eruptions, excessive hotness or coldness, rashes, scratches, or slow blood refill when finger pressure is applied and then released or pain, soreness or sensitiveness, indicates that the organ related to that region is in a dis-ease or having problems.

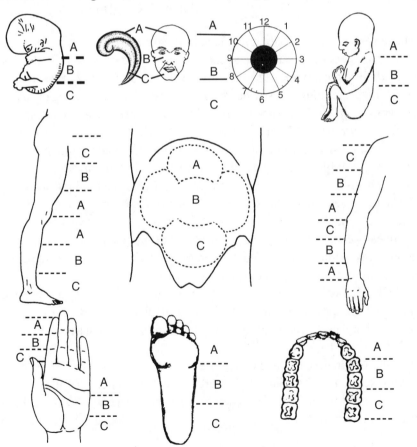

ORGAN REGIONS (continued)

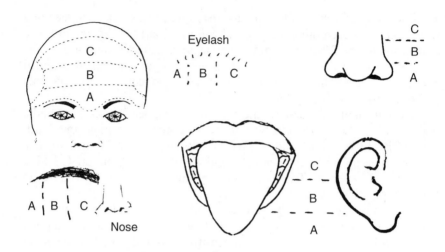

Eyelash

Nose

MUSIC AND SPEAKING SOUNDS

Music is used to calm patients in hospitals, stimulates sexual arousal and to get shoppers in the mood to spend money, excite crowds at football or basketball games, was used to communicate to soldiers in battles, and in rituals and ceremonies, festivals, dances and religious rites. African chants (i.e., rap songs) were used to motivate slaves to work —slave work songs. African rhythms and harmonies were sung for religious songs, stress or emotional release and story telling. African melodic and rhythmic form is present in the blues and jazz. The rhythm for African dance music is in three. This is based on the beats of the heart. Africans count three beats: (1) the heart valves open is the first beat; (2) when the heart pauses is the second beat; and (3) when the heart valve closes is the third beat. The Europeans count only the beats heard and not the rest (pause) beat. They count it two while Africans count in three. This causes Caucasians to be out of step when attempting to dance to Afro-centric music.

Music holistically affects crystals, colors, metals, oils, food, incense and internal organs. Musical notes holistically heal dis-eases, of the spirit, mind, body and organs. Specific music notes can be emphasized in a song in order to heal an organ.

The original scales and harmonies of the so-called blues have been acknowledged as African. The natural tuned instruments of many tone varieties are African. The Caucasian piano is merely a harp that is mechanically hit by drum sticks (hammers) when the fingers touch a piano key. The

AMINO ACIDS BODY CHART

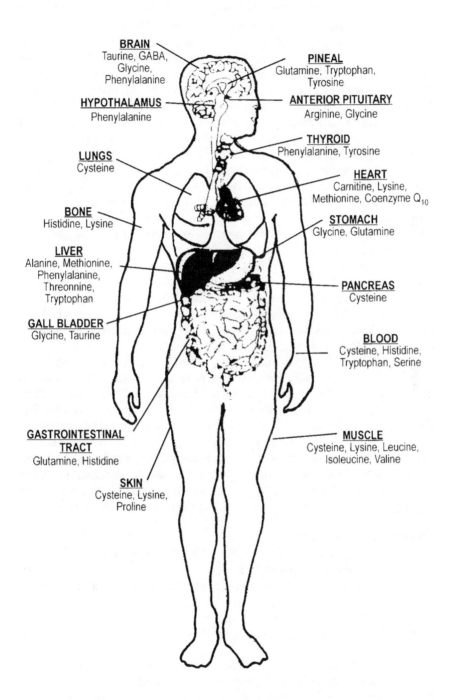

BRAIN
Taurine, GABA,
Glycine,
Phenylalanine

PINEAL
Glutamine, Tryptophan,
Tyrosine

HYPOTHALAMUS
Phenylalanine

ANTERIOR PITUITARY
Arginine, Glycine

THYROID
Phenylalanine, Tyrosine

LUNGS
Cysteine

HEART
Carnitine, Lysine,
Methionine, Coenzyme Q_{10}

BONE
Histidine, Lysine

STOMACH
Glycine, Glutamine

LIVER
Alanine, Methionine,
Phenylalanine,
Threonnine,
Tryptophan

PANCREAS
Cysteine

GALL BLADDER
Glycine, Taurine

BLOOD
Cysteine, Histidine,
Tryptophan, Serine

**GASTROINTESTINAL
TRACT**
Glutamine, Histidine

MUSCLE
Cysteine, Lysine, Leucine,
Isoleucine, Valine

SKIN
Cysteine, Lysine,
Proline

African drum language was stolen by the Caucasians, called the Morris Code; this language rhythm or pulses became the telephone and computer.

The oldest instrument in the world is an African Harp (2500 B.C.), which usually had 22 strings of differing tones. In any case, the Harps had complex tonal system, complex harmonies and required a written musical notation language while the Caucasian seven note scale indicates a static and primitive music language. The contemporary tempered tuned instruments are a European device to make music sound more mechanical, left minded and civilized (caucasoid). Ironically, classical (European) music is also African. In fact, the first Philharmonic (Euro-Classical) Orchestra in America was formed by Blacks in New Orleans before the War of 1812. Many of the slaves were hired out as musical entertainers. The African slaves were educated in African schools of music before coming to the Americas. What is called classical music is a denatured African music. Some of the history of African harmonics in Euro American (jazz) music is in the book, *The Bluesmen* by S. Charters. The only new art form is jazz. The pioneers of this music are Louis Armstrong, Charlie Parker and John Coltrane.

African music is derived from a wholistic Maat cultural foundation. Music is culturally confined and a language of culture. Music is culture. Caucasians without a knowledge of and respect for African culture cannot truly understand African music. Music (African as well as European) is not a universal language. For example, Caucasians cannot distinguish the difference between a happy or sad African rhythmic pattern and melody. Consequently, Caucasians label all fast African melodies or rhythms as happy music. There are sad blues with fast rhythms and happy blues with slow rhythms. Musically, Caucasians do not understand or appreciate all of their own cultural music. Most Caucasians do not understand other Caucasian ethnic music or classical European music. European music is not universally understood by Caucasians. Music transmits and translates culture. It is a language of a culture. It is not a universal language anymore than Bantu the language is a universal language. Music is culturally confined. Music sounds are another form of healing energy. Music enters the human body by way of the skin, eyes, ears, and foods. The healing notes can be sung, played on a musical instrument or heard.

The Effects of Musical Notes

D	For digestion and assimilation, dis-eases involving the lungs and the respiratory system.
G	Stimulates tranquility, peace, eliminates infections and increases immunity.
C	Blood dis-ease and purification.
E	Purification, assists in healing diabetes, intestinal and bowel dis-eases.
B	Nervous systems, eye and brain injuries, and insomnia.
F	The nervous system, circulatory system and heart.
A	Dis-eases of eye, ear, nose, dental, and emotional disorders.

Neutral Note   Treatment of all injuries and dis-eases.
Musical Notes for the Weekdays
Musical notes have optimum days for radiating energy. The predominant music note for each day of the week is as follows:

Sunday	D	*Thursday*	B
Monday	G	*Friday*	F
Tuesday	C	*Saturday*	A
Wednesday	E		

Action of Music Notes
The action of music depends upon whether musical notes are classified by the Male Principle— concentrated (contracted) like the sun or the Female Principle—expanded like the sky and outer space. These two actions have specific notes.

Male Principle (Contractive)   C, E, D
Female Principle (Expansive)   G, B, F

Speaking Sounds (Music in Phonics)
The vibrations of the ear, chest, sinus cavity and organs can have healing properties. In the body, the sound of spoken letters is heard and then turns into an electrical signal and then into a chemical that has a healing, emotional and spiritual affect. Inhale deeply and slowly fill the lungs and exhale slowly while pronouncing a letter.

A	Healing the lymphatics, digestions
AH	Respiratory system
HAH	Heart, gall bladder, liver
KAH	Pineal, kidney, bladder, sex organs
E	Pineal, pituitary, nasal passage
O	Pancreas, spleen
U	Stomach, large and small intestines

African Music Theory
Blacks hear, sing and play music superiorly because of the high amount of Melanin in the inner ear bones and greater bone density and in the Melaninated hair of the cochlea receptor. The high amount of Melanin causes the African ear to absorb more sound (overtones) in the sound.

The African scales start on the high note and end on the low. This is owing to the anatomy of the body. The breath makes a high sound coming into the body and a low sound leaving the body. African scales follow the laws of the body's breath. African scales focus on the heart's rhythm. The heart rhythm is three beats as the second beat is silent. Whites do not count the silent beat and as a result they dance out of rhythm to Black music. They dance in two beats while Blacks dance in three beats.

African instruments were traditionally naturally tuned (all notes different) while European instruments are temper-tuned (all notes, such as the note "A" are the same cycle per second, varying only in pitch).

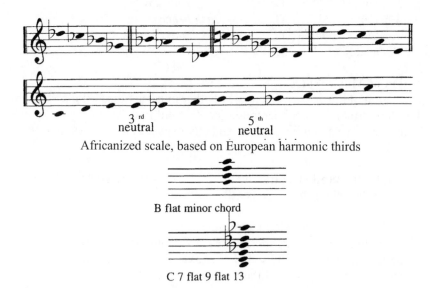

Africanized scale, based on European harmonic thirds

B flat minor chord

C 7 flat 9 flat 13

Music Scales (descending, consists of 5 notes) omit the 4th and 7th interval of European diatonic scale and alter the third.

Africanized European Scale. The third and fifth notes are partial overtones and not found on the temper-tuned European piano. African singers and instrumentalists use these notes. The European minor scale with lowered (flat) 5th is nearest to the African scale (can have a flat 9th and augmented 11th note). There are no major or minor scales in African music, just a communal type scale (a marriage of the European major and minor scale—C major combined with C minor).

Melody. In African music, the melody is dependent upon the harmonic structure and rhythm. Two types have hexatonic-gapped scale:

- Impango: female melody, high and fast
- Ziya Bilo: male melody, slow

GEMS OR CRYSTALS

Crystals (gems) are holistic and used for the treatment of dis-ease and bio-chemical stressors. They are also used to stimulate mental and spiritual energies. In addition, they are used in religious ceremonies or worn on garments, fingers, toes, as bracelets, necklaces, hair decorations and placed on acupuncture related meridians.

Caucasian invaders misinterpreted the ancient African cultures' therapeutic usage of holistic gems and called the gem therapy system jewelry or vain decorations. The Papyrus of Nun (18th Dynasty), which dates back to King Heser Ti (4300 B.C.) mentions crystals. Furthermore, gems can be used to treat a variety of dis-eases. Gems are crystallized plants or minerals (metals) and possess the fossilized energies of the plants and minerals. They can transmit and receive energies. They can be programmed just as a computer is programmed. For example, the juice of an herb (medicinal herb tea) can be poured over the crystal and this will cause the crystal to have the aura (power) of that herb. Further, a piece of colored cloth can be placed over a crystal and the gem will retain the aura of that color. This same principle can be used to program a crystal with a healing music note. In order to deprogram or erase the previous program of a crystal, water can be poured over it. There are many ways to program and deprogram a crystal.

TYPE OF CRYSTAL	PURPOSE USED
Amethyst	Purifies the blood; an appetite suppressant.
Aquamarine	Vital as a preventive; kidneys; heart.
Coral	Stimulant for digestion; blood purifier, prevents stomach cramps.
Diamond	Increase emotional intensities; increase willpower.
Emerald	Increases wisdom; good for glands; prevents diabetes; improves memory.
Garnet	Purifies tissue; good for rheumatism and arthritis; cleanses glands (e.g., pineal, prostrate, pituitary, etc.).
Jade	Has a calming effect on tension; migraines; balances thoughts; aids wisdom.
Moonstone	Effective for edema, kidney, bladder, and menstrual discomforts; helps intuitive thoughts.
Opal	Acts upon the reproductive system; generative properties; immunitive properties.
Pearl	Effective as a cleanser of blood; good for higher thoughts; wisdom.
Quartz	Balances thinking; relieves insomnia, prevents mood swings; combats infections.
Ruby	Stimulates the removal of internal plaque (e.g., varicose veins); swollen arteries, strengthens eyes.
Sapphire	Curative for skin diseases; heart diseases; helps prevent and cure depression.
Topaz	Good for liver diseases; digestive problems; nervousness for mental illness; a sex depressant.
Turquoise	Effective for increasing energy; accident preventive.

Crystals

The shape of crystals such as tetragonal, zircon, and double pyramids, attracts and radiates healing energy that has an affect on the health of the spirit, mind and body. Ancient Egyptians made khat cake (bread) into various curative crystal shapes such as conical and isosceles triangles. Crystals' shapes can be classified as; crystals are right-minded, left-minded, right-handed, left-handed and translate reverse motion. This science is African in origin and is mentioned in *The Book of the Dead;* in King Unas' (3500 B.C.) pyramid and in the papyrus of King Tutankhamen—Tut (3266 B.C.). Crystals are fossilized energy and have color harmonics, which have curative powers.

Crystals were worn to elevate the spirited mind and stimulate the Melanin and master gland—Pineal. Melanin makes the brain cell for all cells in the body. When Melanin is active, the higher thought is active. Therefore, Africans stimulated Melanin with crystals. In many ancient Egyptian pictures, we see crystals worn for healing and spiritual elevation. However, Caucasians thought crystals to be decorative jewelry. All art and artifacts in Africa were functional.

Crystals were also known by the Egyptians to be used to radiate fields of form, mass and gravity. The crystals were programmed and used to make objects decrease in weight. This knowledge may have been used to build pyramids.

Usage	Crystal	Usage	Crystal	Usage	Crystal
Abundance	Citrine	Depression	Topaz	Maat	Rhodecrosite, Rose Quartz
Addiction	Kunzite	Detoxification	Covellite	Meditation	Phenacite, Rose Quartz
Alcoholism	Amethyst	Diabetes	Bloodstone, Amethyst	Memory	Hematite
Allergies	Chrysocolla	Eloquence	Blue Tourmaline	Mental Clarity	Amber
Anger	Carnelian	Envy-Jealousy	Carnelian	Money	Malachite, Aventurine
Appetite	Kunzite	Female Health	Moonstone	Nervousness	Watermelon Tour
Arthritis	Malachite	Family, Children, and Relationship Violence	Jet	PMS	Moonstone
Blood Pressure	Bloodstone	Fidelity	Jade	Protection	Black Tourmaline
Broken Bones	Calcite	Games of Chance	Amazonite	Women	Snowflake Obsidian
Broken Heart	Chrysophrase	Grief	Obsidian	Self-Awareness	Labradorite
Calming	Sodalite	Harmony	Sodalite	Self Love	Rhodochrosite, Rose Quartz
Confidence	Tiger Eye	Happiness	Citrine	Sex	Garnet
Commitment	Garnet	Headache	Sugalite, Ruby	Sinus	Ulexite
Common Sense	Hematite	Immune System	Malachite	Sleep	Jade, Lepidolite
Concentration	Flourite	Indigestion	Citrine, Gr. Tour	Stress	Spectrolite
Cooperation	Smoky Quartz	Leg Cramps	Bloodstone	Tension	Lepidolite

USAGE	CRYSTAL	USAGE	CRYSTAL	USAGE	CRYSTAL
Courage	*Aquamarine*	**Loneliness**	*Jade,* *Pink Tour*	**Transition** *Lepidolite*	
Creativity	*Azurite*	**Luck**	*Green* *Aventurine*	**Wrinkles**	*Lepidolite,* *Rose Quartz*

CRYSTAL (GEM)	USAGE I	USAGE II
Amazonite (*Virgo*)	Love, Balance, Soothing	Eliminates stressors in emotional process. Enhances love. Nerves.
Amber (*Leo*)	Healing, Strength, Protection	Stimulates correctness in decisions and handling all of life's situations skillfully.
Amethyst (*Pisces*)	Spirituality, Contentment, Meditation	Enhances intellectual-emotional-physical bodies. Stability, strength and peace.
Aquamarine (*Gemini*)	Courage, Protection, Awareness	Refines spiritual awareness and thought process. Protects against pollution.
Aventurine (*Aries*)	Balance, Healing, Alignment	Balances Male-Female Principles. Harmonizes in working with spirit guides.
Azurite (*Sagittarius*)	Creativity, Meditation, Release	Resolves indecision and worry. Helps enter meditation mind state.
Bloodstone (*Pisces*)	Courage, Balance, Healing	Revitalizes and renews relationships. Centers and grounds heart energy. Blood circulation.
Boji Stone (*Scorpio*)	Regenerates, Healing	Balances Male/Female Principle. Cleans and charges Aura. Removes energy blocks. Cell growth.
Calcite (*Cancer*)	Amplifier, Refraction, Healing	Different colors of Calcite placed on Chakra amplify energy. Healing bones.
Carnelian (*Taurus*)	Protection, Strength, Stabilizing	Eliminates negative energy and sorrows. Protects against fear and rage. Energy stabilizing.
Chrysocolla (*Libra*)	Alignment, Balance, Meditation	Balances Chakras, ethereal planes and Male/Female Principle. Broken Heart.
Chrysoprase (*Libra*)	Alignment, Balance, Meditation	Balances Chakras, ethereal planes and Male/Female Principle. Broken Heart.
Citrine (*Leo*)	Optimism, Wealth, Cleansing	Stimulates Aura fields. Stimulates intuitive self. Promotes optimism. Abundance.

CRYSTAL (GEM)	USAGE I	USAGE II
Coral (Pisces)	Intuition, Regeneration, Connections	Stimulates intuition, visualization and communication with past masters. Circulation and tissue.
Covellite (Sagittarius)	Dreams, Rebirth, Healing	Converts dreams into reality. Releases the past. Stimulates cells to purge.
Diamond (Taurus)	Strength, Innocence, Abundance	Stimulates, endurance and a loving nature. Abundance in all areas of life.
Flourite (Aries)	Order, Balance, Healing	Elevates energy to bring order in mental-emotional-physical and spiritual realms.
Garnet (Leo)	Health, Commitment, Purification	Dissolves negative energy from Chakras. Adds commitment to purpose. Circulation.
Hematite (Leo)	Order, Balance, Mental	Helps utilization of mental capabilities. Balances Male/Female Principles. Dissolves negativity. Blood
Jade (Aries)	Fidelity, Harmony, Confidence	Helps actualize and attain devotion to purpose. Inner peace, self-reliance and self-sufficient. Loneliness, sleep.
Jasper (Leo)	Nurturer, Protection, Healing	Communicates morality and joy to others. For travel and against negativity. Internal organs.
Jet (Aquarius)	Protection, Healing, Psychic	Dissolves negative energy, guards and protects. Strengthens psychic aware ness. Health and Healing.
Kunzite (Taurus)	Balance, Healing, Meditation	Stimulates heart Chakra to 2nd and 3rd Chakras to produce loving communication. Compulsions.
Labradorite (Leo)	Transforms, Healing	Generates intuition and thought. Clears and balances Aura. Brain.
Lapis (Sagittarius)	Awareness, Connection, Creativity	Harmonizes physical and celestial realms. Expands intuitive and physical. Creative potential.
Lepidolite (Libra)	Transition, Healing, Honesty	Gives solutions to negative old patterns. Assists openness and honesty. Stress, tension, BP.
Malachite (Aries)	Intuition, Balancing, Transform	Transformation of spirit. Activates all Chakras to stimulate and enhance psychic abilities.
Moldavite (Scorpio)	Astral travel, Amplifier, Healing	Stimulates higher dimensional energy. Amplifies vibrations of other stones to enhance healing.

CRYSTAL (GEM)	USAGE I	USAGE II
Moonstone *(Cancer)*	Cleansing, Attainment, Healing	A cleanser of Chakra negative energy. Destiny fulfillment. PMS, female health and birth.
Obsidian *(Sagittarius)*	Reflection, Grounding, Shielding	Dissolves one's inadequacies and grounds energy to earth. Shields against negativity. Grief.
Onyx *(Aries)*	Protection, Projection, Defensive	Protects from social and spiritual conflict and psychic attack. Reduces sexual impulses.
Opal *(Pisces)*	Psychic Vision, Purifier	Helps utilization of intuition and higher power to invoke visions. Enhance dreamtime. Purifies blood, kidneys.
Peridot *(Virgo)*	Protection, Cleansing, Stimulates Healing	physical protection. Stimulates and cleans heart and navel Chakras. Heart, lungs.
Phenacite *(Gemini)*	Meditation, Knowing, Healing	Stimulates deep meditation. Brings the way of love and heavenly being. Cleanses.
Quartz *(All Signs)*	Elevates beneficial energy.	Modifies available energy for user. Balance.
Rhodochrosite *(Scorpio)*	Love, Balance, Purifier	Harmonizes love on all levels, physical. Purifies root and sacral Chakras.
Ruby *(Cancer)*	Dreaming, Teaching, Protection	Diverts psychic attacks. Intense and vivid dreams. Ancient knowledge.
Sapphire *(Gemini)*	Prosperity, Clarity, Healing	Dissolves unwanted thoughts. Brings joy and peace. Fulfills dreams, brings wealth. Blood.
Selenite *(Taurus)*	Awareness, Flexibility, Clear focus of mind, awareness Healing	of self, surroundings. Flexibility in one's nature. Skeletal system.
Sodalite *(Sagittarius)*	Mental, Fellowship, Healing	Stimulates logical conclusions and manifest trust in self and others. Digestive disorders.
Sugalite *(Virgo)*	Love, Energy, Healing Regenerates Maat.	
Tiger Eye *(Aries)*	Grounding, Balancing, Psychic .	Utilizes balanced thoughts Balance of both brain hemispheres. Psychic.
Topaz *(Sagittarius)*	Love, Success, Creativity	Focus elevates individuality and creativity. Replaces negativity with love. Success in all endeavors.
Tourmaline *(Libra)*		Cleanses, maintains and stimulates Chakras. Attracts inspiration and confidence. Lessens fear.
Turquoise *(Scorpio)*	Protection, Healing, Balance	Balances and protects. Dissolves negativity.

ANATOMY
(Differences Between the Black and White Races)

	BLACKS	WHITES
Melanin	-high content	-Least amount-causing albinism.
	-Increase color absorption in eyes	-Least ability
	-Increase sound absorption in ears	
	-Acts as a polymer	
	-Converts energy	
	-Acts as a computer	
	-Controls cyclical rhythms of all organs	
	-Controls sleep	
	-Controls growth (rate of puberty)	
	-Reacts to gravity (electromagnetic forces)	
	- Highest storage of information	
	-Processes largest amount of information in mid-brain	
	-Processes left-mind thoughts in right and left hemispheres of brain	
	-Processes right mind thoughts in left and right hemispheres of brain	
	-Can taste full range of flavor of foods due to melanin in cells	
	-Can smell the true aromas has the broadest range of smell identification	
	-Highest psyche ability	
	- Absorbs most electromagnetic energy	
	-Highest civilizing ability due to high melanin content	
	-Increased memory to memory transfer of stored information	
	-Process most information in corpus colostrums	
	-Evolve highest spirituality due to melanin content	
Skin melanin (Black Pigmentation)	-Allows protection from sun's ultraviolet rays	-Least of all races, causing white skin
	-Allows protection from extreme hot and cold temperatures	
Buttock (Stetobygia)	-High muscular development	- Flat, limited mobility
	-Allows extensive hip and thigh movements	
Legs	- Longer in proportion to upper body	-Short

	BLACKS	WHITES
Blood	-Allows better movement for walking and running -When heated (burnt) forms complex pyramids -Allows better storage and transmuting of energy	-Less pyramidal
Liver	-Slightly large -Allows increased cleansing and energy storage	-Slightly smaller
Hair	-Least amount of body hair caused by heat insulating effect of melanin -Broadest color spectrum bands in hair	-The most hairy of all races
Hair type	-Curly and brown -Allows quicker transmission and receiving of electrical and magnetic energy similar to an antenna -Hair shaped like galaxy (cross section shape)	-Flat and limp, weak antennas -Least color bands. -Hair is closest to fur -Hair has a kidney shape, slightly divided appearance
Alcohol	-Higher amount naturally made by body. Helps to cool body.	-Lowest amount.
Ammonia	-Lowest amount naturally made by body	-Highest amount, makes then slightly warm when in cold temperatures and problems in hot temperatures -Sun can cause cancer
Eyes	- Farthest apart -Allows increased field of vision (peripheral) -Eyes are brown, due to Melanin content -Allows better reception of Sun's color light heat which results in higher stimulation of pineal and pituitary glands - Absorbs full color, can see the true color of objects	-Closer together, narrow field of vision -Eyes blue, gray and green because veins are seen in back of eyes -See paler colors
Nose	- Broad and flat -Allows angular contour to air columns causing it to vibrate at higher frequency Thus, stimulating electromagnetic energy. -Allows wider field of vision for each individual eye	-Raised chiseled bridge blocks field of vision and separates and divides images (sees world divided) limited field of vision
Women's physique	-"T" shape similar to men, broad shoulder fossils indicate superior muscular structure. -Allows more independent muscular movements and counterbalance for hips and pregnancy weight	-No "T" shape, narrow shoulders, hips wider than shoulders, poor counterbalancing ability
Nerves	-High melanin content in nervous system -Allows nerve messages to travel faster and protects against disease	-Least amount of melanin of all races
Jaw	-Wider arch - Indicates diet high in vegetables	-Narrow; similar to flesh eating animals

	BLACKS	WHITES
Arms	-Longer in proportion to body -Allows better counter balancing	-Short, limit balancing ability

Lips	-Thick
	-Allows wider face muscular field
	    and better extraction of juices
	    from plants
		-Thin

Voice	-Wider range of speech tones; high and
	    low sounds
	
	-Melanin allows melodious and
	    rhythmical speech
		-Limited range with flat speech tones,
		    tones no rhythm, lacks melodious
		    sounds

Ears	-Small and stationary -Allows better center of sounds -Fluid different in weight inside air	-Large- can move them

Stomach	-Has the most flora (Fungi, Yeast and
	    bacteria that live in stomach, entire
	    digestive tract, uterus, vagina,
	    eyes, ears, etc.)
	- Is specific and unique only to Blacks,
	    have slightly more than 3 pounds
	-Allows food to be broken down
	    (metabolized) at a greater
	    nutritional level
		-No vast variety of flora, limits
		    food metabolism. Tends to
		    have a worm population

Vagina lips	-Larger -Allows tighter seal and increases flora lifespan	-Smaller
Vaginal shaft	-Longer -Allows increased muscular activity	-Short
Penis	-Length slightly longer	-Shorter
Skull	-Sagittal contour flat (top of head)	-Round
Face Height	-Low	-High
Eye	-Orbital opening rectangular	-Angular
Nasal	-Opening wide (nose)	-Narrow
Lower Nasal Margin	-Wide base	-Sharp
Facial Profile	-Downward slant	-Straight, no slant
Palate Shape	-Wide	-Narrow
Skin	-Absorb greatest percentage of colors	-Reflect colors
Color	-Eyes darken with age	-Extremely rare
Sacral Spot	-Birthmark on lower back and/or buttocks)	-Extremely rare

Breath	-Deeper (characteristic of
	    right-minded thinking)
		-Shallow breath
		    (Left-minded)

Skin	-Processes more Vitamin D (high amount owing to melanin)	-Poor processor of Vitamin D

Calcium intake	-Lower (High amount of
	    Vitamin D created by
	    melanin stabilizes calcium,
	    reduces need for high intake)
		-High Calcium intake required

**Sternoclavicular
muscle**
	-Allows mobility for swinging
	    from one tree limb to another
	    similar to monkeys; rare
		-Found abundantly

	BLACKS	WHITES
Pores of skin	-Widen with age	-No change
Muscle	-Fast twitch, highly responsive to stimuli, fast action, muscle is light in color, body has lowest salt content	-Slow twitch, less responsive, slow in action, muscle is dark in color, body has high salt content
Skin	-Has the most skin pores of any race	-Least pores
	-Better cooling	-Inadequate cooling
	-Most skin surface in relationship anatomy	-Least
Nutrients	-Highest nutrient density (most vitamins, minerals and amino acids per square inch)	-Least

There are differences in the Black and White Races explored in the books: *The Races of Europe* by C.S. Coon, *Genetics and The Races of Man* by William Boyd, T*he Encyclopedia Britannica* under Races of Mankind, *Diet and Nutrition* by Rudolph Ballantine and in pamphlets titled *Black Dot (Humanities Ancestral Blackness, the Black)* by R. King and *The Cress Theory (Racial Confrontation)* by F. Cress Welsing, textbook of *Black-Related Diseases* by R. A. Williams, *Estudios Sore Las Auithaminoses Y Las Perturbaciones Del Crescimento En Los Ninos Avitamonosicos* by R. A. Agillar.

CAUCASIAN SLEEP PATTERNS
(Measurable, Observable, etc.)

Steps		Electrical Current in Brain
1	**Low Beta**	13 to 16 cycles per second (c/sec)
2	**Alpha**	9 to 13 c/sec
3	**Theta**	6 to 9 c/sec
4	**Delta**	below 6 c/sec
5		REM (Rapid Eye Movement)

Steps	Sensations
1	See pictures (eyes closed)
2	Feel like body is floating
3	Dream (illusions, violence, sex, psychotic withdrawal, stimulation of Melanin may cause nightmares, etc.)
4	REM
5	Dead Sleep (senses do not react to stimuli, can sense the spirit)
6	Arousal (semiconsciousness of body and mind)
7	Awake (consciousness)

AFRICAN SLEEP PATTERN

Steps	Electrical/Magnetic
1	Male Principle, decrease in electricity
	Female Principle, increase in Magnetism
2	Male Principle generates magnetism, regenerates electricity
	Female Principle regenerates magnetism, generates electricity
3	Third Eye/Pineal Gland electromagnetic balanced vibrations

Steps	Sensations
1	Holistic pictures of spirit and physical life
2	Feel earth, lunar, solar and galaxy cycles
3	Emotional movement in body, psyche dream trance
4	Dream about life in timeless state
5	REM – Pineal Gland Vibrations
6	Reverse Order (Steps 5, 4, 3, 2, 1) and returns to physical body existence

AFRICAN SLEEP
Sleep is the Inactivity of the Conscious Mind.
Rest is the Inactivity of the Body.

ENTER SLEEP				EXIT SLEEP		
Body	**Mind**	**Spirit**	**Black Dot**	**Spirit**	**Mind**	**Body**
Inactive	Voluntary Inactive	Voluntary Active	Enter-Exit	Voluntary Inactive Involuntary Active	Voluntary Active	Active

CYCLIC SLEEP SEQUENCE

CYCLES			
Earth	**Lunar**	**Solar**	**Celestial**
Physical Inactive	Conscious Emotion, Inactivity	Electrical Decrease See Pictures	Magnetic Increase Floating

SLEEP SUPPLEMENTS

Calcium	3,000 mg	Magnesium	1,500 mg
Vitamin B Complex	100 mg	Vitamin B$_6$ (Pyridoxine)	300 mg
Vitamin B$_5$ (Panthonenic Acid)	300 mg	Melatonin	1-3 mcg
Tyrosine	500 mg	Nutritional Brewer's Yeast	3 tbsp
GABA	As Directed		

HERBS
Catnip, Passion Flower, Hops, Skullcap, Chamomile, Lady's Slipper, Valerian

PSYCHOLOGY
(Difference between Black and White Races)

BLACK RACE **(African-Centered Thought)**	**WHITE RACE** **(European-Centered Thought)**
-Equally uses right and left hemisphere of brain and mid-brain. -Characterized by right-minded spiritual concepts, love, affection and sharing. -Mid-brain characterized by equal balances of rational thought and creative thought.	-Characterized by unholistic Egotism, illogical use of left mind, non-spiritual individualism, rationalizations and non-creative. -Rationales based upon conflict between evil subconscious and good conscious. Military logic and predator nature.
-Time exists in the "now" and is eternal and cyclic. Future, past and present are combined. -Time is based on the beginning and ending of an event and is composed of the seen and unseen (spiritual, God manifested) causes of an event. Commonly called colored people time. Time is fixed by the event. For example, the seasons of spring, summer, winter and fall start according to nature's (unseen) clock.	-No present tense of life. Life exists in the past and future; this results in time conflicts and places no value on present. -Time is a fixed abstract measurable duration. The seasons start according to a fixed calendar date and not according to nature.
-Thoughts are concept oriented. The meaning of thoughts as well as of words are based on the story (situations) they are used in. For example, the word "bad" can be meant as good, modern, intellectual, excellence or bad. Consequently, this gives rise to statements such as "that's a bad car."	-Thoughts are linear oriented. The meaning of words are fixed and based upon static logic rationales. Consequently, a "bad car" means a car unacceptable instead of the Afri-Centric meaning of an excellent car.
-Culture is based upon Maat, the family (extended) marriage, ancestors, harmony with nature, spirituality.	-Culture is based upon creating evil to control good and creating good to control evil. -Have a pride-type family (similar to animals). -Control of nature. -Religions are political systems used to manipulate the powerless.
-Communal. Family-centered.	-Self-centered.
-Property owned by society; shared resources.	-Property is owned by individuals; no sharing of resources.
-Marriages: Predominantly polygamous included polygyny and monogamous marriages.	-Monogamous and the practice of polygamous relationships as sexual recreation (illegalgamy).
-Sex is reproductive, regenerational and spiritually used to serve Maat.	-Sex is a physical activity, recreational and reproductive.

BLACK RACE (African-Centered Thought)	WHITE RACE (European-Centered Thought)
-Individual's value in society is based upon what the individual contributes to society or "you are what you do."	-"You Are What You Own."
-Economics. Abundantly sharing your goods, talent, labor, child rearing, knowledge with society.	-Economics based upon scarcity, consumerism, or the creation of shortages. Thus, only an elite few can gain access to goods, resources, talent and knowledge.
-Science is wholistic and controlled by Maat.	-Science is rational and abstract based upon one group (the elite) controlling a system.
-Religion. Monotheism (belief in one God).	-Belief in many Gods. God created the Devil. (Evil type God).
-A person is born to achieve their highest level of humanism.	-A person is born in sin.
-Life is based on sense (seen) and non-sense (unseen) and is beyond the power of the mind.	-Life based upon seen, measured, touched or abstracted knowledge.
-Humans belong to God (no slavery).	-Humans are owned by man (Full Slavery).

AFRICAN WHOLISTIC ZODIAC CHART

Body	Zodiac	Music Note	Color	Zodiac House
Pituitary, Eyes, Cerebrum, Nose	Aries	D^b	Red	1
Neck, Cerebellum, Throat, Lower Brain, Thyroid	Taurus	E^b	Yellow	2
Heart, Thymus, Spleen	Leo	$A^\#$	Orange	5
Kidney, Adrenal, Bladder	Libra	D	Yellow	7
Breast, Veins, Arteries, Stomach	Cancer	$B^\#$	Green	4
Intestine, Liver, Pancreas, Lower Abdomen	Virgo	C	Violet	6
Sciatic Nerve, Thigh, Hips, Buttocks	Sagittarius	F	Purple	9
Genitals, Gonads, Rectum	Scorpio	E	Red	8
Para-thyroid, Lower Leg, Colon, Ankles	Aquarius	A	Indigo	11
Feet, Circulation, Pineal	Pisces	B	Indigo	12
Knees, Teeth, Bones	Capricorn	G	Blue	10
Arms, Fallopian Tubes, Thymus	Gemini	$F^\#$	Violet	3

ACUPRESSURE MERIDIANS

Meridians are pathways that carry energy to and from specific organs. Bumps, rashes, scratches or a change of skin texture, color or temperature; as well as a change of hair texture and/or color on a meridian indicates a disorder with that organ. These meridians are reviewed in *Acupuncture for Americans* by L. Wensel.

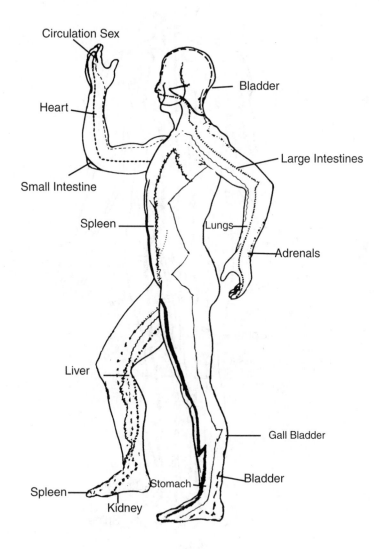

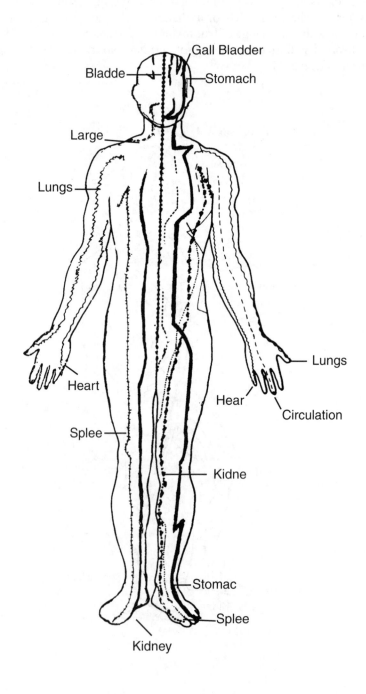

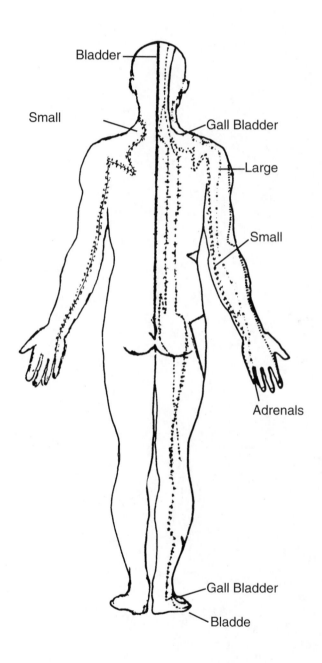

Section 16

Wholistic Perspectives

Science

Wholistic science is a science, which asks wholistic questions and receives wholistic answers. Non-wholistic science views man as a machine without a spirit. It separates science as a non-cultural, non-racial, or non-religious body of knowledge, while African wholistic science is a functional part of the culture, astrology, religion and racial identity of Black peoples.

AFRICAN SCIENCE	EUROPEAN SCIENCE
All things (organic and inorganic)are living; these living things are placed in kingdoms.	There are two living things— plants and animals These living things are in two kingdoms. There are non-living things called organic.
Kingdoms: Mineral, Plant, Spirit (Deities), Ancestral, Animal, Human.	**Kingdoms:** Plant, Animal
Organic, all things in nature are alive and give and receive energy and they eat a type of food and produce a type of waste.	Organic things (living); Inorganic things (not living)
African science states that all things are controlled by seen and unseen forces. Accidents are controlled by the law of Accident. Subsequently, there is no use of the word "accident" in this science.	European science—uses the words accident coincidence or undefined. All things are caused by seen forces or it is accidental or due to random selection (by chance).
Man is three things (body, mind, spirit) that occupy one space at the same time. No crude limited earth laws can apply to man or define man's life, health, diseases, death, and spirituality.	No two things can occupy the same space at the same time. Local earth laws can explain all things.
The earth has its own heat and excites the earth's heat. For example, you cannot give energy to a dead person. It takes energy to receive energy. Only the living can give to the living. Therefore, the earth has its own living energy.	The sun gives the earth sun heat.
The earth was made whole.	The earth was made in layers.
The layers of the earth indicate the age of the layer, not the age of the earth.	Each layer of the earth can indicate the total age of the earth.
Science is based on Male and Female Principle.	Focus on the Caucasian male principle.
Science uses trances, astrology, divination and ancestors.	Science is abstract and only uses biology and chemistry.

AFRICANSCIENCE	EUROPEAN SCIENCE
Studies the past, present and future as one. To study the past is to study the future.	Studies the past (standard formulas) and future (theories) separately.
Science is a language of culture and Maat.	Science is non-cultural.
Science is combined with Art. (Science is Art, Art is science)	Science is separate from art.
Time, space and distance are mixed together as one.	Time, space and distance are separated.
Males, Females and Children express diseases differently.	All disease diagnosis, signs and symptoms are based upon the white male's expression of disease.

Holistic Science
    Part + Part = New Part (Not a Sum)
	Particle Science
	    Part + Part = Sum of Parts

Vitamin A + Vitamin D = New (Synergistic) Vitamin >To combine, they both have to alter themselves and change into something new.	Vitamin A + Vitamin D = Vitamin A, D > Combine without changing is a contradiction in logic and science
Human Cells Grow = Corpuscles Divide Human cells grow from a Melanin template called a Stole.	Cells Divide (Corpuscles and Cells are the same).
Science myths are a part of the Art of Science.	Science myths (theories) are believed to be facts and are used as facts.
Science is spiritual.	Science is not spiritual.
There are many different types of air, water, vitamins, minerals, cells, molecules and atoms—too numerous to label. These various types are similar to the many different types of humans, water, plants, language, insects and cultures. Every race has a unique biochemical personality and breathes in a unique form of air (metabolizes a specific ratio of gases to air). The lungs digest air, then the liver synchronizes the building of the form of air needed by the individual. The gases are put in the right combination for the individual.	There is one type of water, air, mineral, etc. Everyone drinks the same water but converts it to their race's biochemistry and the biochemistry of each race is different. Each race has a different Melanin content and a different biochemistry. Races metabolize food differently Water and air is food. These obvious facts are defined in ethnomedicine. Caucasians ignore these facts and say that all races are the same.
Each particular plant and animal converts the air they breathe into the unique	

AFRICAN SCIENCE	EUROPEAN SCIENCE

structure they require before it is absorbed (metabolizes a specific ratio of gases) air. Each human requires a unique biochemical form of air, water and color light heat (sun rays). We breathe in the air then the body converts the substance into the right molecular/elemental combination for our biochemical personality. Air is digested differently by different races.

Scientific proofs are wholistic and found only in nature.	Scientific proofs are performed in an artificial environment (laboratory) under controlled conditions. These scientific proofs are experiments (science rituals and ceremonies) which force nature to give answers to questions devised by man. Science proofs are not totally valid. For example, Vitamin A is tested in a room with light, air and a temperature of 72°F. Vitamin A in the body is digested in the dark and at 98.6°F. Consequently, the laboratory proofs of Vitamin A's actions and reactions within the body are based upon the wrong conditions. The laboratory proof of Vitamin A is at best 60% accurate. It does not reflect the intelligence or spirituality of Vitamin A. The proof is a science guess about Vitamin A— mythology.
Food is medicine and medicine is food. The African concept is that food (medicine) stimulates the body towards health(has enzymes) or disease (cooked, has no enzymes. Foods cannot create health. Health is created by God. Whole food can stimulate good health. Junk food (processed) can stimulate poor health. Food cannot create you. Food cannot uncreate you. Food stimulates the wellness in you. Processed foods and drugs drain the body's energy. The body can spend all its energy defending itself from enzymeless junk foods or drugs. Eventually, the energy is lost and the health is lost—disease.	The basic difference between African and Caucasian medicine science is in concept. Hippocrates believed that food (herbal medicine) is a fuel that provides energy that operates the body. If you give the body the wrong fuel (processed food or drug medicine), it will get sick. This Greek concept is the foundation of Caucasian health and biological science.
What is morally wrong cannot be scientifically or rationally correct.	What is scientifically correct is rationally correct.

VIOLENCE AND CHILDREN:
BEATING, HITTING AND SPANKING CHILDREN

Acts of physical violence against African children is a Caucasian socially engineered behavior (seasonin). Beatings teach the child that violence is the solution to problems. Beating a child should have a relationship to Maat. Beating should connect the child to Maat. Beating a Black child is usually done in the same way as Caucasians. Beatings connect the child to Caucasian culture. Beatings usually imitate the slave and slave master relationship. The adult is the slave master and child the slave. If the beating does not define Maat—don't do it. Historical evidence validates that physical violence was not used by ancient Africans. In fact, Incas, Chinese, Japanese, Indians, Eskimos and other races of color do not beat children. Even among African headhunters and cannibals, the beating of children was not used for discipline. Spanking or lightly hitting the child to get their attention is needed (i.e., a child getting ready to touch a fire or wander into the street). The elders called it slaptime and laptime (nurturing, Maat).

The Maat social conditions are not available for the child and parents. The beating of children lacks a cultural definition. The beating of children does not transmit or translate African culture. The elders and ancestors have no involvement in the child's beatings. The child can use the parents' violent beatings as a way to manipulate their parents by behaving or talking disrespectful. The parent responds to the child's disrespect toward them with a beating. The child may then cause the parent to feel guilty for lacking control over the parent/child relationship. The parent may feel angry because they lack parenting skills and do not have the social skills needed to control the child. The child can use the parent's guilt or anger at themselves to manipulate the parent into letting them go to a movie, eat pizza, play a computer game, etc.

All intelligent thinking stops the moment violence begins. Violence is the beginning of social ignorance in solving a problem. The Caucasian practice of beating (violent physical attacks) children was and is used because children are considered selfish, have subconscious animalistic traits, have deep evilness in their soul and/or have need to have sex with the parent or have a violent nature. While in African culture, children are considered endowed with the spirit of the ancestors, striving to achieve Godliness, are raised to reach their highest level of humanism, mirror the village's soul, are God's property, the future of the village and Maat. Subsequently, in African culture violent attacks upon a child were considered a violent attack to destroy the culture, God, Maat, ancestors, spirits, society, tribe and individual.

Child abuse, beatings and sexual abuse (minors watch or listening to pornographic R rated videos and/or movies) perpetrated upon Black children by Black adults is justified by excuses (rationales). For example, one of the popular excuses for beating a child is the saying "spare the rod and spoil the child." The rod is misinterpreted to mean a stick, spanking or physical beating. Historically, the rod (or scepter) referred to in this saying is the divining rod or staff of a shepherd. The rod is the symbol of authority. The rod was not used to beat the sheep. The rod was used to guide the sheep. The rod is a symbol of the ultimate authority—God. The guiding force is Maat. The rod is symbol of Maat and God. In other words, do not spare Maat or the spirituality of God or else the child will perish (be spoiled). A rod was believed to be guided by God. Parents without adequate parenting skills or the village support can be physically violent with children and use fists, switches, baseball bats, shoes, belts, hollering, verbal abuse, screaming, cursing and threaten the child with torture and violent punishments. The Slave Master beating the slaves did not stop slave revolts. In any ease, the sparing of the rod meant to ignore God's wisdom and cause the child to decay (spoil). The non-violent Civil Rights Movement of the 1960s was used to teach love, justice, harmony, democracy, peace and understanding to Caucasians. However, Blacks used violence in their male/female relationships and beat their children. Blacks were teaching their children to solve Black problems with violence and White problems with non-violence. Beating children must stop and alternative solutions used. The culture, Maat, spirituality and the control of rewards and punishments and shaming the child can be used in place of beatings. Only take away rewards for specific behaviors. Do not tell the child they are bad. Tell the child the behavior was bad. Take away a reward as punishment. The child is not the sum total of bad behaviors. Many unacceptable behaviors were learned from the parent and medias. Correcting the child means to correct a parenting skill. Punishment of the child can be taking away privileges (i.e., CDs, videos, television, play time, telephone usage).

SMOKING AND CHILDREN

Is smoke (tobacco, marijuana) a natural food for the body? No! The human body was not designed for the inhalation of smoke in the lungs. Lungs are only anatomically structured to inhale clean (unpolluted) air. The cancer-causing and mood altering drugs are in droplet form in the smoke. The burning of tobacco and/or marijuana creates a drug. Fire (heat) creates a synthetic poisonous chemical combined with a transoil (synthetic) drug. Smoking in the presence of a child is child abuse. The drug droplets in the smoke cause liver damage, DHEA hormone imbalance, addiction, decreased oxygen to the child's brain and cancer. An adult who smokes in the presence of a child causes the child to be a passive smoker. An adult smoker forces the child to be a passive smoker. This kind of forced smoking is child abuse, a crime and is destructive to the child's health. Passive smoking is indirect and drugs in the smoke have a higher cancerous content of toxins and tar. The thick oily tar contains drugs and is addicting. Ironically, the tobacco companies lowered the tar in a cigarette. This caused smokers to smoke more cigarettes in order to reach the drug level they use to get from the tar drug of one cigarette.

The drugs in smoke weaken the lungs, liver, kidneys, skin, immunity and destroy Vitamin C. The smoke from a single cigarette destroys the Vitamin C content of an average orange. Vitamin C is vital in protecting the child against dis-eases.

Smoke deprives the child's (and adult's) skin of clean air (oxygen). This causes premature aging. The chemicals in smoke aggravate asthmatic and allergic children. It irritates the sensitive mucous membrane (inner skin surface) of the nose. Children have an immature immune system; smoking is twice as destructive to the child.

The chemicals in smoke can cause skipped heartbeats, palpitation of the heart, nervousness, rapid heart rates, paralysis of the cilia (hair) in the lungs; toxins are absorbed, dizziness, shortness of breath, headaches from rises in blood pressure and pains of distress over the front of the chest. Smoke decreases circulation to the hands, feet and legs. The nicotine causes the veins to constrict (close) and this limits the blood flow to the heart, sex organs and other vital organs. The female passive smoker undergoes menopause at a younger age.

Children learn by example. They imitate adult behavior. Historically, the original smoke eaters (nicotine drug addicts) were Caucasians. Blacks who are nicotine drug smokers are socially conditioned (engineered, seasonin) to do so.

The non-smoking adults and children can be partially protected from smoke by using a high efficiency particle air (hepa) filter or the electronic precipitator air cleaners, which can remove a few of the cancerous chemicals. The immunity can be protected from smoke with supplements such as Glutathione, Chaparral, Pau D' Arco, Cysteine, Vitamin A, C, E, B_1, B_6, Pantothenic Acid, PABA, Echinacea, Selenium, Bee Propolis and Zinc. Alkaline minerals, Phenylalanine, Betaine Hydrochloride and the herb Kudzu and Quassia can help curb the craving for the smoke. Tobacco and marijuana is processed with steroids, excessive amounts of estrogen, white sugar, ammonia, etc. Consequently, Vanadyl Sulfate, Progesterone and Milk Thistle need to be added to a treatment protocol.

SHOULD WE EAT FOOD?
(Breathatarian Concept)

In African sciences of chemistry, physics, and biology, it is understood that only God can create life and energy. Energy is in the atom (life). Trees do not eat dirt for energy and atoms do not eat food for energy. All things are composed of atoms. You do not need to eat food. The atoms of energy (food) are electromagnetic and biochemical. A positive (clockwise spin) and negative (counterclockwise spin) atom rubbing together generates electromagnetic and biochemical energy. Food stimulates the atom to spin fast or slow. The food atoms (particles) cause the body's atoms to lose their synchronized spin; the body's atoms try to regain their synchronized spin—this regaining of spin creates energy.

Humans are composed of atoms. The body's atoms are capable of adapting. The current diet and social situation of Africans is an adaptation to White Supremacy. The African's life is not a normal African life. It is a dysfunctional life and not normal. The current biochemical and electromagnetic behaviors of atoms is an adaptation that is erroneously assumed to be normal. For example, the Ice Age caused the land in Europe to freeze. This freezing destroyed vegetation and contributed to the Caucasian cannibals using animal meat for food. The Caucasians' dietary adaptation eventually became a normal diet. Caucasian scientists justify their scavenger diet as optimum, despite scientific proofs that humans can exist as vegetarians and despite proofs that atoms do not eat food for energy. The atoms that compose the skin, nerves, brain, bones and organs are wholistic and use another source of energy. Thoughts create thoughts, emotions create emotions and energy generates energy. Energy is already present in the atom. The atom did not create itself. It was created with its God-given energy supply. Food was used as an offering to the Holy Temple (human body). Food has mental and spiritual intelligence. The atoms that compose the tissue of plants are spiritual and intelligent. Digestion (eating) separates the food's spirit and mind from the tissue of the food so that the body's atoms can use it. The course matter (tissue fiber, minerals) residue of the food lessens the vitality of the body. The ancient carnoptic jars have figures and paintings on them that indicate the spirit and intelligence of the organs. Today, the spirit and intelligence of the organs are not used because the Caucasians have forced Africans to believe that organs (atoms) are only a physical (mechanical) structure. Africans no longer have the cultural program needed to access their own intelligence or their spiritual relationship to food, organs and atoms.

Eating earth minerals in plants and/or animal minerals causes the life span of humans to decrease. The minerals (electrolytes) are stressors. They rust (oxidize) the cells and atoms. Oxidizing ages the cells and atoms, destroys immunity, causes disease and eventually death. All ancient books and religious books (Indian, Chinese, African, Incas, European) indicate that humans lived from 400 to 1,000 years of age. Human beings once grew to heights of 10 to 25 feet tall. Ancient Africans' fasts (food abstinence), and used whole foods spiritually and as part of rituals and ceremonies. Food is passive. The digestive system acts upon the food; food does not act upon the body's cells (atoms). The body's atoms action upon the food is called energy.

The stomach is a protrusion of a pipe. It is not a separate organ like the heart. The stomach is not technically classified as inside the body. The stomach is a bulging out of a hollow tube that runs from the mouth to the anus. The tube is inside the body. It is protected similar to the way the skin on the hands, arms, legs, chest, etc. We do not think of our skin eating food. Particles of food are sucked into the blood by the straw-like hair (villa) of the small intestine. Once the food particles (atoms) are in the blood, they are electromagnetically and by smell guided to where they are needed. The food atoms cause an imbalance and the body's reaction to the imbalance is called energy.

The Caucasian practice of eating animal flesh (J. A. Rogers, *100 Amazing Facts About the Negro*) is dysfunctional. The Caucasians use a science myth to define the hollow tube called the stomach as an organ and/or gland is questionable. In any case, the spirit and mental energy of food excites the body's cells in a negative or positive manner and does not give or create energy. Humans are not created by food nor are humans the ancestors of food, and they cannot be uncreated by food. Food stimulates energy already present in the body. In ancient dietetic practices, food was used to excite the energy the body accumulated after fasting. The ancient wholistic African could move the spirit and intelligence of the body's atoms and generate energy. This is called free will. Willing the atoms to move means food is not necessary. Spirit does not need food. Spirit manifests mind and mind manifests the body. The key to energy is spirituality. The spirituality of the African biochemical and electromagnetic body can only be accessed with the African Maat cultural program. A Caucasian program (acculturated diet) eaten by an African de-programs the African biochemistry, spirit and intelligence and creates a diseased and culturally castrated African. Atoms (Atun) are spirits seeking higher levels and by passing through the human body (as food), they hope to obtain it. It is their spirit that wants communion with a spirit. The food atoms seek communion. In books such as *Proper Food of Man* by J. Smith and *Principles of Science* by W. Jevons, this subject is raised.

RUN OR DON'T RUN

Running is an isolated activity. The body requires a natural whole food diet; spiritual, mental and physical activities to be healthy. An isolated, unholistic activity cannot achieve wellness. Running is an isolated activity and needs to be part of a wholistic lifestyle in order to benefit the health. Exercise tones and/or builds muscles. Exercise requires fuel and that fuel is obtained from a good digestive system, the correct combining of whole foods. The diet provides the fuel. A junk food diet and exercise increases the degeneration of the body. A natural foods diet and exercise increases the wellness. Exercise (running) that includes affirmations, chants, prayers, drums and African music (i.e., jazz, positive rap, gospel, etc.) African physical games put the act of running in an African cultural context, which results in wholistic exercise. This form of exercise benefits the spirit, mind and body.

EXERCISE

Exercise does not help the lungs and heart. George Shoehart, M.D., cardiologist, runner and author of many books on running has said "Exercise does virtually nothing for the lungs; that has been amply proved by pulmonary specialists. Nor does it especially benefit your heart. Running, no matter what you have been told, primarily trains and conditions the muscles. Leg muscles can improve as much as 300% in work capacity with minimal changes in heart capability." The strengthening of the heart after a heart attack is not achieved by developing leg muscles (running) rather than heart muscle. Cardiologist Paul Dudley White (a bicyclist) examined legs and considered good muscular structure and tone as a measure for surgical risk. Cardiologist Gordon Cumming of Canada research has indicated that improvement in metabolic muscle processes and peripheral circulation could account for increased heart stroke volume.

Exercise does not prevent heart dis-ease. Heart disease is a systemic (bodily) illness. The elimination of processed foods and drugs can cure heart disease. Running has little effect on the wellness of the heart.

Reasons for Exercise

- Decreases stress
- Increases self-esteem
- Increases digestion
- Increases oxygen supply to cells
- Relieves tension
- Relieves constipation
- Increases flexibility of muscles and bones

- Decreases depression
- Increases sexual energy
- Increases the efficiency of the body
- Helps burn off fat
- Increases creativity
- Increases endurance

Exercise Tips

- Exercising all muscle groups or the whole body at one time is a more healthy holistic workout for fitness, rather than the fragmented and isolated workouts of fitness trainers, gym body toning exercise and body building

- Schedule time daily to do light workouts or light exercise. On your days off from work, exercise (i.e., work, jog, ride a bike, swim, play a sport). Acquire more knowledge about nutrition, African culture and spirituality and consciousness (i.e., read, listen to health lectures on CD or tape, watch health television programs, attend health seminars or lectures).

- Drink at least two glasses of water one to two hours before you work out. Drink water on a schedule. It is a food and too much at one time stops its digestion. Drink as much water as you need to while you are working out, then one or two glasses after the workout.

- To prevent the loss of muscle during exercise, eat a small whole grain (starch) carbohydrate meal within two hours after you work out.

- Experience your spirit and feel each muscle as you are working it. Recite positive affirmations and/or prayers while you are exercising.

- Keep all movements fluid and smooth. No sudden jerky movements.

Exercise Warm-Ups

1st   5 – 15 minutes on stationary bike, rowing machine or treadmill
2nd   5 – 15 minutes on rowing machine or cross-country ski machine
3rd   5 – 15 minutes of stretching
4th   Sit-ups (crunches only). Three sets of 5 – 15 repetitions
5th   Vertical leg raises. Three sets of 5 – 15 repetitions

EXERCISE	MUSCLES EXERCISED
Calf Raises	Calf Muscle
Chest Press/Pec Deck	Chest, Shoulders
Forearm Curls	Wrist, Forearms, Fingers
Lat Pull-down	Lats, Biceps
Leg Curls	Hamstrings, Calves
Leg Extensions	Front of Thigh
Leg Press or Squat	Thigh, Buttocks
Shoulder Press/Lateral Raises	Shoulders, Triceps, Traps
Tricep Push Downs	Triceps, Forearms
Two-arm Curls	Biceps, Forearms

Exercise Work-Out Schedule

Monday, Wednesday, Friday   Weights
Tuesday, Thursday, Saturday   Cardiovascular Exercise (running, Low intensity and long duration Exercise)

Walking

- You can walk with two to five pound hand weights and/or five to ten pound leg weights

- You can walk with a variety of arm positions (i.e., side lateral-front, circle positions, raised arms, rotate arms while walking, flexing arms [contracting and relaxing muscles, etc.])
- You can walk up steps or steep hills. This will exercise your thighs and buttock muscles.

Walking Schedules (Three to Four Times a Week)

Weeks 1 & 2   Walk two miles at normal walking pace, three times a week for 30 minutes
Weeks 3 to 5   Walk three miles (mile one at normal pace, miles two and three at brisk pace, three times a week for 30 minutes

Weeks 6 – 13	Walk three miles briskly four times a week for 30 minutes
Schedule Weekly Walks *(intermediate and advanced walkers can use any combination of walks*	• Walk at normal pace for one minute
	• Walk briskly for one minute
	• Walk normally for one minute
	• Jog lightly for two minutes
	• Walk normally for one minute
	• Walk briskly for two minutes
	• Jog lightly for one minute
	• Walk briskly for one minute
	• Walk normally for three minutes
	• Walk briskly for three minutes
	• Walk normally for three to four minutes (total time, 18-20 minutes).

SUN EXPOSURE

Get sunlight exposure daily and use full spectrum artificial lights. Sunlight is food for the body and emotions. Exercise outdoors.

SUNLIGHT INCREASES	SUNLIGHT DECREASES
Pineal Gland Activity	Free radicals
Endurance	Respiratory rate
Vitamin D	Bone loss
Energy (increased glycogen stores in the liver)	Lactic acid in the blood following exercise
Melanin Secretion	Diseases
Strength	Blood pressure
Melatonin and Serotonin	Fatigue and depression
Balance of Stress	Blood sugar
Sex Hormones	
Oxygen Supply of Blood	Diastolic (Resting heart rate)

WHOLISTIC FEMALE/MALE PUBERTY
(Teenagers, Herbs, etc.)

In African culture puberty is a phase of a spiritual, mental and physical growth. In Caucasian culture, puberty is the juvenile male and female becoming fertile. Puberty is a word derived from the French language and it means "grown up." During puberty, boys between ages 14 and 18 years start to have the ability to ejaculate sperm and girls between ages 12 and 14 start to ovulate and menstruate. During puberty, the boy's voice lowers, facial, underarm and genital hair starts to grow. The male hormone cycle starts to influence moods, behaviors and thoughts. In uncircumcised boys, the penis foreskin protects the penis head and secretes a moist fluid, which lubricates the penis head. This fluid increases during intercourse. There is no medical or health hygienic validation for the surgical butchering called circumcision. Circumcision is a religious and/or cultural ritual. In some cultures, females are circumcised. In any case, girls in puberty start to grow mammae (breasts), larger labia (vaginal lips), underarm hair, genital hair, more fatty tissue under the skin and the hips (pelvis) expand.

The pubescent growth is physically caused by sex hormones. Sex hormones are made by the ovaries, testicles and adrenal glands. These hormones stimulate and cause growth. The sex hormones cause fertility and spiritual, mental, emotional and physical changes. The spiritual, mental and emotional energies increases and fluctuates and changes in order to help the wholistic transition into adulthood.

Adolescence or pubescence is the wholistic, hormonal and cyclical preparation for adulthood.

Rites of Passage rituals, ceremonies and academic classes that teach Maat, the Human Cycle, Male/Female Relationship, proper sexual intercourse, obligations to the village, ancestors, children and your mate, spiritual duty, mental duty and physical duty were structured holistically. The purpose of the Rites of Passage is to transmit and translate Maat culture.

Herbs & Health

The male/female child, in puberty, requires specific nutrition and sex hormone balance. A natural foods diet is the optimum diet for this growth phase. This diet requires the complete elimination of synthetic (man-made) foods, preservatives, conservatives, soaps, toothpastes and deodorants and should include the use of cotton underwear.

The female child should use the unbleached sanitary napkin, not tampons. Tampons cause the reabsorption of decomposed (putrefied) flesh and take moisture out of the skin of the labias and vagina, causing skin disease. Additionally, the girl should be given herbs such as Red Raspberry Leaves, Chaste, Black Cohosh, Wild Yam, Catnip, Saw Palmetto, False Unicorn, Don Quai, Damiana, Cramp Bark, Bayberry, Gotu Kola, Rosemary, Ginger, Ginseng, Sarsaparilla and Lady Slipper. In the case of suppressed menstruation, Pennyroyal and Black Cohosh should be used cautiously (if it is desired to cause hemorrhaging). Progesterone Crème/Lotion can be applied to fatty tissue areas (i.e., hips, thighs, stomach, etc.)

The male child should be given herbs such as Maca, Muira Puama, Tribulus, Dopa Bean, Saw Palmetto, Pygeum, Wild Yam, Fo-Ti, Gotu Kola, Ginseng, Damiana, Yohimbe, Echinacea, Sarsaparilla, Catnip, Goldenseal and Rosemary. Progesterone Crème/Lotion can be applied to bony areas in order to correct hormone imbalances caused by junk foods, meat, eggs, dairy, commercial fruits and vegetables.

Supplements can aid passage into pubescence. Supplements such as Pregnenolone (Progesterone tablets), Vitamin E, C, A, D, and B Complex, Coenzyme Q10, Vanadyl Sulfate, Lipoic, Wheat Germ Oil, Lecithin, Kelp, Histidine, Phosphorus, Selenium, Calcium, Potassium, Magnesium, Manganese and Iron are beneficial for puberty.

Ideally, the child's puberty education should start before the puberty transition starts. It should be viewed as the Maat training of the new ancestors and elders of the society.

MEDICAL MIRACLES

Caucasian Orthodox medicine takes the credit for scientific miracles and modern advances in health. This medical science assumes that it has saved mankind from disease. Caucasians claim that their vaccinations are miracle cures. However, vaccines can cripple and cause many diseases and death. Polio Vaccine has cancer-causing Simian Virus 40. Many vaccines have cancer-causing formaldehyde, poisonous aluminum and DNA and RNA from rotten pork, beef and monkey tissue. No vaccine improves immunity; they destroy immunity. Chicken Pox vaccine is totally unsafe; the ingredients are white sugar, Thimersol (poisonous mercury), fetal bovine serum (cattle pus), EDTA, neomycin, Varicella Zoster Virus (herpes), hydrolyzed gelatin (pork, beef), MRC-5 cells, sodium chloride (salt), potassium chloride, monosodium glutamate (cancer), potassium phosphate monobasic, sodium phosphate dibasic, protein (pork, beef) and unspecified chemicals.

The diseases that Caucasian medicine claims to have eradicated has nothing to do with the use of drug medicine or vaccinations. The diseases that the Caucasian medicines claim to have eliminated were eliminated by cleanliness, soap and water, toilets usage and basic bodily hygiene.

European cities were kept filthy with human, dog, cat, rat, bat and insect waste; discarded remains of butchered animals, urine, dead bodies, garbage and stagnant waters. Unsanitary conditions and filth created an environment for disease. The Caucasians' Bubonic Plague was caused by fleas biting diseased and dead rats then biting humans; malaria is caused by anopheles mosquitoes (they used stagnant, polluted water); yellow fever is caused by stegomia mosquitoes and typhus fever is caused by body lice. The failure of surgeons to clean incisions caused many deaths until 1865 when Lister introduced antiseptics. African Egyptians used antiseptic herbal wines over 3,000 years before the Caucasians' miracle discovery of antiseptic. Lister observed that foul smelling sewage was treated with carbolic acid, so, he applied carbolic acid to foul smelling, pus-filled surgical wounds. However, the Caucasian medical scientists of that century thought that an antiseptic was another superstitious ritual. They failed to recognize that antiseptic procedures were related to cleanliness until much later. The Caucasians were defecating and urinating on the dirt floors of their homes and in their drinking water. This caused diseases. The miracle cure for this was John Harrington's invention of the toilet bowl (water closet), in 1500. In 1865, Semmelweis stopped childbed fever by having hospitals wash sheets, utensils and floors and having health practitioners wash their hands after touching dis-eased patients wounds and corpses. A simple matter of cleanliness and hygienic care ended many illnesses. However, the pus peddlers (vaccinationists) teach the public that miracle of vaccinations solved the problems of diseases.

The pus peddlers operate on the theory that a disease attack can be stopped by injecting diseased pus into the veins. The fleas that caused the Bubonic Plague inoculate people when they bite; the mosquitoes that cause yellow fever and malaria inoculate people when they bite. The fleas vaccinate and yet the public gets the diseases. It is assumed that man cannot withstand a small insect's inoculating dosage of disease but can withstand a large hypodermic needle's large inoculating dosage of disease. Many people get vaccinations (inoculations) or initial attacks of influenza, colds, headaches, syphilis, gonorrhea, herpes, yeast infections, smallpox, chickenpox, fevers, polio, athlete's feet, tooth decay, and toothaches and yet continue to get a second, third and fourth attack of the same disease. Many of these diseases are blamed upon an evil enemy attack of bacteria. This bacteria theory was first recorded in European history by John Astrue, a physician to Louis XIV, and is still used today to justify Caucasian medical mythology, ignorance and practices based upon superstitions.

The bacteria theory (mythology) assumes that evil bacteria are always trying to attack people. Unsanitary conditions, ignorance, superstitions, medically-caused diseases, vaccinations, poor hygiene and uncleanliness cause the accumulation of toxins in the body. The body is well equipped to control and eliminate impurities if good hygiene is followed. However, science mythology and the religious belief that evil (devil) is out to destroy people's health keeps this widespread paranoia alive.

The rampant paranoia about catching colds, viruses, bacterial infections and dis-eases, is organized ignorance. Vaccinationists and drug peddlers stimulate, create, recreate and manufacture this germ theory paranoia to sell mouth washes, antihistamines for the nose, disinfectant sprays, douche solutions, feminine hygiene sprays, deodorants, antibiotics, bottle sterilizers, eye washes, soaps, toothpaste and foot sprays. This massive paranoia leads one to live in fear of an attack from a predatory dis-eased bacteria. Bacteria reside in the body at all times. An imbalance of bacteria caused by dis-ease. Bacteria do not cause disease; they react to disease.

Bacteria can get out of balance when faulty dietary habits are present. Disease causing bacteria are an exception. The body maintains a bacteria balance (symbiosis). A sick bacteria can live in a sick body. A sick bacteria produces exotoxins, which may resemble gram-negative bacteria. A sick bacteria in the human body is in more danger of being attached by the body's enzymes and immunity than can be imagined. The bodily defenses against sick bacteria are tantamount to a full-scale nuclear war and criss-crossed with complex defense mechanisms, which are more dangerous to the human body than to the bacteria. A gram-negative bacteria resembles healthy or friendly bacteria.

The body confuses the exotoxins produced by sick bacteria as a gram-negative bacteria. Gram-negative bacteria have look-alike bacteria with lipopolysaccharide endotoxin in their walls, which are misinterpreted as gram negatives. Once this misread signal is transmitted to the brain, leukocytes (killer police) activate enzymes that phagocytically (eat the enemy) and secrete lysosomal enzymes that become sticky, cluster together blocking the blood supply. Next, the secondary defense activates more leukocytes and more phagocytic leukocytes (killer attack police) come to the area where the sick bacteria are. This stress reaction activates the sympathetic nervous system's epinephrine. The blood vessels overreact to epinephrine, which results in an abundance of high concentrations of death dealing necrotizers (defense army of killers). Further still, heat is used to attack the bacteria and pyrogen (hot flames from germs) is secreted from the suicide leukocytes, adding fever to hemorrhage and death to the bacteria. All this defense reaction tends to be over-reactive and overkills the bacteria when there is nothing poisonous about the endotoxin of the sick bacteria. Caucasian science is aware of the body's defense reactions and continues the science propaganda. The propaganda is based upon mythology, superstitions and lies. It teaches the public to be in fear of bacteria.

The religious belief, science mythology and scientific propaganda about evil bacteria helps the medical profession to convince the public that medical miracles have cured disease. Again, the use of soap and water and good hygiene caused the medical miracle. The only thing that can be cured is ham.

The miracle working medical profession overlooks the obvious. For example, if two people have the same disease that erroneously means the disease had spread or is infectious or contagious. This medical definition means that flus, headaches, coughs, sneezes, cataracts, flatulence, gas, menstruation cramps, stuttering and stammering, insomnia, diarrhea, smallpox, cholera, Bubonic Plague, leprosy, measles and the common cold are contagious. The vast majority of contagious evil bacteria (microbes) caused diseases cure themselves.

The microbial (germs) diseases such as plague, typhus, leprosy, and malaria had basically ceased before the time of medical miracle drugs, vaccines, serums and nutritional supplements. Microbes (bacteria) are blamed for all illnesses and yet bacteria have behaviors, which escape interpretations.

There are many types of germs, which can kill the human. However, they merely cause self-limiting diseases such as the flu. Why these germs are resistant to killing themselves or being killed by other germs is not explained. Why germs do not fight battles between each other as to which germ should kill the human is not explained by medical science. Why healthy germs do not attack and cause health is not explained. Caucasian science explains the relationship between the host (human) and the germ such as virulence, resistance, toxicity, attenuation, homeostasis or imbalance. Why microbes exist in the body despite escalating bodily immunity is beyond Caucasian science. When Caucasians link a germ with a disease, it is called the Doctrine of Specific Etiology. In African wholistic science, germs are symptoms of disease. Bacteria (germs) are similar to flies attracted to garbage (cellular waste). Caucasian allopathic medicine kills the flies (bacteria) and leaves the garbage. Consequently, the body remains in a diseased condition. Added to this, vaccines cause a secondary disease while drugs suppress the illness and cause a different disease. This is pointed out in the book *The Doctor's Dilemma* by G. Shaw.

The *Doctrine of Specific Etiology* links a specific germ as causing a specific disease. Yet, the doctrine has failed to theoretically explain or get rid of cancer, headaches, stress, mental illness and arteriosclerosis. Caucasian medical failures are blamed on the lack of research and/or a lack of a new vaccine. In other words failures are blamed on the future. Technology has to be developed very soon in the future to cure the disease. Caucasian science does not explain why the germ enters the body and then kills some people while not killing others. It seems probable that some other factor converts the germ in the body to a deadly killer.

Junk foods, drugs, radiation, synthetic hormones and vaccinations alter fungus, yeast and bacteria, which causes biochemical imbalances. The alteration causes altered microbe flora (fungus, yeast, bacteria), which alters the biochemical ecology. It can be clearly seen that instability occurs (fungus, yeast, bacteria) when the health sustaining biochemical ecology is altered. It can be clearly seen that instability occurs when Caucasians make alterations in large animal life (smaller animal life germs are just as imbalanced) such as the mongoose. For example, in 1872, Europeans brought the Indian mongoose to the island of Jamaica to control the rats. The mongoose not only destroyed the rats but also multiplied and destroyed birds, reptiles and other small animals. The body's and environment's ecology are similar. When the microbes are destroyed by drugs, antibiotics, synthetic sex hormones, steroids, radiation, air and water pollution, the body becomes diseased and accumulates waste. The bacteria multiplies because they have an abundant food supply of waste.

In Caucasian science, the evil microbes are used as a scapegoat and blamed for the disease. The effects of miracle drugs altering the body's electromagnetic balance and biochemical germ population must be paid for by degenerative diseases or by the health destruction of future generations.

The increase in world populations is not due to the discovery of antimicrobial drugs nor is it due to the Caucasian discovery that filth caused diseases. The world population was estimated to be over 450 million in the Seventeenth Century. It is now estimated to be five billion—an over tenfold increase. This increase in population started in the 16th century during periods of famines, hunger, plagues and pestilence. The increase occurred in countries without Caucasian allopathic medicine. Populations increase whenever the lives of the public is threatened with extinction. Nobel Prize winner, K. Lornz' research has documented this finding. However, Caucasian science takes the credit for nature's disease defense reactions, their medical science takes credit for diseases eliminated instead of the use of sanitation and hygiene (use of soap and water). The introduction of easy to wash cheap cotton underwear allowed for better personal hygiene among Caucasians. Further, the introduction of the African method of making transparent glass, which allowed sunlight to enter the dark cave-like homes of Europeans improved health. Sunlight stimulated more cleanliness in homes. Sunlight, soap and the end of the taboo that forbade bathing decrease filth and disease more than medical miracle drugs. The Africans introduced soap to Caucasians after the 11th century. Soap eliminated diseases until the belief that bathing opens the pores and causes dis-eases (plagues) to enter the body. This superstition stopped the Europeans from taking baths and diseases began to increase.

Filth caused diseases directly and indirectly. The Caucasian homes were filthy with human and animal waste and pollution and they had a diet that consisted of rotten food (parasite infected). This caused diseases. *(Conditions of the Working Man in England* by Engels, *Treatise on Diseases of Tradesmen* by B. Ramazzini). The poverty of the workers and the filthy and polluted environment caused many illnesses. The rich created the poverty and exploited the poor and land *(Mediziniche Polizei* by Johanna Peter Frank). The usage of hygiene and cleanliness stopped childhood diseases, not modern medical miracle drugs.

In cities, rats have to eat the rotten foods of the people. The Caucasian food supply is limited and this limitation does not meet the nutritional requirements of the rat, cat and dog diets. These animals ate poor diets, became diseased and then the Caucasians ate the rats, cats and dogs. This caused their diseased conditions to worsen. Caucasians on a nutritionally limited diet have weak immunity, which causes diseases. Diseased rats bit immune weak people resulting in diseases. Poverty, nutritional lacking diets, filthy overcrowded polluted cities create cities of diseased and mentally ill Caucasians.

The overcrowded Black slave and free Black's concentration camps (slums) had no sanitation. This provided a disease atmosphere for Blacks in European slave colonies in the Americas, West Indies and in colonized Africa. Whites in similar circumstances of filthy, nutritionally starved, overcrowded slums suffered from disease*s (The Deserted Village* by Goldsmith). These overcrowded dis-eased atmosphere's murdered many Blacks. Caucasians were infested with diseases that were transmitted to immune weakened Africans. Caucasians carried many diseases such as in the 14th century leprosy, 15th century plague, 16th century syphilis, 17th and 18th centuries' scarlet fever, tuberculosis, measles and pox to their slave colonies and colonialized Africa. Caucasian diseases added to force overcrowding, filth, hunger and mono-diets that served to weaken the health and immunity of Africans. The total deaths of Blacks caused by Caucasian slavery, disease, abortions, vaccinations, surgery and drug mutilations has not been estimated.

Caucasians believe they are immune to disease only after they have been vaccinated with an animal's diseased pus mixed with poisonous chemicals. They do not believe the body can build immunity without catching a disease. Immunity and infection research was done by Nobel Prize winner Metchnikoff, and he concluded that constipation is the cause of degeneration and disease, not bacteria. Immunity is the new medical fad that cannot explain why people do not have immunity to poison oak, dirt, polluted water and air and poison ivy despite centuries of exposure. Cleanliness and sanitation has stopped Caucasian diseases. For example, stagnation of low salt brackish water causes an increase in germ (flagellate) population, which in turn poisons fish that die and decay resulting in polluted water which results in disease carrying mosquitoes.

Measles, chickenpox, smallpox, and scarlet fever, etc. are the cleansing of toxins out the body through the skin. Toxins, poor nourishment and unsanitary practices cause the body to be diseased by cellular waste. For example, from 1825 to 1923 scarlet fever deaths decreased from 135 per 100,000 to one per 100,000. This decline occurred without serums, vaccines and medical intervention. Clean air, hygienic care, and improved sanitation were on the increase so diseases such as scarlet fever decreased. Despite obvious evidences, the Caucasians believe that their medical science cured these diseases. Caucasians believe their science's ability to destroy evil bacteria and destroy cell particles (virus) stopped contagious diseases. They claim their medical miracles, pus and poison chemical inoculations have saved civilization. Ironically, a case of smallpox with a vaccination scar is classified as chickenpox while a case of smallpox without a vaccination scar is classified as smallpox. *Smallpox: Its Differential Diagnosis* by A. Honey, M.D. points out the absurdity of vaccinations.

The vaccinations are a medical superstitious ritual based upon science myths not facts. Vaccinations introduce a disease into a person in order to cure a disease. Vaccine is pus from a sick animal. Pus is the diseased fluid from a suppurating wound, which is injected into the blood resulting in disease. Secondary diseases are caused by intravenous vaccinations such as syphilis, AIDS, herpes, cerebrospinal meningitis, lockjaw, etc. The accumulation of various pus and chemical toxins causes a vaccination load which biochemically poisons. The chemicals create new toxic chemicals and destroy immunity. Subsequently, one vaccination leads to another vaccination. If the paranoia of evil bacteria myth fails to manipulate the public then an evil dead cell particle (virus) myth is blamed for causing a disease.

Virus means poison. Consequently, arsenic is a virus, DDT is a virus, vaccine is a virus, penicillin and all drugs are viruses. It is medically defined as dead as well as living, and can spread disease. Whenever a germ or bacteria cannot be blamed for the cause of a disease, a virus is recruited to be the cause. A virus can be in one's system and not cause an illness and at the same time it is believed to cause an illness. Caucasian science uses laboratory animals (rat or monkey) and injects them with a virus. The animal may react to the virus within a few weeks, months, or not at all. How a virus (polio virus) enters the body is unknown. What is known is that radiation, drugs, vaccinations and overfeeding on denatured foods and cooked foods cause weak immunity and diseases, which inflames and destroy nerves causing crippling polio. Caucasian science has claimed to have cured the world of polio with vaccinations, yet polio still occurs among vaccinated children and adults.

Ancient Africans practiced inoculation first. In northern Africa, the Ashantes used arm-to-arm inoculation. For example, the Ashanti health practitioner would have a sick person rub their arm's kidney acupuncture meridian against the kidney acupuncture meridian of a healthy individual's arm. This arm to arm rubbing transferred the disease's aura to the healthy individual and transferred the immunity against that disease through the spirit, psyche and then the physical body. The Baris tribe, of Lado, used the breasts for inoculation. The Nubians were believed to use inoculation for smallpox.

In India, the Vedic father of medicine, Dhanwantari (1500 B.C.), used inoculation and vaccine. However, these colored cultures used inoculation and vaccination on a psycho-spiritual, spirit-psyche, auric and acupuncture scientific level. These scientific healing levels and curative devices may be loss forever and/or disguised in the many healing papyrus stolen by Caucasians. Caucasians call this higher knowledge a mystery system. It is a mystery to them, but not to African wholistic healers.

The diseases caused by contagious evil bacteria myth are numerous. A review of a few of the dis-eases that destroyed European populations and the diseases Caucasians carried into Africa and all parts of the world indicates the path of superstitions, science myths, ignorance, greed, White Supremacy Psychosis, poor hygiene and uncleanliness. In fact, the European diseases were a useful tool for stealing land and resources, destroying their enemies and African peoples. A few of these diseases claimed to be cured by Caucasian science's medical miracles (science) are as follows.

DIPHTHERIA

Diphtheria is the over-consumption of animal flesh, which causes protein degenerative diseases and deteriorates immunity. Constant overeating, which occurred in European cultures between food famines or in fear of famines causes constipation, fermentation and decomposition of food in the digestive system, putrefied food forms toxins in the stomach and intestines. Ironically, diphtheria's so-called bacteria is present in individuals with "colds," and throat infections. The bacteria is present at all times in healthy individuals according to the book *The Principles and Practice of Medicine* by William Osier, M.D. Diphtheria and other evil diseases are not found among strict vegetarians or diets that are at least 80% raw or in diets that include small amounts of animal flesh. The Caucasian's medical science adds this cured dis-ease claims to have cured this with a medical scientific miracle cure. This dis-ease was cured by Europeans having a steady food supply and good hygiene.

TYPHOID FEVER

The mosquito can be a carrier of typhoid disease if it has unclean water available. Unclean water has decomposed animal flesh, trash, manure, filth and septic sewage. Mosquitoes that populate the polluted water get it into their body and transfer the polluted water directly into the blood of people by biting them. The body's reaction to the pollution is called Typhoid Fever. The typhoid vaccine cannot replace cleanliness, good hygiene and pure water. For example, the British Army (1918) and French Army (1914) were both vaccinated for typhoid. Yet, they had outbreaks of typhoid and deaths at a high rate. If the natural defenses of the body are allowed to function it will take an individual three to seven days to rid the body of typhoid. However, the continued living in a septic sewage environment with a mosquito population coupled with an under-nutritional diet weakens immunity, which causes disease and death. The Caucasian medical scientists take credit for ridding the world of typhoid and never suggests that cleanliness solved the problem.

CHOLERA

Cholera is a disease caused by poor hygiene and faulty eating. Food ferments and putrefies in the stomach and intestines, causing toxic poisoning of the body and the destruction of immunity. The body tries to eject the poisons by vomiting. Vomiting requires the body to use large amounts of fluid (blood serum) and lose water resulting in dehydration. Dehydration causes electrolyte stress, oxidization of tissue, bone deterioration, mood swings, weak immunity and disease.

The limited diet of Europeans, plus poor sanitary treatment of foods, along with bakers adding clay and other non-foods to bread, caused this disease. The Caucasian had a tendency to overeat when food was available because of the fear of starvation. Overeating is a mental illness called an Eating Disorder. Caucasians with a fear disease have an eating disorder and are obsessed with eating and tend to be violent toward others and live in constant fear of starvation. Overeating causes constipation, toxic poisoning, immune fatigue and systemic weakness. During the famine era, Caucasians would greet each other by saying "have you eaten today" as starvation was a constant threat. Periods of overfeeding and stuffing food in a constipated system and Eating Disorders produced cholera. A steady food supply, sanitary storing of food and preparing food hygienically caused cholera to end—not a medical miracle.

SCURVY

Scurvy is a vitamin C deficiency. European sailors on long voyages with inadequate nourishment would get scurvy. The general state of health in

Section 16: Wholistic Perspectives

early European culture (as well as today) is in a mild state of scurvy. The modern diet of white sugar, bleached white flour, processed grains (cereals), cooked foods, canned meats and cow's milk causes scurvy or near scurvy-like states. Again, medical science is credited with curing this strictly undernutritional dietary related dis-ease.

The cost of medical miracles requires huge amounts of monies for research. The Food, Research and Disease Industries cannot make high profits if inexpensive good hygiene, soap, water, and cleanliness are used instead of vaccinations and drugs. The Research Industry uses an ancient African science of testing cures on animals. For example, in African cultures a patient with a disease is treated by giving that same disease and treatment to an animal. A patient with a broken leg has the leg set and herbs are given. Simultaneously, a chicken's leg is broken in a similar location and treated with herbs. If the chicken recovers, the patient recovers. Ironically, in European culture, a disease is given to an animal and the curative drug is given to rid the animal of the disease. If the test animal recovers, the drug is safe and the human will be given the same drug. However, if the curative drug does not work, the human will be given the drug at a lower dosage. In Caucasian culture, the use of test animals is classified as a scientific laboratory test. While in African cultures, the Caucasians label the animal test as superstitious ignorance of primitive savage Black people. The success standard for a drug's animal and/or human test can be altered. For example, during a research drug test trial, the drug given to an animal or human volunteer may cause harmful side effects on the fourth day of usage. The drug researchers base the drug's success upon the first three days of use and omit the results of the fourth day. Consequently, the drug companies can legally sell the drug as a successful remedy. Research is a form of pagan Caucasian rituals and superstitions.

The Caucasians' beliefs in their pagan rituals, ceremonies, science myths and superstitions are used to reinforce and perpetrate the hoax of medical miracles. There are plainly no medical miracles. Soap, water, good hygiene, and cleanliness and the reduction of superstitions and myths are the miracles. Caucasian illness is and was the result of filth.

The diseases of Europeans were caused by their filthy cultural lifestyles. It is a their deeply embedded superstitions, White Supremacy Psychosis, Eating Disorder, cooked food, pagan rituals and ceremonies and a loss of the instinct of health due to unwholistic lifestyles, which causes disease *(L'Hygiene Philosphique,* by Virby).

Europeans made disease a sin and convicted people to death for having colds *(Erewhon* by S. Butler). Caucasians believed diseases to be sexually appealing. The iconographic and literary references have indicated that in the 16th century in many parts of Europe a goiter was considered attractive among females. In fact, the plants they liked were dis-eased. In Holland, in the 16th century, tulips infected by a virus (made it have a unique color pattern) were expensive. This diseased plant was very popular in many European countries until it was recognized as a weak flower. The degeneration of a man's body, which caused it to appear like a woman's body, was considered attractive during the Florentine Renaissance.

Disease was present in the Middle Ages, in Europe, due to the cave homes and wooden and loam houses with straw roofs. Their caves and homes were infested with fleas, lice and rats. Black rats are more home-oriented and favored cave homes and wood and loam homes while the brown rats favored brick homes. Brown rats invaded the home for food and then would leave because they nest outdoors. Food particles and meat pieces on the floors caused the rats to be attracted to the filthy European homes and caves. Ironically, the healthy rats bitten by plague bacilli carrying mosquitoes usually do not get plague, while the rats eating under-nutritional cooked human food get the plague. The diseases, of Caucasians, were (and are) caused by a deviation from nature, and, it is doubtful that the Caucasians can ever be free if disease or rid themselves of White Supremacy Psychosis *(Hygiea or Essays Moral and Medical on the Causes Affecting the Personal State of Our Middling and Affluent Classes* by Thomas Beddoes). The Caucasians try to diagnose and treat disease because they want to know the nature of disease not the nature of the person who has the disease. However, the Caucasians' symptom treating therapies views the body's cleansing reaction and adaptive ability to a disease as a disease. (*The Story of Man, From the First Human to Primitive Culture and Beyond* by C. Coon). Trust in nature's ability to heal seems to be the foremost tool of cultures in communal African society *(The Descent of Man* by C. Darwin, *Mutual Aid, A Factor of Evolution* by Kropotin). The African healers believed a sick spirit, sick mind, sick family and sick village was spiritually, mentally and physical responsible for an individual's illness. This is why the Asclepian (African Imhotep medical science) cult in Rome believed that to consult a doctor after 30 years of age meant that the sick person was a fool who did not understand that the village, family and ancestors keep you healthy. European hunger, White Supremacy Psychosis, lack of human technology, lack of a healthy village (society) and lack of human and natural resources combined with diseases and uncleanliness caused them to invade Africa for disease remedies (so-called Fountain of Youth).

The Europeans on explorations (invasions) followed a sequence of sending navigators, missionaries, soldiers and then merchants. It was the rich who sponsored the merchants that invaded Africa. The increased spread of the news that the Africans had no diseases, plenty of food and a good life was published in books and articles such as the semifactual book *Voyage Av Bresil* by De Lery in 1556; Captain Samuel Wallis, in 1767, reported his invasion of Tahiti and spoke of the glorious life of the Blacks; Philibert Commerson, a physician and naturalist on the Ship La Bouneuse, published an account of the journey to Tahiti comparing life there with Utopia; Captain James Cook's invasions were commercially written in many languages and published widely by journalists in London, New York, France, Germany and many other

European countries. The articles spoke of plenty of food, herb medicine, excellent health and wealth of African peoples. This caused the rich power elite Europeans to sponsor invasions of Africa in search of human and natural resources, wealth, food and health. However, they also brought diseases and death to Africans.

African trypanosomiasis (sleeping sickness) was brought to the African Ogowe Region by the Europeans in the late Eighteenth Century and recorded by Albert Schweitzer. It killed one third of the population that had contact with it. It killed 200,000 out of 300,000 Blacks in Uganda. In upper Ogowe, it killed 1,500 out of 2,000 in one village. In tribes that were isolated from Caucasians or with minimum contact with Caucasians, the total amount of deaths (millions) was never calculated by the Europeans because Africans were considered animals and savages. Diseased Caucasians made physical contact with isolated tribes. And, these tribes went deep into the African interior and carried Caucasian diseases to other tribes. This caused dis-eases to spread widely in Africa. For example, an isolated tribe such as the Tupari, natives of Brazil, one third of the population was killed by Caucasian measles. European measles killed 99% of the Eskimos of the Canadian Arctic in 1952. Diseases of Europeans had a profound effect on Africa because the African diet was made under-nutritional. Caucasians stole land and used it for their food crops. This left poor nutrient soil for the Africans to grow their food. African food crops grown on poor soil produce crops of inadequate nutritional value. Africans who ate these inadequate foods developed inadequate immunity and diseases. Many tribes and farmers were constantly moving in order to avoid the predatory Caucasians. The African agriculture became unstable and the health of Africans deteriorated. The Caucasian invaders disrupted the harvest season of crops and storage of foods and caused soil erosion, polluted wells and streams and spread filth. The Caucasians indirectly and directly caused millions to die and caused others to become physically, mentally and spiritually ill.

Mental illness and psychosis are associated with certain cultural patterns. The Caucasian mental disease rate has been on a steady increase. For example, Caucasian neurosis, psychosis, Eating Disorders, Depression, suicides, alcoholism, sex addiction and violence addiction has spread just as the tarantism and dancing mania mental illness of the Middle Ages. The village fool, senile dementia of the old and other mental defects have been part of their culture. The Kirghizes and Kalmuks Tribes that were isolated from Whites until 1850 had an abrupt epidemic of mental illness when they socialized with the Caucasian civilization. European civilization is dysfunctional and creates mental illness within itself. The Caucasian workplace is dysfunctional and has created mental illnesses among workers who have monotonous work. Studies have indicated that monotonous work causes impaired thinking, hallucinations, talking to oneself, changes in brain wave patterns, childish emotional response and distorted visual perceptions. The Caucasian that worked on plantations, ships, farms, factories and peasant jobs were mentally ill. These mentally

Caucasians made contact with Africans and caused not only physical diseases but also mental diseases. Caucasian art reveals their diseased state.

The art of Caucasian culture reflects the health and diseased condition of their race. Drawings, paintings, functional artistic furniture, pottery, games, statues, jewelry, cosmetics are indicators of the health of ancient Africans. Art pictorially reflects facts which written history often overlooks; in *Plague and Pestilence in Literature and Art* by R. Crawford (1914) this is eloquently revealed. Europeans made disease into a gift from God or God's way of getting rid of the ungodly (African savages and American Indians). Caucasian women and men with diseases (such as tuberculosis) were considered as attractive, spiritual, beautiful and romantic. This indicates how dysfunctional Caucasian culture is. They have a psychosis that is escalating because their dysfunctional culture compliments psychosis. A confused mind seeks confused (dis-eased) answers. The mentally confused Caucasian is nurtured in a dysfunctional society that creates a diseased subconscious and psychotic mind. However, in the midst of European cultural confusion the Africans die in untold numbers. The total death of Africans can be deduced from the percentage of Caucasian deaths. The same percentage of deaths' figures can be correlated to equal the African death toll.

Europeans had plagues in the 14th century. Plagues killed one-fourth of the people. Plagues attacked England with repeated epidemics from the Fourteenth to Seventeenth Centuries, destroying the entire villages and towns *(History of the Plague, 1722* by D. DeFoe). The death toll for the African population is greater or at least equal to that of the Europeans. Aside from plague deaths, there were deaths caused by the under-nutritional diet that Africans ate. Africans were forced to eat the disease-causing European mono-diets and cooked foods because of colonialism, land colonialization and slavery.

The teeth of African mummies indicate that cavities were rare in Egypt before the dynastic era. However, cavities increased especially among the rich elite African groups. Ironically, the poor African families and workers who had kept their original whole food diet were cavity free. In the African tribe of Luo, the children who lived in the cities and ate European junk foods had a 28% cavity rate. However, Banyarvanda children who ate white sugar, cooked foods, and very few European foods had an 11% cavity rate.

The colonialization of African diets, land and cultural castration had far-reaching effects. Anthropologists have found that sudden shifts in diets cause severe gastrointestinal (digestive) illnesses and constipation. Diets that are acculturated naturally (without European influence) can be balanced despite being limited. African civilization introduced yams, peanuts and corn into China between A.D. 1550 and 1600. New foods caused the population increases of 60 to 100 million in 1578; in 1660 it increased to 110 million; in 1741 to 140 million; in 1850 to 300 million. These foods were acculturated by the Chinese; they were not forced upon the Chinese like the Europeans did to the Blacks.

South African Zulus replaced millet with corn. Corn yields larger crops than millet. Unfortunately, corn required cultivation of large amounts of land; resulting in the destruction of sweet fruits and berries, and other foods. The European food merchant colonialization and cultivation of the land had destructive effects on Africans health. White racism was very destructive. Added to this, White Supremacy Psychosis dismantled African culture causing populations of Africans to be dysfunctional. Corn caused the Zulus to become dis-eased. The Zulus eventually believed that they always ate corn and could not fathom that it was a recent addition to their diet. The Caucasians' poor health and diseases caused their invasion to stop in Central Africa *(Health, Culture and Community* by B. Paul).

Central Africa was the White man's grave and he did not penetrate it. Malaria in Algeria left many Caucasians dead in the Mitidja Plain. The tsetse fly, carrier of trypanosomiasis (sleeping sickness), stopped the Caucasians and stopped them from raising cattle crops in Central Africa. In many cases, the unskilled, ignorant, superstitious European doctors were unaware of Africa's medicinal herbs and curative clay.

The word chemistry is derived from the African medicinal clay treatment system and clay. One of its oldest names for Kemet (Egypt) is Kamt, Qemt or Keme, which means Black. This word often referred to Egypt because black clay (mud) is found on the banks of the Nile. Coptics or Christian Egyptians distorted the word as Kheme and it was further distorted by the Greeks, Romans, Syrians, and Arabs. The Egyptians used combinations of medicinal herbs and clay as well as medicinal metals. These medical combinations were called Khemeia because clay was the main curative ingredient and the catalyst. The Caucasian Arabs further distorted Keme and prefixed the word with "Al" and it became Al-Khemeia or Alchemy.

MEN'S CYCLE, ORGASM, REPRODUCTION, IMPOTENCY

The reproduction system of men is often mysterious and crudely explained. Men have emotional fluctuations triggered by monthly hormonal changes, monthly periods of sexual excitation or impotency influenced by emotions. Men are erroneously believed to be sperm production factories, non-cyclic and unfeeling creatures.

The man's cycle is hormone controlled. Sperm takes between 60 to 72 days to develop into a mature organism. Female sperm has two heads (black dots) and male sperm has one black dot. Male sperm moves fast and female sperm moves slowly owing to its two heads. Sperm is stored in a coiled 20-foot long tube (epididymides) during incubation until it matures. During the incubation (maturity) the sperm must be regulated at a constant temperature, which is three to four degrees below body temperature. The temperature regulation of the sperm in the epididymides attached to the testes (ball-like organ) that are encased in the scrotum (sac-like). The testicles go up and down in order to regulate the sperm's temperature. The scrotum moves the testicles close to the body when sperm is too cold and droops down away from the body when the sperm is too warm. Sperm production is triggered by the estrogen and progesterone sex hormones. Egyptian men would sit in very hot baths to kill the sperm. This was a crude birth control method. This method is safer than the pill but has become outdated.

The men's cycle closely duplicates the women's cycle. During a 28-day cycle, the man's sperm is triggered for ejaculatory by pheromones and testosterone hormones. The hormone ratio changes between the 14th and 28th days to stimulate sexual intercourse. Additionally, during female ovulation and male testosterone spurts, the body temperature slightly increases during this period. The sex hormones stimulate arousal, emotions and fertility. The increased body heat of estrus speeds up the action of the sperm causes the lubrication of the uterus vagina and penis and the increased heat allows for better protection of the sperm. If the males' hormones are imbalanced, then the estrus hormone shift may trigger unemotional sex (spiritually detached), irritation or petty arguments with females. The males unbalanced hormone ratios can trigger moodiness, hysterical tantrums or arguments that tend to be resolved by his conclusion that he is right and the woman is wrong. Most men are unaware of their hormone shifts or they are in denial about their cycle (periods). A high level of testosterone can trigger hysterical (irrational) behavior or sexual energy can be misdirected, causing strong emotional attachments to sports activity or aggressive sexual acts, monthly temper tantrums, a need to be catered to or babied or the Testosterone Syndrome (PMS) monthly conflict. These are a few of the many monthly emotional irrational mood behavioral actions. Some men, on their monthly, tend to be overly rational. However, their rationalism is emotionally motivated. Mineral imbalances or inadequate minerals in the diet can cause the male's moodiness and cycle problems.

Minerals have a cycle and any organism that contains minerals has a cycle *(Biological Rhythms in Human and Animals* by Gay Gaer-Luce). Consequently, the internal organs such as the testicles, prostate and epididymides have a cycle (sequence) of activity and inactivity. These cycles are influenced by sex hormones, pheromones and the predominant mineral that the organ contains. Males have a cycle because the minerals within the testicles, prostate and sperm have a cycle. The cyclic nature of plants, insects and the Mineral Kingdom was confirmed in Pre-Egyptian and Egyptian science. A Hindu physicist Jagadis Chandri Bose presented scientific proof (year 1901) of the mineral cycle to the Royal Society of Physiologists. The Caucasian scientists denied that the minerals have a cycle and declared the research was done on muscle tissue instead of minerals. However, today, the Caucasian scientists have done electronic monitoring of minerals, which has verified that minerals have a cycle, respond to drugs, stimuli and music. Minerals have a reaction similar to vegetables and animal muscle tissue. The minerals zinc and selenium are highest in the semen and each of these minerals have a cycle. The male cycle can be correlated with the phases of the moon. The moon influences water (tides), blood flow (surgery is not advised during a full moon) and mental illness (the mentally ill are more bazaar during full moons). The male body has a higher water content than the female body.

At the end of the sperm cycle, the sperm deteriorates. In other words, sperm dies (just as the egg of the ovary dies) and its mineral nutrient content is recycled in the body. The multiple deaths of the sperm trigger another hormone shift towards progesterone. This shift causes a stress reaction and activates the thyroid gland. The hormones progesterone, estrogen and testosterone fluctuate and this causes the male mood to fluctuate. A new ratio causes the development of new sperms and the male cycle starts over again. The sperm cycle is ignored and men constantly ejaculating sperm are exhausting the supply of vitamins and minerals needed to re-supply sperm. Hypersex and ejaculations deplete the trace minerals. Each ejaculation causes the loss of the same amount of nutrients needed to run twenty miles. Multiple ejaculations without proper supplements and herbs result in mood swings and reproductive diseases. Excessive ejaculatory sex decreases immunity and decreases thinking, sensitivity and spirituality. Sexual abstinence and injaculations (sex regeneration) increases the trace mineral accumulations in men, increases the quality of sperm and increases access to higher spiritual growth.

Sperm is ejaculated in a fluid base. The sperm in the fluid may amount to a teaspoon (2%), while the major portion of fluid is 60% seminal and 38% prostrate fluid. Prostrate fluid is clear, seminal fluid is yellow and sperm is clear. The fluid that is first released from the penis is from the Cowper's gland and it neutralizes the acid of the urine residues. The fluid quality and quantity is dependent upon the natural nutrients used to compose it. These natural nutrients are derived from a natural diet, Maat thinking and spirituality and the ancestors. Drugs, alcohol, droplets of drugs in marijuana and tobacco smoke, salt, vinegar, junk foods, cooked foods, excess estrogen in non-organic meat, eggs and dairy reduce the sperm count and destroys hormone balance.

The Male Cycle is complex. There are zodiac signs, earth, moon (lunar) and sun (solar) influences on both the male and female cycles. The Male Cycle is usually 10% physical and 90% spiritual, mental and emotional. It is a holistic cycle. The cycle is dependent upon the state of health and regulated by sex hormone levels and ratios. Without proper sex hormones, the cycle, moods, thoughts and behaviors are abnormal. When the male hormones decline, he grows long hairs in the ears and/or nose. When female hormones decline, they grow long hair on the chin, upper lip or facial areas. Hormones stimulate the Estrus sex drive (reproductive urge) and improper hormone levels make sex unholistic. Estrus (sexual arousal) can be triggered by the male's imagination; physical stimulation; female pheromones; drugs; pornography; electronic inducement; sexual songs, music videos and movies; sex gestures; flirtation; sexual dancing and synthetic sex hormones in foods. Abnormal triggers deregulate Estrus and make it non-cyclic (uncontrolled). The following charts briefly summarize a few factors involved in the cycle.

MALE and FEMALE HORMONE 28-DAY CYCLE
(Approximations)

Day of Month	Sex Hormone	Nerve Hormone	Behavior
1 to 12	Estrogen	Serotonin	Stress, Action
6 to 16	Testosterone	Mixed Ratio	Sexual Arousal (Estrus)
12 to 28	Progesterone	Melatonin	Growth, Development, Relaxation

MALE SEXUALITY

Symptom	Reaction
Testosterone Syndrome	Behavior, Moods and Thoughts similar to PMS (often masked with hypersex).
Andropause	Behavior, Moods and Thoughts similar to Menopause. Lack of sexual desire, impotence, long hair growth in nose and/or ears (often masked by forcing self to be overly sexual)

MALE PERIOD
(Duration of Cyclic Symptoms)

Symptom	Starts	Period (Duration)	Cause
Testosterone Syndrome	Puberty	3 days to 2 weeks.	Intermittent and/or sporadic High Estrogen, Low Testosterone, Unstable Blood Sugar, Undernutrition, Disease, Drugs, Liver Stress.
Andropause	50-years-old	6 years or less.	Intermittent and/or cyclical High Estrogen, Low Testosterone, Low Progesterone, Weak Adrenals, Unstable Blood Sugar, Liver Stress

SEX HORMONES (Can be purchased)

Hormone	Chemistry
Testosterone	Made in testicles (men) and Adrenal Cortex (Men and women)
Progesterone	Derived from DHEA . Changes to estrogen, testosterone
DHEA (Dehydroephi-androsterone)	Changes to testosterone, estrogen, progesterone. Made from Adrenal chemicals.
Estrogen	Made by conversion of chemicals from Adrenals.

SEXUAL AROUSAL (ESTRUS)

Phases	Behaviors
Proestrus	Tends to want to socialize with females, sexual hunting, flirtation
Estrus	Desires intercourse, wants orgasm, attachment
Metestrus	Wants to be left alone following intercourse, detachment

The Estrus phases can be clustered and occur within one day or the duration of phases can be unequal and vary (i.e., one to three days for each phase).

HORMONE AFFECTS

LEVEL	EMOTIONS
Estrogen	
Normal	Nurturing, kindness
High	Fear, threatening, doubtful (increases fat to hips and breasts in women, prostate and breast disease in men)
Low	Depression, Moody, Alters Leptin Hormone (Appetite control) Imbalances Tends to like crunchy snack foods
Progesterone	
Normal	Acceptance, willingness, caring
High	Selfishness, Aggressive (increases fat to breast in women and causes breast disease in men)
Low	Nervousness, depression, anxiety
Imbalances	Tends to like creamy snack foods
Testosterone	
Normal	Protective, wants to be in control, macho behavior, flirtation
Imbalance High or Low	Uncaring, wants to have way, aggressive. Tends to like symbols of penis and testicles (i.e., cars, erect nipples, guns, ball games). Tends to like salty foods, alcohol, vinegar and stimulants

SEX PHEROMONES (fer-o-mons)

Pheromones
- Non-offensive, undetectable hormone stimulating fumes (odors) secreted from pores
- Stimulates sexual arousal (Estrus) in Heterosexuals
- Influences behavior, moods, thoughts, PMS, Andropause, Testosterone Syndrome, Menopause, etc.
- Alters chemical, electrical and magnetic balance of the body
- Testosterone odor and secretion in the blood stimulates estrus

Male Pheromones
- Highest levels during estrus
- Triggers estrus (biochemically) in females
  (May not trigger feelings for physical sex but instead stimulate emotional and spiritual aspects of sex)

Female Pheromones
- Highest levels during fertile days of cycle (ovulation)
- Triggers estrus in males (may trigger sexual ideation and/or sexual conquests without emotional spiritual bond)

Pheromone Imbalance Symptoms
- Unstable male cycle
- Mood swings
- Mixed messages in conversations

- Unpredictable behavior and/or moods
- Distorted/confused rational thoughts
- Lifestyle of excess emotional sexual stimulation causes hypersex (sporadic and fluctuating constant sex appetite)

EXCESS ESTROGEN

Estrogen and steroid hormones are added to non-organic fruits, vegetables, milk, eggs, dairy and meats causes excess estrogen.

Excess estrogen causes:

- PMS
- Bone loss
- Early Andropause

- Loss of sex desire
- Early menopause
- Arthritis
- Vaginal dryness

- High blood pressure

- Diabetes
- Dry Skin
- Low Sperm Count (Sarsaparilla increases)
- Baldness
- Split ends on hair
- Prostate disease
- Weight, water and/or fat increase
- Premature ejaculation and/or dribbling of urine (both sexes)

Take supplements to balance hormone level and blood cleansing herbs to first out estrogen (Echinacea, goldenseal, Burdock, Chaparral, Red Clover, etc.).

REMEDIES
(Cycle Problems and Excess Estrogen)

Suggested remedies for hormone and cycle problems:

DHEA	50 mg. in the a.m.
Pregnenolone	100 to 150 mg. in the p.m.
Progesterone (Cream)	Use from 12 to 26 days of cycle
Wild Yam tablets	Follow label directions
Histidine	2,000 mg. before bedtime (promotes erection the next morning)
Growth Hormone (Arginine and Ornithine)	Follow label. (Regulates cycle)
Melatonin	3 mg. (Helps relax and aids erection)

Herbs
These herbs cleanse and strengthen the prostate and are used for prostate diseases: Saw Palmetto, Yohimbe (can increase blood pressure), Pygeum, Tribulus, Maca, Wild Yam, Muira Puama, Wild Oats, Damiana, Dopa Bean.

TENTYRA TEMPLE CIRCULAR ZODIAC
WORLD'S OLDEST ZODIAC
(Cycles of Plants and Stars)

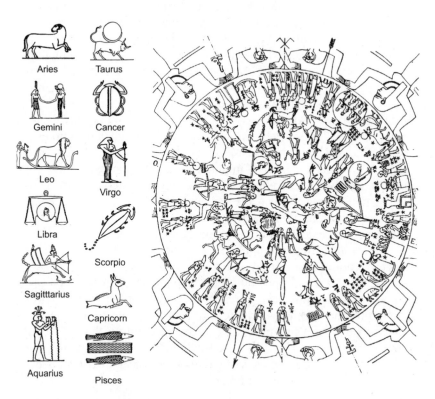

Aries

Taurus

Gemini

Cancer

Leo

Virgo

Libra

Scorpio

Sagitttarius

Capricorn

Aquarius

Pisces

Can be found in V. Denon's *Description de l'Egypt 1809* and *Rediscovery of Ancient Egypt* by Peter Clayton (1982). For enlarged chart, see page 525.

About the Illustration

Ancient African history and astrology (Zodiac) indicates that the earth is presently upside down and off its axis. The Ptolemy Greeks who had sculptured at the Tentyra (Dendera)—"Middle" Annu—city temple, the famous Annu Mystery School's circular/concentric zodiac. The ancient Annu's 36 astrological/astronomical star "decans" are divided into twelve "signs." It indicates millions of years of African culture, history and science.

The Circular Zodiac has three Virgos between the Lion and Libra. African priests told this to Herodotus (Book II).

The ancient African Priests knew that the poles of the Earth and the Ecliptic had formerly coincided and that the Poles have been three times within the plane of the Ecliptic. The ancient African Initiates (students) were taught this (M. Blavatsky, *Secret Doctrine II*). All ancient African health practitioners used astrology as part of diagnosing and treating disease.

IMPOTENCY REMEDIES

Impotency is the failure to maintain or achieve erection.

Impotency is caused by diseases. Disease that interferes with circulation, stress and emotions can cause impotency. Men that have mental or emotional causes for impotence will have erections in the morning or during sleep. Men that have impotence caused by disease or medication will not. The emotional causes of impotency are multiple. Emotionalism is usually based on a woman's behavior and not upon the man's own emotional acting out. For example, impotency amongst women takes on another behavioral pattern. Women generally refuse to have sexual intercourse or are emotionally not involved in the intercourse and these behaviors are not directly labeled impotency. Impotency is caused by genital diseases, drugs, heart disease, high blood pressure and diabetes medicine causes impotence, antihistamines, nicotine, anti-depressants, sedatives, hardening of arteries, clogged arteries, ulcer medicine, poor circulation, excess estrogen, electrolyte stress, alcohol, smoking, degenerative disease, poor nutrition and poor health.

Impotency is basically a defense mechanism of the body. The body protects the woman from extremely poor quality sperm by temporarily or permanently ending sperm usage. This poor quality sperm is not allowed to leave the man's body. Impotency is not a spontaneous event. It takes an accumulation of poor physical, psychological and spiritual health. A bodily reaction to poor health is impotency. This symptom of a dis-ease is warning the body of a far more serious dis-ease within the total body. Impotency can be caused by a dis-eased state in the entire body. However, when the body has no other means of warning the man to alter his dis-ease producing behavior it resorts to impotency.

Supplement	Dosage	Remarks
Vitamin B Complex, B_{12}, B_{15}, C, E, Folic Acid, Para Aminobenzoic Acid, Zinc, Selenium	Follow label directions.	Nourishes and enhances sperm and vitality.
See Prostate Problems, page 97, for additional supplements.		

AMINO ACIDS

Histidine	Follow label directions.	Taken at night on an empty stomach can cause erections.
Arginine	As indicated.	Stimulates sperm growth.

HERBS

Damiana, Dopa Bean, Ginseng, Gotu Kola, Horny Goat, Maca, Mucuna Purine, Muira Puama, Sarsaparilla, Saw Palmetto, Tribulus, Wild Oats, Yohimbe.

HOMEOPATHIC

Kali. Phos.	As directed.	Enhances nutrients to organs.

FOODS

Bee Pollen, Brewer's Yeast, Dates, Lecithin, Pumpkin Seeds, Raw Nuts, Royal Jelly.

GLANDULARS

Orchic, Adrenal Pituitary	As directed.	Stimulates sperm production.

PROSTATE REMEDY

Prostrate problems are caused by the weakening, hardening, inflexibility or swelling of the gland. The glandular function of the prostatic fluid is usually altered in smell, viscosity (thickness) and color. The prostate fluid inadequately nourishes and transports sperm when the prostate is diseased.

Enlarged
Cranesbill, Shepherd's Purse, Witch Hazel

Problems Urinating
Gravel Root, Juniper Berry, Uva Ursi

Inflammation
Cat's Claw, Feverfew, MSM

Pain
Boswella, White Willow

Cancer
Chaparral, Echinacea, Goldenseal, Horsetail, Red Cover

Infection
Cranberry Juice, Grapeseed Oil, Lysine

Promote Erection

Histidine	2,000 mg. 1 hour before bedtime on an empty stomach	
Niacinamide	As directed.	Relaxes glands
Testosterone	As directed.	Stimulates Sexual arousal.

Overall Health
See Prostate Problems, page 97, for foods.

Avoid White Sugar, Salt, Vinegar, Alcohol, Fried Foods, Junk Foods, Non-organic Meats, Eggs and Dairy.

Man:
The Sexual Aggressor and Other Lies

The Caucasian belief that the man is physically the sexual aggressor has contributed to a distortion in women's health concepts and relationships. Penis penetration is caused by the hip movement of the man. Women equally have hips and can be by anatomical definition, the sexual aggressor. Anatomically, the man's penis is composed of sponge tissue while the woman's vagina is composed of muscle tissue. The penis is passive (lacks muscle activity) and the vagina is active (is a muscle). In other words, a man (male penis) that enters a cave (vagina) in which he is attacked by thousands of women (vaginal muscles) could never be considered an aggressive conqueror of the woman. This belief is based upon rape. During rape, the erect penis can be forced into the vagina. However, during the normal sexual intercourse the male and female hips are both active. The penis is stimulated by the muscular structure of the vagina. An erect penis is classified under the Female Principle, while a flaccid penis comes under the Male Principle. Sexual aggression is culturally defined and based upon the sex rituals and ceremonies of a culture.

Orgasm and Ejaculation

Men associate orgasm with the good physical sensation of ejaculation and women believe it is the same as a climax. Orgasm is the pleasant holistic sensation caused by a physically stimulating climax caused by the elevation of mind and spirit. Orgasm can be achieved without ejaculating sperm. Orgasm is a holistic expression of mental and spiritual balance. Orgasm is achieved by men and women when their Male and Female Principles combine to stimulate the Pineal. The female has the genetic code of her father (Male Principle) and the male has the genetic code and physical characteristics (nipples) of his mother (Female Principle). During holistic heterosexual intercourse, the Male and Female Principle combine in a holy union—they become one. The pleasant physical sensation of this union reaches its highest height—orgasm during sexual intercourse. Each feeling (touch, hearing, etc.) and emotion (happiness, anger, etc.) has a threshold. A threshold is the lower limit that triggers a sensation and the upper limit whereby the sensation reaches its maximum level. For example, a finger will get burnt (upper limit). Stimulation (real or imagined) of the glans penis (head of the penis) reaches threshold and sends a signal to the frenulum (sensation center on the underside of the penis). The frenulum then triggers a climax and/or ejaculation. A climax is not an orgasm. An orgasm can only be achieved by the holistic union of the complementary sexes of male and female. A man with a man or a woman with a woman (homosexuals) can sexually masturbate each other to achieve a climax but they can never have an orgasm or sexual intercourse. Men have a Female Principle or gentle or feminine (i.e., gentlemen) quality. The Male Principle has feminine emotionalism (not to be confused with effeminate). Men should consciously and emotionally accept the female portion of their Male Principle. They were created by their mother and father, so they have half of each parent's sexual, emotional and physical characteristics.

A man can switch to the woman's frequency during intercourse with the woman. A woman can switch to the man's frequency. This dissolves and harmonizes the female/male division. This dissolution returns the woman and man to a non-sexual holistic energy level. This non-sexual energy is orgasmic because it is spiritual purity. Spiritual purity is culturally defined and has no beginning and no end. Orgasm is a holistic energy, which is beyond the pleasant sensation of a woman's climax and a man's ejaculation and climax. It is safe to say that very, very few men have had an orgasm. Orgasm is culturally defined. It may be similar to having a special talent. Very few have the talent (holistic cultural sex rituals and ceremonies) to achieve orgasm. They have had a physically pleasant climax and pleasing sensation from ejaculation and not an orgasm.

An orgasm by African cultural definition is achieved by complementary sexes. It is a unit of two different sexes (male/female), which results in the man and woman joined together to form a complement—one unit. The physical being, psyche being and spirit being join together to form one complementary human being. Man's spirituality and mentality and woman's spirituality and mentality join and form one spiritual human complement. Orgasm is the expression of wholism. Wholism is the expression of culture. The Caucasians believe men and women are opposite sexes and can achieve a climax by masturbation, homosexuality, rape, sex with children or electrical devices, masochism, sadism, anally, orally and through necrophilia (intercourse with a dead person). These are Caucasian ways in which a woman can climax and a man can climax and ejaculate. Climax and orgasm are two different things. Orgasm is God-centered. A prayer should be said before sex. Orgasm requires Maat cultural sexual rituals and ceremonies. An African who is not free to practice their culture at all times and in all situations is in some form of slavery (i.e., psychological, religious, physical, oppression, sex colonialism, etc.). A Black person that uses Caucasian sexual rituals and ceremonies cannot access the intelligence needed to have an orgasm. They are sexually colonized.

CONDOMS—THE SIDE EFFECTS OF SAFE SEX

Condoms are a synthetic product with many dangerous chemicals. The side effects of condoms and the talc powder and spermicidal chemicals should be printed on the label and the public made aware of them just as they are made aware of the side effects of prescription medicines.

The chemicals used in Latex condoms cause the same allergies as latex gloves, nipples and pacifiers, contraceptive cervical caps and diaphragms, underwear, waist and leg bands, tennis shoes, etc. Condom allergies increase with each use and have been linked to causing food allergies. The Allergy Analysis Center, in Birmingham, England, has reported that 7.7% of the population can have latex allergies while The Henry Ford Hospital, in Detroit, Michigan (USA) reports 6.6%. The AIDS Alert (February 1995) reported that there might be a latex condom allergy epidemic occurring. Latex allergies can cause inflammation of the vagina, uterus and penis, hives, allergies, difficulty breathing, rashes, mood swings and immunity problems (U.S. Food and Drug Administration).

The talc powder used as a lubricant is dangerous. It contains magnesium silicate, boric acid, zinc oxide, coloring agents and other chemicals. The American Medical Association reveals that talc is toxic. It has caused poisoning when swallowed and when applied to open skin (abraded). Zinc oxide has caused blocked hair pores and Zinc Pox skin eruption with zinc workers. Talc contributes to cancer of the uterus and prostate, hardening of the fallopian tubes, cancer of the ovaries and if inhaled it can cause pneumonia, lung irritation, vomiting and coughing. Talc is chemically similar to asbestos and has the same poisonous effect and can cause cancer of the reproductive organs. (*Consumer's Dictionary of Cosmetic Ingredients* by Ruth Winters; *Nutrition Review* article, "Dangers of Talc Use for Women," Summer 1995; *Times* article, "Danger of Talc Used on Condom" March 15, 1995; *Journal of Obstetrics and Gynecology*, May 1996).

Condoms' sperm killing chemical, p-nonylphenol, is called a spermicide. Phenol, the chemical base for nonylphenol is derived from cancer-causing coal tar. It causes skin to die (necrosis) and is a poison. Nonylphenol is a poison that causes a low sperm count and uterus and breast cancer, birth defects, prostate problems, reproductive abnormalities (i.e., Fibroids, Chlamydia, Pelvic Inflammatory Disease, etc.) Talc weakens the immunity. Condom spermicide is an Endocrine Disrupter Chemical (EDC). In other words, it causes hormone and male cycle imbalances and perverts glandular function (i.e., Pineal Gland). Endocrine Disrupters cause female animals to act like males (*Our Stolen Future* by Theo Colborn).

The polyurethane transparent condom can reduce sperm count and cause cancer. The chemicals used to make polyurethane and latex condoms as well as the talc and spermicide are absorbed into the skin of men and women and carried by the blood to organs, nerves, bones, tissue, sperm, eggs, cells and the brain with dangerous consequences. There are other factors to consider aside from the chemicals.

Condoms have a 13-31% failure rate, which has resulted in unwanted pregnancies (*Family Planning Perspective*, Vol. 24, 1992). Condoms cannot totally block the passage of sperm. Condoms have holes in them, which are created during their manufacture. These holes can be five microns in diameter, which allows bacteria and viruses (dead cell particles) to pass through. The condoms can be abrasive to the vagina, resulting in sores. They are often contaminated by bacteria growth (lycopodium), which results in tumors. Condoms fail to prevent nearly one in every three HIV infections. (*Rubber Chemistry and Technology* by C.M. Roland, June 1992; *Sexually Transmitted Disease,* R.F. Carey, et al, July/August 1992; *Manual of Clinical Micro-biology,* 4th Edition, University of Texas, Susan Weller, Ph.D.).

The public should be warned of the possible side effects of condoms, talc and spermicides. Prescription drugs, cigarettes, pillows, appliances, household cleaners and toothpastes warn the consumer. Condoms present more of a health hazard yet carry no warning or list of possible side effects. The consumer without any type of condom warning or side effect listed assumes that they are totally safe and 100% protected. This assumption may prove to have disastrous results.

Health food stores sell safer condoms.

WHOLISTIC FEMALE/MALE RELATIONSHIPS

The female/male relationship is microcosmic of the culture. The relationship serves Maat and transmits and translates culture. Black female/male (woman/man) relationships (monogamous polygyny and polygamous) is the smallest functional unit of the culture. Sex reflects the culture, the sexual rituals and ceremonies are an outgrowth of the culture (*Sex, Custom and Psychopathology: A Study of South African Pagan Natives* by B. Lambscher; *The Science of Human Regeneration* by H. Hotema; *Sexual Secrets* by N. Douglas and P. Slinger).

The Black wholistic female/male relationship is for the upliftment of the culture and creating a technology (children) that advance the culture. The culture (i.e., village) serves the relationship and the relationship serves the culture. It takes a village to have a marriage. In other words, it takes African centeredness to have a holistic African cultural marriage. Contemporary Black folks' relationships are based upon Caucasian rituals and ceremonies, Caucasian psychology and Caucasian group dynamics. They all have a chattel slave mentality that Negro men must love Black women as if they were White women and Negro women must love Black men as if they were White men. Caucasian-type relationships further Caucasian culture. African relationships further African culture. African cultural relationships solve African problems. African female/male relationships serve Maat. Caucasian cultural type Black relationships serve White supremacy. Consequently, relationships between Black men and women are deteriorating just like relationships between White men and women.

In the wholistic Black woman/man relationship in Pre-Egyptian and Egyptian culture, the involvement of diet was of primary importance. The importance of foods in the maintenance of spiritual, mental and physical health is well established (*Sex, Nutrition* by P. Airola). In fact, research by Konrad Lorenz (Nobel Prize) revealed that people act like the animals they eat. Those domesticated and chemicalized animals no longer adhere to their natural mating rituals and ceremonies and selection processes. They are forced into sexual activities based upon eroticism, sensuality, mass breeding and the animal rituals and ceremonial aspects of the mating process are discontinued or changed to meet the needs of the animal factory. In other words, they have sex but none of their animal rituals and ceremonies (culture) is attached. The animal breeders (and slave breeder) cannot afford the large amount of time that the animal naturally dedicated to the mate selection rituals and ceremonies. These domesticated animals become divorced from their culture and people who eat these animals duplicate their denatured cultural behavior.

The quality of food and physical vitality has a direct and indirect effect on the quality of the woman/man relationship. Food (nutrition) is the fuel that feeds the body. Denatured foods such as bleached white flour and white sugar are depleted of nutrients. They weaken the body's ability to defend itself and makes, the body an excellent host for dis-eases. A body thus weakened cannot be at its best. It cannot think at its best or produce good quality sperms or eggs. A body that uses poor quality fuel operates poorly. This lowered function and weakened vitality may not be noticed because the body has energy reserves and a resistive strain and will tolerate all types of abuse. It will tolerate drug addiction, radiation, alcoholism, smoking marijuana, polluted air and water, and noise pollution. These types of tolerated abuse and poor quality foods produce a poor quality life, even though the quantity (age) of life may be long. Foods are chemicals and chemicals (natural or synthetic) alter the health, spirit, mind, mood and state of consciousness. The healthier people are; the more able they are to serve the relationship. The male/female serves Maat. And, Maat serves the culture. The culture nurtures and is nurturing to the relationship. The relationship is the seed that the culture grows from.

Wholistic sexual relations between Black women and men were specific. In wholism, an orgasm was and is the sublime state of the uplifted spiritual, mental and physical being expressed with sex. A wholistic orgasm cannot be achieved without mutual spiritual and mental harmony based upon the Maat. This wholistic cultural view was often expressed in the communal lifestyle of Africans. The culture uses "rites of passage" to teach the female to understand the male portion of herself. The woman has a man (not to be confused with homosexuality) component because she is anatomically structured by male sperm. This component gives the woman the ability to communicate with and feed the emotions of the male. The acceptance and utilization of the whole self (man/woman parts) in sexual relations is by definition wholism.

The man's cycle, hormonal mood fluctuations and monthly sperm cycle coincide with the woman's cycle (period). These cycles are a physically dominant part of the relationship. The man's emotional and behavioral responsibility during menstruation, pregnancy, birth and menopause is culturally defined and taught to him during his "rites of passage."

The wholism of the Black relationship is based on concept (whole interrelationship) thinking. In this wholistic state, the woman/man has to use every thought, action, emotion and sexual episode as a vehicle for reaffirming Maat. Reaffirmation of Maat dissolves the Caucasian cultural influence on sexuality and relationships. In a relationship, the couple must see a connection between their behavior and Maat, their sexuality and Maat and see their behaviors as African Maat sexual rituals and ceremonies. Otherwise, they will not see God and spirituality in their sexual intercourse. Without God and spirituality involved in sex; sex becomes a feel good behavior, lust and sex acrobatic eroticism.

Spirituality and God involved in a Black relationship makes it African centered. In African cultures, an understanding of Maat, the unseen, invisible worlds, unmanifested, immortal and spiritual intelligence was the only criteria for a relationship. Sexual spiritual enlightenment acquired through "rites of passage" education earned the individual's title of God or Goddess. The fundamental African belief was, if God created man, then man would be called God just as the offspring of a chicken are called chickens. In Caucasian culture, a person whose behavior is according to the teachings of Jesus Christ is called a Christian. In African culture, a person's behavior that follows God's Maat principles were called a God or Goddess. This was not confused to mean Almighty God, The Creator, etc.

The true essential meaning of these titles of Gods and Goddesses found in African history has been distorted by the religious bias of the Caucasian writers. Spiritual growth and a Maatian life aimed towards achieving spiritual upliftment was the primary objective of all Black woman/man relationships. Individuals in a relationship were regarded as spirits and treated as spirits. Spirit is the unified energy that moves intelligence and the world and should not be confused with ghosts or dead ancestors. In an African centered relationship, each person was viewed as a sacred presence of God (or Creator God or One and Only God). An individual served God by serving their mate. If an argument would arise, it was resolved by one asking themselves "How is what I am saying benefiting me? How is my mate listening to me benefiting them and how is this argument benefiting God and serving Maat?" Who is right and who is wrong was not the standard for resolving arguments. Arguments were resolved according to how they benefited Maat, the culture, God and the ancestors. Finding out who is right or wrong in an argument or who is the victor and which person is wrong or the victim does not serve Maat. Being "right" must serve and benefit of the person who is wrong and benefit the village, ancestors, Maat and God. In the "Negro Dialect" (African speech accent), Maat logic is quite noticeable. There are words, which have many meanings. However, Maat selects the "right" meaning. The meaning most "right" for the whole sentence at the time of the sentence's usage in a conversation determines the best "right" definition. "Right" is judged by correctness, justice, harmony, balance, reciprocity, truth, propriety and order (Maat).

Relationships between Black women and men founded on correctness, justice, harmony, balance, reciprocity, truth, propriety and order (Maat) are

African centered. The male/female relationship is a union of God that is the balance of the spirit, mind and body. The couple is Maat and the living will of God. Maat means the couple will not destroy their health with junk foods. Because, to destroy the health means destroying the relationship.

Relationship, water, air, love, children, plants and culture were created by God and will always exist. People do not create relationship. People participate in something made by God called a relationship. Relationship is a sacred creation of God. To dishonor, abuse, misuse or morally pollute a relationship means disrespecting God. Relationship is given to African peoples as another way to serve God.

WOMEN'S HEALTH DISTORTIONS

Women's health is surrounded by many Caucasian scientific opinions, myths and distortions. These distortions have an impact upon the dis-ease and destroys the health of women (*Every Woman's Book* by P. Airola).

The standards of health for a woman's body is based upon scientific myths and opinions. For example, science assumes that the moon influences menstruation. Actually, the moon is used to correlate menstruation (hemorrhaging/bleeding). The moon does not induce or cause menstruation. Caucasian science's cannot explain why fertile women do not menstruate each month or why women miss their menstruation cycle. A missed period indicates that the body has powers within itself to regulate itself and does not depend on the moon. Ironically, the moon is composed of various types of minerals (dirt) and this dirt is many miles away. If one wants to believe that the dirt called the moon has a stronger influence upon their bodies than the earth (dirt) under their feet, then they are using a scientific myth, not factual science.

The African Art and Science of anatomy and physiology reveals many facts and many distortions in Caucasian science. Caucasian science assumes that the planets (dirt), floating thousands of miles away have a stronger influence than the earth (dirt) under the feet. Caucasian science has knowledge about the rotation, orbits, vortices, galaxies and constellations and little knowledge of the rotation, orbits, vortices and galaxies of the dirt (Minerals such as: calcium, magnesium, potassium, copper, zinc, lead, silver, etc.) under their feet. African art and science of chemistry place dirt (minerals) in a special category called the Mineral Kingdom.

The woman's menstruation cycle does not have a defined beginning or end (other than menopause). The cycle of ovulation is controlled by hormones and menstruation is not part of the ovulation cycle. The hormonal cycle ends when the women's body has no hormones — this would mean death.

Menstruation, ovulation and the hormone cycle have a wholistic meaning. Contemporary menstruation occurs when the uterus is deteriorating and hemorrhaging (loosing fresh blood). Menstruation is a period when the spirit and the nutrients from the cellular deterioration of the egg recycles in the body, while conception is when a spirit (a child) enters through the woman.

The hormonal cycle (period) occurs when thought cycles complete themselves and the thoughts spiral to upper levels of mental growth. In ancient African culture, menstruation (the loss of a few drops of blood from the decayed egg, not hemorrhaging of uterus), was viewed as a spiritually uplifting holistic occurrence. The male hormones react and respond to the female hormone cycle, menstruation and menopause. Caucasians view the fetus' movement in the womb as accidental movements. The fetus was created by God's laws and moves according to laws. The laws of conception (marriage of sperm and egg) produce a child. A fetus is a product of laws. The fetus' movements press the acupuncture meridians of the placenta and uterus. The unborn child's kicks stimulate the organ related sections of the uterus and abdomen (See Acupressure and Body Region Charts). The abdomen and uterus is divided into a circular section composed of the upper region: heart, small intestines; lower region: kidney, bladder; right region: lungs, large intestines; left region: liver, gall bladder and the center region is the stomach and spleen. The child, stimulates these regions and influences the nutrients that the mother's blood feeds the placenta. This determines the nutritional menu of the unborn child.

It is generally noticed that during pregnancy women appear more physically healthy. The pregnant woman is cleansing her body in order to produce good quality nourishment for the fetus. The baby's cells and body are basically pure. The mother's cells become pure in order to maintain the health of the unborn child. This prevents her body from rejecting the child.

Postnatal Depression may occur as well as the newborn baby's rejection of the breast milk. Both activities are related to the placenta. The newborn baby and placenta are one. The placenta helps to convert the nutrients and oxygen of the mother to the baby's biochemistry. The placenta belongs to and is attached to the baby. The baby communicates biochemically and electromagnetically with the placenta. After birth, the placenta supplies the baby with oxygen, nutrients and the hormone it uses to trigger breathing. The placenta stores the oxygen the baby needs to make the transition from breathing through the mother to breathing on its own. When the umbilical cord is cut before it stops pulsating (supplying oxygen and nutrients) it cannot receive messages (biochemical and electromagnetic) from the baby to eject itself. The cutting of the pulsating cord causes the blood and nutrients for the baby to stay in the placenta and become toxins. The mother's hormones trigger the destruction of the toxic placenta instead of her hormones triggering the ejection of the placenta out the uterus. Rejection of the placenta hormonally gets confused with rejection of the baby and this causes Postnatal Depression.

The mother's colostrums milk with vital enzymes, nutrients and bacteria flora are needed for the baby's stomach to have the ability to digest the breast milk that follows colostrums. However, the mother's rejection (Postnatal Depression) of the baby as well as the baby's rejection of the mother causes problems. The baby finds the mother's milk difficult to digest and rejects the milk. The baby subconsciously confuses breast rejection with mother rejection. Pregnant mothers that are given antibiotics and drugs that destroy the bacteria flora needed for the baby to digest the milk. The baby rejects breast milk it cannot digest. In this situation, rub vegetarian bifidus acidophilus on the breast's nipple so the baby can get the bacteria flora needed to digest breast milk. Vaccinations, medical drugs and synthetic chemicals given to the mother and/or baby can cause the rejection of breast milk and hormonal changes cause Postpartum Depression. Cutting the umbilical cord before it stops pulsating causes the loss of oxygen to the baby's brain and lungs. This can result in the baby not breathing properly at birth (absence of deep breaths). Slapping the baby on the buttocks in order to force it to deeply breathe is a criminal offense that amounts to an assault and battery. It causes a permanent emotional scar. The abrupt cutting of the umbilical cord causes the baby to have a decrease in the emotional and mental ability to bond to the mother, bond to the culture and bond to itself. The mother and child, in some way become subliminally and/or subconsciously dysfunctional—either spiritually, emotionally and/or mentally.

Lactation (milk) production is generally distorted. Sexual intercourse and work (job) should be abstained from during lactation. These activities interfere with the quality of milk because they alter the nutritional quality of cells in the mother's body and in the case of sexual activity, alter the hormone level. Incidentally, the lumps (bumps and clogged areas on the breast) correspond to the acupuncture organ regions. The breast gets bumps, lumps and clogs due to a weakness or overexertion of the internal organs.

The mammae (women's breasts) are not seen as food vehicles (milk) and their purpose is distorted. Breasts are viewed as sex objects and locked up in breast nozzles, harnesses and straightjackets to make them appear sexy. These brassiered breasts harness and weaken the pectoral muscles and cut off circulation. They stop the breast skin from breathing. Nylon and/or synthetic panties stop the proper air and ventilation of the vagina. This results in vaginitis, yeast infection, and other types of diseases.

Caucasian facial features and limp hair is the standard of beauty for Black women. Beauty for Black females is based upon spirituality and Maat behavior. Today, women's beauty is based upon muscular development, breast size, the curvature of the hips, Caucasoid facial features, painting colors on the lips and face and the mutilation of flesh (earrings, nose rings, vaginal lip rings). Caucasians use makeup to add color to their pale pink skin. Black women's skin has color. In African culture, makeup has spiritual and cultural meanings. It was not used to make colored women colored.

Another type of distortion is the wearing of high heels. High heals and pointed toes on the shoes of Caucasians was created as symbols of the penis. Ancient Greek homosexual men used them for masturbation. Wearing high heels cause the spinal column to become misaligned, forces body weight upon the uterus, shifts weight to the toes, tilts the body against gravity and is dis-ease inducing. Misalignment can result in back pain, decrease the circulation to the uterus, cause pelvic tilt, poor posture, and nervous system disorders. High heels increase the height of the female by sacrificing the anatomical balance of the body. This off-balanced and poor posture is misinterpreted as beauty.

The iron deficiency anemia of female blood content is another distortion. This junk food research conclusion was based upon an iron deficiency found in less than 30% of those women used in the survey. The deficiency can indicate that the kidneys are weakened and unable to recycle and concentrate minerals. This anemia justifies the prescribing of high levels of synthetic toxic iron to women. This distortion has caused women to have biochemical imbalances.

The women's' orgasm has been vastly distorted. Proper sexual stimulation of the clitoris can be achieved by adequate pelvic-to-pelvic pressure exertion, which can result in the woman having an arousal climax. This pressure has to be applied with a pelvic-to-pelvic, up-and-down sliding motion in order to have an orgasm. Women and men have to be conscious of God's presence during sex know their spirituality and understand how sex serves Maat. Otherwise, sex is reduced to a sensual erotic activity and/or a breeding activity of Caucasian socially engineered slaves.

MENSTRUATION IS NOT NORMAL

Menstruation is not a normal in a healthy woman. Menstruation is the hemorrhaging and flow of fresh blood. Hemorrhaging, whether it occurs in the brain, eyes, lungs or uterus, is not normal. Wholistically, Black African females on a diet of natural foods do not menstruate. Anthropological studies on African women have verified that ancient African women did not menstruate (See cultural clowns, Black folks and sex).

Wholistic women follow natural breeding cycles. These natural breeding (mating) cycles have strict laws. Ancient African women did not have sexual intercourse while pregnant or while breastfeeding or menstruating. Breastfeeding traditionally lasted from three to five years. Intercourse while pregnant causes the body to alter its nutrient and hormone level. This alters the ability to create healthy cells for the baby's body. Sexual intercourse while a woman is pregnant or breastfeeding decreases the health of the unborn child. Excessive sexual intercourse and out-of-cycle sexual intercourse causes the woman to menstruate. Sexual intercourse at night is abnormal and out-of-cycle and weakens the sex organs and health. No animal or insect that eats during the daylight hours has sex at night. Sex during the daylight hours follows the Circadian rhythm of the body. Nighttime sex exploits the female emotionally and spiritually and contributes to the hemorrhaging called menstruation.

The vaginal fluid discharge (not vaginal lubrication for sex) of the female causes menstruation. Vaginal discharge is very high in hormones, vitamins and minerals. It is a highly concentrated mixture equal to the nutritional concentration of semen. The nutrition that is lost due to this milky discharge causes the endometrium (uterus skin) tissue to lose its vitality and deteriorate. This cellular deterioration is known as hemorrhaging and is commonly called menstruation.

All women do not have moon cycle menstruation. Eskimo women menstruate on a sun (solar) cycle, every three years or more. Their menstruation is very light and not the gush of blood of today's hemorrhaging menstruation. Menstruation that occurs among women that are on a natural diet and are not wholistic in sexual practices always occurs on a solar (sun) period. Lunar (moon) periods are a new occurrence among females.

Lunar menstruations (periods) may be socially engineered and/or genetically transmitted (passed on from generation to generation). The lunar period may have been caused by the consistent and persistent habitual lunar sex orgies and raping of women and the nutritionally inadequate diet of the women. The lunar sex rituals and ceremonies modified Caucasian culture and modified the women's hormonal cycle and menstruation. Eventually, the socially and sexually engineered Caucasian women passed the hemorrhaging trait to future females. The Caucasian men's fertility rituals involved groups of men raping Caucasian women has caused them to develop a predisposition for romance, lust and lunar hemorrhaging menstruation. African women in slavery, colonialism and Caucasian oppression were forced to follow Caucasian sex rituals and ceremonies and the lunar hemorrhaging cycle as well as sex lust and romancing of Caucasian culture. The Caucasian religions and medicine believe this abnormality is necessary. Often, blood thinning herbs that help induce hemorrhaging are taken by women because the women believe in menstruation. They herbally make themselves menstruate.

Menstruation is the loss of fresh blood, not dis-eased blood. It was (and is) commonly believed in religions that the woman is purging herself of sinful blood. This Caucasian myth is subconsciously promoted by women and men. It is not a biological or anatomical fact that hemorrhaging is normal or that this blood is sinful and unneeded—it is science mythology.

In nature, menstruation among female animals occurs whenever the female is enslaved. Female animals such as wild wolves, bears, gorillas, goats, pigs, kangaroos, cats, monkeys, sheep and other female mammalians (animals that feed their babies milk) will menstruate when enslaved. Enslaved animals are those domesticated by Caucasians such as those that are in a zoo, circus, breeding farm or kept as pets. Enslavement causes the behavior, hormonal level and nutritional diet of the animal to be altered according to the needs of the enslavers. Female animals put in a Caucasian socially restricted and controlled behavioral situation will menstruate, while so called wild (free) female animals do not menstruate. Aside from this, diet contributes to female menstruation. For example, female and male gorillas given a so-called modern diet (junk food, cooked food and animal flesh) will masturbate, menstruate, become violent have excessive sexual intercourse and do homosexual activities.

Menstruation can be irregular, cramping and of long duration owing to manganese, iron and calciums deficiency. A female, at any age with a brief period of manganese deficiency can biochemically cause a menopausal episode. A fertile woman's Menopausal episode can be hours or a few days of duration. It usually goes unnoticed by young females because they still have a lunar period. Stressors (i.e., emotional, oppression, dietary, social, relationship, etc.) can cause hormonal imbalances that decrease oxygen and nourishing blood to the uterus and increase waste and carbon dioxide in the uterus. This weakens the uterus and contributes to menstruation hemorrhaging. Hormonal imbalances caused by estrogen and steroid hormones in non-organic eggs, dairy and meats causes the uterus to oxidize (deteriorate) and this contributes to infertility and uterus hemorrhaging. Unless the male's frequency is constant and synchronized with the frequency of the ovaries and holistic, there will be infertility. The sperm has two frequencies and the ovaries (eggs) have two frequencies. They must be both on the same frequency for fertilization. A weak uterus and ovaries have unstable frequencies. Hemorrhaging weakens the uterus, fallopian tubes and ovaries.

Menstruation is not normal; however, menstruation is not necessarily caused by an abnormality in Black women alone; this unnatural condition is shared by Black men as well. Caucasian science teaches Blacks to be unaware that the woman's brain (according to body weight) is larger and more convoluted than the man's brain. Women have two "X" chromosomes. The "X" chromosomes carry the genetic immunity factors while the "Y" chromosome does not. Men have one "X" and one "Y" chromosome. Women's eggs determine the below waist characteristic (sex of the child). Men's sperm determines the above waist characteristic (personality traits). Women have a greater endurance capacity and fossil relics verify that women have had muscular development equal to men. Additionally, women have three lobes on their thyroid—this increases cell growth and rejuvenation ability and men have two lobes, women have two generative (sex) centers in the brain and men have one—this increases intelligence states. The myths, lies and bias in Caucasian religion, science, and social institutions influence the way the female anatomy is interpreted.

Caucasian men use menstruation to control women. And, at one time a woman who did not menstruate was murdered because she was considered to be a witch. Menstruating women are in a weaker physical, spiritual and mental state and easier to dominate. In ancient African cultures, women who menstruated were isolated and given herbal medicine because menstruation was considered a problem and a disease symptom of the village. Women were not isolated because they were sinful or evil, but because they were in a diseased condition and needed the dis-ease to be holistically corrected. The ancient Africans realized that menstruation is not normal and that it reflects a tribal or cultural disease. Today, it is a symptom of Caucasian oppression.

Menstruation has many aspects that affect the totality of African peoples lifestyles. Menstruation by Black African women is a recent occurrence. No anthropological research, or research from medical science or veterinarian science can validate that hemorrhaging is normal for women.

Menstruation is often justified by a culture's lunar zodiacal rationales. The zodiac concepts are a cultural language that varies in each culture. In African cultures, zodiac science if applied to an individual, was applied at conception. In other words, the zodiac sign starts at conception, not birth. Ironically, 90% of all wholistic African births occurred between May and June. Consequently, the other signs of the zodiac were rarely applied to Africans. Today the majority of births in countries such as those in France, Germany, Australia, Canada, America etc. still occur during May and June. This further validates that a natural mating cycle still exists among humans. Africans followed this mating cycle of every three years and had classical menstruation that lasted a few hours or a day. It required no sanitary napkin. Tribes and cultures, which lost great numbers of people due to Caucasian wars and dis-ease, would increase sexual intercourse and have out of cycle sex to regain a population. However, this procreation was a temporary mating practice and abnormal. Excessive sexual intercourse causes nocturnal emission, prostrate problems, impotency, and decreased thinking among men. Excessive sexual intercourse always causes menstruation among women. In fact, women prostitutes have longer bleeding (menstruation) due to excessive sexual practices. In any case, the children conceived during non-mating cycles have behavior, emotions, thoughts and spirituality that has adapted to the biochemical oppression. Hemorrhaging (bleeding) among Black African women represents a deterioration of the African culture and race and is a form of genocide.

Fruitarian and vegetarian women, normally, do not menstruate. If they do menstruate it consists of two or more drops of blood (about the size of a pea) from the unfertilized egg. The lymph glands absorb the non-fertilized egg atrophy (waste) and remove it out of the body. A blood flow (dead egg waste) of a few hours or days or no blood flow is normal. Menstruation in African cultures must be treated as a cultural imbalance and a form of genocide and the hormonal and biochemical effect of White Supremacy.

THE 9 TYPES OF MENSTRUATION

Types	Symptoms	Causes
1.	Cramping, nervous tension and pain during menses with not discomfort before cycle.	Low Estrogen can be related to antibiotics, not enough raw food in diet, etc. High Progesterone (related to tender breasts and acne on cycle), liver distress.
2.	Excessive bleeding.	High Estrogen (heavy flow two to three days) blood unable to clot (weak liver, kidney and/or adrenals) uterine fibroids, anemia, thyroid problems, drugs, junk foods.

Types	Symptoms	Causes
3.	Bloating, swollen ankles, headaches nervousness, premenstrual tension and/or nausea.	Mineral imbalance (losing Calcium, Iron, etc,)., Iron, etc.) Potassium, High Estrogen (Caused by caffeine, chocolate, meat, eggs, dairy, processed soy), liver stress.
4.	Cramps after PMS, bloating, swollen, ankles, headaches, nervousness and/or nausea.	High Estrogen can be related to a short period of heavy bleeding and edema, low Zinc, Manganese and Magnesium.
5.	Rapid heartbeat during menstruation, nervous, dry mouth, digestion and/or sensitivity to light.	Loss of Iron, Iodine, Calcium and/or Potassium, Low Estrogen.
6.	Menstruation and fatigue, heavy or bearing down feeling in pelvic area, weakness, exhaustion, loss of energy.	Anemia, liver stress, amino acid imbalance, (protein), stress (adrenal gland exhaustion).
7.	No menstruation – Amenorrhea.	Mental, emotional and/or spiritual stress, athletic overtraining (low body fat), inadequate female gender type exercise and/or spiritual dancing. Anemia, high protein and saturated processed fat. (Not to be confused with classical amenorrhea.
8.	Pain	Endometriosis, ruptured follicle, fibroid, rheumatism, varicose veins, clogged arteries and/or veins of the uterus and or pelvic areas. Waste congested uterus.
9.	Hormone imbalance (mood swings, bone loss, hunger, etc.) related to heavy bleeding, fibroids, cramps, breast lumps, low systolic blood pressure and pulse, aborted pregnancies, bloated swollen ankles during cycle, bleeding more than three days, swollen breasts, vomiting and toxemia of pregnancy, premenstrual nervousness, edema, nausea and headaches.	**Estrogen Imbalance** (hormone produced by ovary follicle) related to heavy bleeding, fibroids, cramps, breast lumps, swollen ankles during cycle, antibiotics. Not enough raw food in diet. **Progesterone Imbalance** (hormone produced by corpus lutetium – egg) liver stress, excess estrogen.

MENSTRUATION REMEDIES

Supplements	Use
Black Cohosh	Hormone balance, vaginal dryness, hot flashes, cramps, estrogen deficiency
Chaste (Viitex)	Hormone balance, breast discomfort, mood swings, menstruation problems
Red Raspberry, Squaw Vine	Hormone balance
Squaw Vine	Strengthens uterus
Cramp Bark	Cramps
Dong Quai	Hormone balance, cramps, irregular cycle (do not use if heavy bleeding)
Shepherd's Purse, Witch Hazel, White Oak Bark, Blessed Thistle, Alum Root	Heavy bleeding
Vitamin K	Heavy bleeding

Gingko	Bloating, swollen ankles, breast pain
Dandelion Root, Yellow Dock	Iron deficiency
Ginger Root	Edema, swollen ankles, bloating, digestion problems
White Willow, Boswella	Pain
Feverfew	Headache, fever
Yohimbe and Damiana Combination, Testoterone Tablets/Gel, Dopa Bean, Tribulus Wild Yam Crème (Progesterone)	Lack of sexual desire
Licorice Root (Deglycyrrhiza for heart, sugar or kidney problems	Energy, fatigue, regulates sugar
Motherwort, Scullcap, St. John's Wort	Depression, nervous tension
Fo-Ti, Ginseng, DHEA, Yohimbe combined with Damiana	Fatigue
Red Clover	Hormone balance, hot flashes
Flax, Primrose, Hemp or Borage Oil	Heavy flow
Beta Carotene, MSM, Lysine and/or MSM Crème/Lotion	Skin outbreak, Acne
B Complex	Irritability, Fatigue, Mood Swings
Chromium and/or Vanadium	Sugar and/or Chocolate Craving
Catnip, Chamomile, Kava Kava, Passion Flower	Nerve Calmative
Cat's Claw, Feverfew, MSM	Inflammation of uterus, endometriosis
Pregnenolone, Progesterone Crème/Lotion	PMS, Menopause, infertility, emotional problems, mood swings, hair loss. Needed if non-organic fruit, vegetables, meats, eggs and dairy are eaten

GARDEN PARTY OF ANCIENT AFRICAN VEGETARIAN WOMEN "SUN PEOPLE"
Tomb painting of Nefer-hetep, Thebes, c. 1350 B.C.

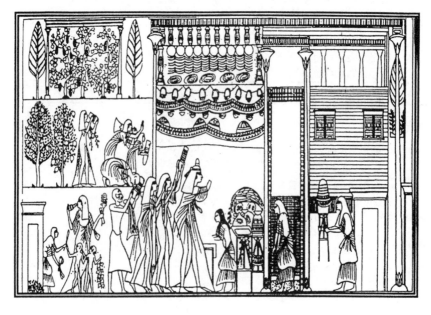

About the Illustration
These "Sun People" are priestesses. They did not menstruate and wore no underwear. Amenses (non-menstruating) women ovulate. They are playing a spiritual musical instrument called a "sistrum" in the shape of Sun Goddess *Het Heru* on top of her personification of *Annu Khet*. It is *Annu Khet's* highest spiritual sound manifestations. It is imitated by European priest when they ring small bells during religious rituals and ceremonies.

The food indicates that the Priestesses are vegetarians (no meat, dairy or eggs) and that they drank fruit juices. The vegetable and fruit garden indicates deep soil beds were used to plant various types of fruits, grapevines and vegetables.The men are the priestesses' servants. These vegetarian priestesses are on the "Aten Path" of the "Earth Goddesses" (deified women).

HUMAN KINGDOM, SEX, MASTURBATION, ORAL SEX

The Human Kingdom is found in African science. In Caucasian science, humans are placed in the Animal Kingdom. In African science, humans are placed in a separate kingdom because they are uniquely different from all animals. *(Studies in Animal and Human Behavior* by K. Lorenz)

The African classification of life forms into five kingdoms is done because life forms have common sets of laws that govern each kingdom. Laws that are common to a particular group are given a common title such as Human Kingdom Animal Kingdom, Mineral Kingdom and Plant Kingdom.

The Human Kingdom is separate from the Animal Kingdom. There is no half animal and half human or animal in transition to become human, which can link (missing link) the Human and Animal Kingdoms. The separation between the Kingdoms is distinct, precise and clear. An animal cannot become a plant. A plant cannot become a human. An apple tree cannot become a peach tree. A bird cannot become a horse. The most intelligent ape cannot become as intelligent as the most ignorant human. An animal cannot become a human (evolution). Humans possess qualities beyond animals, humans can create machines, religions, languages, art and books while apes cannot. An ape in "estrurn" (lust, sexual heat) will starve or kill until it has satisfied its sexual desire. A human does not place sexual desire above its own life. There are many myths and scientific contradictions used to promote a Caucasian science theory (fantasy) that says man evolved from apes.

The Caucasian scientists who promote the science myth (theory, fantasy) that man evolved from the ape must look at themselves. The Caucasians have short legs as compared to the body trunk—the ape has short legs as compared to body trunk. Caucasians have straight limp hair—the ape has straight hair. Caucasians have underdeveloped buttock muscles (flat behinds)—the ape has the same. The ape has white skin—Caucasians have white skin. There are many similarities between the ape and the Caucasian, which could mean that the Caucasian came from the ape. The Orangutan, Gorilla, and Chimpanzee of today are absolutely a separate species from those that it is projected that Caucasian man evolved from. If man evolved from the ape of today then sexual reproduction between man and today's species of the monkey would be possible. If it were possible that man could have sex with monkeys, there would still be a species of ape interbreeding with man. There would remain some form of sexual intercourse between Caucasians and apes. Caucasians and apes would have a common mating (heat) cycle. In contrast, Black Africans are anatomically the direct opposite of the ape in hair structure, buttock muscle development, leg length, skin color, etc. Again, the Human Kingdom is separated from the Animal Kingdom. There are some similarities between the Animal and Human Kingdoms, but the differences between the two kingdoms far exceed the similarities. One of the main differences in the Human Kingdom is in the original or perfect state for humans.

Humans were created, by God, in a perfect state; the female and male have complementary sex organs. Caucasian science mythology believes that humans were bisexual (possessed both female and male functional sex organs of equal development) and later evolved into two separate sexes called man and woman. In the book *Physical Life of Woman* by G. Napheys, this is reviewed. This science myth believes that the separation in the sexes occurred in order to create a variety of human beings. This myth was created by Caucasian culture. This myth is in Caucasian religions that believe that the separation occurred because of sin. In any case, the similarities do not mean the same function. Men have similarities in sex organs such as a uterus (prostrate), ovaries (testicles) nipples and mammae glands (milk producing breasts). The women possess similarities in sex organs such as the clitoris (penis) and two testicle glands on the sides of the clitoris. These sex organs are similar because the sexes are complementary. In the book, *Children of Mu* by J. Churchward, the subject is overviewed. In nature, organs have adaptability. Adaptability of organs is misinterpreted as degenerated (dormant) organs.

Nature is very strict and wastes no energy. Every raindrop is used and recycled in nature- nothing is wasted. The similarities between female/male sex organs in humans are not a wasteful mistake of nature. The similarities were developed to serve a purpose and that purpose is to make them complementary sexes, not opposite sexes.

Dermoid cysts (undeveloped babies in the womb) are found in females and males that have degenerated. A dermoid cyst is a fetus. There is scientific evidence of this in the book *The Awakening of Woman* by J. Kellogg. Dermoid cysts have been found in girls who did not ovulate and boys who did not produce sperm. Religious science mythology states that men were created male and female and a dermoid mutation is used to justify the self-fertilization myth. Caucasian history mythology supports the culture's mythology, which supports the science mythology.

Black folks using Caucasian sex behaviors and perversions have been culturally castrated and sexually colonized; they have degenerated. The Caucasians have degenerated the air (polluted), water (polluted), soil (depleted of minerals) and degenerated Africans (health has deteriorated and lifespan has decreased). Therefore, the Africans' ability to visualize and have holistic sex has degenerated.

A higher human development comes from a higher humanism, intelligence comes from intelligence, water comes from water, air comes from air, God comes from God, humans come from the Human Kingdom, life comes from life, and light comes from light. These African truths are the basis for the African art and science of sex. In African religions, God is called Mother-Father (man and woman) God. God is a complete complement. Man and woman together are a complement.

Man and woman are created to reach their highest level of humanism —perfection. A human cannot create a perfect state unless a perfect state already exists within the human. In other words, you cannot get something from nothing. In African science, this is and was the primary law. In Caucasian science mythology, they believe that the earth was created out of nothing. They believed that you can get something from nothing. This Caucasian science myth assumes that you can get water from an empty glass. In unwholistic Caucasian science, dualism is considered in conflict or in opposition to each other. For example, in order to describe light you say it fights darkness. In order to describe an apple you must also describe an orange. Subsequently, you can say that an apple tastes better than an orange. Caucasian opposite logic is different from African logic. For example, in African science, light is described by comparing it to other types of light. Apples are described in comparison with other types of apples. There is no need for the opposite sex logic in wholistic logic. Consequently, humans are considered created sexually as complements (female and male). The use of Caucasian antagonistic dualism leads to the belief that man and woman are opposites. The antagonistic dualism belief leads one to assume that there must be the rich against the poor, slave against master, and superior against inferior people. In wholistic African logic, there are many types of rights and all rights (privileges) are the expression of Maat in a different form. Perfection of the human is a right. This right is exercised by using African culture's health practices, sexual rituals and behaviors, religious concepts and Maat.

Good health is a human right. Good health can only be obtained by using whole foods (unprocessed) and following the natural laws of the body. For example, it is natural to squat while having a bowel movement; it is natural to squat to birth a child; it is not natural to mutilate parts of the body (circumcisions, earring holes in ear), it is not natural for a child to urinate and defecate on itself in African culture (babies learn to have bowel movements and urinate without diapers or wetting the bed); it is not natural to chew gum (causes the stomach to secrete too much mucous), etc. There are many Caucasian thoughts and behaviors, which have distorted the Africans' understanding of the body and sex.

Sex is derived from sexus. Sexus means to cut off, separate, take a part of and amputate. Sex is part of the Tree of Life. You give a part of yourself (genetic code) when conceiving a child. Therefore, excessive sex gives away a lot of nutrients and shortens the lifespan. Fruit trees that produce large crops year after year have short lifespans. In men, excessive ejaculation of sperm causes impotency, weakens thinking, causes prostrate problems and decreases quality and quantity of the life of the offspring. In the book *Sexual Knowledge* by W. Hill, further information on the subject is revealed. In women, producing many babies causes the reproductive organs to deteriorate. Excessive sex causes a hormone drain, nutrient depletion and decreased thinking ability. This is discussed in *Sexology* by Clements.

Male animals (bulls, horses) and humans are weak after sexual intercourse. In *Evolution of Sex* by Geddes and Thompson, this is discussed. Male insects usually die or are eaten after sexual intercourse. Moreover, the woman's vagina pulsates and uterus pulsates making rhythm for the sperm to travel through—the vagina's convoluted muscles pulsate, the uterus opening is small and the sphincter muscle pulsates, the sperm in the uterus can be destroyed by vaginal acid, discharge and fluid moves in tidal pulsating waves, which are in harmony with the sperm motion and the egg is further concealed in the pulsating fallopian tubes, making the path for the sperm one of rhythmaticity. The sperm route to the egg is full of pulsations. The egg has pulsating aura, vibration and radiation, which help the egg to develop. The contraction and relaxation of muscles and electrical impulses create pulsations. Pulsations create rhythm, colors, sound (music), language, dances (geometric shapes), types of light and magnetism. The movement of the sperm and egg are a harmonious symphony of holistic creation. Each act of sex creates either a child, a spirit or a thought because it is a creation activity. Sperm and egg unite to form the Tree of Life. The Tree of Life —of Spiritual Life—was designed to feed the Tree of Physical Life. The recycling of orgasm energy to the Pineal is called sexual regeneration. This feeds the Tree of Life. The brain and spinal nerves resemble an upside down tree (Tree of Spirit Life) while the glands resemble a tree (Tree of Physical Life).

Black women have been socially engineered by Caucasian culture to accept sexual lust, Caucasian dating and sex rituals and ceremonies. Black women tend to feel unfulfilled and unsatisfied by unemotional and non-spiritual Caucasian sexual intercourse. In the book *Woman and Superwoman* by A. Raleigh, this is discussed. Their holistic negative reaction to Caucasian type sex is called frigidity. For example, an individual who initially inhales cigarette smoke coughs to reject the smoke. The throat and stomach, of an individual who initially drinks alcohol, will burn. These are natural rejections similar to a woman's spiritual, emotional and mental reaction to Caucasian perverted sexual intercourse is a naturally negative (naturally frigid). The repetition of Caucasian sexual rituals and ceremonies of creates Black sexual puppets (Africans' acceptance of Caucasian sexuality as normal). Sexual lust (sex without the spirituality, Maat, God or the purpose of procreation) between

Black men and women is a form of slave sex. The loss of the fruits (sperm, egg) of the Human Tree of Life through masturbation and oral sex results in the Black race's genocide on a spiritual and cultural level.

A human that exercises wholistic sexual control over a longer lifespan. Rigid sexual intercourse codes (laws) combined with spirituality, Maat and God and cultural meanings are normal for African people. Sexual intercourse for reproduction occurred three to four times in an African woman's lifespan. Sexual intercourse for Sexual Regeneration occurred more often. It involved using the orgasm energy to stimulate the Pineal. Males would not ejaculate for Regenerative sex. Whenever sexual intercourse was performed, it was never at night. A woman would have between one and four children in her lifetime because sex was abstained from while she was pregnant (ten months) and during breastfeeding (three to five years). In fact, 80% of the births occurred between May and June in many African cultures because human mating laws were followed.

Sexual intercourse, for reproduction, was indulged in from one to four times in a monogamous man's lifespan and 12 or more times in a wholistic polygamous man's lifespan (based on number of wives). In the case of a polygamous woman with two or more husbands, reproductive sex was from one to four times in a lifespan. Sexual regenerative sexual intercourse had no limit. These natural wholistic sexual intercourse practices caused the lifespan to be long. Regeneration and sexual reproduction increased the lifespan. Excessive sexual intercourse was caused by slavery and the social engineering processes of White Supremacy. An excessively refined or processed food diet, excess estrogen and steroids in foods, genetically modified foods and radiated foods can cause masturbation and confusion. Masturbation is socially engineered into African peoples lifestyle.

Venereal dis-ease only occurs in civilizations where there is weak immunity, processed foods, cooked foods, drugs, junk foods and excessive and noncyclical sexual intercourse. The reproductive organs have a natural cycle of activity, building, cleansing and rest. Excessive sexual activity decreases the building, cleansing and rest of the organs, which causes toxins to accumulate. Toxins cause skin eruptions (herpes, cysts, tumors, etc.). The signs and symptoms of the deterioration of the reproductive system is called venereal dis-ease.

Masturbation and Oral Sex

Masturbation is the self-stimulation (sometimes to the point of climax) of the sexual organs. It is a common cultural practice in Caucasian societies and is socially engineered into Black folks' lifestyles. This is discussed in *The Science of Life* by Fowler.

The lust for sexual intercourse is culturally taught by Caucasian media, science and sex rituals and ceremonies. Lust is a characteristic of the Animal Kingdom not the Human Kingdom. The desire for sexual lust is socially taught to be satisfied by sexual intercourse with the opposite sex, with same sex masturbation (homosexuality), with a beast, child, electrical device, plastic penis or vagina or by masturbation. Lust, like estrum (sexual heat), is thought to need immediate satisfied. The procreation of the human species is not a part of masturbation or lust. In other words, it is an abnormal and perverted activity that is deliberately taught to Africans. Each episode of masturbation can lead to masturbation addiction and cause hormonal emotional, mental and spiritual imbalances. This abuse or addiction causes the reproductive organs and spirit to deteriorate. A predisposition for masturbation is passed on to a child by its parents' emotional, social and philosophical positive attitude about masturbation.

A pregnant woman who has sexual intercourse with a man is creating a lust desire in the fetus. A father who has excessive sexual intercourse with the child's mother or with another woman may genetically pass on the predisposition for lust. The father and/or mother's lust, masturbation and/or oral sex (mouth masturbation) and anal masturbation attitudes are passed to the unborn child. Lust is the primary cause of masturbation. Masturbation causes ejaculation and the murder of sperm. In the woman, it causes the deterioration of the mother instinct. The parenting instinct to nurture is misguided and discharged during hand, mouth and/or anal masturbation.

In wholistic African science and religions, oral masturbation is considered against life. Oral masturbation (or oral sex) is another Caucasian taught sexual lust degenerative behavior. It is practiced in the animal kingdom primarily by males only. Among animals, oral sex is only performed for a few minutes (if not less) and only occurs during heat (breeding cycles). Female animals use their tongue to sense fertility in male animals. Oral sex among ancient Caucasians was used to preserve virginity. Caucasian men used it to compete with the female's homosexual lover. And, it was used to help sex climax challenged women achieve an arousal climax. Males with inability to make the female achieve a climax use it. The oral masturbation (sex) act performed by women upon men is a Caucasian learned behavior.

The oral tasting of the female animal's genitals is used to test the pH level, estrum level, availability for mating, dis-ease or health status of female reproductive organs. Oddly enough, oral sex performed by highly active female prostitutes upon men is believed to cause sterility among prostitutes.

Homosexuality or sexual intercourse is physiologically impossible. Only a man and a woman can "enter-the-course" = entercourse (The male sex organs enters into the canal [vaginal shaft; course]). A woman's tongue is not anatomically made to be inserted into another woman's vagina. A man's penis is not anatomically made to be inserted into the anus and bowel movement (feces) of another man. The penis is not made for masturbating in manure stuck in the rectum. The mouth has no sex glands or reproduction function, the anus has no sex glands or reproductive function. Sex in nature can cause reproduction. Homosexuality is also another form of masturbation. This form of masturbation uses another person (of the same sex) as the masturbating device. Moreover, in nature each gender (male or female) has its own peculiar type of sexuality (foreplay, petting, kissing, mating ceremonies) and specific sex organs. In nature, the act of sex can lead to reproduction. Therefore, homosexuality is anti-sex and anti-nature. If there were a homosexual gender then homosexuals would have their own uniquely different sex organs and sex mating rituals and not a borrowed heterosexual one. Consequently, void of gender and sexuality the homosexuals become two parties of the same sex that masturbate each other. They are homo-masturbators (same sex).

Sex

Females, in general, have a higher percentage of positive lipids than males. Females are anabolic; males are catabolic. Sexual intercourse increases fatty acid. FA activity (catabolic) in males and increases sterols (anabolic) in females. The changes have an effect on the pulse, temperature and blood pressure.

Types of Sexual Personalities

In male and female sexual relationships, each individual brings their emotional vocabulary. Emotions influence sexual likes and dislikes. Sexual likes and dislikes are determined by your genetic code, parents, sexual experiences, culture, emotional sexual wounds (hurts), spirituality, dysfunctions, physical structure and personality. Sex, just like foods, motor vehicles, races, planets, music, animals, languages, water (i.e., spring, ocean, distilled and polluted) and seasons are classified. The classification of sex behaviors is called sexual personalities.

Having an understanding of your sexual personality and your partner's sexual personality produces more harmony in the relationship. Understanding your partner's sexual personality gives you the knowledge you need to sexually adapt. You are only sexually compatible or complimentary if you can adapt. Therefore, adapting, adjusting and being flexible is the key to sexual harmony. If you are not sexually compatible or complimentary, then adapting will make you have sexual harmony. Adapting is the key. The following are general descriptions and not precise classifications of sexual personalities. They were taught during the African holistic academic classes called a "rites of passage."

Type One: Warrior (Challenger) Sexuality
Birth Date between March 22 and May 12
Warriors like sex to be a struggle, sport and/or a psychological game of chess (mind game). They tend to find sexual delight in a hunter and prey scenario or the now you can have sex and now you cannot have sex (mood game). Sexual rejection is a challenge to their romantic tactics and merely arouses them more. Warriors want to sexually out-perform their sex partner. They tend to want to have a better orgasm than their mate or their mate's previous

partner. They feel sex is enhanced if it is mixed with wit, sexy words, and flirtation. They get excited by dominating sex activities.

Female Warriors
These females are passionately sensual more than nurturing. They have a need for material security—the more security, the more sexy they are. They feel that the energy the males get from sex with them should contribute to his emotional and intellectual well being. They require emotional security and positive comments. They like their sexual abilities, positions, and foreplay praised or else they will criticize the male's sexuality. Warriors do not like criticism about their eroticism. They like the male to perform sex in a nurturing manner.

Male Warriors
Warriors like to feel as if they are in control of the choices of sexual positions and petting. They tend to like females that have a passive outer sexual personality and an aggressive inner sexual personality. They are willing to let the female achieve an orgasm first only if they feel that the female is not their sexual equal. If the female presents too much of a sexual challenge to arouse to orgasmic levels than he may escalate his eroticism as a means to subdue her and be victorious. He tends to imagine himself as a sex idol that is too sexually complicated to be satisfied by any woman.

Type Two: Innovator Sexuality
Birth Date between May 13 and July 3
Sex tends to be based upon their changeable mood. They don't have fixed sexual positions or foreplay styles. They are sexually spontaneous and will attempt offbeat sexual maneuvers and eroticism. They enjoy innovating and experimenting with various types of sexual feelings, touches, moods, words, and positions more than they like physical sex.

Female Innovators
These females tend to use a nurturing approach to sex. They prefer sexual partners that encourage her to explore sex techniques. They like males that are sure of their ability to sexually please her. Sexual servitude to her sex needs excites her to be more erotic. Innovators' moods for sex are influenced by the ups and downs of her social life. Sex tends to be a fun-loving activity and more of a dream sensation than a physical activity. They like sex positions and petting to be an adventure of surprise.

Male Innovators
Males tend to use a nurturing approach to sex. They have a vivid sexual imagination and don't like limitations set on their sexual conduct. Innovators seem to be involved in the emotional temperature of the female's sexism. These men are sexually moody and don't like to feel emotionally obligated. They don't

like questions about their sexual behaviors or thoughts nor do they want to show that a woman's sexual personality has changed them. Innovators become sexually bored if sex constantly demands them to redefine themselves or their feelings or sexual motives.

Type Three: Leader Sexuality
Birth Date between July 4 and August 24
Leaders have an emotionally explosive sexual nature and like to be sexually in charge. They feel that they must completely sexually satisfy themselves and their partner and challenge themselves to do so. Once they have won the sexual challenge, they emotionally withdraw until a greater orgasmic challenge presents itself. During sex, they may talk foolish, use foolish positions and foreplay moves. Leaders know what sexually pleases them and are determined to be satisfied. Leaders can resort to emotionalism and emotional manipulation to create sexual episodes. They tend to enjoy the idea of sex more than sex. They enjoy turning ordinary words, sounds, positions, or body movements into eroticism.

Female Leaders
These females are sexually charismatic, charming, and flirtatious. They tend to be slightly rough and yet gentle in sexual positions and activities. They are sexually assertive and make sex into a battle of ego satisfaction. She may not compromise with the use of sexual positions and tends to block her own sexual satisfaction. They tend to be sensual and enjoy the physicalness of sex.

Male Leaders
Males like to dominate sexual intercourse activities and positions. They prefer sex positions that have them in control. These males can be aroused by associating mysticism with sex rather than physical lust. They act as if they know all their sexual feelings and have a superior sex stud mannerism. They seem to require a sexual take-charge female who can pretend to be submissive to his sexual desires.

Type Four: Idealist Sexuality
Birth Date between August 25 and October 15
They are emotionally withdrawn with their sexuality and mentally pretend to teach and preach about sex while engaged in sexual intercourse. They tend to have a lesson plan for sexuality. They may feel bad after having sex because they did not follow their sex positions and foreplay plan. After sex, they mentally review their failed sexual lesson plan. This allows them to emotionally extend the feeling of sex. The Idealists are in denial about feeling good during sex and set extraordinary high standards for orgasms.

Female Idealist

These females tend to be romantic and have a nurturing sexual mannerism. They seem to hold back their sensual nature and submit to the sexual maneuvers of the male. In their mind, they organize the sexual episode and require the male to be assertive and aggressive during sex. Their imagination allows them to be emotionally engaged in the sex act. Sex must be ideal, romantic, poetic, and the male a smooth talker. She tends to reject sex if her previous sexual episode did not meet her romantic desires or sex lesson plan. She sets high standards for orgasms and fails herself for not transcending above the human sex level.

Male Idealist

Males tend to have a nurturing mannerism towards sex. They desire the sex to be surrounded with romanticism and flirtation. They tend to feel good about themselves if they think their previous sex was rewarding. They may have an erotic appetite for sex that conflicts with their need for spiritualized sex. A female's innocent behaviors and dress, lace on brassiere, or slip, crossing of the legs, facial expressions and/or breathing can excite him sexually. They have pre-set ideals and high standards for sex. They want to sexually elevate themselves beyond the human existence.

Type Five: Organizer Sexuality
Birth Date between October 16 and December 6

They tend to connect seemingly irrelevant and disconnect body movements and activities with sex. They have a complex sexual desire and character logic. Organizers tend to want to manipulate you into having sex. They can have many sublime sexual related rituals. They use sex rituals to organize sex. They get more excited about organizing sex than having sex.

Female Organizer

These females tend to be sensual and enjoy erotic sexual gestures and foreplay. They tend to begin sex with very simple movements but as their passion increases, they demand more complex positions and series of foreplay and petting. Their sublime sex-related organized rituals may hinder sexual ecstasy. This can result in her becoming manipulative in order to feel that sex has a logical organized meaning.

Male Organizer

Males are chauvinistic about sex and must feel like the hunter capturing a prey. They tend to have difficulty exposing their true sexual desires to females. He tends to want females that use their sexuality to challenge or confront him rather than their mentality. They approach sex either hot or cold because they do not trust sex to fulfill them. Organizers tend to be sexually rigid and prefer the same organized positions and foreplay. He has favorite sexual foreplay, petting techniques, and positions but won't let the female know them. He wants you to ask questions about how and what to do to sexually please him but feels confronted if you ask the questions.

Type Six: Counselor Sexuality
Birth Date Between December 7 and January 27
They tend to have sex on a spiritual, healing, emotional, entertaining, and therapeutic level. They are physically sexy, but choose to base sex upon spirituality. Their sexual spirituality can be hidden or obvious. They like to be creative and unconventional during sex. It does not matter how physically fulfilling a sex episode is; they still can become bored with sex because it did not meet therapeutic standards. While engaging in sex, they enjoy sex in their imagination more than the act of sex. They counsel themselves to be better at sex.

Female Counselor
These females are sensual about sex and are not aware of when they are flirting or their partner is flirting. They enjoy romance, but deny enjoying it. During sex, they emotionally give all or none or partially of their passion and yet expect their partner to always give totally. They can be creative and erotic during sex, petting, and foreplay. They don't like sex to be a routine and expect it to have therapeutic results.

Male Counselor
Males tend to accent sexual creativity. If it is difficult to figure out how to sexually satisfy the female, they will pretend that they can selfishly be satisfied when they are not satisfied. Sex tends to be an artistic and spiritual activity. They have sex moods and don't like them interrupted with sexual intercourse. These males dislike being manipulated into having sex or restricted to ordinary sexual positions. They avoid questions about their sexual nature, desires, and/or fantasies. They secretly feel that they have a way to make sex therapeutic.

Type Seven: Visionary Sexuality
Birth Date between January 28 and Mar 2
Visionaries are fixed in their sexual wants, moods, and needs. They tend to enjoy sexual spirituality. Sex tends to begin in an emotional systematic way with step-by-step arousal, and then it becomes physically exciting. They are sexually rigid and enjoy their sexual rigidity on a spiritual basis.

Female Visionary
Females tend to evaluate whether they should engage in sex on the correctness of the morals and spirituality of the male. They have a vision about sex and deep sensual passionate desires but tend to withhold fulfilling their sexual appetite. Visionaries over-analyze the males' sex comments, sexual positions, and romantic activities to the point of taking the enjoyment out of sex.

They find sex to be erotic and repulsive simultaneously. They engage in sex in a lofty manner, but emotionally are erotic. Visionaries enjoy creative sex, but must be gradually aroused into the pleasure of it.

Male Visionary

Visionaries approach sex in a nurturing manner. They tend to place morals and ethics (rules) of sex above their own physical sexual pleasures. He tends to be critical of females' sexual comments, taste, and desires. They tend to feel following sexual rules means the same as getting sexually satisfied. They do not like to take chances with new sexual positions or activities. During sex, he does not like to hear emotional comments or criticism of his lack of sexual passion. These males have good sexual erotic instincts, which can enhance sex, but they are too sexually strict to follow them. He hides his true sexual passion by using step-by-step sexual activities and a vague outer shell of spirituality.

SEXUAL MATCHING
(Do not confuse with Personality Matching)

SEXUAL TYPE MALE / FEMALE			TYPE OF MATCH				
			COMPATIBLE		COMPLIMENTARY		
Type One Warrior March 22 to May 12	Aries ♈	Taurus ♉	Type Seven Visionary January 28 to March 2	Aquarius ♒ Pisces ♓	Type Two Innovator May 13 to July 3	Gemini ♊	Cancer ♋
Type Two Innovator May 13 to July 3	Gemini ♊	Cancer ♋	Type Three Leader July 4 to August 24	Cancer ♋ Leo ♌	Type One Warrior March 22 to May 12	Aries ♈	Taurus ♉
Type Three Leader July 4 to August 24	Cancer ♋	Leo ♌	Type Two Innovator May 13 to July 3	Gemini ♊ Cancer ♋	Type Four Idealist August 25 to October 15	Virgo ♍	Libra ♎
Type Four Idealist August 25 to October 15	Virgo ♍	Libra ♎	Type Three Leader July 4 to August 24	Gemini ♊ Leo ♌	Type Five Organizer October 16 to December 6	Scorpio ♏	Sagittarius ♐
Type Five Organizer October 16 to December 6	Scorpio ♏	Sagittarius ♐	Type Six Counselor December 7 to January 27	Capricorn ♑ Aquarius ♒	Type Four Idealist August 25 to October 15	Virgo ♍	Libra ♎
Type Six Counselor December 7 to January 27	Capricorn ♑	Aquarius ♒	Type Five Organizer October 16 to December 6	Scorpio ♏ Sagittarius ♐	Type Seven Visionary January 22 to March 2	Aquarius ♒	Pisces ♓
Type Seven Visionary January 28 to March 2	Aquarius ♒	Pisces ♓	Type One Warrior March 22 to May 12	Aries ♈ Taurus ♉	Type Six Counselor December 7 to January 27	Capricorn ♑	Aquarius ♒

For enlarged Sexual Matching chart, see page 526.

Sex and Colors

Violet	Spiritual Sexual Passion
Indigo	Harmonious Sex
Blue	Peaceful Mood Sexuality
Green	Sex Inspired by Love
Yellow	Sexual Physical Stamina
Orange	Sexual Passion
Red	Physical Sex, Lust

The Deities of the Sexual Types

Below are names of characters. Each character (deity) represents a personality type and a specific type of energy, spirit, or language.

Khemitic	Yoruba	Hebrew/Canaanite
Seker	Babaluaye	Zadkiel
Maat	Aje Chagullia	Jophiel
Herukhuti	Ogun	Chamuel
Heru	Shango	Michael
Het-Heru	Oshun	Uriel
Sebek	Elegba	Raphael
Auset	Yemaya	Gabriel

WORDS

The average number of words spoken and heard each day in general (non-intimate) conversations is approximately 20,000. Of these words:

3,000 are slang (can be misinterpreted and have double meanings)
2,000 are used to hurt others
    500 are profanity, obscene, abusive and/or curse words
2,000 are mispronounced
2,000 are grammatically incorrect
2,000 are not heard
4,000 are misunderstood or misinterpreted
2,000 are unnecessary

Total 17,500 wasted words

20,000 words per day
17,500 wasted words
2,500 words actually clearly communicated

Of the 2,500 words, 80% of them are forgotten in six minutes. Therefore, the words you use need to be selected according to Maat and carefully used.

MALE/FEMALE RELATIONSHIP
CONVERSATION CONSIDERATIONS

In a conversation, you must consider…

- How does what you say benefit you?
- How does what you say benefit the other person?
- How do your words/behaviors benefit Maat?
- Did you say it to hurt your mate?
- What did you think you were saying?
- Did you say it because you wanted to argue, you were angry with yourself, your mate, your relationship, or because you do not have enough intelligence to say it another way?
- What was your attitude, facial expression, tone of voice, and body language?
- How did you feel while you were saying it?
- In an argument, do you pause between short sentences? Do you raise your voice, cry, get nervous, get tense, point your finger, constantly interrupt, feel hurt, upset, etc.?
- Do you argue as a way to punish or manipulate or to gain Maat?
- Do you argue to get attention?

TALKING GUIDELINES

- Compromise/adapt your behavior or activity. Never compromise or pervert your morals, will spirit (Maat).
- Never say that one idea/behavior is better than another.
- The idea/behavior that furthers Maat (Justice, Order, Balance, Harmony, Reciprocity, Correctness) is the best.
- Never allow a Third Party (friend, parent, couple, religion) to get between you and your mate.
- Communicate directly to each other. Don't refer to he/she said, they said, according to, etc.
- Try not to use slang words and unnecessary words in order to keep communication clear. Sentences should be short and to the point.
- Do not use your mate for entertainment.
- You should be your best entertainment.
- Do not try to convert your mate from their religion/idea/diet/behavior.
- Do not constantly rephrase/restate your position.
- State your position and your reasons/feelings for your position and how it serves Maat.
- Do not constantly put down, criticize and make unfavorable remarks about your mate's feelings/behavior. Slaves/colonized, traumatized mates have a low tolerance for frustration, failure, pain, conflict and have low self-esteem, patience and attention.

- Slavery Trauma has taught Black folks to view failures/conflict as indicating that something is spiritually, emotionally or karmic wrong with them. The failure/conflict is built into Caucasian society. It is used to manipulate and control. A Slavery Traumatized Black person tends to want to be punished or seek approval and translate everything to be emotional.
- Direct anger towards a specific negative situation or feeling, not toward your mate.
- Do not argue about how you are arguing.
- Only a behavior or idea can be wrong. Your mate is not wrong. Say you are talking/angry about the wrong behavior/idea of your mate.
- You can be mixed up or upset about your thoughts on a situation, subject or person. This does not mean that the point you are making is not valid (Maat).
- It is all right to be upset or confused as talking can help you get rid of anger and confusion and arrive at a clear point.
- You can be upset while talking about a problem, but clear about the answer to the problem.
- You give power to words and then feel powerless.
- Words take on a different meaning based upon the tone, attitude and emotions while using them. Therefore, you may need to translate an obvious "word" definition.
- If you are intelligent enough to ask a question, then you are intelligent enough to accept an answer. You may not understand or agree with the answer.
- Pause after you say something. Allow the person to answer to say "uh huh," etc.

CHANGING THOUGHTS AND FEELINGS

Step	Action
1.	Before giving your opinion, remember to…
	a. Put yourself in the other person's place
	b. Pretend how it feels hearing what you are about to say
	c. Choose one specific attitude/behavior that the person is capable of changing. Expect slow change
	d. Choose an appropriate time to give an opinion or advice; usually you cannot say it in the moment it occurs or is needed.
	e. Ask if you can discuss something that you feel will bring more togetherness (Maat).
2.	Give your opinion
3.	Make sure your opinion is understood
4.	Offer solution
5.	Commit yourself to change and participate
6.	Allow the person to offer their response and solution
7.	Use a compromised solution
8.	Give positive encouragement

Practice these steps by picking something the person is already positively doing. Ask them to do it. Show by your attitude/behavior that you feel good about the change. Give encouragement each time. Practice allows you to get used to asking and allows the others to get used to change.

FEELINGS AND THOUGHTS CYCLES

- Everything follows laws, cycles, patterns, rhythms—the planets, tides, wind, sun, moon, plants (growing fruits and flowers) and seasons, as well as feelings and thoughts.
- Feelings and thoughts belong to the Universe, feelings cycle to high points and low points and passes through males and females.
- Feelings and thoughts have a Galaxy, Solar, Lunar and Earth cycle. Cycles can be 23 to 30 days and influenced by the Planets.
- Allow the feeling or thought to pass through you. Realize you do not own a feeling or thought.
- Witness each other's cycles. Do not get angry or upset with someone's cycle any more than you would get angry with the tide, wind, moon, etc.
- You are taught to react to your feelings and thoughts by your culture, family, experiences, religion, mate, slave/colonial trauma.
- A feeling (i.e., anger) can add to or take away from your life.
- Unhappiness cycles to happiness, upset to calm, mania to depression, action to rest, positive to negative and negative to positive because they are complimentary pairs.
- A feeling is neither good or bad, it is how the feeling is used (one can love violence or love peace, love is neither good or bad; it is its usage that can present a problem).

FEMALE AND MALE EMOTIONAL CYCLES

Puberty, Testosterone Syndrome, Andropause, PMS, Menstruation and Menopause have an effect on cycles.

1. JANUARY	1	2	3	4	5	6	7	8	9	10	11	12	13	14	15	16	17	18	19	20	21	22	23	24	25	26	27	28
2. JAN/FEB	29	30	31	1	2	3	4	5	6	7	8	9	10	11	12	13	14	15	16	17	18	19	20	21	22	23	24	25
3. FEB/MAR	26	27	28	1	2	3	4	5	6	7	8	9	10	11	12	13	14	15	16	17	18	19	20	21	22	23	24	25
4. MAR/APR	26	27	28	27	30	31	1	2	3	4	5	6	7	8	9	10	11	12	13	14	15	16	17	18	19	20	21	22
5. APR/MAY	23	24	25	26	27	28	29	30	1	2	3	4	5	6	7	8	9	10	11	12	13	14	15	16	17	18	19	20
6. MAY/JUN	21	22	23	24	25	26	27	28	29	30	31	1	2	3	4	5	6	7	8	9	10	11	12	13	14	15	16	17
7. JUN/JUL	18	19	20	21	22	23	24	25	26	27	28	29	30	1	2	3	4	5	6	7	8	9	10	11	12	13	14	15
8. JUL/AUG	16	17	18	19	20	21	22	23	24	25	26	27	28	29	30	31	1	2	3	4	5	6	7	8	9	10	11	12
9. AUG/SEP	13	14	15	16	17	18	19	20	21	22	23	24	25	26	27	28	29	30	31	1	2	3	4	5	6	7	8	9
10. SEP/OCT	10	11	12	13	14	15	16	17	18	19	20	21	22	23	24	25	26	27	28	29	30	1	2	3	4	5	6	7
11. OCT/NOV	8	9	10	11	12	13	14	15	16	17	18	19	20	21	22	23	24	25	26	27	28	29	30	31	1	2	3	4
12. NOV/DEC	5	6	7	8	9	10	11	12	13	14	15	16	17	18	19	20	21	22	23	24	25	26	27	28	29	30	1	2
13. DECEMBER	3	4	5	6	7	8	9	10	11	12	13	14	15	16	17	18	19	20	21	22	23	24	25	26	27	28	29	30

For enlarged chart, see page 524.

KEY

1	Anger	18	Mistrustful	**Additional Categories**	
2	Anxiety	19	Talkative	36	_____
3	Cramps/Pain	20	Spend too much money	37	_____
4	Cheerful	21	Want to fix things for people	38	_____
5	Depressed	22	Menstruation	39	_____
6	Energetic	23	Back Pain	40	_____
7	Food or Snack craving	24	Sexually Aroused	41	_____
8	Forgetful	25	Swelling		
9	Headache	26	Tenderness		
10	Hopelessness	28	Water gain/Retention		
11	Impatient	29	Weight gain		
12	Insecure	30	Lack energy		
13	Insomnia	31	Nervous		
14	Irritable	32	Moody		
15	Lonely	33	Jealousy		
16	Worried	34	Tend to cry		
17	Want to sleep	35	Stressed		

Put the number that coincides with your emotion on the date it occurs. You may have to use a different color pen (red, green, etc.). At the end of two or three months, you will see an emotional pattern (cycle). This will be your emotional cycle (Personality Cycle).

Example of Moon Calendar

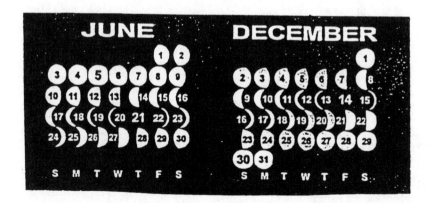

Every individual has emotional and behavioral ups and downs. This is their emotional cycle. People have rituals and ceremonies that they do before, during and after a type of emotion or behavior. Aside from this, the individual performs his family's rituals and ceremonies for emotions and behaviors. We commonly say "the whole family acts that way," which means they have the same rituals and ceremonies. Emotions spiritually, mentally, emotionally and physically pass through each person in a pattern (cycle).

Emotionally triggered behaviors do not belong to the individual, they belong to the universe.

The purpose of doing an emotional cycle chart is to give you control over your emotions. To do the chart, use the above calendar and a moon calendar or a calendar with the phases of the moon. Some people are not aware of their fluctuating emotions, so they may need someone else to identify their emotions. The moon allows you to predict your emotions and/or behaviors before they happen to you. This empowers you to have control over your emotions instead of your emotions controlling you. It also allows others to adjust and adapt to your emotions. When you become aware of your cycle, you modify your life in a positive direction. For example, on your energetic days—take Chamomile, Catnip or Kava so you won't exhaust yourself; on sleepy days, take Ginseng or Fo-Ti; on food craving days, take Chickweed, Phenylalanine or Cravex; on depression days, take St. John's Wort, etc.

CONVERSATION DO'S AND DON'TS TO SAY

Do's	Don'ts
Say "I cannot answer your question at this moment. I may need time to sort out an emotional and/or intellectual answer Tomorrow (or specified time), I will tell you how I am dealing with it."	-Say "You are stupid, stubborn, opinionated, hardheaded, crazy," etc. - You never consider my feelings - You wont' change your ways! - You don't care about our relationship.
Be quiet after you state an opinion as your mate may need silence to to sort out the issue.	- I know you only listen to what others say or what your friends say, but…I appreciate you listening to me. You don't care about anything but sports, Jesus, Muhammad, Moses, Ra, your friends, what you want to do, etc.
I feel good knowing you will listen to me and share my feeling.	- I know you won't believe me, but… - I told you so - You don't understand
I do not understand. I want to, but right now, I do not.	- You can do better - The trouble with you is
When talking a lot, pause and tell mate "I feel good knowing you listen."	- You don't forget to do things for others
Compromise/adapt and follow Maat.	- You ignore what I say
I care about your feelings.	- I don't care (say it is your choice)…
Let's discuss the negative and positive behavior and not discuss each other.	- No problem (I have no problem solving my problems)
You do not have to be perfect to get my Kupenda (Love).	- I am fine (I am dealing with my ups and downs

Do's *(Continued)*	Don'ts *(Continued)*
I am sorry to upset you.	- Stop nagging, fussing, talking, etc.
I do not know what to say or do when you say or do .... Can you help me?	- You should have known better
Share feelings without trying to fix or repair feelings.	- This relationship is a bad mistake
Let each other know when or how you did something for them.	- If you do as I say, we would be happy
Never go to bed angry or upset with your mate. Seek harmony, apologize, pray, etc.	- Everything is left up to me
In case of mutual split decision or voting tie, use Maat to break the tie.	- I don't get any help from you
I love being with you.	- How could you do that?

Relationship Considerations...

- A relationship is a process, changes, develops, makes mistakes, etc.
- Require spiritual ritual (prayer, etc.)
- Men usually *talk* to express *ideas,* then *feelings*
- Men growth sequence:
  - Childhood (sensation), Youth (thinking)
  - Manhood (Refinement of thought and feeling)
  - Adulthood (Group/cultural refinement)
- Women usually *talk* to express *feelings* then *ideas*
- Women growth sequence:
  - Childhood, Womanhood, Youth, Adulthood
- Communicate, listen, respect each other's thoughts and feelings
- Behave in public. Only criticize and/or argue privately
- Arguments or criticism is used to gain closeness and Maat
- Watch words in argument. Do not curse or interrupt.
- Your mate is your companion, not your clone
- Your mate is not perfect, has wounds, good and bad habits that may never change. If you accept the best, you have to accept the rest.
- Your mate is not psychic
- Say "Please," "Thank You," "Good Morning," etc.
- Forgive each other and compromise
- Love yourself, recognize talents, gifts, faults, etc.
- Have a hobby, life purpose
- Witness each others insolubles
- Have family meetings, activities, a budget

Do Not...

- Say "You never listen," which means "I know who you are and don't need your version."
- Combine a series of past arguments. Stay with one issue at a time.
- Assume.

- Think your mate is totally aware at all times of their own behavior or yours.
- Feel you know your mate because of intimacy
- Think love will give you everything
- Become an expert psychotherapist for your mate
- Go to bed angry. Apologize.

HUMAN ENERGY FLOW

Energy is processed in stages and/or cycles differently by the female and male. When the female is in the feeling stage, the male is in the thinking stage. Their brains are slightly different. Female language skills are in the Frontal lobe and males' are in the Parital lobe of the brain. A 2-3 month old male infant has a testosterone rise, which makes his thought/feeling pattern different from a female's. Males talking to females should say what they "feel," then what they "think." Females talking to males should say what they "think," then what they "feel." Females tend to feel then see, hear, touch and taste while males tend to think then see, hear, touch and taste.

	Female Principle			
Stage	**1st**	**2nd**	**3rd**	**4th**
Sends and Receives Information	Senses it	Feels it	Thinks it	Maats (Balance, Adapt) it
Element	Earth	Water	Air	Fire
	Male Principle			
Sends and Receives Information	Senses it	Thinks it	Feels it	Maats it
Element	Earth	Air	Water	Fire

FEMALE PERSPECTIVES

- Practice Maat and Kupenda (Love).
- Listens with the Third Ear. Sees with the Third Eye. Feel with the Third Emotion.
- Be a companion and witness/acknowledge problems with no right solutions or wrong solutions.
- Tends to believe that if something works, it can work better.
- If she feels bad about herself, may feel bad about relationship and achievements.
- Usually cannot overlook their mate bonding spiritually, intellectually with another female. But, with much difficulty, can overlook sexual adultery (physical attachments).
- More committed; the more sensitive you are and the easier you are to be hurt.

- Most committed. Usually compromises (gives in) to their mate.
- Change behavior by complimenting positive behaviors. Not by criticizing negative.
- Judges attitudes and emotions of the word spoken, then words.
- When talking to friends or family, is emotionally processing information.
- Prefers to socialize and talks in order to solve problems with mate.
- Talks for closeness and to bring more Maat into relationship.
- Talks in intellectual and emotional details.
- If upset, will socialize.
- Must feel good in order to be positive about giving and receiving in relationship.
- If a female has problems receiving positiveness and feels unable to have positive relationship, she may develop uterine fibroids or an attitude of negativeness.
- Her feelings cause the behavior of love.
- If a female is made to feel special, she feels Kupenda (Love).
- Rewards and/or punishment are similar to taking in or letting out a dress. She may do many good things and still get no benefit from actions. If you take in or let out a size 6 dress in her mind, it is still a size 6 while to men, it is made into a size 5 or size 7.
- Gives until empty.
- Bad feelings are like a cold. Treat it until it gets better.
- Trust your mate to change.
- Your mate has the right to experience their good and bad emotions.
- Do not punish your mate with many questions during a cycle of silence.
- Has to have a feeling to talk.

MALE PERSPECTIVES

- Practice Maat and Kupenda (Love).
- Listen with the Third Ear. See with the Third Eye. Feel with the Third Emotion.
- Do not argue with females about their feelings.
- Do not give intellectual advice or solutions for females' feelings. They have the right to feel good or bad.
- Be a witness to emotions.
- Be a companion and a witness and acknowledge feelings and problems that do not have a solution.
- He believes that if something is working badly or poorly, it is working. So don't fix it.
- If achievements or accomplishments that day are inadequate, then he may feel inadequate about himself and the relationship.
- He usually overlooks his female bonding with male friends on a spiritual or intellectual level. But, he cannot overlook sexual adultery.

- The person committed the most to the relationship is more sensitive and more easily hurt.
- Has to have a reason to talk.
- His feelings can be changed by complimenting the positive, not by criticizing the negative.
- He usually judges the words, then the attitude of female.
- When he is mumbling or grumpy, he is processing information.
- He prefers to be by himself, other male friends, engrossed in an activity to solve problems (does not require mate's help to solve problems).
- Talks for answers.
- Solves details or parts of problems before the whole problem.
- If upset, will be alone.
- Must be aware of the positive giving and receiving in relationship to feel good about his mate.
- If he has a problem talking about his true feelings and does not feel valued in relationship, he can develop prostate disease.

AFRICAN-CENTERED FAST
Fasting (A Guide for Beginners and/or the Advanced)

A fast is a diet consisting of water. Fasting causes the spirit, mind and body to regenerate and restore its purest state. Fasting has been used and abused by religious groups, medical practitioners and mind expansion (psyche) groups. A fast follows the laws of nature. It is a give and take reciprocity diet. Consequently, an African traditional fast was and is used to create balance. In other words, a person gives wholistic energies to the fast and the fast gives wholistic energy to the person. The purpose of a typical fast would be to create balance, not to become more positive in thinking or spirit, but to become balanced (Maat).

Part 1
Water consumption is important for the balance of the body. The first meal of the day should be at least one quart of water. The average person requires one ounce of water for every two pounds of body weight. For example, a person weighing 100 pounds should drink 50 fluid ounces of water. In other words, divide the weight in half and that will be the minimum amount needed to prevent dehydration. It is advised to drink as much water as possible—one to three gallons daily.

Part 2
The wholistic person should gradually prepare for a fast by using a liquid diet before fasting. For example, each day of a fast requires two days of liquid diet in the orthodox African system. A liquid diet is highly cleansing and could be used singularly as a health treatment.

BREAKFAST	LUNCH	DINNER
	1ˢᵗ Day	
1 quart of water	Vegetable	Fruit Juices. Add sesame butter
A variety of fruit juices		almond and/or soy protein isolate
		to juices for protein
	2ⁿᵈ Day	
Repeat 1ˢᵗ day* (add ¼ part water to ¾ part juice)		
	3ʳᵈ Day	*Dilute all juices
Repeat 1ˢᵗ day* (add ¼ part water to ¾ part juice)		
	4ᵗʰ Day	
Repeat 1ˢᵗ day* (add ¼ part water to ¾ part juice)		
	5ᵗʰ Day	
1 quart of water	Restricted to 3 types	Restricted to 3 types
Add 3 part water to juices	of fruit only	of fruits only
	6ᵗʰ Day	
1 quart of water	Restricted to 2 types	Restricted to 2 types
Add 2 part water to juices	of fruit	of fruit
	7ᵗʰ Day	
Quart of water add 3 parts	Restricted to 1 type of	Restricted to 1 type of
water to 3 parts juice	fruit only	fruit only

Part 3

A fast was used to give balance to nature and receive balance from nature. The system of likes treating likes caused the usage of drinking the body's naturally distilled water (urine). Baby's urine was used to wash babies because of the urine's homeopathic qualities. Consequently, ancient African fasters would drink their own urine. They would add a small amount to a glass of water.

The water fast system is based on nature. In nature, the humans live in an atmosphere, which contains distilled water vapors. In fact, we walk and breathe in a cloud of distilled water vapor, which we call atmosphere. The body absorbs distilled water. The water in the vegetables and fruits that we eat is distilled. If you drink spring water, the body will distill it before it uses it. Spring water is alive and has to have microbes, very small plants, particles of rocks and soil, small insects, soluble and insoluble matter in it to qualify as spring water. The dead spring water, sold in stores was obtained from a spring, and then filtered to remove soluble and insoluble matter and the life in it. It is not technically spring water, just processed water from a spring. If you truly wanted spring water, you would have to go to a spring and drink from it. Aside from this, the body cannot metabolize the minerals in mineral water. The body can only use minerals when they are in a plant. In other words, you cannot eat dirt (minerals) and only minerals in plants can keep you alive.

Your kidneys are stressed by the inorganic minerals added to water and this water makes you acidic.

The salt in the water in your body is in it to help you to keep the water longer. It is not seawater. It is distilled water with electrolytes in it. There is a similarity between the mineral salt water in your body and sea salt water, but they are not the same.

Ideally, you could live without drinking water. However, you would need to be able to get plenty watery-type organic plants (i.e. melons, coconut water, fruits, etc.). The current Caucasian politics of food vegetables has had a negative effect upon our diets. Caucasians dictate what and when large food supplies are available based on business reasons. Therefore, various types of fasts are presented to reflect the reality of our dietary oppression. Most (99%) of us cannot afford distilled water or organic foods for our fasts. Boiled water is only water available for most folks. That is why taking cleansing herbs daily is a must on a fast or for those who live in or near ecologically polluted cities.

The first water introduced in the fast is distilled water. Distilled water cleanses the body of waste. The body distills the water you drink before it uses it. Atmospheric distilled water is rain and snow and creates freshwater streams and rivers. This is the distilled water we drink. Once the water enters the body, mineral salts are added. Therefore, this water diet (fast) begins with distilled water, then spring water and finally mineral salts in seawater. However, in this fast the seawater will be made by using sea plants (spirulina or blue-green algae and chlorophyll). In drinking water in this sequence, the natural water rhythm of the body is conformed to.

WATER FAST

First to seventh day:	Distilled water
	Water and Raw fruit and vegetable juices
	For one week distilled water plus juices
	Distilled water and pasteurized juices for one week.

It is optional the length of time you can fast. Those who work may want to fast on the weekends. Some find it best to fast one day out of each week. If you live in a city with air, water, soil, noise and radiation pollution, I strongly recommend that you take a cleansing herb each day, regardless to the type of fast you choose. Cleanser herbs can be taken individually or in combination. Some cleansing herbs are Red Clover, Echinacea, Goldenseal, Chaparral, Pau D'Arco, Burdock Root, Dandelion Root, etc.

You can add a few drops of concentrated oxygen and/or chlorophyll to your distilled water.

Some need to curb their hunger craving while on a fast. Chickweed is recommended for this. Others need to take a calmative herb to help them relax (i.e., Catnip, Kava, Chamomile, Valerian, Passion Flower, etc.) or White Willow, Feverfew or Scullcap for headaches.

WATER SCHEDULE OF FAST

1st Day
Distilled water all day

2nd Day
Combine equally distilled and spring water

3rd Day
Spring water

4th Day
Spring water. Add 1 to 2 eye drops of liquid kelp or trace mineral liquid concentrate or blue-green algae. **Note:** adding the below ingredients is optional; distilled water can be used. Add 1 to 2 drops of liquid chlorophyll to each gallon of water.

5th Day
Repeat 4th Day

6th Day
Repeat 4th Day
Discontinue adding spirulina or blue-green algae coupled with chlorophyll. Add teaspoon of seawater to each gallon of water.

7th Day
Repeat 6th Day

The transition from a fast to solid foods should be made with a liquid diet.

1st Day
Repeat 7th day of liquid diet

2nd Day
Repeat 6th day of liquid diet

3rd Day
Repeat 5th day of liquid diet.
Follow the diet in the reverse order. The transition from a liquid diet to a solid diet should be gradual.

SOLID FOOD SCHEDULE

1st Day
Eat one type of solid fruit

2nd Day
Eat 2 types of solid fruit

3rd Day
Eat 3 types of solid fruit

4th Day
Drink 1 quart of water

5th Day
Breakfast: Fruits
Lunch: Vegetables
Dinner: Fruits

You should begin to eat foods according to hunger and use simple food combinations.

Exercise
Light exercise during the fast is essential. For example, deep knee bends, walking while swinging arms briskly, crawling, massaging abdomen daily, deep breathing exercises, leg stretches, etc. Additionally, chew a string of saffron, as this will remove lactic acid waste from the muscles and increase energy endurance.

Herbs
Herbal medicine before air, water, radiation and food pollution was taken for not more than six consecutive days and none on the 7th day. Then, resume herbals for six consecutive days with one day of abstinence. Further, specific herbs' therapeutic effectiveness diminishes in strength after one to two months of prolonged usage. Subsequently, another herb with the same therapeutic value can be substituted.

1st Day
Appetite Suppressants: Chickweed, Bilberry, Bitter Melon, Gymnema Sylvestre, Guggilipid

2nd Day
Repeat 1st Day
May need Calmative: Catnip, Kava, Chamomile, Passion Flower, Valerian (Strongest)
May need Energizers: Ginseng, Fo-Ti, Kola Nuts, Damiana, Yohimbe. Do not use Ephedra or Guarana, they drain the body of energy.

3rd Day
Liver and Blood Cleansers: Oregon Grape, Yellow Dock, Prickly Ash, Red Beet Root, Chaparral, Mullein

4th Day
Kidney Cleanser: Juniper Berry, Uva Ursi, Buchu, Orris, Gravel Root

5th Day
Brain and Gland Herbs: Gota Kola, Red Raspberry Leaves Fo-ti

6th Day
Nerves, Cartilage: Skullcap, Catnip, Comfrey, Bayberry Bark

7th Day
Blood Sugar Levels: Cedar Berries, Primrose, Gentian

Part 4: Enema

Enemas are used to cleanse the body of the large amounts of toxins that accumulate during a liquid diet and/or a fast. The enemas cleanse the inner skin of the colon and feed the colon vital nutrients.

No more than three enemas should be taken a day and at least one a day. Use two quarts of water. The standard measurement is usually fi ounce of herb to 10 ounces of water or 1 ounce of herb to 20 ounces water. Enemas can also be taken every other day (three a week or two a week).

1st Day
Cape Aloe, Cascara Sagrada

2nd Day
Comfrey (1 cup), Molasses (1 cup)

3rd Day
Cramp Bark, Indian Hemp

4th Day
Valerian, Catnip

5th Day
Repeat 1st day

6th Day
Repeat 1st day

7th Day
Repeat 2nd day

Part 5: Baths

Cleansing Bath

Epsom salt should be used in the bath water—3 cups to 3 pounds. Add fi cup of baking soda. Apple cider vinegar or raw lemon juice could be used to help cleanse the pores (Use one to three cups in the tub of water). Additionally, herbal baths of lavender, burdock, elecampane can be used (½ cup of each, prepared in 1 gallon water).

A sponge bath of aloe Vera juice can be used daily. Those who desire a highly escalated cleansing herb bath can make a tea of the below herbs and add to bath water

Mustard Powder:	3 tablespoons
Horseradish Powder:	3 tablespoons
Ginger Powder:	3 tablespoons
Clove Powder:	3 tablespoons
Hyssop:	1 cup

Eye Drops

You can purchase homeopathic and/or Herbal Eye Drops from a health food store or you can make them.

    For example: ½ tsp Eyebright
                    ½ tsp Goldenseal Root

Let Golden Seal Root simmer one hour in 2 cups of distilled water, then turn off heat and add Eyebright. Let mixture steep for an hour or more. Then strain. Pour into a glass container and put in refrigerator. Let sit overnight then strain mixture again through cotton gauze or cheesecloth. Pour into a brown (amber) eyedropper bottle. This you can purchase from a commercial drug store or health food store. Use herbal eye drops as often as desired to give your eyes a cleansing bath.

Ear Drops

You can purchase from a health food store or buy garlic capsules. Punch a hole in the capsule with a needle; squeeze the oil in the ears. You may need to put cotton in the ears to stop the oil from leaking out. Use the drops as often as desired as an ear bath.

Underarms and Teeth

Deodorant and toothpaste should be natural. Clay can be eaten daily while on the fast (up to 3 teaspoons a day).

First Day

Few drops of Chlorophyll to two glasses of Pau D'Arco. Take 3 times daily. An energy herb such as Gentian, Fo-Ti, Astralagus, Ginseng or Yohimbe can be taken as needed.

Technically, the fast does not begin until the body has completely rid itself of food in the digestive tract. This complete evacuation of food takes approximately three days of food abstinence. Usually, on the third day the food craving disappears because the food has left the body. The fast begins when the colon and rectum have no manure in them.

There is an abundance of information on fasting in books such as *Save Your Life* by *Fasting* by H. Carrington, *Fasting Can Save Your Life* by H. Shelton, *How to Keep Slim, Healthy and Young with Juice Fasting* by P. Airola, *Fasting for Renewal of Life* by H. Shelton, *How to Fast* by K. Jaffrey and F*asting: The Ultimate Diet* by A. Cott.

HERPES, WHOLISTIC TREATMENT

Herpes is a name given to skin eruptions. Skin eruptions (bumps, acne, chicken pox, measles, blackheads, etc.) are a part of a cleansing process in which impurities, toxins and contaminants are ejected through the skin. The skin eruptions are not the disease but a reaction to a disease. Herpes, like all other skin eruptions, is caused by impurities within the body. Herpes is a symptom of a dis-ease, not a dis-ease in itself.

Herpes has been known for well over 2,000 years. The Romans recorded it. Herpes literally means creep. It was believed to creep into the body. There is no cure for the body curing itself. Herpes are bumps that appear because the body is cleansing and using the skin for a bowel movement.

Herpes is not caught primarily from other people or a dead cell particle (virus). In an unhealthy state or disease state, the immunity is too weak to protect the body from herpes' contamination. The body can create herpes as a way of cleansing.

The key to understanding dis-eases and symptoms such as herpes lies in answering a question. How did the first person on the earth contact (catch) herpes? There must have been a first person to have herpes in order to transmit it to another person. The first person to have herpes created this dis-ease symptom in the body. The body will always produce herpes or rashes or bumps to get rid of waste or biochemical imbalances. Poor health that causes herpes is created by eating synthetic foods, cooked foods, eating late at night, improper food combining, vaccinations, drugs, radiation, junk foods, sexual intercourse during menstruation, pregnancy and breastfeeding and non-natural human mating. Additionally, faulty exercising, excessive estrogen, using chemically treated tampons and non-cotton underwear and taking antibiotics that alter vaginal flora (fungus, yeast, bacteria), all cause dis-eases.

Symptoms and Definition
Herpes has been associated with an abnormal dead cell particle (virus). The onset of the dis-ease is usually swelling of the lymph glands in the genital groin area. This swelling is often associated with pain, itching and/or burning. The swelling and pain may be accompanied by fever, headache, increased discharge in female and urethral discharge in males.

Herpes usually appears in moist areas above the waist (Simplex I) and below the waist (Simplex II). Herpes Simplex II can be transmitted from below the waist to above the waist. A scratch, cut, abrasion, open area on the skin or sore on the eye or lips (mouth area) can absorb the herpes bump fluid and transmit the disease. Herpes can be transmitted via kissing, oral sex, having an open area on your hand while touching a herpes dis-eased person's open bump as well as your open skin contact on an open Herpes bump during sexual intercourse.

The first attack of herpes is usually between one to two days after a person makes contact with the disease. After the initial contact, there may be approximately three weeks of cold-like or flu-like (mucous congestion) symptoms. The subsequent herpes attacks are usually triggered by stress, cooked food, allergies, drugs, junk foods, disease or hormonal, spiritual, emotional and physical imbalances. Herpes has a 10 to 14 day cycle. The skin eruptions (bumps) take three days to fill with fluid. The impurities in the bump are ejected when the bumps burst. Once the bumps burst, a scab grows and heals the skin. This takes seven to ten days. If the health status is not holistically improved, the dis-ease can be triggered again and again. There are some physical remedies for this wholistic (spirit, mind, body) dis-ease.

Apply to Skin
- Aloe Vera Gel or oil, Camphor oil
- Gentian Violet — anti-fungus (color from flower can stain). Make a strong tea, 2 tbsp. to a cup and apply with cotton balls.
- Ice bag can be applied to relieve itching.
- Clove oil, Aloe Oil, Witch Hazel Oil (or 2 tbsp. to a cup, apply with cotton balls).
- Apply Wheat Germ Oil, Vitamin E, Peppermint Oil, Calendula Oil or Eucalyptus Oil.
- Tormentil tea or commercial tea — apply to area (2 tbsp. to a cup).
- Clay toothpaste — apply to area.
- Ointment — 3 tbsp. of Marigold, Aloe, Gentian Flower — add to 2 pints of spring water. Let stand 14 days (shake everyday). Add 8 Calendula. Apply to skin.
- Bee Propolis (Fights bacteria)— apply to area.
- Lysine crème (Skin infection) — apply to area.
- MSM lotion (Skin inflammation and infection — apply to area.

No remedy is perfect for all individuals, in that dis-ease attains to the biochemical personality of the individual. The dis-ease has a personality, which is directly related to the nutritional debt of the individual. Further, one herb, vitamin or douche is effective for one biochemical personality, while other herbs, vitamins may be effective for another. By trying various combinations, you may find the effective holistic remedy for you.

Baths: hot or cold (See herbs)

Douche: Acidophilus capsules — open 3 to 4 capsules and dissolve in 6 ounces of water. (Two small containers of yogurt can be substituted).

Douche Solution
Tbsp. Vitamin C (strengthens tissue) — ascorbic acid powder
Tbsp. Garlic powder (antibiotic)
Tbsp. Hops (helps release impurities)
Tbsp. Clay (helps stabilize skin and purify)
Tbsp. Sea Salt (aids absorption of nutrients)

Combine, use 1 quart of water, prepare herbs separately in 3 cups of water.

Juices: Cranberry

Open Lesions (Sores)

Sprinkle or apply directly to the sores: Zinc powder, Dolomite powder, lysine powder (or cream) mixed with aloe gel.

Supplements	Suggested Dosage	Remarks
Vitamin A	10,000 I.U.	Anti-viral properties. Large quantities of "A" are found in apples, apricots, carrots, avocados, spinach, pumpkin, prunes, papaya.
Lecithin	1,000-3,000 mg.	Helps maintain healthy skin.
B Complex	50-100 mg.	Maintains healthy skin.
Potassium	50 mg.	Enhances skin nourishment.
Magnesium	500 mg.	Prevents skin weakness.
Pantothenic Acid	1,000 mg.	Helps heal and relieves stress.
Zinc	50-60 mg.	Heals and stabilizes skin.
Calcium	80-100 mg.	Maintains skin health.
BHT	1,000 mg.	Inhibits the growth of bumps.
Selenium	1,000 mg.	Cleanses and improves skin.
Caprylic Acid	1,000 mg. (Bump eruption — 2,000- 4,000 mg.)	
Lipoic Acid	100-200 mg.	Helps nourish the skin.
Plant Sterolins	As directed.	Enhances the growth of healthy skin.
DHEA	As directed.	Helps prevent skin problems.

AMINO ACIDS

Lysine	1,000 mg., three times daily.	Prevents skin disease and eruptions.
Glucosamine and	2,000 mg.	Repairs skin and provides nourishment.
Chondroitins	2,000 mg.	Maintains healthy skin and increases skin circulation.

HERBS

Black Willow, Burdock, Chaparral, Elder Flower, Goldenseal, Myrrh, Pau D'Arco, Red Clover, Sanicle, Thuja, Witch Hazel.

HOMEOPATHIC

Nat. Mur.	As directed.	Maintains healthy skin.
Kali. Phos.	As directed.	Cleanses skin.

GLANDULARS

Adrenals	As directed.	Aids healthy skin.

FOODS

Almonds, Avocado, Bananas, Brown Rice, Brussels Sprouts, Carrots, Celery, Green Vegetables, Lemons, Mushrooms, Oranges, Papaya, Pecans, Pineapple, Sesame Seeds, Strawberries, Tomatoes, Raw Nuts

Diagnosis

Herpes fluid can be visually diagnosed by the naked eye. The fluid contained in vesicular (thin-walled bump) has many characteristics.

Prevention

A natural whole food diet and healthy mind and spirit is optimum for the prevention of herpes. Wear cotton underwear (boxer trunks for males). Do not wear while sleeping in bed. Do not have anal and oral masturbation or masturbate. Do not use birth control pills. The birth control pills contain chemicals that may cause another attack and they do not stop conception. They actually cause embryo abortion and are fetus killer pills—death pills.

Herpes dis-eased individuals should warn all potential sex partners and abstain from sexual contacts during attacks and while herpes sores are open.

> **WARNING:** An open herpes sore can transmit the dis-ease from a pregnant woman to a child during delivery—the child may die, as the dis-ease attacks the baby's entire body. A child or teenager with an open sore can receive herpes from an adult herpes carrier without having sex with that adult.

CULTURAL CLOWNS:
BLACK FOLKS AND SEX

In nature, there are specific laws for mating (sexual intercourse) and a mating season for all animals, insects and plants. All animals, insects and plants follow mating laws except the Caucasian race and those races that follow Caucasian cultural sex behaviors. Following Caucasian non-cyclic sexual rituals and ceremonies is the primary reason why humans have the highest reproductive failure rate of all animals. All animals that hunt and eat during the daylight hours have sex during the daylight hours except Caucasians and Africans that follow Caucasian sex rituals and ceremonies. Caucasians and those Black folks who follow Caucasian sexuality are the only animals that have venereal dis-eases. Sex is the political and social language of a culture. Mating, petting, intercourse position and erotic areas of the body are culturally specific. Sex should reinforce the culture and spiritually elevate the individuals. Sex should be based upon Maat principles of rewards and punishment. There are many ways that Black folks violate their African culture's sex laws and mating rituals and ceremonies. An understanding of the culturally defined sex laws are needed in order to avoid sexual violations.

The natural rhythm of the body indicates that between the hours of 10:00 a.m. and 2:00 p.m., there are increases in the body temperature, depth of respiration, taste bud sensitivity, hearing and seeing activity, responses, respiration, eye blinking, pulse, etc. The peak physical performance time for the human body is reached during the day hours, not the night hours. The influence of the moon on sex and menstruation is often used to justify mating at night. Lunar periodicity does not affect sexual mating of other mammalians. The influence of the moon upon rituals, ceremonies, customs, physical activity, habits and emotions is a culturally learned response. The cosmic force acts upon the moon. The moon is react-ing to a force and is not the originator of force (energy). The moon is not proactive but reactive and it reacts to this force cyclically. Africans can absorb and radiate the earth, lunar (moon), solar (sun), and galaxy cycles that are harmonized by their high melanin bodily content. Caucasians' melanin albinism allows them to only feel the earth and moon (lunar) cycles. They believe that a ball of dirt called the moon is more powerful than the holistic forces that the move the moon and created the moon. The dirt worshippers think that the moon is the originator of force (energy). This is similar to believing that the hands of a clock cause the mechanism inside the clock to work. The reacting moon is an indicator that the nerv-ous system and emotions are being cyclically aroused and this stimulation is translated to mean sex. The diet and not the moon can influence the lunar periodicity of women and men as indicated by Professor Ehert's works (i.e., *Mucousless Diet*). This lunar (moon) mating corresponds to the sexual erotic behavior of cultures, which had festivals, religious rites, and sex orgies during full moons. Female and male animals in the wild (natu-ral state) do not become sexually excited or controlled by the full moon.

In a natural holistic state, the periodic mating season occurred accord-ing to a solar (sun reacting to force) rather than lunar periodicity. The sun cycle influenced people to have sexual intercourse once a year during springtime in monogamous and polygamous cultures. Among the polyga-mous (one wife, several husbands) Eskimos, the solar (sun) cycle of repro-duction was quite evident until 1940. Eskimo sexual breeding conformed to the normal estrum (sexual arousal) of animals and the human accultur-ated sex cycle. Humans have a reproductive (procreation) drive, not a sex drive. The "sex drive" is a culturally taught physical behavior. There are only reproductive drives in animals, plants and insects. The African culture defines the sex organs as having two functions, reproduction (sperm ejac-ulation) and regeneration (injaculation—no sperm release). Regeneration was/is used to stimulate energy centers (chakras) and the pineal gland.

The higher birth rate still occurs at a regular cycle. Statistics collected from France, Germany, Russia, Scotland and England, indicate that the largest number of births occurs in the month of February. This would indi-cate that human breeding occurred in May or June. The largest number of conceptions in Holland and France correspond to May-June; in Sweden to June; Greece to April, and in Spain, Italy and Austria to May. The further south in the hemisphere, births occur earlier in the spring and reproductive sex occurs earlier for conceptions. These births indicate that sexual arousal for reproduction (estrum) occurs at the end of spring or beginning of sum-mer.

Fragments of the reproduction and natural sex cycle still remains to a lesser extent within various human races. This natural sex cycle indicates that in so-called primitive times races had only two mating seasons, one in spring and one during food harvest time. The procreation impulse was aroused at these times and had cultural symbolic meanings with arousal zones, rituals, ceremonies, petting and sex positions. When sexual intercourse became less spiritual and more sensual and acrobatic and the diets denatured, the birthed children became denatured, less spiritual, morally weak, emotionally motived and physically weak.

In some so-called primitive peoples, the remnants of a human mating cycle are still evident. Children of the Semang, or Aboriginal tribes of the Siamese State of Jalor, are usually born in March or immediately after the wet season. This indicates conception in June. Among the Native Americans, certain tribes in Hindustan, among the Esquimas, and the native Australians, the breeding occurs in the spring. In the book titled *History of Human Marriage b*y Westermack, the human mating season reveals evidence of occurrence in spring or early summer.

Mating occurred in tropical countries at the beginning of the rainy seasons. The sexual mating cycle has been altered by the domestication of people by Caucasian kings and governments, by hyper sex stimulation, in music videos, movies, dances, language, clothes, songs, television, books, commercials and religions, excess hormones in junk foods, high protein diets, by forced breeding people to believe there is no sex cycle and by the artificial separation of the body, mind and spirit.

The human mating cycle is instinctively high in February, March and April. This is the beginning of the season when fresh vegetables and fruits are abundant. An abundance of fresh fruits and vegetables assures the child and mother that there is enough food for their survival.

Children born out of the natural breeding cycle are less intelligent and have a deteriorated health status. A study in the 1950's at Teachers College in New York City by Professor Feriano and K. Pinter, which used 17,500 children, indicated that children born in the winter months in that latitude had a lower I.Q. than children born in the summer months. Children and animals have poor health and the a shorter lifespan when born outside of the natural mating cycle. Children's poor health is caused by many factors. Caucasian predatory military governments, capitalist multinations' corporations, the power elite and disease industry constantly need laborers. They emotionally, socially and psychologically train their citizen population to constantly breed children, so they can constantly have laborers for the factories, armies and secondary support industries. This elite class creates a breeding labor peasant class. They are socially engineered to stop breastfeeding the children. The stopping of breastfeeding, causing bonding disease and makes the mother and child available for work. The elite need consumers to exploit economically. Women and child labor is needed for factories.

Cattle milk decreases and/or stops the nursing period and the child's dependency on its mother. The use of processed or raw cattle milk has not reduced the physiological nursing period of children. Nursing periods lasts from two to five years. Pasteurized cow's milk is a cooked slimy white pus. It is denatured because it is exposed to air, light and temperatures above the temperature of a cow's body. Cow's milk, sucked from the teats, is not homogenized, pasteurized, saturated with harmful antibiotics, chemicals and estrogen or exposed to light and air and it is drunk at the cow's body temperature. Breastfeeding averages three years in all colored cultures. Vegetable milk substitutes and cow's milk makes the mother available time for work. Working stops the baby's bonding, emotional learning and cultural learning. In nature, a baby attaches to the mother and the mother attaches the child to the culture. The introduction of vegetable and cow's milk (goat's milk in Africa) destroys the cultural influence of the mother upon the child and allows the child to attach to Caucasian culture. No woman would think of breastfeeding a cow. A woman frowns upon the thought. An infant gets subtle acculturation with the rituals and ceremonies of breastfeeding and being with the mother. The mother's skin texture, conversations, emotions, behaviors and movements are ways in which culture is transmitted. Cultural transmission stops when vegetable and cow's milk are given. The baby loses a vital means of being physical and spiritually taught language and thought by the emotional language that contact that breastfeeding provides.

The time of day that sexual intercourse occurs is another holistic factor in mating. After 2:00 p.m. the bodily functions begin to decrease, so nighttime is the worse time to have sex or do physical exercise. During slavery, this acculturated daytime sex activity was broken because labor was needed during the day. The breeding (sex) activities were done at night for the slave masters' convenience.

The circular cycle of the organs reveals which organs are producing energy and which are receiving energy. Organs' circadian rhythm (cycle) is built into the body and it dictated daytime sex. Violation of the cycle causes weakness. All plants, insects, planets, oceans (tides) follow their cycles. Procreation or sex at night can weaken the reproductive organs and causes the glands and organs that help reproduction to deteriorate (kidneys, prostrate, pineal gland, pituitary gland, etc.) These weaken and/or deteriorated glands and/or organs lose full function and immunity defense ability, resulting in diseases. The Mammalian cyclic laws are non-compromising and cannot be changed

The Mammalian breeding cycle was explored in the book titled *The Sexual Season of Mammal* by Heape. Heape's research revealed that the estrous (sex excitation) cycle has stages: The coming of sex desire (heat) pro-estrum; sexual, mating-estrus; conception metestrum; and anestrum, the period between mating. The spiritual and cultural functions of sex are not mentioned. Sex is the language of a culture. Sex transmits and translates culture through its rituals and ceremonies (sex positions, petting, dating, touching, talking before, during and after sex).

The body chemistry changes, hormone smells are given off, sensitivity of senses increases and blood increases to sex organs during the mating (breeding) phase called estrum. Wild animals, such as tigers, lions, etc. have one estrum a year. However, when the wild cat is enslaved by a circus or zoo, it has three or four estrums. This abnormal sexual mating practice irritates the sex organs and causes them to be overused and weakened. The nature of the human body causes a weakness in one organ or organ system to affect other organs. In humans, the kidneys work under pressure and the kidneys help regulate hormones and excrete waste created by the overexcited sex glands. The prostrate gland gets overused and abused by excessive sexual intercourse. In nature, once an organ or muscle tissue becomes weak, it also becomes stiff. This stiffness (not to be confused with the penis sponge tissue being filled with blood resulting in erection) is called "nature's cast." For example, if you sprain your ankle, the ankle becomes stiff ("nature's cast") and this stiffness immobilizes the ankle while it is under repair. The same reaction occurs in the uterus and prostate. The prostrate becomes weak which results in "nature's cast." This "nature's cast" is a defense reaction of the body and is used to immobilize the prostrate gland so it can be repaired. In females, the menstruation cramps are another example of "nature's cast." The weakened uterus, which was caused to be weakened by excessive sex or menstruation is stiffened while the body tries to repair the damages. However, breathing, walking, stress, fibroids and sex stimulation exerts pressure on the uterus and causes pain (cramps). Sitting, breathing, bladder pressure and other bodily activities cause the stiffened uterus to move and this movement is called cramps. A stiff muscle and/or organ collects more waste, has decreased oxygen and decreased nutrients and looses its flexibility and this loss causes stiffness. The movement of a stiff uterus is painful and called cramps. The kidneys try to eliminate the cellular waste created by worn out tissues and dead cells. Consequently, the kidneys become overtaxed and weaken. The kidneys' hormone function, cleansing action and ability to help recycle minerals (iron) cause it to be related to the two ovaries and testicles. Weak sex organs can weaken the kidneys and pituitary gland.

The ancient African and Pacific basin cultures were aware that organs that function in pairs are interrelated and share activities. Chinese medicine such as that in the ancient medical text *The Yellow Emperors Classic* used the dual function of organ principle. The oldest medical book in the world, written by an African named Imhotep (See Cover), is called the Ebers Papyrus. Organs such as the liver and gall bladder function together; the large intestines and lungs function together (complimentary); and the uterus (male uterus-prostrate), ovaries and testicles function with the kidneys, pituitary, and pineal. The kidney and sex organs go into the descend stage (non-energy generating state between 3:00 and 5:00 p.m.). Nighttime sex stresses and weakens the sex organs and kidneys. It is advised that additional supplements (male and/or female formulas) be taken as each sex act is equal to the energy needed to run twenty miles. Without supplementation, the sex organs get weak and deteriorate. Weakened and/or deteriorated sex organs result in mucous discharge known as venereal dis-ease, prostrate problems, menstruation, tumors, warts, unbalanced hormone (i.e., progesterone), mood swings, bone loss, loss of hair (baldness), etc. Ironically, excess estrogen can cause sex addiction and reproductive diseases. Hypersex or having sex in order to feel normal is a sign of sex addiction. In other words, having too much sex is a sign of sex addiction disease.

The laws of the human body are fixed rigid laws. Similar other laws, such as you are either dead or alive, pregnant or not pregnant, healthy or diseased, having healthy holistic African cultural sex or Caucasian dis-eased sex and you are either sleep or awake. These laws, the cyclic (circadian) laws, and the sperm maturity cycle can be found in books such as Stedman's *Medical Dictionary*. The body and its laws are ancient and have not changed. Historically, selfish Kings demanded that people in their kingdoms violate bodily laws. Kings (African and European) demanded that the only daytime activity would be manual labor because labor produced monies for their empires. Kings made people breed more children in order to increase the labor force and thus increase their monies and armies. Today, the Caucasian predatory military multi-national governments and corporations continue this socializing process. Historically, Black folks subjected to slavery and/or colonialism were made to breed (mate) out of cycle and have sex at night because it meant monies to the White slave master. Ironically, Black folks are still having sex and indulging in sexual lust because they were mentally (not physically) owned by the White slave masters (Caucasian government and/or multinationals). They are having too much sex. Excessive sex and sex addiction weakens the physical body as well as the mind and spirit. Birth control pills and devices and prophylactics contribute to hypersex and massive reproductive failures, impotency, venereal diseases, weak and poor quality sperm and eggs, all of which result in poor quality children with short lifespans. Black folks are masturbating and homosexually and heterosexually intercoursing the race to death (extinction).

There is much evidence to support African mating cycles. Europeans such as Hippocrates (European Father of Medicine) upon visiting Africa stated that Africans had very rigid sex laws.

In the *Boulek Papyrus* (1500 B.C.), an Egyptian sage, Kneusu-Hetep, states that his son was breastfed for three years. Additionally, in the "Moral Precepts of Ancient Egypt" as recorded by Ptahotep, a government official in the reign of Assa, a king of the Fourth Dynasty (3360 B.C.), stated children were breastfed for three years. In traditional cultures (non-Caucasian), during the breastfeeding period of time sex was not allowed. In fact, no animals (i.e., rats, dogs, elephants, pigs, etc.) have sex while pregnant except traditional Caucasian culture. Sex while the female is pregnant changes the hormone and nutrient of the fetus, alters the biochemistry of the female and causes sympathetic stress. This rule of sexual abstinence protects the species and creates a sexual system that sustains a culture. Incidentally, wild vegetarian gorillas when in captivity (zoos, circuses, laboratories) and fed junk/synthetic foods and meat become violent. Animals put into captivity (i.e., oppression) by Caucasians indulged in excessive sex, practiced homosexual activities, violently beat their young children, masturbate and the females begin to menstruate. Animals or a race (Africans) in Caucasian captivity develop dysfunctional behaviors. Dysfunctional behaviors are a symptom of oppression (captivity).

Sexual systems are altered and created by each individual culture. A sexual system is those behaviors performed before, during and after copulation (sexual intercourse). Sex is the language of a culture. Sex behaviors are icons that reinforce culture. In some cultures, the act of sexual intercourse is a mixture of a series of rituals and ceremonies such as courting, petting and necking, dancing, singing, alcohol consumption, and finally the sex act. While in other cultures the parents of the mating couple get together, perform rituals and ceremonies that include communicating with deceased ancestors and God. After this formal socializing, the day and time of marriage and/or sex of the mating couple is arranged by the parents. In other cultures, a test of virginity is given to the female and if she passes the test, she is allowed to have sex with her mate. The net result of the sex system is to transmit, translate and reinforce the culture and be in spiritual communion with God and then reproduction.

The Caucasians' colonization of sexual behavior and systems by chattel slavery and social engineering is far reaching. In addition to slavery, sexual engineering has been caused by Caucasian created African Wars on the continent, by interracial marriages, intercultural marriages by sex inspired media (movies, computer games, music videos, clothes, books, songs, etc.), menstruation, perversions, pornography (dehumanization of sex), forced intertribal marriages, rape, venereal dis-eases, the cessation of breastfeeding, sex exploitation, forced monogamy and Europeanized illegalgamy (polygamy practiced as deceit), etc.

Black folks are sexually cultural clowns with no idea of what acculturated holistic sex means. Ancient African families got married and had a couple, the couple got married and then dated each other, the husband/wife loved their mate until their mate became the person they desired to love, non-homosexual marriage between two or more women that selected a male to marry (polygyny), it takes a village (community support, culture) to have a marriage and to raise a child. Holistic sex sustains a culture while Caucasian type sex erodes the African cultural basis for sex and equates sex to an acrobatic fun event. The natural laws can be condensed as follows: The sex is communion with God and the ancestors, sex is a spiritual activity, sex transmits and translates culture and natural mating cycle (season) for humans is approximately every three years. This cycle is a solar cycle (the uterus is on a solar cycle and ovaries are on a lunar cycle). The majority of the births among all peoples around the world occurs between the months of June and July. This places the human mating time in September or October at approximately three-year intervals. In nature, all mammalian (milk drinking animals) females do not have sex while the female is pregnant (one year of sexual abstinence). Mammalians do not have sex while the female is nursing (two to three years of nursing and sex abstinence). Sexual intercourse at these times destroys the quality of cell spirituality, mentality and alters the hormone and nutrient quality of the milk. Holistic laws, if followed, would mean that a man with one wife would have reproductive sex every three years at the most. While a man with two or more wives would have reproductive sex every two years at the most. Aside from this, the women and men abstain from sex for one year after the end of nursing or a miscarriage. This period of time allowed the woman to revitalize the reproductive system. In any case, many Caucasian sexual lust standards, chauvinistic medical science principles, religious laws and social standards are created by men to benefit men and sexually exploit females.

There are two types of sex-regenerative (injaculation—do not release sperm) and reproductive (ejaculation—release sperm). Sexual regeneration (non-ejaculation) is a method of transferring the orgasm sensation to the pineal (third eye). An orgasmic feeling is reached without female or male having a climax (penis is withdrawn out of the vagina). The climax sensation is sent to the pineal. This is called sexual regeneration and this type of sex can be performed often.

Chauvinistic African and European men contribute to the deterioration of a woman's body. Men are responsible for half of the births, abortions, fibroids, miscarriages, venereal dis-eases, morning sickness and difficult menstruations. Incidentally, pregnant females without male holistic support and nurturing develop emotional, behavioral and holistic problems. Menstruation only occurs when a female animal is put in captivity (oppression) such as a circus, zoo, farm, domesticated as a pet or enslaved. In nature, no female animals (so-called wild animals) menstruate. In other words, only oppressed (enslaved) women will menstruate. Oppression can be manipulation and control on a spiritual, social, physical, emotional, intellectual level and in the form of sexual servitude or sexual excess. Menstruation, impotency, reproductive failures such as still births, deformities, retarded children, children born with hyperactivity or attention deficit, gender confused, infant addicts, miscarriages, premature babies, etc. are signs of hypersex, Caucasian sex customs, poor quality sperm and/or egg and sex oppression.

In cultures where women were not inferiorized and sexually exploited by men, the women did not menstruate. Menstruation is the loss of thirty times the amount of calcium found in systemic blood. Thus, the bone structure is smaller and degenerated due to menses. Healthy menstruation was the blood from the egg and the superficial endometrium tissue that the egg was attached to. It was a very light blood flow and lasted from one to three days. A sanitary napkin may or may not be required for this healthy type of menstruation. Contemporary menstruation with a heavy blood flow that has to have a sanitary napkin is caused by the hemorrhaging of the uterus. In fact, menstruation's definition in today's books is defined as hemorrhaging.

The earlier cultures such as the ancient Gauls had women who were physically equal in physique as men and they did not menstruate. In Ammian and Diodorus writings, women were reported as being stronger than men and were able to fight side-by-side in combat with men.

The Andombis women of the Congo had splendid physiques. The Papuans, women were taller and stronger than men. Ancient Teutons' female skeletons revealed that they were seven feet tall.

Menstruation, petty rape, inferiorization, sex exploitation, female homosexuality, pedophile rape of girls and female prostitution is built into the Caucasian civilization. It causes the uterus to react by deteriorating and menstruating. In the booklet, *Special Instructions to Women* by H. E. Butler, menstruation and genital mucous discharge (leukorrhea) are indicated to be pathological (a dis-ease) and it disappeared when women are in a socially unexploitative sexual environment. In the book *Regeneration for Women* by K. S. Guthrie, M.D., menstruation is documented as the deterioration of the uterus, caused by the loss of vital nutrients in the mucous discharge. The cells lose their biochemical structure due to mucous discharge, deterioration and hemorrhage (menstruate). Caucasian religions say that menstruation is caused by the original female sin. Menstruation means to purge the body of sin. In *Man and Woman* by Havelock Ellis, the anatomical structure of women is scientifically verified to be superior to men. However, the social freedom that women enjoyed in the ancient agricultural communities in which collective families were the norm, menstruation was unheard of and holistic mating cycles were followed. The Caucasian colonization of sex rituals and ceremonies, seasonin of slaves (domestication), the labeling of African culture's sex laws as evil and primitive, the colonization of Africa and slavery destroyed African holistic sex. Ironically, the sexual position of the man on top of woman during intercourse is called "the missionary position." This restraining sexual position was used by Caucasian male and female missionaries to rape African slaves. The missionary position identifies that there are problems in African relationships, sex and menstruation. These problems are engineered into African folks' lifestyle and are believed to be normal. It is not normal for a Black person to adopt Caucasian culture and behave like a white person.

Black folks are exploited and enslaved by unholistic sexual behavior. A purely sensual approach to sex is the approach that breeding slaves were forced to use. An example of this is kissing. Kissing is a European sexual and friendship custom while the rubbing of noses is an Eskimo custom. Kissing has been found to exist in African literature, pictures and hieroglyphics. However, Caucasians have redefined kissing and used it as a way to keep Africans attached to Caucasian culture. African men kiss each other and African women kiss each other because kissing is a spiritual custom. Caucasian kissing between men and women is primarily sexual.

Unholistic Black folks quote Black literature, speak about the greatness of Africa, wear African clothes, some have African names, reclaim a natural food African diet, wear African hairstyles, talk about being Black and Proud and go to bed at night and have sex just like they are still owned by the white Slave Master. They probably have sex in the Master's bedroom. They are psychologically owned by the white master (Caucasian culture) if they do not say a prayer and ask God to guide and spiritualize their heterosexual sex.

Not only must Black folks do away with the illusion of being able to access African holistic sex, but with it, Blacks must do away with the illusion that recovery of lost holistic sex is our main hope. Culture defines sexual rituals and ceremonies. To be sexually free of Caucasians, you would have to be culturally free. Freedom means being able to practice your culture at all times and in all situations. You must first have your culture in order to have sex rituals. Recovery of African holistic sex means freedom from Caucasian control (mental and physical). The African culturalized sex is currently hidden by nature, time, events, history, and obscured by a slave mentality. English and other Caucasian languages must be Africentrically translated as those languages have locked away the information needed to translate Black holistic sexual heritage.

The retrieval of our sex system requires the use of all types of thought processes. The "deductive" (left mind—Male Principle) reasoning process requires fragmenting, isolating and analytical taking apart of ideas. The "reductive" (right minded—Female Principle) reasoning process requires the putting together and building of ideas. The "circular" reasoning process requires the uniting of ideas from any and all sources that tell the same story. All these reasoning processes are used simultaneously from a spirit centered spiritual focus. If we use our left mind with a spiritual base and all reasoning processes, we can retrieve lost "aboriginal" holistic African sex and reinvent sex from our preslavery memory (genetic code).

Reinvention takes into account that we are a mixture of an ancestral kingdom, cultural kingdom and spiritual/deity kingdom that can reinvent sex and African cultural in a contemporary language that our children can hear. Our African sex system must be shaped in contemporary behaviors that our youth can connect to and feel. It is available in ancient rituals and ceremonies, but needs to be translated holistically so our youth can use it. We just have to extract it. We have to extract it from an African holistic view. Thus, our sex will benefit spirit, mind and body. We do not need physical sex, as we are not slaves breeding slaves. The African cultures' mixture of the past, present and future has preserved our methods for liberation. In other words, the "past" is in the "present." The present sexual fragments of cryptic and/or icon behaviors need to be holistically retranslated. The positiveness in the behavior has to be psychospiritually surgically removed. Sex solutions are contained in the present sex system in some altered distorted form. The various codes of the continuation of matter and energy of DNA, of sexual cultural traditions, create and insure that holistic ancient sex modes are interwoven into current good, bad, distorted and perverted sex modes of behavior. They are somewhat superficially contained at the perimeter of the behavioral surface or by simple behavior parallels.

Sexually domesticated peoples are bred to reproduce their own kind just as in chattel slavery slaves were bred to reproduce their own kind. The field niggers bred (mated) with field niggers in order to produce a better quality of field niggers. Caucasian culture socially engineers college graduates breeding with other college graduates and the wealthy upper class breeds with the wealthy upper class. This results in a massive sexual domestication of peoples. People are domesticated to believe that there is only one way to mate and that is the Caucasian culture's way. This is sexual colonization and the domestication of sex.

History can reveal much of the sexual nature of undomesticated man. However, history does not repeat itself any more than you can repeat your yesterday. Cultures develop habits and these cultural habits are behaviors, which repeat themselves. Cultures develop bad habits and good habits and a reporting of cultural habits, racial habits and/or human kingdom habits are repeated in history. The original context of how the habit began is locked in time and events and astrology. In a natural state sex is a holistic encounter practiced during the day hours (preferably between 10:00 a.m. and 2:00 p.m.). The bad cultural habit of night time sex is locked in the social engineering scheme of the power elite, feudal kings, Caucasian barbarianism, etc.

There is a tendency to overlook the natural breeding hours of African peoples and to equate Caucasian sexual behavior as the same as African sexual behavior and, at the same time, to define African culture's sex system, on the evidence of Caucasian anthropologist. Caucasians defined African Maat culture as primitive sex mixed with rituals, taboos, and magic. The Caucasian definition is taken as correct by African peoples because they are addicted to Caucasian culture and/or have a sex addiction. The Circadian rhythm of the body, mating cycle and moon and sun cycle of the reproductive organs define sex as a daylight hour holistic God-centered activity.

Victor Turner's writing on African societies, especially of the Ndembu Lunda of Zambia by European academics. He is a White Supremacist who is considered a fairly unbiased sympathetic observer. He observed that Africans had sex during the day hours and he deduced that African sex was full of delusions, hocus-pocus and unsound rituals. The undeveloped Caucasian linear thought causes them to believe and then see. In other words, they do not see and then believe. Their mind tells them that their eyes are lying. They have a Bipolar White Supremacist Psychosis and see with their beliefs, not with their vision. What their eyes witness was African culture and African sex in the context of African culture. Sex mirrors culture, reinforces culture and transmits and translates culture. The holistic nature of sex and the religious and cultural influences upon sex are lost to the naked eye of an alien Caucasian cultural observer, and, they are lost to contemporary unholistic Black folks. The vast majority of Blacks are socially engineered (seasonin) to follow a strict monogamous marriage form, and Caucasian sex rituals and ceremonies. Within the Caucasian culture's sex practices include pedophilia, pornography, homosexuality, masturbation, incest, necrophilia, sex with animals and has Freudian hidden subsconscious meanings.

A seasonin Black with a slave mentality never supports polygyny, inferiorizes African polygamy as a sex playground and seasonin Blacks follow Caucasian sexual appetites as normal. Nonetheless, monogamy, polygyny and polygamy were practiced side by side in Africa,and in unity with God and spirituality sex was the focus. The sexually polygamous woman acted out her sexual and/or social need for companionship within her monogamous, polygamous or polygynamous African marriage. Within African culture, she had socially acceptable events and ceremonies that allowed her to have the liberated freedom to have sex with more than one sex partner or have more than one companion. In contemporary Black society, she is considered sexually unfaithful and without morals. African society is unilineal, patrilineal and matrilineal with sex rituals and ceremonies for each. In patrilineal African societies, the sex culture adjusted to support it. Sexuality and mating is different in matrilineal as well as unilineal African societies. Today, sexuality is strictly defined upon patrilineal sex, rituals and ceremonies. The sexually polygamous woman in matrilineal African society is not sexually unfaithful nor a cultural mutation but a reality within African definitions. Monogamy as moral and polygyny and polygamy as immoral is forced upon Africans (seasonin, socially engineered) and causes cultural abrasion and a deep conflict in the cultural psyche.

Created by our culture, our culture defines our diet. Our beliefs are influenced by what we eat. If we eat a diet of cloned, genetically modified, hybridized, chemicalized and hormone treated the domesticated plants then our thoughts are influenced by the Caucasian culture that freaked the vegetables and fruits. When Africans eat Caucasian domesticated plants grown on slave plantations, they develop the aura and/or chemicalized domesticated nature of the tame plants. In other words, we are what we eat. Sex has become colonialized and domesticated and Caucasian. A sexually colonialized and Caucasian domesticated African is called a citizen. Every African citizen of a puppet African country or so-called independent country or European country is a trained tamed sexually controlled puppet of the Caucasians. A slave's sex is never a holistic sex or natural sex. Blacks do not know true holistic sex any more than a clown can know life outside a circus. African holistic sex ceremonies (systems) of petting and necking sexual regeneration, caressing, sex positions and sexual spirituality are icons that build, sustain and maintain culture. Sex is neither physical nor mental. It is a melaninated harmony of the earth, lunar, solar and galaxy cycles of the body that is ancestral, Maat, Godly and spiritual. Sex with an African program (acculturation) allows you to access your higher Maatian glory. Sex using a Caucasian sex program will never allow an African to access his own intelligence.

The African sexual culture is icons and small keynote devices that store extremely vast complex data about nature, culture and destiny. True African sexuality creates a cultural learning device that is void of Caucasian cultural contamination.

The quest for holistic African cultural sex should start with a few guidelines such as:

- Saying a prayer and asking God to bless your sexual act;
- Sex during the day (when possible);
- Sexual Regeneration as well as Sexual Reproduction
- Sexual abstinence during pregnancy, menstruation and breastfeeding;
- Breastfeeding of children;
- Men participating in the birth ceremony/ritual and a placenta ceremony/ritual;
- Emotional, mental and behaviors that indicate participation in pregnancy, menstruation and menopause by men;
- Passive sexual roles during sex by men and dominant roles for women, and a mixture of roles;
- Thinking about procreation and enlightenment for sex;
- After sex petting, caressing, prayer, conversation and necking;
- Use more (non-sexual intercourse) behavior of sharing;
- Eating a natural foods diet.
- Do not eat one hour before or after sex.

The holistic sex view should not look to ancient history to solve today's sex problems. African sexuality must look more internally, eliminate cultural contradictions and translate ancient sex rituals and ceremonies into a contemporary behavior that youth can understand, feel and use. Men should learn to accept their Female Principle (African woman in them). In other words, his gentleman. This is not to be confused with homosexuality. The woman should be sensitive to their Male Principle (African man in her) and learn to use and share this emotional, mental and physical energy with her mate. This is explored in the book, *The Secret of Regeneration* by Hotena.

The holistic perspective (spiritual, mental and physical), which can help to sustain Black folks, can be found in books such as *Sex and Nutrition* by Airola, *Sexual Secrets* by Douglas and Slinger and *Native African Medicine* by G. W. Harley. In the pamphlets "Black Dot (Humanities Ancestral Blackness)" by R. King and "The Cress Theory of Racial Confrontation" by Frances Cress Welsing, the significance of melanin in the unique anatomy of Blacks and cellular creation is academically explored from a scientific position. *Diet and Nutrition* by Ballantine, M.D., points to some racial and cultural differences needed to become more enlightened about culture and holistic sex.

Until Black culture gets rid of nighttime slave sex and other Caucasian sexual distortions, they will produce poor quality eggs, sperm and a distorted sexual cultural language for their children. They will be the Caucasians' cultural clowns (cultural misfits).

BIRTHDATE AND BIOLOGICAL DISPOSITIONS

Births were cyclically planned by the parents or the food supply. Many times, astrological charts were cast to help the couple plan children. Number one represents January, two represents February, etc. A person born in number six (June) was conceived in the tenth month (October).

Spring and summer births may be prone to respiratory disease bronchitis, tuberculosis, kidney, heart and circulatory disorders.

Autumn and winter births may be prone to digestive disorder in the liver, gallbladder, spleen, pancreas and small intestine, illness of diabetes, constipation, stomach ulcers, diarrhea, and nervous disorders.

WOMEN'S WHOLISTIC HEALTH

Physiology of the Women's Reproductive System

The woman's reproduction system is primarily internal and is not more complex than the man's cycle. The man's cycle has temperature drops in the middle of the month that corresponds to the ovalutory mid-cycle temperature drop. In addition, a man's temperature rises to a high level, which corresponds to that of the woman's temperature after ovulation. The specific hormonal causes of the man's temperature cycle are the same as the woman's. He has the same hormones as females (estrogen, testosterone and progesterone). They are made by conversion of one hormone into another. The man's sex organs are external and internal and the female's are internal. The woman's internal reproductive organs consist of the ovaries, fallopian tubes, uterus, cervix and vagina.

The uterus is located approximately three to four inches below the navel. There are two ovaries, one on each side of the uterus and located on each side of the lower pelvic area. The uterus is considered a body with four appendages — two arms (Fallopian Tubes) and two legs (ovaries). In African science, the uterus' fallopian tubes' health is reflected by the arms and the health state of the ovaries are reflected by the legs while the health state of the torso and internal organ is related to the uterus. The ovaries secrete the hormones estrogen and progesterone and the adrenal glands convert hormones into testosterone. One of the primary functions of estrogen is to aid in the maintenance and development of female bodily characteristics such as breast development and body contour. *(A Textbook of Gynecology* by Cowper Thwaite).

There are five aspects to women's sexuality. Menstruation, pregnancy, childbirth, nursing and menopause. Conception bonds life and a menstruation inhibit natural life *(Maternal Emotions* by N. Newton).

The first day of menstrual bleeding is called day one of the menstrual cycle. Whether the intricate hormone feedback system of the endocrine glands, starts with bleeding, is unlikely. The pituitary is part of the hormonal cycle and not its co-worker hypothalamus. The hypothalamus reacts to changes in the Earth's magnetic field and the effects of solar activities and this has an effect on the hormone activity. The hypothalamus has a connection between astrological conception and birth control. Aside from the pituitary and hypothalamus, effects upon menstruation, the hormones estrogen and progesterone can cause mild diarrhea and weight loss when out of balance *(Astrological Birth Control* by S. Ostrander).

During the first five days of the cycle, the progesterone increases and estrogen which decreases causes a release of Follicle-Stimulating Hormone (FSH) from the pituitary gland. The FSH stimulates the follicles in the ovaries. When the eggs are in the ovaries they cause the production of estrogen.

The estrogen stimulates the growth of the skin inside the uterus (endometrium). The skin gets thicker and richer in blood and the walls of the uterus prepare for the fertilized egg. The egg implants in the endometrium whether fertilized or not. The mucous plug of the cervix becomes thinner and more slippery, which assists the sperms travel through the cervix. During this part of the cycle, one of the undeveloped follicles begins to outgrow the others, becoming the Graafian follicle that produces the egg for the month. As the Graafian follicle grows toward the surface of the ovary, preparing to eject the egg, the fallopian tube on the same side reaches under the ovary to receive the expelled egg. The increasing estrogen level starts to block the FSH from the pituitary *(Anatomy and Physiology* by E. Steven and Ashley Montagu).

The Graafian follicle has a higher amount of prostaglandins, which causes the ovary to contract and eject the egg. While this occurs, the ovary turns to the side close to the hair-like (fimbriated) end of the fallopian tube that engages the egg and its protoplasm.

Inside the tube, the egg travels slowly to the uterus, propelled by fimbria (hairlike fingers). The ruptured Graafian follicle develops into the corpus luteum (yellow body) and secretes progesterone and estrogen to stimulate the uterine lining which becomes spongy. This causes an increase in resting (basal) body temperature. It is usually one-half to four-tenths (.4) degree temperature increase or more and is a sign of ovulation. A decrease of body temperature occurs after ovulation. However, if a pregnancy does not occur, the increase in uterus skin hemorrhages and passes out of the body through the vagina. This is called menstruation. The menstruation cycles continue month after month until a woman is in her late forties or fifties. When the ovaries cease to produce an egg each month, the woman has begun menopause and her childbearing period has ceased *(Review of Medical Physiology* by W. Ganong).

The external genitals are known as the vulva. The vulva is not one specific organ. It is the name given to the entire outer area of the genital urethral organs. This includes the clitoris (female penis), the urethra (urine outlet) and the opening of the vagina. These are encompassed by the labia (lips) minora and majora. The vagina is a tubelike structure consisting of smooth muscle and lined with soft mucous membrane tissue. Sperm is ejaculated into a cuplike area near the mouth of the uterus. This vaginal area and mouth (cervix) of the uterus are lubricated by the secretions of the Bartholin gland, which are two small glands located near the opening. The urethra is a part of the urinary system. The uretha is a tube that urine passes out. It is located between the clitoris and the vagina. The anus and pubic hair area are not, technically considered part of the vulva even though most discussions of the vulva inevitably mention them because of their close proximity to the vulva.

The internal organs of the urinary system are the kidneys, ureter and bladder. The kidneys are behind the abdominal organ near the lower ribs, resting against the muscles of the back. They are protected by a cushion of fat, which assists in retaining them in position. Urine is drained from the kidneys by a narrow tube called the ureter. The ureter connects the kidneys with the bladder. The bladder is a sac that stores urine. The urine leaves the bladder through a tube called the urethra. Because the external female reproductive and urinary systems are very close, a disorder of one system will often affect the other. For example, a vaginal infection (reproductive system) might cause a burning sensation during urination (excretory system). The majority of health problems that women have are related to the reproductive and excretory systems (*Cyclopedic Medical Dictionary* by C. Taber).

DISEASES AND PATHOLOGY

Leukorrhea

Disease
Leukorrhea is the white uterine discharge that contains white blood cells and excreted dead or damaged vaginal cells. The white blood cells indicate that it is a disease condition.

Normally, the vagina has a balance of bacteria, flora (plants), microorganisms and yeast. Doderlein bacillus bacteria helps maintain the pH of the vaginal flora. The normal vaginal flora is slightly acidic. This is caused by the fermentation of lactic acid from natural sugar (glycogen) by the Doderlein bacillus (bacteria). Antibiotics kill the Doderlein bacillus (bacteria) and weaken the immune system. Antibiotics cause the acidity of the vagina to be low, which causes yeast to multiply, creating a yeast infection.

Normally the uterus' leukorrhea (mucosal skin cellular deterioration) remains very slight. A slight leukorrhea is secreted by the mucous membrane skin that lines the genital tract. This slight leukorrhea protects the mucous membrane skin lining the genital tract. The cellular quantity and mucousal quality of uterus secretions changes before and after menstruation, sexual intercourse and the birthing of a child. All forms of stress caused by exhaustion, chemicals, hypersex, drugs, fatigue, catarrh, junk foods and emotions can cause changes in the color, odor, thickness and amount of leukorrhea secreted. Secretions are also altered by estrogen, when the estrogen level rises prior to ovulation, the uterus secretions are clear, slippery and watery. This is called the wet days. However, as long as the secretions remain normal during stressors (chemical, emotional, disease, etc.) and ovulation estrogen increases, the discharge cannot be classified as pathological. When leukorrhea mucosa discharge becomes chronic or severe and the color, odor and thickness changes, it is a type of leukorrhea disease.

Pathology
Leukorrhea is primarily an abnormal catarrhal condition (mucous secretion) similar to nasal catarrh (runny nose) and epidermal catarrh. The classification of the mucous discharge (catarrhal) disease depends upon whether it is caused by cellular waste congestion of the mucous membrane or severe inflammation. Emotions, anxiety, tension, fatigue and stressors can nutritionally drain the cells of the mucosal skin causing it to deteriorate, get infected and discharge leukorrhea. Extreme tension can cause the muscle that separates the vagina and anus (perineal muscles) to contract and block the drain of vaginal secretions. The secretions blocked in the uterus can become septic, irritate, infect and/or inflame the skin causing leukorrhea.

The vaginal catarrh discharge varies, based on both the dis-ease and the diet. Both can cause a disease variation in leukorrhea consistency, which depends on the type of skin (derma) involved and the origin of discharge (fallopian tubes, uterus, ovaries, vagina). Vulva leukorrhea, which occurs primarily in adolescents is principally oily (sebaceous) in composition. It is usually caused by excessive sexual intercourse, excess estrogen and/or sexual stimulation of the mother during pregnancy. Adolescent girls can have poor hygienic practices, resulting in worms traveling from the anus to the vagina's vulva. Hygienically, a female should clean the vulva area at least once a day. After a bowel movement or urination, females should wipe with unbleached and unscented toilet tissue from front (vagina) to back (anus). This will prevent bacteria from traveling (migrating) from the anus to the vulva. The sebaceousness (oiliness) leukorrhea is caused by immature sebaceous glands in adolescents. This type of dis-ease of leukorrhea can also be found among older women and is caused by hypertrophy (exhaustion) of the sebaceous glands. Girls and young women can exhaust the sebaceous glands and cause dryness of the vagina. A Vitamin E suppository can solve this condition.

The leukorrhea of young adult women (preceding sexual intercourse and pregnancy) usually has an acid pH, contains plasma, blood, fatty matter, pus and epithelial scales. Pus in the leukorrhea indicates a disease process.

Leukorrhea with cervical and uterine mucosa is predominant in women during the childbearing period. Cervical leukorrhea is ropy, thick, tenacious, and similar to raw egg white. Uterine leukorrhea is water, contains blood and pus, which causes it to have a yellow color. Both of the leukorrheas are alkaline and indicate a dis-ease process.

When there is a combination of various leukorrhea types, the septic leukorrhea fluid can indicate the part of the reproductive system and severity of the disease.

The secondary cause of leukorrhea is usually the deterioration of the sex organs while the primary cause is a disease in the body. The same diseases that occur to other parts of the body can occur to the reproductive system such as rheumatism, poor circulation, hardening of arteries, clogged arteries, etc. *(The Physiological Basis of Medical Practice* by C. Best).

The Bodily Generated Causes

High blood pressure/hypertension causes the uterine and vaginal muscles to be tense resulting in waste accumulation—deterioration. Stress causes the pH to be too acidic. This can alter the bacteria, yeast, fungus and pH of the uterus. The seminal acidic ejaculation fluid of men alters the pH balance of the woman's genital tract. Frequent sexual intercourse and/or sex stimulation inhibits the protective balance of the vaginal milieu from recuperating its normal pH. Contraception devices (invented by men) contribute to excess sex, they rub and weaken the skin of uterus, pinch the nerve meridian and cause infections.

Physical traumas, disease, junk foods, drugs, excess estrogen, excessive physical activity, and negative emotional states cause the sympathetic nervous system to decrease the blood flow (and cleansing) to the reproductive system.

The symptoms of a sympathetic nervous system stressed reproductive system are:

- Vital (the residual toxins of bacteria) and fungal (candida)
- Bacterial (venereal dis-eases such as gonorrhea, syphilis)
- Inflammation of the endometrium, salpingitis, ovaritis, vaginitis, cervicitis. All are signs of deterioration of the uterus
- Displacement of the uterus by a physical trauma, strenuous exercise, an accident, sex or work (introverted or front position is normal, retroverted or tilted and mid-position are not normal)

The majority of herbs prescribed in herbal books are allopathic and geared towards suppressing symptoms. They usually have astringents such as Wild Alum Root, Witch Hazel, Blood Root or herbs with tannic acid. The herbs may contain oily (resinous) astringents (Myrrh) or an astringent alkaloid (Goldenseal) instead of tannic acid. The herbal astringents usually are safer than the synthetic astringents. The herbs may have estrogen (i.e., Black Cohosh, Chaste, etc.), which is a stress hormone that reduces blood to the uterus and this stops leukorrhea. Herbs are often used from an allopathic perspective and based upon the triage military approach to symptoms. Excess use of allopathic tannic herbs (tannin is predominantly used in the manufacture of leathers), particularly in douches can cause the formation of scar tissue in the uterus and/or vagina. Scar tissue is basically dead tissue that is leatherized. Strong astringent and tannic acid herbs can cause the sensitive uterine and vaginal skin to leatherize, get weak and degenerate resulting in uterine skin problems. The scar tissue may prevent the fertilized egg from embedding in the endometrium and may cause difficulty in conceiving and/or infertility (*A Study on Matera Medical* by N. Choundhuri).

Treatment of Leukorrhea
Proper rest, nutrition, exercise and sleep is of primary importance. Sleep helps the secretion of the hormone Melatonin as well as promotes healing. A type of cyclic healing of the body takes place during the sleep cellular cycle (anabolism). During the sleep cycle, growth hormones are released which stimulate cell repair.

Herbal tinctures/extracts can be used such as Witch Hazel, Shepherd's Purse, Saw Palmetto, Burdock Root, Echinacea and Devil's Claw. Combine equal amounts (mix together) and take 30 to 40 drops daily or until a leukorrhea crisis subsides. These herbs stimulate, cleanse, regenerate and decrease excretion plus they are beneficial to the lymphatic system.

The health history of the female also determines treatment. If in the past there were episodes of venereal dis-ease, then the homeopathic herb of Thuja 6X should be used as indicated on the label. In addition to Thuja, a woman whose physical activities are sedentary should also use the cell salt drug of Natrun (sodium) Sulphate.

The non-wholistic immuno-suppressive orthodox treatment of venereal diseases focuses upon suppressing the symptoms, changing the biochemistry, destroying helpful bacteria and alteration of vaginal flora. It does not focus upon the cellular waste, electrolyte waste, fungus, yeast and bacterial debris, cell particles (viruses) and plasmids that may congest the sex organs and deteriorate the tissue.

In 85% of infected women, their weak immunity caused them to develop gonorrhea. If the body's defenses are weak, then they may not have symptoms. Gonorrhea can be a hidden cause of leukorrhea. The typical early symptoms in men are pain when urinating and a discharge of pus from the penis. There are typically no early warning symptoms in women. The women's symptoms can be detected between two and thirty days. Gonorrhea does not cause external skin sores or eruptions; it is a dis-ease of the mucous membrane. There are, however, some detectable symptoms such as warts in perineum and vulva and/or profuse green leukorrhea. The leukorrhea may not have a color but will have the aroma of fish or cheese. Other symptoms are severe pain in the left inguinal section (groin) and left ovary, excessive perspiration before menses and the periodic fleshy growths of polyps.

If the health history reveals syphilis, the leukorrhea could be the result of having sex outside of the normal one birth per three-year cycle, hypersex, synthetic douches, chemicals from condoms, excess estrogen, stressors and/or degeneration of the sex organs. A bloody and greenish burning discharge, burning in the genitals and itching, which increases after urinating and breasts that fill with milk during menstruation and become sore are symptoms of a venereal disease such as syphilis.

A wholistic approach is of the utmost importance in understanding reproductive organ deterioration and its effect on uterus dis-ease and leukorrhea. In a disease process, the diseased can alter the senses (taste, smell, touch, etc.). Therefore, alterations in sensations are a way in which the body tells the woman that it is ill. A dis-ease uses symptoms to call attention to an illness. The modifications and alterations of the senses was analyzed by ancient African healers. The ancient healers believed that dis-eases were messages from the Gods and Goddesses. Diseases such as leukorrhea can indicate social and/or spiritual problems in the African village as well as the male and female relationship. Disease can be a physical expression of an emotional illness. Sex organs create (reproduction). Sexual disease can indicate that Africans are losing their ability to create or recreate African culture due to Caucasian cultural castration of African sex laws and African civilization. We, as an oppressed people, are taught to be sexually dysfunctional (non-African in sexuality). This means we are taught to destroy each other—sexually sterilize each other. This subconscious crime causes us to torture our emotions and punish ourselves. A woman may emotionally and spiritually punish herself via her reproductive organs. She may punish herself with fibroids and the male may punish himself with prostate disease. Spiritual, emotional and health problems can cause the uterus to deteriorate resulting in V.D. (Venereal Disease). Venereal Disease, such as leukorrhea can be the result of a prolapsed colon (loss of muscle tone and ligament tone), insufficient exercise, lack of Maat, deficient spirituality, synthetic foods, etc. Yoka, African uterus healing dances and Afri-Aerobics for women have many postures and muscle movements, which deal directly with rejuvenating and maintaining intestinal and uterus tone and health. Massage (popular in Northern Africa) can unblock energy in the body particularly in the pelvic area. Being massaged brings the breath up to touch the hands and Pineal. The masseur can place one hand on the abdomen while the woman breathes deeply from the abdomen through the hands. This allows the body to be grounded and protected. The masseur's other hand is placed on the woman's head and they visualize the leukorrhea being removed out of the dis-eased body. Wanting to become healthy, thinking health and claiming health is necessary for healing. Sometimes women can create dis-eases of the reproductive organs on a subconscious level. A woman must visualize green light bathing the dis-ease condition, as well as consciously breathing healing energy through the uterus—this produces a soothing effect.

During a yeast infection, the female body is in an acidic state. Alkalinity of blood is helpful. The body's growth and repair takes place in alkalinity while a high acid state causes deterioration, disease, addiction and triggers yeast. The female and male have to be simultaneously treated for yeast infection or they will re-infect each other. The herb Pau D'Arco cures yeast infection. The diet has to be changed. The infected persons cannot eat mushrooms, yeast (read labels), sugar, dried fruit, fermented foods (soy sauce, wine, beer, cheese, vinegar), bleached white flour, wheat, white rice, grits or potatoes, honey and chocolate. A broth of zucchini, celery and parsley can prove effective. Supplementing the diet with foods and vitamins is helpful. Stress can cause a yeast infection. Stress makes the body acidic. Daily yoga balances the body, pH level, blood and the emotions and helps remove dis-ease. Yoga can provide the energy necessary to correct the imbalances in the woman's life. A massage to the back of the leg just behind the ankle is beneficial. Massage pressure on the ankles stimulates circulation and relaxes the fallopians ovaries. *The Handbook of Alternatives to Chemical Medicine* by M. Jackson and T. Teague and *Yoga and Medicine* by S. Brennan).

Do-In exercise can be used to treat leukorrhea. It consists of exercises that can help maintain and develop self. The exercises are wholistic and focus upon the spiritual, mental and physical by using various types of chanting, Yoka (Yoga), exercise, meditation, the martial arts, spiritual rituals and other forms of self-development.

Do-In alters the atmospheric charges that enter the inner part of the body through "Entering Points." Once the energy enters the body, it can charge the dis-eased organs. The energy enters the back, gathers at the front for each organ, and can be directed to correct the dis-ease state. Do-In is an African science that is claimed by the Japanese.

Leukorrhea can also be treated where the Melanin forces in the body cluster together or intersect (Chakras). These places of Melanin energy convergence generate an electromagnetic flow toward the external atmosphere while receiving energy flow from the internal atmosphere *(The Chakras* by C. Leadbeader).

Excessive charge to the Sacral or Second Melanin Cluster (Chakra) can cause leukorrhea.The stimulation of the Chakra areas on the fingers, palms, toes, and soles, shiatsu massage, moxibustion, acupuncture, yoga and exercise can help to treat leukorrhea.

Leukorrhea can be painful. Pain can be associated with muscle and bone alignment (Myofascial). A healthy woman can recuperate from poor myofascial alignment and recover emotional equilibrium. A woman body's alignment has been distorted or weakened by stressors, poor nutrition and emotional issues cannot recuperate without some type of healing protocol.

Rolfing, which is a type of massage that balances the physical alignment. Rolfing requires moving the tissue that holds muscles and bones in alignment. It is a painful type of rubbing massage. It can be effective against leukorrhea. Women's leukorrhea can cause a negative response, which precipitates movement away from myofascial (tissue that attaches muscles to bones) balance and myofascial ease. Negative relationships, social conditions and emotion cause stress and tension (hypertonicity) in the tissue that holds bones in alignment (myofascial flexors). Stressors (emotional, mental, chemical) can cause muscle attachment tissue (myofascial) stress, which can pull the body out of alignment. This causes somaticpsychi—bodily misalignment caused illnesses. Misalignment blocks circulation and the cleansing of internal organs (i.e., uterus). Rolfing reduces stress and blockages. Rolfing helps the glands to function and harmonizes the chemistry of the body. It has a positive effect on the negative chemical and physiological changes that the cells make during a disease process. The emotions can cause the body to be ill (psychosomatic). Physical changes in the body and posture influences emotions, which in turn influences the glands and sex organs. Rolfing can positively influence the restoration of physiological flow.

The outer expression of the dis-ease and pain reflects the Male Principle (acidic, fast) and the Female Principle (alkaline, slow). Pain expresses itself quickly (Male Principle) and/or slowly (Female Principle). Pain is transmitted from sensory to receptor endings (pain sensors) in the skin (derma). There are two types of fibers—myelinated and unmyelinated. The myelinated conducts nerve impulses rapidly (Male Principle) and the unmyelinated slowly (Female Principle). This indicates the neuro-physiological complexity of pain. Consequently, the type of pain, such as sharp (Male Principle) or dull (Female Principle) and speed of pain can indicate if the disease (i.e., leukorrhea) is caused by stressors on the sympathetic nervous system (Male Principle) or parasympathetic nervous system (Female Principle) as well as being caused by an alkaline imbalance (Female Principle) and/or acid imbalance (Male Principle).

The treatment of women's leukorrhea has to be holistic. The goal of structural integration is to achieve correct posture (verticality of the body). The massage technique involves pressing deep and hard on the elastic soft tissue structure (myofascial) of the anatomy in order to align it correctly. Correct alignment lessens the force of gravity on the body and reduces the amount of energy spent. The primary focus of treatment is retraining the muscles and tissue and balancing the movements of the body. Rolfing helps bodily equilibrium and the realignment of joints. The realignment will help the pain to subside and leukorrhea to be altered *(Rolling the Integration of Human Structures* by I. Roll).

The criteria for choosing a health protocol/treatment should be based upon the following:

Characteristics of Symptoms
Is there a burning sensation, itching, pain or painless? Is the vaginal/uterus discharge offensive, greenish, bloody, brown, stringy, thin, watery, thick, flesh colored (non-offensive), slimy, black, gushing, pus-like (purulent) and/or milky?

Occurrence of Symptoms
Do the symptoms occur in the daytime, night, after sex, menses, urination and/or bowel movements? Do they occur instead of menstruation or with menopause symptoms?

Accompanied Symptoms
Do I get backache, abdominal pain, diarrhea, bleeding, weakness, urinary irritation, digestion problems (liver), cramps, depression, nervousness and moody? Before the symptoms, did I have any miscarriages, abortions and stillbirths?

There are over fifty herbs used for the treatment of leukorrhea. The usage of an herb such as False Unicorn root is specific for offensive discharge and the prolapse of the uterus. If in addition to the offensiveness, there are chills in hot weather, then the primary cause is weak immunity. Accordingly, Psorium is the treatment remedy. The use of cooked (burnt) marijuana will cause a purulent (pus), yellowish discharge. The usage of salt (table salt, sea salt, etc.) can cause a water acrid discharge coupled with dryness and sensitiveness of the vagina. Nat-Mur 6x will be the remedy. Consequently, in both cases marijuana, sugar, fermented foods, salt, mushrooms, honey, dried fruit, non-organic dairy, eggs, milk, processed oils and junk food should be avoided.

Fibroid Tumors: Cause and Cure
Fibroid tumors of the uterus are a modern-day plague of African-American women. More than 60% of the Black women are afflicted with the disease.

Tumor is a word describing a bump rather than naming a disease. The muscle fiber of the uterus weakens and develops a bump-like ballooning-out, similar to a hemorrhoid or varicose vein. Fibroids can grow with or without a capsule. Inside the fibroid capsule, there can be rotten blood, trapped veins, arteries, cellular waste, and a mass of muscle or fluid pus. The tumor can be the size of a bean or as large as a grapefruit. It can have various shapes, such as flat, oval, spider web-like, mushroom, needle-like, or even grow like a tree. Fibroids are usually benign and non-cancerous and typically do not require surgery. They tend to shrink during menopause due to decreased estrogen production.

The Three Layers of the Uterus

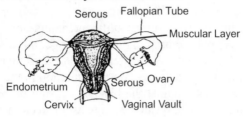

The Various Types of Fibroid Tumors.
Fibroids can grow anywhere, including on the ligaments of the uterus.

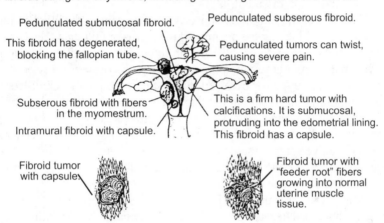

For enlarged chart, see page 530.

A stressed liver cannot neutralize waste and therefore contribute to the growth of fibroids. A stressed liver is caused by junk foods, drugs, dairy, meat, and inadequate Calciums and Manganese. An ovulating female who temporarily cannot metabolize Manganese can cause her uterus to weaken and put her body temporarily in a menopause state. This temporary menopause state can cause fibroids and it can occur whether the female is a teenager or a young adult. Hormone imbalances can cause fibroids. It is indicated by facial hair, hair growth on the upper lip and /or chin, brittle nails and/or white spots on the fingernails, split ends on the hair, thin hair, white spots on the skin, pica (eating clay, starch or ice), hot flashes, night sweats, mood swings, hyper-sensitivity to smells, insomnia, loss of energy, etc. This disease-causing imbal-ance results in cellular waste accumulation in the uterus, which can lead to fibroid tumors.

Fibroids can hamper the ability of the uterus muscles to contract and expand. The plant-like roots of fibroids can choke the uterus muscle fibers, veins and arteries. This stops vital nutrients from nourishing, cleansing and pro-tecting the uterus. Waste becomes trapped in the uterus—fibroids. The fibroids can trap blood and waste and cause blood vessels to leak. Uterus muscles can

pull against the fibroid and its roots causing pain. Tumors can block and interrupt menstruation; stop fertilized eggs from implanting in the uterus; decrease
organism quality; cause sterility, painful intercourse, bleeding after sex, lower
back and pelvic pain, cramping, mood swings, miscarriages, urinary tract
infections, kidney problems, numbness and/or tingling in the legs, excessive
bleeding, hormonal imbalances, poor circulation to the uterus and legs, etc.
The tumor can press against the bladder causing problems with urination
and/or retention of urine. It can press against the rectum causing constipation.
Fibroids can hamper digestion in the intestines and stomach. They can distort
the natural shape of the abdomen causing a pregnant-like figure, which can
cause social embarrassment.

The size of the tumor is not nearly as important as the location (against
the bladder or blocking the opening of the uterus or fallopian tubes) since the
uterus can accommodate a nine-month fetus. The conventional treatment is
to watch the tumor grow (monitor) and then give a hysterectomy or block the
blood flow to the tumor by inserting plastic in the tumor vessels (death by
strangulation). This is similar to tying a newborn's umbilical cord in order for
it to fall off. The tumor or tumors can be removed surgically, in which case
the uterus and pelvic area must be reconstructed in order to conceive a child.
Reconstructive surgery that leads to conception is successful in over 80% of
the women who choose it. The tumors can also be dissolved with natural
remedies and spiritual cleansing.

Many factors can contribute to fibroids. The chemicals that make
polyurethane or latex condoms cause chlamydia, pelvic inflammatory dis-
ease, sterility, cancer and endometriosis. The spermicide gel in condoms can
cause cancer while the inner powder coating causes cysts and tumors. Estrogen
based birth control pills can also cause cysts, cancer and tumors. Melatonin
based contraceptive pills are safer. However, they can contribute to fibroids.
Norplant, radiation (x-rays, ultrasounds, microwave ovens, computers, etc.),
and irradiated foods can cause fibroids. Stress and hypertension cause the
uterus muscles to hold tension and waste, which can lead to tumors. Stress,
emotional and/or Slavery Trauma can decrease Melatonin levels, which result
in disease and fibroids. High blood pressure and diabetes cause cellular waste
congestion and weaken the uterus. The synthetic chemicals in cough suppressants and deodorants get into the blood and hold (suppress) waste in the
uterus. Skin bleaching concoctions, synthetic hair relaxers, douches, vaginal
deodorants, conscious dioxin bleach in sanitary napkins and tampons cause
disease. Super absorbent tampons pull the moisture out of the vaginal skin
causing cracked skin and skin diseases (ie., tumors, cysts) and poisonous artificial nail glue enters the blood and result in the deterioration of cells (uterine). High levels of the Pineal gland's Melatonin hormone caused by the
rebound effect of taking legal and illegal drugs cause infertility. The high
level can cause amenorrehic (absence of menstruation) as well as toxic waste
in the uterus—fibroids. Toxic waste and/or acid sperm harms the tissue of the

vagina and uterus. A man's sperm is only as healthy as he is—sick man, sick sperm. All of these are contributing factors for fibroids.

There are many natural remedies for fibroid tumors, such as a natural foods diet, herbs, exercise, colonics, dancing, massage, meditation, herbal cleansing baths and spiritual rituals. A natural foods diet is one free of synthetic estrogen found in cow's milk, meat and eggs; and free of foods that dehydrate tissue (uterine), such as white sugar, vinegar, alcohol, sodas, salt, bleached white flour, polished white rice and caffeine. Caffeine causes the uterus to develop fibroids by decreasing the blood flow to the uterus, which causes waste to accumulate—fibroids. Fibroids are waste isolated in a bump form called a tumor.

FIBROID TREATMENT

Supplements	Suggested Dosage	Remarks
Glutathione	1,000 mg.	Shrinks tumors.
Pregnenolone	100 mg.	Shrinks cysts.
Manganese	50 mg., three times daily.	Improves health of uterus.
Potassium	99 mg. daily.	Aids bodily functions. Excretes cellular waste.
Vitamin K	50-80 mcg.	Stabilizes bones. Stops bleeding.
Herbal combination (equal parts) Witch Hazel, Shepherd's Purse, White Oak Bark, Thuja and Burdock	2 – 3 cups daily.	Shrinks tumors.
Herbal combination (equal parts) Red Raspberry, Chaste [Vitex] or Dong Quai, Black Cohosh, Squaw Vine, Damiana and Blessed Thistle	2 – 3 cups daily.	Cleanses blood. Strengthens uterus.
Herbal combination (equal parts) Red Clover, Dandelion Root Chaparral, Echinacea and Goldenseal	2 – 3 cups daily.	Cleanses blood. Eliminates cellular waste.
Cramp Bark, Boswella and White Willow	As needed.	Pain relief.
Feverfew and St. John's Wort	As needed.	Relieves tension and stress.
Saw Palmetto and Pygeum	½ dosage.	Reduces estrogen level, which reduces fibroids.
Yohimbe, Tribulus, Dopa Bean and Damiana	As needed.	Increases sexual desire.
Progesterone/Wild Yam	As directed.	Balances hormones.
Comfrey	As needed.	Reduces bleeding.
Alum Root douche	As needed.	Causes blood to clot naturally. Reduces bleeding.
Can-X (Black Salve) Tablets	1 – 2 tablets, twice daily after meals.	Dissolves tumors.

Dancing centered upon the Female Principle stimulates the parasympathetic nervous system, which is used for repair. This type of dancing focuses on pelvic rocking motions, side-to-side hip motion, circular and flowing motions performed at a walking pace with music or drumming. Dancing can be accompanied with a healing prayer or meditation, which can be done before, during and/or after the dance. The dancing can incorporate healing colors (blue, green, etc.) and/or purifying colors (yellow, white, etc.), along with incense, candles and/or a healing altar. There are many spiritual, mental and physical or holistic causes of fibroid tumors and many holistic variations for their treatment.

The failure to freely use the spiritual regeneration creative force, or Female Principle, self doubt and Slavery Trauma all contribute to the cause of fibroids. It is not just the fibroid tumor that is the issue; it is the health of men and children and the African culture that the uterus mirrors. Fibroids are a male and female problem that indicates a disease in the village (African society).

Cell Civilization

The cell civilization is important in understanding fibroids. The cell is the basic unit of the human body. Cells do not divide, only corpuscles divide. Cells have a nerve attached to them and a blood supply attached to the nerve (arteries). A melanin template grows and the mass (body) of the cell grows from the stole (melanin template). The cell gets old and dies, then a new stole grows and a new mass (body) grows from it. Cells are the foundation upon which tissues are formed. Tissues comprise organs, organs work collectively to form organ systems and the culmination of this cell progression is the human body. Subsequently, an understanding of the cell can improve the scope of comprehending fibroid tumors (abnormal cells) in the female body.

There are specific cell social behavior patterns which defend and control the cell community. Every cell defends itself against chemicals, waste or dangerous cells. The ability of the cell to defend itself is decreased by junk foods, drugs and poor nutrition. Defective weak cells develop due to biochemical imbalances. A defective cell is one which behaves contrary to the normal cell society. It makes the cell society (body) weak *(Beyond Reductionism* by P. Weiss).

Immunologists have revealed that the ability to develop cells that attack and destroy tumors (antibodies) and malignant tumor development (fibroids) have a close relationship. Animals that live a long time (humans) and eat junk foods, take drugs and vaccinations can cause a defective (mutated) cell to grow. Complex animals (humans) have many corpuscle divisions and cell growths. With each multiplication of cells comes the possibility of a cell defect. A natural whole foods diet helps to develop cell police that can destroy asocial cells (defected). (The *Logic of Scientific Discovery* by K. Popper).

Cell immaturity is one of the primary characteristics of a malignant tumor growth. When a cell loses the specific characteristics that make it a member of a particular tissue or organ such as the intestinal epithelium, mammary gland, endometrium or the epidermis, it regresses to an uncontrollable juvenile state similar to an ontogenetically or phylogenetically earlier growth phase. The cell begins to develop behavior similar to a unicellular organism or an embryonic cell and begins cell multiplication without consideration for the tissue it is supposed to be part of. The further the cell regresses, the more the newly developed tissue becomes asocial and defected the more malignant the tumor. Severe growths of malignant tumors depend on weak immunity and the inability to defend the healthy cells from defected asocial cells. This growth culminates when malignant cells are treated by the surrounding tissue cells as their own cell type and are nourished and protected by them. This is when the deadly infiltrative growth develops into a fibroid tumor (*Studies in Animal and Human Behavior* by K. Lorenz).

Types of Fibroids

(Internal Bumps), Types
Fibroids are also designated as myoma, fibro-myoma and fibrous tumors. Fibroids are a localized hypertrophy (Male Principle) or hyperplasia (Female Principle) within the uterine tissue. Hypertrophy is excessive growth of tissue without multiplication of its cells and can be due to sympathetic stress (Male Principle), acid imbalance and electrolyte insufficiency. While hyperplasia is the excessive growth of tissue due to excessive multiplication of its cells and can be due to parasympathetic stress (Female Principle), alkaline imbalance and electrolyte deficiency. These abnormal growths occur within the uterine wall as well as in the connective tissues, especially the fibrous. Abnormal growth in the fibers is called fibroids. When fibroids include amounts of muscular tissue growth of a pale fleshy color and do not feel like growths, but are more similar to an inflammation, it can indicate biochemical problems with the Male Principle. When fibroids are pale in color, more firm and dense in texture, almost cartilaginous and feel similar to a foreign body embedded in soft muscular tissue it can indicate biochemical problems with the Female Principle. According to their locality, they are given the names of subperitoneal, interstitial and submucous. All fibroids are interstitial in their early stages of growth and are caused by biochemical imbalances within the Male Principle or Female Principle.

The intramural or interstitial, fibroid tumor is located in the middle of the uterus muscular wall. This type of tumor predominantly develops entirely in the wall, and is painless. Occasionally, large intramural tumors will obstruct the birth canal and/or the fallopian tubes.

Fibroids are also located in the subserosal area of the uterus, beneath the peritoneum- the outer lining of the uterus. These tumors are classified as subperitonal (beneath the outer skin) or subserous (beneath the skin). They freely grow on any area of the uterus outer wall. The subserous fibroids sometimes achieve massive proportions and cause no other symptom except feelings of heaviness. If they grow in front of the uterus, they press against the bladder and cause urination difficulties. If they grow on the lower portion of the uterus, they can cause blockage of the birth canal. Enlarged or bloated veins on the surface of the subserous fibroids can rupture and bleed.

The subserous fibroids often develop to pedunculate (stalk like)—grow similarly to a tree on the outer portion of the uterus. They then attach themselves to the uterine wall by a stalk-like protuberance (growth), pedunculated subserous myoma (muscular type tumor) usually do not initiate pain until it twists around its own stalk. This causes the blood supply to the tumor to decrease. This decrease causes severe pain.

The submucous (beneath the inside skin) fibroid develops inside the uterine wall beneath the endometrium and protrudes into the uterine cavity. Submucous fibroids consist of about 5% of the various types of fibroids. They are the type that cause the most problems and severest difficulties. Submucous fibroids will enlarge and cause the uterus lining to break, thereby causing severe bleeding which can cause a woman to bleed to death. A submucous fibroid can also interrupt and disturb pregnancy. When the placenta begins to develop inside of the uterus, it can grow in the area of the myoma. This will stop the inner uterus skin from having an equal supply of blood as the other sections of the uterus starve the placenta of nutrients and blood. Subsequently, the placenta will not be able to bond to the endometrium area. This can result in hemorrhaging and miscarriage.

Submucous fibroids can also become pedunculated as they increase in growth. Consequently, the uterus then regards the fibroid as a foreign body and contracts in order to expel the fibroid. If the uterus successfully expels the pedunculated fibroid through the cervix, the myoma will remain attached by its stalk. This self-aborting tumor then becomes infected, ulcerated (develops sores) and bleeds. Fibroids are not an immediate threat to life and are not associated with cancer, although in rare cases there may be a secondary cancerous involvement.

In general, the symptoms of the interstitial and subperitoneal tumors are few. The physical difficulties, infertility problems and pain are associated with submucosal fibroids.

Subperitoneal fibroids
When they are massive, they give a sense of bearing down in the abdominal area and the abdomen as well as constipation, dysuria (painful and difficult urination), malnutrition (nutrients are diverted to and absorbed by the tumor) neuralgia (pain) of the lower extremities, back pain and shortness of breath.

Submucous fibroids
These have the same symptoms as the below interstitial fibroids but with increased severity. In addition to the excessive hemorrhage and menstrual colic, they are characterized by severe leukorrhea. The leukorrhea is caused by the bloating (distention) of the skin of the endometrium, resulting in mucous secretion. The colic is the primary result of labor-like muscle contractions by

the uterus in its efforts to expel the stagnated (rotten) blood in the dilated (bloated) vessels and/or may be the cause of irritation by submucous polypi (stem-like tumor).

Interstitial fluids
- Can cause forward or backward tilting of the cervix, uterus, etc.
- Can cause menstruation pain (dysmenorrhea)
- The primary symptoms are menorrhagia (excessive bleeding during pregnancy) and metrorrhagia (uterine hemorrhage between menstruations) accompanied by severe pain. The hemorrhaging (or menstruation) is caused by excessive dilation, which weakens the blood vessels of the uterine wall. A woman in this condition is usually anemic, which may cause hemorrhaging, which is considered natural. The herb Yellow Dock combined with Dandelion Root can supply the iron needed in anemia.

The treatment of fibroids by the orthodox medicine consists of monitoring them, which means to let them grow. The increased growth of the fibroid allows the woman to be easily persuaded and emotionally manipulated to have surgical removal of the fibroids by removing the uterus (hysterectomy). In menopausal women, the fibroid may degenerate, undergo softening, fatty degeneration, followed by induration (hardening) and finally calcification. The primary danger with surgery is that the cutting allows diseased cells to spread into the blood and tissues and the fibroids can suppurate (discharge pus), which can cause severe blood intoxication. Suppuration of subperitoneal fibroids can result in fatal peritonitis (inflammation of the skin inside the abdominal cavity).

Fibroids that are not treated can cause obstructions of the uterus and/or fallopian tubes, unnatural relocation of the uterine organs that result from tumors, tissue degeneration, interruption of the ability to bear a child or conceive and severe complications. The biochemistry of the female becomes imbalanced, immunity weakens and the moods fluctuate because of excessive blood loss and diversion of nutrients to nourish the tumor.

Treatment Modalities

Lemon
The lemon (alkaline energy) can be used to increase the elimination of toxins and for assisting in the fixation of useful elements. Treatment can consist of two to six fresh lemons a day based on individual tolerance. The lemon is the only food verified as having a juice (fresh) that is completely anionic. It is anionic because the electrons in orbit are spinning in a clockwise direction. All other scientifically verified foods are cationic. Subsequently, their electrons in orbit spin in a counter- clockwise direction. Fresh lemon juice inside the system can be converted into various types of

enzymes. Its conversion into enzymes requires less chemical change than any other natural substance scientifically known. However, there are females who have an allergic reaction to lemons. Women allergic to lemons can convert calcium into anionic substances. The herb Fennel, as well as the supplement Betaine Hydrochloride can help alkaline the system *(Health Guide for Survival* by S. Kirban).

Clay

The planet earth receives its vital life force energies from the air, sun and waters. The earth and its soil has the energies necessary to act as a healing agent of physical regeneration. The earth's skin of muds, sands and clay participate in the life generating, restoring, cleansing and protecting process of the earth. Clay, one of the earth's greasy dirt skins have a regenerating, cleansing, restoring and protecting quality when wet and impermeable. Analysis of clay reveals that it contains the following chemical elements and oxides in compound: Aluminum, Titanium, Silica, Potassium, Sodium and Magnesium. It is effective in treatment beyond the substances it contains, because it can stimulate healing (a catalyst) rather than acting as the agent of change (healing).

There are precautions that must be observed for internal and external clay treatments. Clay does not adjust itself to the presence of synthetic medicines and homeopathic remedies. It is recommended that internal clay treatment be preceded by drinking herbal purifying teas and/or antioxidant or immune enhancing supplements.

Clay is a beneficial remedy for fibroid tumors. Internally, the ingestion of 1 teaspoon of clay in a glass of distilled water, once a day on an empty stomach is beneficial. Clay and/or herbal poultices and/or rubbing clay over the uterus and abdomen can reduce (shrink) and dissolve cysts and uterine fibroids. The poultices can clay applications can be used until the cyst or fibroid is eradicated. The herbs White Willow, Arnica and/or Boswella can be added to poultices or clay applications in cases of pain. The clay application and poultices should be stopped during the period of menstruation. The poultice should be applied for at least two hours. It can be applied nightly and can remain on the body overnight. The poultice can be approximately 10 to 12 inches in length and one inch in width. The clay must be close to the skin, cheesecloth can be placed between the clay on hairy areas of the body only. Initiate the treatment with cold clay. Warm clay can be used in instances where tolerance is low towards cold clay. Put plastic or Saran wrap over the poultice and tape the poultices to the skin. In cases of bleeding tumors, alternate the clay with the application of a wheat bran-ivy poultice.

Herbal douches and synthetic douches can be replaced by Clay, Walnut Tree Leaf and Wild Alum Root douches. The treatment should consist of four tablespoons of Clay or Wild Alum Root powder in two quarts of tepid water, or two tablespoons of Clay and Wild Alum Root powder. Walnut leaves should be placed in two quarts of water, approximately two handfuls of leaves. They should be steeped for approximately 30 minutes. Douche temperature should be slightly tepid. The douche injections should be rapid. *(Our Earth, Our Cure* by R. Dextreit).

Autolysis, or self-destruction of tissue by its own enzymes, can be applied to the treatment of fibroid tumors. This treatment relies on the principle that the body, when anabolic (building) nutrients are below the optimum level, will maintain vital tissues and will not nourish the diseased tissue (fibroids). Tumors, when treated through autolysis, can be eradicated and seldom have recurrences. Rigid diet restriction and fasting are positive factors in autolysis. *(Every Woman's Guide to National Health* by G. Whitehorse).

Transmutation
Biological transmutation or conversions of one substance into another substance demonstrate that higher levels of energy can cause lower energy to change. Animals and plants have the ability to change one vitamin into another. The body has the biochemical ability to change unhealthy tissue (fibroids) into healthy tissue—transmutation.

Human beings have the potential to create the nutrients, which are missing from the diet. Optimum holistic health is required to do this. Many people are deficient in specific minerals because they cannot change (transmute) the nutrients they have into the nutrients they need. The body's inability to create the necessary nutrients for metabolic functions is the true essence of imbalance, ill health and dis-eases such as tumors. The utilization of transmutation of fibroid tumors should not be overlooked in a wholistic treatment approach *(Biological Transmutations* by Kervan).

Colonic Irrigation
The woman's body loses its immunity and ability to function optimally because the colon is impacted with waste. An impacted and diseased colon weakens the body and allows fibroids to form. A healthy colon is an essential ingredient in maintenance of wellness. Colonic irrigation can cleanse the colon. A colonic requires approximately twenty to thirty gallons of water injected into the colon through the rectum. Irrigation the plaster-like manure coating that accumulates within the colon as a result of junk foods. The pain that is experienced due to fibroids can be reduced by the use of colonics. A colonic frees the colon from the weight of the 5 to 10 pounds of impacted feces. This weighty manure coating of the colon affects the uterus, urinary bladder and the menstrual cycle. Colonic irrigation can aid the body in recuperating health and getting rid of fibroid tumors. In the colonic water can be cleansing, strengthening and laxative herbs. *(Colon Health* by N. Walker).

Herbal Treatment
Herbs offer a solution to fibroid tumors. Herbs should be used to cleanse the blood of the impurities in the system, nourish the body, build immunity and correct constipation.

Sage, Sanicle or Thuja poultices can eradicate the external tumors. A Slippery Elm poultice is also an excellent herb for tumors.

Internal tumors can be treated with the combination of two or three of the following herbs, from an allopathic, homeopathic or naturopathic perspective: Bayberry, Slippery Elm, Shepherd's Purse, Thuja, Witch Hazel, Mugwort, Chickweed, Wild Yam, Cranesbill, Burdock Root, Saw Palmetto, White Pond Lily. Red Clover, Dandelion Root, Goldenseal, Blue Violet, Yellow Dock, Rock Rose, Sorrel, Blue Flag, Virgin's Ower, Poplar and Comfrey, Blue Violet (combined with Red Clover Blossoms), Cleavers, Coral, and Poke Root (can be used as a poultice or tea).

The above herbs can also be used for the treatment of cancer. Cancer of the woman's reproductive organs can begin as fibroids (*Back to Eden* by J. Kloss).

Cell salts such as Kali Mur (potassium chloride), Silicea and Calcium Fluoride can be used for fibroids. Phosphoric acid, 3x can nourish the nervous system and circulatory system and can reverse bleeding. China 30x can be taken for leukorrhea and bleeding. In chronic bleeding and recent acute blood loss, Calcium Phosphate is helpful. The use of a heating pad with natural oil (i.e., Castor Oil) can be applied to the area between the anus and the coccyx bone for approximately twenty minutes. This treatment can be used on alternating days for the duration of a month. Do not use while menstruating. The heat application treatment is a technique that can be used to increase the hemotacrit index as well as other anti-anemia factors. Fibroids are associated with a decreased hemoglobin concentration or a low blood volume, which can be raised with a heating pad. A low blood volume can cause hemorrhaging, leukorrhea and fibroids. (*Mental and Elemental Nutrients* by C. Pfeiffer).

The dis-ease state of dysmenorrhea (painful menstruation) can also cause pain in the head, back and abdomen. Menstruation pain that can cause doubling over (momentarily bending over) which seems to lessen pain with pressure to the area can be treated with Colocynthia 12x. Five drops of Asafetida every three to four hours can be effective. After the pain has subsided, stay on a maintenance dose of five drops daily until the dysmenorrhea is eradicated. Colocynthia and Asafetida are not primarily relievers. Colocynthia, which should be continued following menstruation (two tablets twice per day) is effective for shrinking tumors. It is effective where high levels of lead have been ingested in the system. Asafetida is effective in eliminating dis-eased vaginal flora and syphilitic toxic residues that can cause tumors. China cannot be taken simultaneously with Asafetida. China antidotes the effectiveness of Asafetida.

Ferrum 2x to 6x tincture and Hamametis can effectively control the excessive bleeding between menses (or protracted menses) and menorrhagia (bleeding during menses)

Calcium Iodide 3x is useful in shrinking tumors and treating females with tumors that have had have a history (beginning in childhood) of glandular enlargements (thyroid, adenoids, tonsils).

Indian Pennywort (hydrocotyle) 1x-6x is useful with dermatological dis-eases such as skin infections. The primary difficulties are imbalanced vaginal flora, excess estrogen and syphilitic residual toxins from past treated or untreated infections. White Ash (Fraxinus Americana) tincture 10-15 drops three times per day.

Thuja (Arbor Vitae) 6x can be used externally and applied locally, particularly in spongy polypi. The treatment of polypi can be facilitated through oral usage with 6x tablets of Thuja. This is usually indicated for women who have a history of gonorrhea. The primary factors that indicate Thuja usage are profuse wart growth on the skin and mucous membrane. A thick, excessive, sometimes greenish color and fish brine odored leukorrhea can indicate Thuja use. Silicea, Savine (Sabina), and Thuja 6x are particularly useful remedies in women who are habitual aborters in their third month.

Synthetic foods and vinegar, excess salt, excess sugar and alcohol can derange connective tissues. The use of tea, chocolate and coffee contain substances that interfere with the RNA functions in cells (intelligence mechanism). This is a contributory factor in the development of fibroids. Alcoholic beverages, caffeinated tea and coffee stops the effectiveness of herbal remedies. Sodas are high in caffeine content, which causes nerve irritability that has pain-intensifying properties. *(How to Use the 12 Tissue Salt by E. Chapman).*

Summary View of Women's Wholistic Health
As women begin to define for themselves their own optimum nutrition, hormone levels and health standards and become aware of the intrinsic nature of their physiology their health will become a true reality. The beginning of this reality starts when the female holistically defines for herself the internal organs and external environment from the Male Principle and Female Principle. If the understanding of health disease remedies, wellness, exercise, spirituality and society is done only from the Male Principle, then dis-ease will destroy the woman. If the relationship between herself and the universe, children, males and life is not holistic, then there is no future for the female because she cannot create herself unless she has the natural energies of Male and Female Principles. If she does not have the natural energies for creating and sustaining herself, the Caucasian culture is going to create her. It will create her to be an enemy to herself, her culture and her ancestors.

What are the natural energies that the woman has for creating herself? Females defining themselves spiritually and spirituality defining them physically is offered as the natural creating energies.

The women's physiology has an energy related organ community (organ systems). The reproductive organs are responsible not only for themselves but to all other organs. The cosmic energy of the galaxy as it affects the moon cycles, menstruation, birthing, vegetables, sun, fruit, organs, menopause, sexual personality, exercise, emotions and male relationships have an effect on the female and defines the female. Additionally, the harmony that the body maintains with melanin means that an insufficient or deficient amount of melanin spells disease (leukorrhea, fibroids, etc.). Determine your melanin level with a pulse rate and respiratory rate ratio.

For example:

P   (Pulse rate for 1 minute) $\dfrac{80 \text{ pulse}}{20 \text{ respiration}} = 4$

RR   (Respiratory Rate for 1 minute)

If the fraction (ratio) reduces to a number above 4 or more, then there is melanin insufficiency. If the number is 3 or less, then there is a melanin deficiency.

Fibroid tumors have a controlling effect on the body, spirit, mind, emotions and actions and help to continue the oppression of the race. Leukorrhea makes the body susceptible to illness and Caucasian medicine. With Caucasian medicine comes Caucasian culture, oppression, exploitation and Bi-Polar White Supremacy Psychosis.

The use of natural wholistic treatment helps the body to defend its most important product—life!

The objective of wholistic remedies is to give the responsibility of health back to the owner. The owner of health is each individual woman.

White Racism Addiction

The Steps to addiction are:
1. Initiate
2. Re-initiate
3. Needs development (craving)
4. Mental dependency
5. Physical dependency

The addiction complex starts when an individual or culture (Black people) is (1) initiated to the object of addiction [behavior servitude or substance (alcohol)]. Usually a friend, peer or relative gives the alcohol to the individual at a social gathering (wedding, party, dance). Next, the individual is (2) re-initiated and given alcohol at a societal function. Then the individual associates an alcoholic drink with a social gathering and (3) needs development or craves a drink at a party. Next, the individual becomes mentally (4) dependent on a drink at parties and uses alibis and irrational justifications for drinking. Then, the individual becomes (5) physically dependent on alcohol and at this point is called an addict. This addicted Black person wants to serve (work for) Caucasians, wants a Caucasian education and awards (Oscar, Grammy), is behaving to be rewarded by Whites. The Black person sees himself and whites as one (we). This type of Black person will kill to protect Caucasian culture. The Black person with Caucasian addiction has a psychosis (total break with reality). This addiction is the only form of democracy whites practice. White Racism/White Supremacy is democratized—equally distributed to Black folks all over this planet. This addiction sustains white supremacy, exploitation, oppression, violence, criminalization, inferiorization and unchained slavery of Black folks. Blacks have co-dependent White Racism Addiction while Caucasians have White Racism Addiction. Blacks that depend upon white acceptance, approval and rewards are co-dependent. A Slavery Traumatized Black person thinks Caucasians are meant to be in charge and will always be in charge. They visualize success in a white world. Caucasians with the addiction are drunk on White Supremacy and assume they will always be in control.

Addictive Steps
The White Racism Addiction defends the psychosis of White Supremacy. It is founded upon the belief that Whites are supreme. It has created the myth that an albinism (deficiency of melanin) is superior. White racism becomes addicting because the Caucasian educational system defines Caucasian education as the best. The Caucasian's science is promoted as the only true science, European limp hair is the most beautiful hair, European music is civilized, Caucasian culture is the highest culture, Caucasian laws and justice are the correct laws and justice, while every aspect of Black culture is democratically made inferior. *(The Cress Theory* by Frances Cress Welsing). Caucasian culture creates and maintains White Supremacy and White Racism Addiction through its medias (television, radio, newspapers, religious books, cartoons, fairy tales, text books, movies, science). Whites create a Willie Lynch mentality in Caucasians and constantly re-initiated Blacks into White Racism Addiction. The White Supremacist is constantly made addicted to White Racism. Their psychosis is made to be normal. In other words, the White Supremacist is never far away from his next White Superiority fix. He begins to crave the White racism because his peers give him mental and emotional support and elevate his self-esteem for being a conformist to the addiction. The addict has a mental dependency and needs to think himself superior in order to feel normal. The addicts have drug parties (social activities and conversations) that reinforce White Supremacy. The White racist addict depends upon Black mammies (i.e., Oprah) and Uncle Bens (Montel, Colin Powell) to solve Caucasian emotional and social problems. They depend upon Black servitude roles such as house nigger jobs (office workers, soldiers, scientists, professional athletes, entertainers, doctors, mayors and elected offi-

cials). Blacks may view the jobs differently. However, the Caucasians militarily and economically own the house (i.e., America, Africa) and the Black race works in the Caucasian house. They serve the owner of the house (slave master). Thus, the jobs serve to better Caucasian culture not Black culture. The White addicts depend on Blacks for physical entertainment (actors, singers, musicians). Black entertainers who entertain White or predominately white audiences are modern-day coons and nigger minstrel characters. It is ironic that the sex fantasies of Whites subliminally requires the African clothes of so-called sexually exotic, erotic, savage and hyper-sexed Black primitives. White women dress in African Egyptian clothing styles called nightgowns. They subconsciously use Egyptian clothing for the enhancement of their sex behavioral fantasies. This reinforces White Supremacy.

Bi-Polar White Supremacy Psychosis uses White Racism to defend the psychosis. White Racism is terrorism. This terrorism makes Blacks fear and stand in awe of Caucasian power, military governments and money. Power and money are words that mean "if you do not accept Caucasian rule, then you get Caucasian violence (war, economic blockage, etc.)." Money is backed by violence, not by gold. Caucasian terrorism is White Racism Addiction, racial profiling, denial of reparations, vaccinations, miseducation, materialistic and sex rap videos, forcing African countries to pay debts, etc. White Racism Addiction is a self-imposed terrorism that has been socially engineered into the Black psyche.

Bi-Polar means the White Supremacy Psychosis uses passive and active (maniac, aggressive) tactics as tools to defend White Supremacy. The psychosis (craziness) uses violence (wars) to maintain peace and uses peace as a tool to control violence. In other words, violence (active) and peace (passive) are one and the same. They are mixed together as one. The American Indians would say that "White man speaks with a forked tongue," which means he lies and tells the truth only to maintain White Supremacy. He is Bi-Polar. White Racism Addiction has the addict believing that they are not addicted while at the same time they are addicted (Bi-Polar).

The English language has built-in rewards for White Racism Addicts. This language has over 200 negative meanings for the word Black. The use of this language by Whites gives them a false sense of superiority similar to a euphoric high of a heroin addict except this high is in the mind. Some of the negative connotations are blackmail (criminal act), black humor (low humor with cursing), black day (sad day), black list (people forbidden to participate in an activity), black clothes (associated with funerals = death), black hat (worn by the bad guy in westerns, white hat by good guy), blacken your name (make your name disrespectable), etc. Further, colors near black are also negative: blues (sad), devil's food cake (evil dark brown color), blue moon (lover separated from loved one), etc. These words and phrases perpetuate White racism. *(Prejudice and Racism* by J. Jones; see Anatomy, Psychology in Chart Section). White Racism

Addiction helps act out the psychosis. Hatred of Blacks is one of the physical manifestations (lynching, judiciary lynching, jails) of this mental illness. The addict's culture has a psychosis. A psychosis is a self-created ill-founded belief held despite obvious facts to the contrary. In this psychosis, Caucasians can stand in front of the architectural miracle the African Giza pyramid and say that the pyramid does not exist. Caucasians see with their mind. They believe then they see. They have lying eyes. They see what their mind tells them to see. Their eyes deny reality. The pyramids are physical evidence that the Black race and culture is the oldest, most highly developed socially, and most scientific of all races on this planet. However, the Caucasian cannot see reality because the psychosis is a break with reality. The addiction craves more unreality (its drug) and usurps and cannibalizes African people and culture in order to maintain the high. They need treatment. An African cannot join the insane (become insane) in order to treat the insane. Black folks cannot join the system in order to change the system. If they do it, it is because they do not know the power of the system. The education, legal, political and economic systems are an outgrowth of the culture. The culture creates and maintains the systems. In order to change the system, the culture would have to change first. It is white culture that is sick (White Supremacy Psychosis). It is a waste of energy and time to try to change the systems. It is Caucasian culture. The culture and systems are one and the same. White Supremacy is White culture, they are one and the same. Only a Caucasian can change Caucasian culture. The efforts of Hippocrates to get his Caucasian culture to change to eating health foods took over 2,000 years and still junk food is king. Caucasians still do not associate White Supremacy as a disease. To be crazy is to be normal.

The White Racism Addiction high is maintained by myths about the founders of health. Egyptian medicine is clearly referred to in writings of Galen, Dioscorides, Pliny, and Hippocrates as pointed out in *The Legacy of Egypt* by S.R.K. Glanville. Egyptian medical knowledge is the foundation of African traditional medicine (this includes herbs, drugs, acupuncture, massage, diet therapy, etc.) of the Songoan culture dating to the Paceolithicus Period about 100,000 years ago. The priest/monk doctors educated through the mystery systems was part of the Lupemban, Stillbay, and Rhodesian cultures of Mesocithic Period dating 30,000 to 8,000 B.C. The culture of the African Zinjanthropus Boise dating 600,000 B.C. was highly developed which indicates medicinal herbal knowledge. This clearly confirms that Africa's medical science was developed long before Caucasian cultures. Despite all this evidence, Caucasians believe the myth that Hippocrates discovered medicine. The African surgical, diagnosis and herb/drug prescriptions are used by Caucasians. They use them to suppress and cut out disease. However, it is an ancient modern science that the Caucasians say they discovered and they say using ancient African science makes this modern.

Wholistic medical science includes psychology, sociology, computer science, meditation, natural birth, music, art, etc. Yet, the addicted Europeans say that they are studying and incorporating Eastern (Chinese, Japanese) medicine into their orthodox medicine. The Eastern medical science was taught to the Chinese and Japanese by Africans. The Caucasians continue to credit the Orientals (at the exclusion of Black Africa) with the African sciences. History continuously contradicts this White Racism Addiction lie. The "lies" are used to maintain the high. The high is used to maintain White Supremacy.

The oldest written therapeutic usage of the science of massage is in the books of Imhotep. He wrote of the cellular nutritive usage of massage, the muscle relaxation dynamics of massage and the increased mobility of the muscular system. In fact, he wrote of the psychosomatic applications and hypnotic usages of massage.

Hipprocrates (called himself an Escalapian = Greek word for Imhotep) learned of some of the basic massage techniques in Africa and wrote about it in 430 B.C. It was Hippocrates used African herb knowledge. Furthermore, one of the oldest drawings of massage, the 2,000-year-old Alabaster Relief, shows a Black African Assyrian named San Herib receiving a therapeutic massage. This drawing can be found in the Bergamon Museum in Berlin.

Reality has no place with the addict. Despite historical evidence, the addicted culture credits their Caucasian usurpers of massage with establishment of massage as a science. The ancient African civilization practiced massage. Their massage knowledge was widespread in the Pacific Basin cultures. The Japanese, Indians and Chinese practiced massage around 700 B.C. In addition to massage, the Ancient Romans used the African massage cylinder roller device known as thermo-massage. Roman artifacts discovered in Herculaneum and Pompeii verifies this. Peter Henry Ling, a Swede, studied the ancient Greek manuscripts on massage, which were derived from the African Medical Records. The Cong-Fou of the Tao-Tee, an ancient Chinese book (contains medical and massage knowledge) and is over 3,000 years old was translated to French in 1830. In the same century after this publication of the translation, Mr. Ling presumably renamed African massage techniques Swedish massage. However, Greek records verify that Hippocrates learned massage from Africans. Hippocrates' African information was studied by Henry Ling via the manuscripts. In fact, Hippocrates stated that physicians must know massage above all else. Aristotle also learned African massage and used African olive oils and water treatments. In the European Middle Ages, massage and massage oil were used as a treatment for many diseases that caused plagues, famines and death. They sought curative African oils erroneously called perfumes, essences and spices. White Racism Addiction can be cured by the Caucasians only. The Caucasian therapist must make the addict analyze their personal and cultural need for White Supremacy. The addict must actively stop all forms (i.e., movies, books, colleges, art, history, medicine, etc.) of participation in White Supremacy or else remain addicted. As long as the addicts says "things are getting better for Blacks," "society is changing," "Blacks are not as bad off," "it is not my fault what my White ancestors did," "Blacks always want a handout," "Blacks sold each other in slavery (overlooking that Whites owned, controlled and created slavery)," "I don't hate Blacks," "Blacks are not trying to lift themselves up," "you people are always complaining and getting emotional about nothing," etc., they will remain addictive. This psychosis is unwholistic and is a disease of spirit, mind and body.

Addiction to White Racism is destroying the ability of Caucasians to participate in the cultural world of people of color.

White racism addicts continuous direct and indirect verbal and non-verbal messages of White supremacy and Black inferiority causes Blacks to be made to feel inferior. For example, Blacks straighten their kinky woolly hair with hot steel combs and grease (hair frying) or straighten their hair with chemical relaxers. This process allows their hair to resemble the White race. White folk's hair is called good hair while Black's hairs is called bad or hard to manage. Straightening Black hair is a form of self-hatred in that Blacks are actively rejecting their own racial characteristics (kinky hair). No matter what the reason a Negro gives for straightening their hair, it amounts to "I hate being Black and African culture." Black men cut their hair very short and shave a hairline around their hair so they can look neat and clean. Their barbershops help them to resemble the nice and neat hair of the Caucasians. This cultural treason causes Blacks to maintain their own inferiority. For example, Black Uncle Tom scientists (biologists, druggists, chemists, medical doctors, nurses, mathematicians, physiologists, etc.) are addicted to Caucasians. They do not use Afri-Centric scientific wisdom and believe the only biology, chemistry and sciences are White. In fact, they reject their own culture's scientific superiority. The White Supremacist Caucasian scientist denounces a Black scientist that arrives at the conclusion that water is wet without Caucasian scientific laboratory testing methods and documentation. Uncle Tom Black scientists are drunk on White science and are practicing cultural adultery upon African science and Africanity. They are too afraid to be Black or African.

Black folks suffering from White Racism Addiction Co-Dependency are mentally ill. They have a psychosis by White psychology standards and psychosis by Black psychology standards. In other words, they are twice as sick and not in their right minds. (See Psychology Chart). Black folks' death, fibroid tumors, prisoners, suicide, diabetes, high school drop outs, high blood pressure, depression, dialysis, prostate disease and tooth decay rate is very high. Black folks solve this very high disease rate by getting high (sex, drugs, marijuana, cocaine, alcohol). What for? They are already high.

LIMITATION: HUNGER

The Caucasian processed food industry is nutritionally limited and disease causing. The industry has sacrificed variety for quantity, limiting the food supply to those moneymaking plants and animal food crops that can easily accept pesticide injections, cloning, hybridizing, genetic modification and that can grow on synthetic (fertilized) soil. They have made seeds that only produce one crop. This creates nutritional deficiencies while the varied African whole food diet is a complex cross of nutrients, which eliminates deficiency. *(Hunger and History by* E. Prentice, *Health From the Ground Up* by Karl Mickey, *Fasting and Undernutrition* by Morgulis).

The Caucasian processed food industry produces limited varieties of food. There are over 350,000 species of edible plants and only 60 are grown by the industry. The meat industry limits their meat diet to 50 animals out of over 2,000,000 known species. In contrast, the typical African on the Gold Coast had an organic whole food diet of over 114 species of fruit, 47 varieties of greens, 46 species of legumes and edible plants not yet known or identified by Caucasian scientists. African people who are forced to abandon their natural food diet for a processed food diet lose their natural instinct specific hunger appetite.

Instinct specific hunger appetite is a desire for nutrients in foods. Today's appetite is created and manipulated by the junk food and meat industry. It is a food craving addiction to eat to fill the stomach, not to fill specific nutrient needs. In other words, Blacks eat what they are trained to eat and not what they nutritionally need. Blacks of equatorial Africa suffering from an iron deficiency caused by Caucasian processed foods are instinctively driven to eat clay (source of minerals). Other colored people such as the Eskimo will eat caribou dung (feces), stomachs of dead animals, and animal bones because the hunger instinct naturally directs them to sources of vitamins and minerals. This instinct specific appetite is lost in Caucasian cultures because foods are the denatured, processed and made into food drugs. These synthetic food type drugs are robbed of nutritional value. Those Africans trained to eat the Caucasian processed diet are no longer capable of using their inherent hunger instinct appetite. Junk foods negatively affects the spirit, mind and body. The Caucasian diet is wheat, potato and meat-centered and created to exploit the consumer for the benefit of the food industry.

In East Africa the *Kikuyu* and the *Masai* peoples live. The *Masai* grow large because they consume cow's milk and the nutrients in cow's milk are geared to grow large cows. The cow's grains are meant to grow large cows and the Masai eat the same grains and grow large. While, the Kikuyu who live the same region grow smaller, they are farmers and live on legumes, tubers and cereals. Further, the Gredanese Blacks, Berber tribes of the Sahara, and cattle raisers of the upper Nile and savannas eat the same diet and grow small. Diets, which are limited to a few plants, are nutritionally dangerous. Moreover, the Blacks who raise a grain food and/or cattle crop for the European market tend to eat a very limited variety of foods. Farmland devoted almost entirely to sugar cane causes other foods not to be grown or be consumed. Manioc flour and cassava supplemented the cane diet causing protein deficiencies. The Caucasians control the crops and land. They indirectly control the diet, appetite and nutrition. African diets are made limited by local environments and the Caucasian control of food crops and natural resources cause the local Africans to have bodily development abnormalities and malnutrition. Protein malnutrition causes AIDS. Therefore, indirectly and directly, Caucasians create disease. Disease means profits for the non-profit businesses and medical industry.

Pygmies (Ashante) of equatorial Africa lose their small physique when they migrate to the plains regions where food is available that is more nutritionally balanced than the rain forest diet. The same type of larger physique occurs with the typically small Chinese and Japanese. When they emigrate to America, it takes two generations before they increase several inches in height.

Another example of nutritional deficiency taken to be normal is the Shetland pony's diet (smallest horse in the world). These horses grow on the Shetland Islands of the British Isles. When the horses are brought to America and fed a better diet, they grew to a normal size after several generations. The nutritional deficient plants grown on a nutrient deficient soil of the Shetland pastures caused the small size of the horse.

When the Caucasians limit the food supply by controlling the crops, land diseases occur. For example, the monoculture (one plant) of sugar cane, mono-crop exploitation of rubber caused beriberi in the Amazon and monocrop cotton caused pellagra. These crops caused distorted hunger sensations because the nutrient range is narrowed by limited crops. A limited nutrient range causes a drug-like craving for a few foods. These few foods have nutritional limitations that caused distorted appetites and diets.

Hunger for specific vitamins, minerals and proteins can produce an appetite that craves the few foods that have the nutrients for the hunger. This deranged appetite causes sexual problems. This subclinical malnourishment triggers the survival instinct and sex. Lack of male hormones due to chronic under nutrition can cause homosexual behaviors, thermal fatigue and development of breasts among men. The lack of hormones can cause male behaviors and characteristics among women. This nutritionally deprived diet affects vital organs. For example, the liver and ovaries are related because the liver inactivates the excess estrogen, which the ovaries pour into the blood. When the liver is weaken and loses its reserve energy (or stored sugar), it can no longer defend the body from the stress hormone estrogen. The body interprets a weakened liver as a crisis and sends out the message that it is in danger of death. Then the adrenal gland sends a message to the pancreas to release enzymes. The liver releases stored glycogen sugar and the pancreas releases insulin to stimulate the break down the stored sugar, so the sugar can be used for the crisis. This sympathetic (fight, flight, protect) nervous system response deactivates the parasympathetic (relax, build, repair) nervous system. This results in liver and adrenal fatigue and may cause mood swings, mental depression and a craving for sugar. In any case, a weakened liver due to synthetic drugs, computers, alcohol, smoking, and an acidic junk food diet causes excess estrogen in the blood. This excess estrogen causes high blood pressure, stress, arthritis, diabetes, bone loss, reproduction problems, eye problems, kidney disease, etc.

Animal hunger is affected by the nutritionally limited animal farming diets. These diets include steroids, estrogen hormones, antibiotics, drugs and chemicals that threaten the lives of the food animals. These animals nervous system interprets this subclinical starvation as a survival crisis and start to reproduce. An animal that is sickly reproduces quickly. The ancient Romans thought that domesticated animals and people were servants designed to for food, labor and to reproduce more laborers and food. The Romans called these offspring proles or proletarians. Later in history, proles became associated with the peasants and working class. Notwithstanding, the soil is the basic foundation of animal, plant and human diets.

European induced soil erosion is a symptom of a bad relationship between them and the soil, just as skin eruptions and tooth decay are symptoms of a poor nutritional relationship with food. Europeans destroy the land and plan for a future that the land will eventually deny. The whole food diet of Africans was based upon a great respect for the soil as a living part of God. Soil is limited such as the black soil of the temperate and humid regions, which is rich in phosphorus and calcium but lacks iodine while red soil (laterite) is poor in phosphorus and calcium. Consequently, plants from various land localities are combined with a cross mixture of plants to avoid nutritional deficiencies in the African diet.

It has to be noted that the absence of varieties of foods in the European diet was overcome by their invasions of Africa. In the book *Foods America Gave the World* by E. Hyatt Verill it is mentioned that the Caucasian limited diet became expanded by the introduction of popcorn, plant sap (chewing gum), *Xictomatl* (tomato), cassava (tapioca), *Cassareep* (basic ingredient in Worcestershire sauce), and over 50 varieties of beans, and five varieties of potatoes, corn, and nuts that they got from Africa and the Americas.

The Caucasian' invasion (Race War) of Africa for food to combat Europe's starvation was necessary for their nutritional survival. Caucasians lacked an agriculture science and wide food varieties and were ignorant of the use of African herb medicine. For example, many ancient Roman recipes were collected by a Roman named *Apicius*. He committed suicide after an elaborate gourmet dinner. Further, in the book *Gluttons and Gourmets* by Betty Wason, extensive use of medicinal herbs are mentioned as part of recipes. Roman foods were usually contaminated, poisoned with lead, overcooked and constipating. The overcooked diets of most Romans consisted of starchy concoctions. The majority of the Romans were on welfare (public relief, homeless and poor). Caucasian civilizations exploit their own kind—reducing the masses to starvation and a general welfare mentality state. The African agriculture and food science and herbal medicine was Euro-centrically acculturated by various Caucasian tribes.

The European tribal laws have allowed the "wise ones" or "learned members," so-called businessmen, to create a privileged group. In former times, this privileged group was called lords, secret societies, elite, feudal kings, popes, merchants or traders. When Caucasian ethnic groups (French, German, etc.), tribes or clans unite, they are called multinational corporations. These corporations have used the time tested colonial systems. They have colonized the concept of God, sex, knowledge, information, people, science and the food industry. Small farmers of vegetable and food animal crops must sell to these huge modern day feudal lords (multinationals). These multinationals privately own the government, money and the militaries. The food regulatory agencies are puppets to protect their colonies. Unfortunately, it is the health of the consumer that is eaten away by the processed synthetic poisonous foods. The multinationals (Caucasian clans and tribes) have exploited Black labor (chattel slavery and wage slavery) and African land until Black labor is no longer economically needed. The Caucasians have continued to exploit Black's health with synthetic drugs and artificial processed food until the remaining Black populations are not only a sick and endangered species but on the verge of termination as a race. Aside from this factor, a limited diet creates diseases.

The orthodox European medical treatments are culturally confined. They involve the need for Caucasian trained or Black schools with a Caucasian Curriculum in the profession of nurses, doctors, specialists and laboratories, X-rays, DNA testing, computers and high priced hospital confinements that follows Caucasian protocols. The Caucasian colonialization of medicine and the food supply has cause a high death rate amongst the poor and forced Black folks to abandon their traditional medicine and culture. Herbal disease healings are cheap in economic cost and holistically viable while Caucasian suppression of disease symptoms, surgical (laser) operations and drugs are expensive—profitable.

There are three types of healings: (1) healing (psychological and spiritual); (2) therapy (homeopathic and naturopathic); and (3) suppressions (allopathic). Drug (poisons) remedies are a relic from European poison lore in that a greater evil is used to destroy a lesser evil. Hygienic cures simply supply the moral conditions so that the body can get well. Basically, they assist the body in its natural tendency to cure itself. Diseases are either mental or physical conditions that tend to cure themselves or physical conditions that do not cure themselves. Eighty percent of the diseases are mental and physical which tend to cure themselves. Ninety percent of the diseases can be treated hygienically (naturopathically), while ten percent can be treated allopathically (herbal allopaths not drug allopaths). Ninety percent of the diseases that get well on their own are relegated to modern medical miracle cures or faith healings.

An individual develops a disease, then gets treated and then gets well. It follows that the treatment cured the disease. Actually the individual got well despite the treatment. However, faith healers and allopaths assumed that their powers cured the disease. In lower levels of civilization, faith healing is the norm while in higher holistic African civilizations, hygienic cures are the norm. Moreover, Caucasian allopathic drug medicine suppresses disease (keep them in the body), soothes the symptoms and does not treat the cause of disease. The processed food industry creates 80% of the diseases and blames all diseases on a bacteria or virus. Processed and cloned foods weaken and deteriorate the health resulting in diseases.

European culture with DNA cloning and its mechanical gadgets and technical developments can create an artificial nature by controlling the weather and using greenhouses that control the climate to grow plants and animals indoors (houses, factories, farms, barns) but Caucasians cannot escape nature forever. They cannot escape nature's revenge and cyclic laws. They can accidentally clone a disease strain that ha no cure or stops reproduction.

AIDS:
A BLACK GENOCIDE GAME

AIDS (Acquired Immune Deficiency Syndrome) was previously called IDS (Immune Deficiency Syndrome). In ancient Caucasian history, it was called the Black Death. The Black Death was characterized by swollen glands, cyst, tumors, bumps, colds, flu, weight loss, skin rot, weakness and eventual death. Today, the Black Death and the common Cold are classified as a loss of immunity. Caucasians define all diseases as a failure of the immune system. Diseases are the body's cleansing process. The body is trying to get well and this is erroneously called a disease.

Diseases of the sex organs arouse fear, emotions and religious issues. It is easier to market a disease such as AIDS if there is sex attached to it. It makes it easier to get the victims to take worthless drugs (i.e., AZT). Taking AZT is like playing Russian roulette with a lethal poison instead of a lethal bullet. It will kill you, but the Disease/Medical industry will always say you die of AIDS and complications of AIDS. If a healthy person takes AZT, they will die within three years (according to Glaxco-Smith, the manufacturers of the drugs). However, they won't prescribe it to a healthy person as this would expose the AIDS genocide crimes.

It has never been clinically proven that a Retrovirus causes AIDS. AIDS is a syndrome with many causes that produces multiple effects and diseases. A syndrome is a collection of diseases. It is not one disease with one cause. It is an effect looking for a cause. Many people that die of AIDS do not have the dead cell particle called a Retrovirus. It has not been proven that sex alone caused the AIDS epidemic. It is more of a political, social and military caused un-disease (non-disease). The fear that AIDS creates causes many people to believe in drug medicines. Fear is used to keep people believing that only drugs (prescription and over-the-counter) will protect and save them. Fear is a marketing tool of terrorists, drug companies, research institutions, religions (fear God and Devil), etc.

AIDS is a syndrome. A syndrome is a group of symptoms and clinical signs that a medical group or insurance companies put together and call a disease. You can add or subtract signs and symptoms from a syndrome as you will. It is a subjective (psychological and emotional) not a objective (chemical test) issue.

AIDS is an arbitrary psychologically and emotionally based collection of signs and symptoms. The ELISA test for AIDS is imperfect but the CDC says it is more accurate than the other imperfect AIDS tests. It will record 200 false AIDS positives (inaccurate/wrong) for every 29 true positives per 100,000 persons.

The ELISA test measures the ability of the body to protect itself. The logic of the test is basically a scientific psychosis. The test shows that your body has an antibody to protect itself. Therefore, if the test shows you have antibodies then that is interpreted to mean you have AIDS. This is crazy and a psychotic conclusion. For example, if you take a mathematics test and pass the test (positive reaction) the teacher would say you passed the test because you failed the test. Therefore, the teacher would put you in Special Education (give you AZT).

There are over twenty-nine diseases and signs that can cause a positive on the ELISA test. Some of them are microbes, malnutrition, Herpes Simplex II, Hepatitis B, Lupus, Myeloma, Hemodialysis, vaccinations, prior pregnancy, silicone implant, cross reaction, alcoholic hepatitis, malaria, tuberculosis, drugs, clotting factors, toxins, cancer, arthritis, cold virus, pregnancy, influenza, semen, another retrovirus, hemophiliac blood products, parasites, infection, worms, etc. This can cause 83% false positives. All positives are indicated as AIDS. There are many diseases on the list that are disease in themselves. They do not need to be called AIDS as they already have a name. Why give a disease a new name? The major cause of AIDS positives, in Africa, is malaria, tuberculosis and malnutrition. These are already diseases. Why call them AIDS?

A retrovirus is present in AIDS victims and is believed to be the cause of the doubling the amount of AIDS victims each year. The early stages of the diseases usually manifest symptoms such as lymph gland swellings, sudden drastic weight loss, prolonged diarrhea, night sweats, extended periods of fatigue and skin diseases. This is usually followed by fungus growth in the mouth, central nervous system malfunctions, tuberculosis, genital warts, Kaposi's sarcoma and finally death. Ironically, venereal diseases such as herpes, yeast infections, gonorrhea, syphilis can be a prelude to AIDS.

Further, AIDS and AIDS Related Condition (ARC) are systemic. Systemic means a weakness or disease of all the bodily organs, tissues, bones, muscles, nerves and all systems. Therefore, it follows, that an AIDS virus (retrovirus) is not the single cause of the disease. This retrovirus is a sign of the health being totally collapsed.

Men and women with AIDS are systemically (entire body) diseased. They do not realize they have AIDS because AIDS can take up to 3 to 14 years before it is defined or has recognizable symptoms that Western (Caucasian) medicine calls AIDS. Meanwhile, the AIDS victims can sexually spread the disease to other people with already weakened immune systems. *(The Truth About AIDS: Evolution of an Epidemic* by A. Fattner).

A disease such as AIDS requires a group of medically defined symptoms before it can be medically classified as AIDS. So it follows that less than the specific number of symptoms (can be less than 6 or 10) means that an AIDS victim does not medically have complete AIDS but partial AIDS called AIDS Related Condition (ARC). This is the absurdity of modern Caucasian medical thought. In other words, if you use this medical model, a woman can be pregnant and classified as not pregnant because she does not fit the Caucasian's subjective signs and symptoms of pregnancy. While in truth, a woman is either pregnant or not. An AIDS victim either has the disease or does not. There is no such thing as having partial (half) AIDS (so-called "Lesser AIDS") or ARC. One either has the disease or does not have it. The fact is that Caucasian modern medicine is ill equipped to do pre-early and early diagnosis of AIDS until AIDS has advanced to the terminal state. While in African traditional medicine, disease diagnosis takes place before the symptomatic signs that Caucasians (Western Medicine) require to make an early diagnosis (*see* Holistic Chart). In African medicine, the defense of the body starts with a natural foods diet. Immunity is built and established by the digestive system, especially the colon. The immunity is only as healthy as the colon. Aside from this, once the AIDS retrovirus goes into the human chromosomes, it has become a living part of the body, so to kill the virus, one would have to kill the AIDS victim.

Immunity begins in the colon. The processed foods (junk foods) diet consists of diseased food. Diseased foods are those foods which are processed, genetically modified, cloned, hybridized, synthetically chemicalized with additives, and cannot grow if once again returned to the soil. The junk food diet includes salt, fried foods, oils, white sugar, antibiotics, hormones, suppressant and poisonous drugs, along with alcohol, recreational drugs, and polluted water. Antibiotics (Tetracycline, Penicillin) are 100% immune suppressive. This means that continuous use of synthetic antibiotics destroys the immune systems. This diet of non-fiber, nutritionless foods alter the friendly relationships of bacteria flora that live in the digestive tract (includes colon). These bacteria flora are necessary for digesting food and protecting the body. However, once they are put in an imbalanced state by junk foods, these same 32 pounds of intestinal flora (yeast, fungus, bacteria) become an enemy of the body and attack it (M. Speck, "Contributions of Microorganisms to Foods and Nutrition, *Nutrition News,* 38 (4): 13, 1975). Consequently, the immune system is destroyed by the biochemical effect cloned and/or synthetic processed junk foods. The orthodox western (Caucasian) medical system has manipulated the health standards so that being ill (from junk and cloned foods) is considered normal. (K. Shahani, J. Uakil, A. Kilara *Natural Antibiotic Activity of Lactobacillus Acidophilus and Bulgaricus II.* Isolation of acidolphilin from L. acidolphilus. Cultured Dairy Products J 12(2): 8, (1977).

The Western medical system, pharmaceutical cartel and food industrial empire have chained together chemicals. They have chained together DNA (cloned plants/animals) and synthetic chemicals to make junk foods that are genetically and chemically unsafe and cause diseases. Oddly enough, they have found that one chemical combined with another forms a new chemical. They know the effects of the individual chemicals, but not the chemical that they make. Individual chemicals can escalate the effect of each other (synergistic). For example, Vitamin C works with bioflavonoids. Further, Western science has found that vitamin C requires the nutritional tribe of nutrients (co-factors) in order for the Vitamin C to work effectively. The Caucasian analytical mind isolates and chains things together (i.e., people-chattel slaves; chemicals). They have chained stores together, radio and television stations, companies, and chained Black folks together in chattel slavery. The end result of all types of chaining and interference with the natural order, cycles, diets or cultures always spells disease. Chaining is forcing an unnatural relationship of chemicals or people. Herbs are natural for the body and have always been recognized and utilized for health in non-Caucasian medicine.

In traditional Chinese, Japanese, Indian and African medicine, the large intestine is synergistically related to the lungs. Therefore, it follows that 83% of AIDS victims have virulent lung infections called Pneumocystis Carinii Pneumonia (PCP). Aside from PCP, herpes, severe yeast infections, toxoplasmosis, cytomeglovirus and lymphadenopathy are also AIDS Related Conditions (ARC). ARC is the body's attempt to fight off the AIDS diseases. AIDS and ARC are present in Africa because Caucasians have socially engineered their processed foods, vaccinations, allopathic medicine and diseases upon Blacks on the Continent of Africa and all over the world. The Caucasian modern diet of processed foods is mucous forming, disease forming, causes slow transient time, and is constipating. This modern foodstuff has replaced the traditional natural whole foods diet of Blacks. A junk food diet, drugs, vaccinations, computers, radiation and polluted air, soil and water can destroy the immune system, resulting in AIDS *(AIDS Fact Book* by K. Mayer, M.D.).

Constipation has many forms; diarrhea, colds, skin eruptions, dandruff, coated tongue, hard stools, three or four bowel movements a week, flatulence, fevers, foul feet or underarm odors, halitosis, straining to have a bowel movement and low water consumption can indicate constipation. Poor nutrition and digestion problems are the indirect result of constipation. Poor health causes a weak colon. The colon becomes too weak to help the body's need for immunity against disease. Added to this, Black scientists do not challenge or expose the Caucasians culture's chemical rituals and ceremonies called science. And the Black population is not aware of African-centered science nor do they know science is the language of culture. And, they do not realize over 500 years of Caucasian culture's domination has socially engineered Blacks to believe that the Caucasian's diet is good for the African biochemistry. They believe Caucasian dietary science is the only dietary science. This indicates that Caucasians have achieved cultural castration and adultery upon Black folks. The Caucasian myth that the bodily rejection of toxins or the body's attempt to get rid of impurities is "disease" is a myth that has become reality. Caucasian medical science uses antibiotics, serums, animal pus, surgery and drug therapies to keep the diseases inside the body. When these diseases make the body deteriorate, they are given the label of AIDS. Their medical treatments of disease symptoms keep the body ill. Failures to cure diseases with drug therapies are not labeled AIDS.

AIDS strikes heterosexual women, men and children in Africa. For example, in Zaire, twelve percent of the population has AIDS. AIDS has been documented in Uganda as far back as 1973. However, the Caucasian horror about AIDS did not develop until 1982 when White gay activists began demanding help.

AIDS statistics in Africa and Haiti are easy to amass because the population uses the Caucasian medical model in their clinics and hospitals. Most diagnosis are subjective—if you look like you have AIDS, then you have AIDS. Whites in America use private doctors, public hospitals and statistical data is not easily amassed. For example, Atlanta, Georgia, with its public hospitals and clinics can easily amass statistics on its Black majority since they use public health facilities. Consequently, Atlanta has the distinction of being a city where Blacks have more V.D. (Venereal Disease) victims than any other city in America. The White populations statistics on V.D. are biased because they do not track Caucasians with the same amount of accuracy. Caucasians are usually treated by private facilities or by private doctors so that their V.D. rate is falsely indicated as low. Caucasian research data and statistics are manipulated in order to make themselves appear superior or more moral. AIDS was scientifically written about in scientific journals after the European tribal war called World War II. Infants (approximately 100,000) in European orphanages had AIDS related pneumocystis due to the accumulated effect of penicillin and protein malnutrition.

The Western (Caucasian) scientific evidence indicates that AIDS is heterosexual in African and homosexual among Whites. It is assumed that the sperm enters the blood during anal sexual intercourse. The sperm can enter the bloodstream during oral sexual intercourse (oral masturbation). Sperm entering any part of the body except the vagina and uterus is considered an enemy and attacked. Thus, oral and anal sperm transmittal may cause the immune system to become nonreactive and can lead to a collapse of immunity reactions. Western evolutionary scientific theory (fantasy belief) bias causes them to relate diseases of Caucasians to lower animals that they evolved from or blame the spreading of diseases on Blacks.

Many animals have similar diseases to humans. Animal biochemistry is totally different from humans. The human body will reject animal cells as well as another human's cells because of biochemical differences. Cowpox is similar to human smallpox but cannot be interchanged or exchanged between man and cow (*The Hygienic Care of Children* by Shelton). They are just similar diseases and nothing more. There are 50 diseases humans have similar to cattle, 35 with horses, 46 with goats and sheep, 42 with pigs and 65 with dogs. Caucasian science has found that the African green monkey has a disease similar to AIDS, which is not AIDS. Animal disease similarities are believed by Caucasians to mean sameness. They believe an animal's disease cells can be accepted and incorporated into human cells despite the fact that human cells reject any cell that is alien. The human body's rejection of alien cells is the main reason why transplanted organs (cells) are rejected and require drugs to force the alien (transplanted) organ to be accepted. Their belief in animal disease being transferred to humans is fortified by another belief that is the theory that Caucasians evolved from a monkey. A belief (theory) based on a belief is a belief. Actually, Caucasians have the sternoclavicular muscle, similar to a monkey. This muscle allows greater mobility when swinging from tree limbs while such a muscle is rare in Blacks. Whites relating themselves to healthy monkeys do not scientifically explain why they evolved to be very unhealthy with disease deterioration and why Africans have escaped AIDS. For example, Ugandan children have developed antibodies to AIDS. This indicates that the AIDS retrovirus has possibly changed to a more deadly killer or perhaps AIDS is merely a mild disease similar to a childhood disease or that only a small portion of the population develops it. Ironically, Haitians develop AIDS in Haiti but not while residing in America. This indicates that protein malnutrition of Blacks in Haiti and/or poor health has caused AIDS in Haiti. Haitians, in America, have better nourishment and better health and good sanitary conditions. Protein malnutrition causes AIDS positives in Haiti. When the Haitians that migrated to America start to eat junk foods, they will soon reflect the American trend for AIDS such as the statistics reported by the Center for Disease Control (CDC).

The CDC statistical hierarchy reflects that 73% of the AIDS victims are bisexual and homosexual males, 17% intravenous drug users, 7% unknown causes, 2% hemophiliacs and 1% heterosexual. Unfortunately, these statistics do not give a true indication of the intravenous (IV) users as the New York City Health Department (NYCHD). They reveal that one-third of the AIDS victims are IV drug users. For example, one-fourth of the cocaine users use IV, one-third of the amphetamine users, aside from this an unestimated percentage of body builders, housewives, herbal users, prostitutes, and heroin users can contact AIDS with unsanitary hypodermic needles. Blood transfusions are the source of spreading diseases and AIDS. A person having physical contact with another person's open sore, bruise, cut, lesion or scratch can also transmit AIDS (Dr. John Scale, *Journal of the Royal Society of Medicine*). Approximately 7% of the people will develop AIDS each year with five to ten times as many carrying AIDS symptoms. According to statistics in San Francisco, California, this would mean that for single men, 205 cases of AIDS will develop for every 100,000 men. AIDs causes the same amount of deaths as cancer and heart disease. In fact, more people are dying from degenerative diseases than AIDS. Poor nutrition and/or a series of diseases or constant disease episodes provide fertile soil for AIDS to develop. Hospital workers have not contacted AIDS from patients. Hospital workers in San Francisco have deliberately stuck themselves with AIDS contaminated hypothermic needles without contacting AIDS. This indicates that the AIDS retrovirus is only active at body temperature and not at the temperature of an exposed hypothermic needle. This indicates that the health workers did not have poor health or protein malnutrition [*Computerized AIDS Information Network (C.A.I.N.)*, DELPHI, General Videotex Corporation].

The victims of AIDS are estimated to be 5 to 10% of the population of the Central African Republic, Zaire, Zambia and Uganda. It is generally believed by Caucasians that the AIDS disease started between 1970 and 1980 in Africa and spread to other countries. However, immigration, tourist and out migration have made the figures about AIDS carriers beyond precision (*Lymphadenopathy-Associated Virus: From Molecular Biology to Pathogenicity* by L. Montagner).

The estimated figures indicate AIDS is an epidemic similar to biochemical warfare. For example, women account for 23% of the AIDS patients in Haiti. Further, 35 to 48% of the women in Zaire and Rwanda have AIDS. Breastfeeding has been suggested as a means of transmitting AIDS. Aside from this, the professional female prostitute has AIDS. The AIDS victim transmits the disease from woman to man and man to woman in a vicious cycle. The scope of AIDS among Black heterosexuals is beyond clear estimates ("Acquired Immunodeficiency Syndrome in Rwanda," *Lancet* 2: 62-5, 1984 by P., D. Rouuroy, P. Lepage, et al.; Seroepidemiology of HTLV-III Antibody in Haiti, *Clinical. Research* 33:414A, 1985 by J., B. Liautoud, F. Thomas, et al.).

Western man (Caucasian man) is the victim of AIDS. Those Black men who follow Caucasian culture's sexual perversions are AIDS victims. Homosexual transmission of AIDS is related to the fact that sexually transmitted intestinal parasites enter the blood through open skin (scratches, sores, etc.) when anal/fecal sex occurs. Intestinal parasites once in the blood weaken the immunity system. Furthermore, sperm that enter the blood during anal sex (or oral) can weaken the immunity. Women with open skin who indulge in oral sex (or anal) with men can also weaken their immune systems. Sperm and fecal matter that enter the blood via open skin through the anus or mouth causes a violation of the natural sequential pattern of immunity because the immune defenses are bypassed, causing the immune system to self-destruct. The Caucasian sex rituals and ceremonies are socially engineered into Black culture and influence and cause diseases and AIDS. The number of AIDS victims in Caucasian society is on a steady increase. The number of those infected with AIDS will probably reach ten million. This increase of AIDS occurs in "high risk" groups (homosexual Caucasian women and men, IV users, blood transfusions, hemophiliacs) as well as, "non-risk" (general public) groups. Risk and non-risk groups have serial sexual relationships and this makes everyone that has more than one consistent sex partner a potential carrier and unprotected.

Condom use is the protection from AIDS and STDs (Sexually Transmitted Diseases). The condom (commonly called "rubbers") can cause AIDS and diseases, and is considered the best choice for men. However, the sexually active person has not used the condom to stop VD in the past or the present and has not used them during the AIDS threat. Obviously, the condom is not used for oral or anal sex by men or women, be they homosexual or heterosexual. Scratches, lesions, or open sores in the mouth or anus allows diseased blood to carry AIDS into the body. Another form of protection is nonoxynol-9, a chemical in some contraceptive gels for women. This chemical agent causes cancer and kills the AIDS retrovirus. Lesbian women and gay men do not use the chemical. The orally sexually active heterosexuals and homosexuals cannot use the toxic chemical. Nonetheless, the gel and condoms are promoted as a form of protection by the AIDS Medical Foundation in New York.

The Black Caribbean population of Belle Glade, Florida has at least one in every three school children infected with the AIDS parasite. This indicates that AIDS can be inflicted among a people by the forcing of processed food, a disease-causing diet, vaccinations, cow's milk, sugar addiction and disease promoting medicine upon Blacks. AIDS in this instance becomes a form of biochemical warfare against Blacks. It is mislabeled a disease instead of a biochemical weapon of genocidal proportions.

AIDS victims are children and heterosexual women and men on the African continent. This clearly means that AIDS is not solely a sexually transmitted disease but a result of degeneration. The fact that sexually inactive children have AIDS indicates that AIDS has its roots in an under-nutritional diet, drug medicine, and unsanitary living conditions. Obviously, poor health and malnutrition are caused by the Caucasian control of land and junk food exploitation, economic and social colonialism, Black Uncle Tom scientists, and cultural slavery. The sum total of these factors results in causing Black folks health to degenerate to an AIDS state.

AIDS cannot be solved by a magic pus (vaccination) or synthetic serum. AIDS, like all diseases, is a result of health that has degenerated and loss immunity. Western science has not solved STD (Sexually Transmitted Diseases) with all of its science and research. Yearly, there are 500,000 victims of genital herpes, 2,000,000 of gonorrhea, 4,000,000 of chlamydia trachomates, 1,000,000 of PID (Pelvic Inflammatory Diseases)—20% of female infertility cases are caused by STDs and infertility among women 20 to 24 years old has tripled in 20 years despite scientific efforts. The Caucasian scientific community has had longer to research these STD diseases and have found no solution. Disease (AIDS, cancer) is an industry controlled by military logic with a predatory mentality with a system of rewards and punishments based on "The Law of the Caves." The only thing that satisfies a predator is more prey (victims) not morality, correctness, death, sex, money, power, etc.

A holistic nutritional approach to AIDS is the basic step in restoring the immunity of the body. (*Herbal Dynamics* by J. Heinerman; *Life Extension* by D. Pearson, S. Shaw and *Mucosless Diet Healing System* by A. Ehret).

AIDS is a sign to all people of African descent that a return to natural whole foods and traditional herbal medicine is the only acquired intent dietetic symbol (a.i.d.s.) for Blacks. Blacks that continue to eat junk foods,non-organic dairy and non-organic meat, use synthetic drugs and/or surgery will find no help for their path to disease death except AIDS. Currently, in the United States of America, 25% of the victims of AIDS are African-American children, women and men. Furthermore, three out of every five children with AIDS are African-Americans; one out of every two women with AIDS are African-Americans, and over 43% of the African-American IV drug abusers have AIDS. This disease is numerically equal to a form of genocide with no controls. It is time Afri-centric scientists help the race, because Euro-centric scientists have not. Caucasians cannot save themselves from a common cold. Therefore, solving the AIDS epidemic is beyond their scope.

AIDS Nutritional Remedies
A disease that goes untreated or treated with drugs develops into a degenerative disease, cancer and/or AIDS. For example, a cold untreated or treated with suppression drugs becomes Flu, Bronchitis, Pneumonia and/or Chronic Pulmonary Disease. These diseases weaken the liver, kidney and large intestines, which causes degenerative diseases, cancer or AIDS to develop. Diseases require money and money demands profit. Therefore, AIDS is no longer just a disease, it has developed into the AIDS industry. It is a profit making industry for drug, herb and supplement companies and the healthcare industry. Like any industry, each year the AIDS industry must have new research findings, new miracle cures and treatments in order to stay in business. The new miracle cures, research and treatments within a year end up on the shelf with last year's unsold miracles.

In Africa, it is easier to get monies for AIDS than nutrition, reparations or debt free technology to become self-sufficient. Therefore, the protein malnutrition, poor health and unsanitary conditions that cause AIDS positives are treated with AZT. The drug AZT causes degenerative diseases, cancer, AIDS and death. Aside from this, most of the AIDS monies given to Africa goes to politicians, bureaucrats, administrators, drug and medical companies and is stolen or unaccounted for. AIDS means free money without strings attached. The AIDS, cancer, vaccination and learning disorders businesses are self perpetuating. They will not go away. They must keep the diseases alive to stay in business. The use of AZT and vaccinations is a medical terrorist attack to destroy health in order to create business profits. AIDS has become a predatory military tool used to keep the Caucasians in control of Africa.

Supplements	Suggested Dosage	Remarks
Mega Multi Vitamin and Mineral	As directed.	Essential nutrients.
Extra strength garlic	As directed.	Purifies, antibiotic.
BHT (Butylated Hydroxytolene)	As directed.	Retards cell destruction.
Co-Enzyme Q	100-200 mg.	Helps purify blood, immune support.
Clay	1 to 2 tsp.	Aids cleansing.
B Complex	100 mg. 3 times daily.	Enhances nerve function, antistress.
PABA	300-10,000 mg.	Helps prevent autoimmune disease.
Biotin	30-150 mcg.	Used for skin disease.
Beta Carotene	25,000 I.U.	Stimulates immunity.
Vitamin A	5,000-25,000 I.U.	Used for infections.
Vitamin C (Acid Free)	500-3,000 mg.	Enhances healing.
Vitamin E	400-800 I.U., 2 times daily.	Protects immunity.
B_{15}	2,000 mcg.	Antioxidant
Pregnenolone	50-100 mg.	Balances hormones.
AMINO ACIDS		
L-Cysteine	1,000 mg.	Protects cells from harm.
L-Arginine	1,000-2,000 mg.	Stimulates immunity. Used for infection.
L-Lysine	1,000-2,000 mg.	Used for infections.
Aspartic Acid	1,000-2,000 mg.	Increases stamina.
L-Tryptophane (5HTP)	50-1,000 mg.	Regulates kidney, respiratory and heart.
L-Ornithine	1,000 mg.	Stimulates tissue repair.
Glutathione	500 mg.	Fights free radicals.
L-Dopa		
GLANDULARS		
Liver Adrena, Thymus, Pituitary	As directed.	Aids immunity.
MINERALS		
Selenium	100-200 mg.	Antioxidant.
Zinc	15-50 mg.	Tissue repair.
Magnesium	200-700 mg.	Antispasmodic, aids metabolism.
Potassium	100-500 mg.	Balances electrolytes and fluids.
Calcium	500-1,500 mg.	Proper nerve, muscle and heart function.
HOMEOPATHIC		
Kali. Phos., Nat. Mur., Silica, Nat. Phos., Kali. Sulph., Calc. Sulph.		Enhances immunity.

HERBS

Pau D'Arco, Echinacea, Chaparral, Red Clover, Burdock, Fo-Ti, Siberian Ginseng, Oregon Grape, Shigandra, Black Walnut, Saw Palmetto, Goldenseal, Cleavers, Wild Cherry Bark, Sarsaparilla, Prickly Ash Bark, Alfalfa.

FOODS

Asparagus, Beans, Beets, Broccoli, Cabbage, Carrots, Cauliflower, Corn, Cucumbers, Currants, Dates, Dulse, Endives, Gooseberries, Grapefruit, Guava, Horseradish, Kale, Kohlrabi, Lemons, Lettuce, Limes, Mamey, Olives, Onions, Oranges, Parsley, Peaches, Peppers, Pilinuts, Pistachios, Pomegranates, Potatoes, Quince, Raisins, Raspberries, Rice, Sesame Seeds, Soursop, Spinach, Strawberries, Tangerines, Tomatoes, Turnip Greens, Walnuts, Watercress, Wheat.

PROSTAGLANDINS

Prostaglandins are vital for the treatment of AIDS and all disease crises. It is necessary to keep the ability to utilize them at an optimum level.

Prostaglandins are fatty acid derivatives with a multitude of physiological functions.

- Help utilize hormones
- Help utilize neurotransmitters
- The inflammatory response
- Platelet aggregation
- Prostaglandins appear to play some role in virtually all biochemical activity

Restore Prostaglandin Balance
- Nutritional doses of Zinc, Magnesium, Vitamins B3, B6, C, and E
- Avoid Vitamin E and other antioxidants in high doses
- Strictly avoid trans fats (processed oils, cooked oils)
- Avoid PUFA: salad dressings, mayonnaise, nuts (except olive oil and coconut oil)
- Avoid excess arachidonic acid: shellfish, mollusks
- Avoid alcohol and vinegar
- Avoid food additives
- Avoid steroids, aspirin and other anti-inflammatory drugs
- Avoid lithium (in therapeutic doses)

DIET

Do not eat processed foods, red meats, pork, bleached flour, white sugar, diary products, fried foods and salt or use alcohol, cigarettes burnt/cooked marijuana and non-prescription synthetic drugs. Get a natural whole foods cookbook. Use Whole Oat, Wheat, Rice or Corn Bran.

Section 17

Herbs, Africa and History

The European Invasion of Ancient Africa for Medicinal Herbs B.C. to 1800 A.D.

The ancient usage of medicinal herbs was established long before Menses combined the upper and lower kingdoms of Egypt in 3200 B.C.

The predynastic cultures of the Amratian, Badarian (cultural ruins found beneath those of Amratians), *Gerzean* (extension of Amratian, 3600 B.C.) and the Nok cultures had medicinal herbs and drugs. In the Berlin *Medical Papyrus,* it is stated that medical schools were established long before Egypt.

The Nile Valley Africans of Egypt came from the southern direction of Abyssinia between 6000 and 3000 B.C. This migration of peoples, knowledge, plants, and medicinal herbs caused a concentration of information. The First Dynasty (3000 B.C.) was ruled by King Mina, then Kings Narmer and Aha. Their relics and coprolith studies (fossil food remains and remains of food in the intestinal tract of mummies) indicate both a primarily raw food diet and medicinal herbs. Various African people such as the Nubians and Hamites of the second cataract (curves in the river) and the Egyptians of the first cataract initiated a cluster of herbal knowledge. Imhotep established holistic medical schools during the regime of Pharaoh Zozer in the fourth Dynastic Era. The medical books produced by Imhotep (20 volumes) spread the allopathic, homeopathic and naturopathic usage of herbs and diagnostic techniques over the continent. His books are presently at Karl Marx University, Leipzig, Germany, where they were given the name of the European who stole them, Ebers and are called the Ebers Papyrus. Historically, he is a science bandit—technology thief. In any case, the rulers of the Fourth Dynasty (3360 B.C.) were Seneferu II and King Asa. It was this dynasty that invaded the Sudan for gold and slaves, and Sinai for copper. With the invasions, the cultural and herb knowledge were exchanged. Medicinal flower essences coupled with medicinal herbs were found in the tomb of Khufu, a ruler during this dynasty. Today's African flower essence treatments are called the Bach Flowers Remedies. Flower essence therapy is given the name of the thief that stole the African science—Bach. The fertile crescent of northeast Africa possessed medical schools. The indigenous herbal medicine and holistic diagnosis and treatments is considered exact. The Nubians had developed the medicinal herb and holistic diagnosis and treatment system of homeopathy. The Caucasians credit Hahneman, the German that stole the system with its invention. He altered and distorted it and reduced it to a mild form of allopathic medicine. Allopathic medicine uses very heavy dosages of homeopathic remedies.

The First through the Thirteenth Dynasties are considered the Old Age Empires. These dynasties had good holistic health. In the tomb of Doctor Skar of the Fifth Dynasty, there were over thirty surgical tools, pictures of scenes depicting activities, a list of the foods he ate and medical information. Mummified remains and coprolith studies indicate that their teeth were cavity-free and that they were free of bone disease, degenerative disease (i.e., Cancer, AIDS), digestive tract illness, had a natural foods diet, and used herbal medicine. The mummies from the dynastic eras after the Thirteenth Dynasty have indications of appendicitis, ulcers, mastoid disease and battle wounds. This indicates that the health began to deteriorate as the diet increased in cooked foods coupled with disease spurred by increased trading and invasions by the Europeans. In addition, the domestication and cultivation of plants caused the nutritional value of plants in the Egyptian diet to decrease. This decreased immunity and weakened the health.

Domestication of plants requires that the plants be taken out of their natural environment and placed on plant plantations. Plantations for plants are a synthetic societal environment, which deteriorates the plant, insect and animal ecology. Plantation plants cause a nutritional alteration of plants. The consumption of nutritionally altered plants alters the health. This domestication or processing of plants is unholistic as cultivated soil becomes drained of nutrients and limits the range of nutrients the plant absorbs. People that eat plants with limited amounts of nutrients develop limited ranges of thoughts, behaviors and moods. They become domesticated. Whatever the Caucasians do to plants, they do to Africans. Plants on a plantation—Africans on a plantation—domesticated plants—domesticated (seasoned) Africans; cloned plants, cloned Africans; the breeding of plants, the breeding of Africans, etc. A distorted picture of plant slaving (breeding, domesticating, etc.), can be found in *The Origin of African Plant Domestication* by Jack Horlan. In this book, the alteration process is delineated. Many valuable herbs were destroyed at the end of the Thirteenth Dynasty. Caucasian Aryans and Semitics invaded and destroyed Egyptian cities, raped women, children and men and stole gold and precious healing crystals. Timaus was a ruler during this invasion period. Many of the African plants were traded (transplanted) to other countries (i.e., Americas, Orient, etc.) during the early (pre-Columbus) African mercantile business. Wherever early Africans traveled to, they brought culture, technology, science, spirituality and plants. They improved other races' civilization. Wherever early Caucasian invaders went, they brought disease, exploitation, war, destruction and undeveloped others' civilizations. Many ancient Africans fought the Caucasians.

During the 15th Dynasty when King Salatis was ruler, the Caucasian Hyksos or shepherd kings invaded Egypt (1730-1580 B.C.) and destroyed wildlife, crops and medicinal herbs. Africans, such as the Black Egyptian Prince, Segenera, died fighting the Hyksos. The Hyksos hated the prince, which is evident by the many wounds on his mummy in Cairo. His mummy reveals a fractured skull, a knife cut over the eye, a bitten tongue and broken jaw. Aside from crops and curative herbs, the Egyptian empire (which included colonies outside of Egypt) had abundant financial wealth and academic knowledge. This made the predatory militaristic Caucasians want to invade and capture Egypt.

Foreign powers in pursuit of Egypt had varying ideas about war. The Caucasian cultures' practice of war has been colonialized and become the only idea of fighting war. However, war ideas often varied within the same culture, with a variety of contrasting organizational structures and sanctions.

War varies from one culture to another. The Caucasian idea of war has become the accepted norm. However, war may also have contrasting objectives in a culture. In ancient Africa, war amongst two groups must satisfy Maat. The victor and defeated must both benefit and preserve each other's honor. There is no precise winner or loser. Maat claims the victory. The end result of war is for both sides to enrich the culture and serve Maat. For example, the Aztecs concept of war had a religious meaning. War was used as a means to get captives for religious sacrifices. The Spanish invasion of the Aztec empire was a shock to the Aztecs because the Spaniards would kill without a ritual and ceremony and the killings had no religious meaning. The Aztecs could not attach any religious principles or cultural purpose to killing in that manner. They did not know how to fight without a spiritual purpose. The Spanish killed to destroy culture. It was savage ideals that Cortez had and used to win the war along with superior weapons. It was a cultural shock for the Aztecs. This same type of senseless killings and use of superior weapons defeated Africans.

The Caucasian war concept is based upon killing the so-called enemy. The African culture's concept of winning a war is based upon Maat and God. In that respect, these war concepts conflict and vary. Often, there are no cultural relevancy factors that can translate a definition of war from one culture to the next. All we really know of these wars is that the Europeans raped the girls and women, stole treasures, destroyed the food supply, dehumanized the defeated and exploited the land. This caused starvation, erosion, famines and diseases. In any case, the Caucasian Race War against Africans continued in Egypt. Two rulers of the Eighteenth Dynasty, from 1600 to 1300 B.C., were Queen Hatshepsut and Ahmes I who fought the Caucasian barbaric invaders, called the Hyksos. The Hyksos persisted in their wars to gain food, wealth, land and herbs. These wars marked the beginning of the long decline of Egypt. The Caucasians' stealing technology, medicinal knowledge, land and destroying valuable treasures were using superior weapons (cannons, rifles, etc.) to capture Africans. It was after this time that the Kush Empire (modern day Sudan Republic) and Queen Hatshepsut united upper and lower Egypt. At the same time, Pharaoh

Thutmosis invaded the land of the Caucasian barbarians and made the defeated European countries his possessions. This cultural contact caused African colonized Caucasians to become more aware of African medicine, wealth, philosophy, agriculture, knowledge, astronomy, mathematics and food.

The Nineteenth Dynasty was ruled by Pharaohs Ramses and Seri (his father) and others. Many invading Caucasian barbaric hordes attempted to capture Africa's technology. The famines and diseases of the Europeans were known to African civilization and attempts were made to give aid to the Caucasians. However, the constant and violent attacks against Africans by gangs of Caucasians may have caused reluctance to help. Nonetheless, Ramses sent vast amounts of wheat to the plagued and famine stricken Europe. Pharaoh Merneptha's priest taught his captured barbaric Caucasian slaves farming, which included herbalism and astrology. African priests were agriculturists, astrologers, social scientists, physicians and chemists. In fact, the priest temples were colleges of learning in art, science and religion.

The Twentieth, Twenty-Second and Twenty-Third Dynastic periods (1085-730 B.C.) had several dynasties ruling at the same time from different capitals in various parts of Africa. Social unrest and strife was caused by the presence of mixed Caucasoid rulers and continued until the Twenty-Fifth (715 to 600 B.C.) Dynasty. Many African cultures were moving away from the invaders and fighting back. This destabilized the agriculture and economy. The Twenty-Sixth Dynasty (663-525 B.C.) was marked by the Egyptians' total loss of independence. The African Egyptians were eventually controlled by the Caucasian Persians.

The Egyptians are noted for their abundant records that reflect their greatness in African medicine and civilization. These records and artwork document a history of fighting against the invading Caucasians, as well as the higher civilization of Africans. Thebes (Greek word) was the greatest city in Chem (later named Egypt). This city was named Wo'se or Nowe by the Africans. This city was the central city of a vast empire, which included Nubia, Cush, Egypt, etc. However, the current study of Africa is mostly of a lesser domain called Egypt and the Caucasians who invaded it.

The early Caucasian invaders of Africa were killed or captured. Caucasian prisoners of wars, learned culture, science, herbal medicine and eventually participated in the African society. Let there be no doubt that these Caucasians contributed nothing to African culture except diseases, land rape and chattel slavery. In fact, Greek society was founded upon the slavery of Caucasians and these Caucasian slaves could not own property. Nonetheless, Black Africans kept Caucasian relatives (sons) of Asian and Mediterranean rulers. These hostages learned culture, philosophy, science and African medicine. The Caucasian hostages and prisoners of war population eventually greatly increased.

Egyptian internal social problems (poverty, high taxes) and Maatian culture gave the Caucasian slaves freedom to participate in society as full citizens and the opportunity to have strikes and rebellions. Weak ineffective kings created a cycle of Black inmigration movements. Blacks migrated below the first cataract of the Nile and a predominantly Caucasian population moved above the second cataract. This resulted in Asian (Caucasian) dynasties and Afri-Asian dynasties mixed with various combinations of races with a few Black dynasties. Periods of social unrest lasted until the Twentieth Dynasty (1200 B.C.) ruled by Sotnekht who was succeeded by Ramses. During these periods, Caucasian barbaric hordes of invaders continuously attacked Africa. Africa's medical science was practiced in African empires that had colonies in Europe and many African trained Caucasian physicians returned to Europe with this so-called new science. A few are indicated in recorded history such as Hippocrates but there were many. In any case, Ramses III fought the invading Caucasian sea merchants and defeated them (1191 B.C.). He captured so many Caucasian slaves (90,000) that he had to colonize them in Europe because he could not transport them to Africa. He eventually had to draft his Caucasian slaves in his army to fight the Caucasian barbarians who were primarily driven by hunger, treasures, freedom from feudalism and disease to Africa. The *Harris Papyrus* makes reference to the career of Ramses III.

The Caucasian invasions, coupled with the Caucasian slaves in Africa, inmigrations, African refugees running from war, in addition to internal African strife (caused by social injustice and feudalistic governments) caused Africa to weaken. With every increase in Africa deterioration, the Greeks became more powerful and eventually undermined and usurped Egyptian culture, agriculture, philosophy, science, banking system, educational system, medical knowledge and religion.

The greatest Caucasian historians Herodotus, Pliny, and Diodorus wrote that the early Black African civilizations were the most advanced of all civilizations in the world. These historians wrote that Europeans borrowed (without permission = stole) Black Africa's sciences, technology, culture and religion. No matter how Caucasians deny this, these Caucasian historians were honest and visited Africa to confirm their findings. Written and pictorial history has confirmed time after time that everything the Caucasians know about hygienic medicine, culture, philosophy, mathematics, astrology, art and politics is unquestionably African.

Greek historians helped to confirm Africa's glory and Egyptian dynasties. The Egyptian dynastic eras lasted over 10,000 years. These dynastic eras saw Egypt dominate world trade, technology, science, medicine, art, science and the herb/drug trade. Much of the era's medicinal knowledge was taught in college (mystery system) by professors who had spiritual, metaphysical, astrology and science knowledge on high levels. They were called god-kings. These mystery-healing systems were taught to priests (so-called monks) in monasteries or temples. The Caucasians called them mystery systems because the knowledge was above anything that they ever learned. For example, if you never heard of or learned mathematics, then the classes on calculus would be a mystery to you. Thus, the Caucasians called African colleges mystery systems.

The succession of Caucasian controllers of Egypt learned at African universities (mystery schools) and they learned from the African monks and transmitted the herb and drug knowledge to Caucasian monks and their native European lands. These monks/herbalists/priests/agriculturists carried the medicinal knowledge intact to Europe and with cultural distortions and modifications adjusted it to a low level of knowledge and limited vocabulary. The successive colonizers of Egypt were the Caucasian Assyrians, Saites, Persians, Greeks and the Romans. The Greeks (invaded Africa 332 B.C.) and Romans (invaded African 201 B.C.). They learned the African medicine system and claimed it as their own knowledge (information thieves) and a discovery of the European culture. They actually learned an introductory level of the medical science and religious philosophy of the spiritual system. (*The Destruction of Black Civilization* by C. Williams, *The African Origin of Civilization* by C. Diop).

Egypt developed monastic living. This type of living required the acquisition of knowledge of Maat, medicinal herbs and spirituality. The Greeks studied on the Upper Nile islands under the religious order at Tabennae founded by Pachomius. These religious herbalists sold herbs, honey and foods at Alexandria. Egyptians lived on these islands and instructed many European religious monks on agriculture, astrology, Maat and industry. This is vaguely mentioned in *The Golden Age of Herbs and Herbalists* by R. Clarkson (1940). The spiritual knowledge was learned and claimed by the Caucasians (Romans) as their own. They transported this system to Europe and built a Benedictine monastery at Monte Cassino in Italy.

Herbology, holistic diagnosis and treatment methods came from African empires such as Mali, Songhai, and Kush. The Kush kingdom was dominated mostly by light-skinned Caucasians and their diet was nutritionally lacking. The Caucasians began to invade the areas southwards, which had plentiful crops, agriculture, treasures, technology, industry and medicine. This area was inhabited by Black Africans and was rich in iron ore and fuel supplies. Areas around the fifth and sixth cataracts of the Nile had vast iron industries. Assyrians were one of the invaders that adopted the African technology of ironwork and a socialized form of medicine similar to the Babylonians, which dated from 2250 B.C. This was around the same period that the Egyptians had traded plants, vegetables, herbs and dry goods with Ethiopia in 2275 B.C. Black Egyptian medicinal knowledge extended across the Sudanic belt of Africa. The Kush Empire began to decline as African empires entering the trade market dominated specific goods such as the Sandalwood, Khat, Hawthorn berry, Cotton, Tropica, Aloe Vera and figs. The Kush decline occurred around the First Century

A.D. Axum, the capital of Ethiopia, was one of the competitors that seized control of part of the Kush trade market.

The desert African empires controlled the aloe vera market. The North Africans controlled such herbs as hawthorn berry, and the forest region controlled coffee, carob, centuary, and eucalyptus. Ethiopia controlled the herb khat, which is a brain stimulant. Axum was typical of the splendid African cities; it had stone palaces, Obelisks, gardens of herbs, indoor water and temples. Meroe was invaded by the Kush; and thus caused Africans to migrate to Lake Chad and beyond. This migration of human resources, technology, farmers and medicinal knowledge helped to weaken Africa.

The internal wars and dispersion of peoples, food, science and herb knowledge helped spread the glory of Africa aboard to Europe. The African mercantile trade industry helped spread information about Africa's human and material resources. Egypt was conquered by Alexander the Great (356-323 B.C.). Then Ptolemy, a general in Alexander's army, ruled Egypt and established the city Alexandria. This gradual decline of Black Egypt is exposed in *African Glory* by J. C. deGraft-Johnson. Other Black races contributed to the decline of Africa. They stole Africa's sciences, philosophy, herbology and holistic diagnosis and treatment systems.

The Phoenicians expanded their trade and colonized North Africa. They invaded northeast Tunisia and established the city of Utica at the mouth of the Majada River around 1100 B.C. They established Carthage in 822 B.C. It was destroyed by the Romans in 200 B.C. Incidentally, St. Augustine, the Black African Bishop studied in the African colonial city of Carthage. This city is where the priest/herbalist monastic system was established and this system expanded herb medicine knowledge all over the European world.

The medicinal herb knowledge was needed in Europe. European civilization's populations were on a massive decline due to dis-eases from their scavenger diet, famines, lack of agriculture, a series of tribal wars, low birth rate, animal flesh diet, poor hygiene and lack of cleanliness. The Roman Empire colonized Northern Africa and used it for grain farms. The continuous European abuse of the land caused the Sahara Desert (Lake) to expand and become a more massive desert. The Apollo spaceship of the National Aeronautics and Space Agency (1982) has validated photographically that the Sahara was at one time an inland lake. Fossil remains validate that the Sahara had vast vegetation and wildlife. Europeans exploited the land for farm crops, herbs and wildlife. Heavy consumption of animal flesh by early Greek, Roman, Arab and Indian civilizations caused destruction to the agriculture, herbs, food crops and forest. Caucasians lacked agriculture skill, did not rotate crops, revitalize the land, compost and were not concerned about ecology. This caused over-irrigation and damage to the land. The over-grazing by cattle gradually reduced the lands to desert and infertile soil. The introduction of European animals such as domesticated cattle, pigs and the undomesticated rat caused ecological imbalances in Africa's wild animal population and plant population. The rape of the Fertile Crescent (present day Iraq and Iran) for food crops and overgrazing by the flesh eaters' animals crops caused damaged that still has not been repaired. The massive amounts of meat that the Caucasians consumed and the method used to insure the supply of animal flesh has reduced north and northeast Africa to vast wastelands. Alexander the Great invaded Africa and India and left the land treeless and barren. An uncontrollable need for White Supremacy and need to own Africa's human and material resources caused the exploitation of plants and the enslavement of Black people. It is estimated that the total land lost throughout the course of European history (predominantly in Africa) is greater than the total land now in cultivation in the entire world (*A Vegetarian Sourcebook* by Keith Akers).

Herb Mercantile Trade among Africans and Europeans

Africa's mercantile system was very successful and involved an abundance of commerce long before the European invasions. Cities, communities, states, African empires and colonies of empires manufactured foodstuff, books, medicinal herbs, metals, crystals, fabrics and dry goods for export. The cost of transporting goods was high especially for the forest regions. Consequently, the kings with wealthy empires and merchants forced smaller merchants to sell to them at lower prices. Inadvertently, this caused large monopolies and competitive power politics in the mercantile system. For example, the long trips to neighboring states required food and supplies for the escort armies, animals of burden, bookkeepers, astrologers, bankers, teachers, children, translators, women and physicians. These inter-country trading trips could only be sponsored by the economically elite individuals or governments. Trading increased the wealth of the monopolist and increased trade.

The Guinea states traded with the merchants of the Sudan. Incidentally, during the Middle Ages the location of Guinea in the tropical forest region of West Africa near the savannas made it inaccessible to Europeans. However, inmigration caused by trading from Guinea to the Sudan brought knowledge of its dry goods, agriculture, treasures and herbal medicine to the Europeans. Items from Africa were sold in Europe and the Europeans were told about houses, wealth, abundance of food, higher civilization and knowledge of the manufactures.

Guinea's merchants were state agencies and increased the wealth of state governments and the kings. Trade from state-to-state required the use of Africa's standardization of money values, measurements, and a commerce law and regulation system. Africa had standardized classification for illnesses, diagnosis and classification of herb and herb treatments by physicians across the continent. Some of the other countries in the mercantile system were Sahara (which monopolized salt and the cactus), Sudan, Maghrib and the northeast African territories of the Mediterranean such as Israel and

Mesopotamia. Kola nuts (stimulants) were sold by the country presently called Ghana. Yorubaland sales were incorporated in the overall mercantile sales of Guinea. There were a few slaves in the forest regions. However, slavery as a human flesh mercantile business was unheard of. The sales of slaves in Guinea were of a social status and they served as servants, porters, laborers, government officials, could be a prince or ruler, teachers and merchants and were a functional part of society. These African slaves were allowed to practice their culture and were not owned. They had full human rights. They could not be raped, beaten or tortured. They could earn freedom from their obligation of labor. Trading in slaves began after the growth of Islam in the Sudan. The kidnapping and exporting of Africans as non-human animal livestock slaves developed from the 16th century by Caucasians only.

Abyssinia resisted the Islamic religious colonialization of their country and remained Christianized. It was from the south and in countries where African names for God was worshiped that the Caucasians started to label Africans as ungodly, pagan and uncivilized heathens and started the slave trade.

The Zagwe warrior kings in the Tenth Century defeated the invasions of the Europeans. The Zagwe people moved southwards from the coastal line to avoid further European attacks and left their Roha rock churches as markers showing their path of retreatment. The Europeans were not dismayed or disillusioned because their motivating force for the invasions was escaping the caves of Europe and horrible primitive lifestyles with famines, starvation, poverty, illiteracy, tribal wars, pandemics, medical ignorance, hunger and tyrannical feudal kings.

The Islamic Muslimized countries expanded from East Africa to Malaysia, Indonesia and India. This included coastal states of Kenya, Tanganyika and Somalia. Islamic colonies traded with the early Ming and late Sung Dynasties of China from which they obtained porcelain. Ironically, the toy of China (the firecracker) was overlooked by the Muslim merchants and it was this toy coupled with disease that was to defeat Africa and end the Muslim reign. The Europeans converted this firecracker toy to the death weapon called the cannon, dynamite and gun. It was the superior weapons of the Caucasians such as guns, cannons and gunpowder bombs that escalated the invasions of Africa and the Americas. These weapons created the ultimate weapon for the exploitation, extermination of peoples, the slave trade, herb trading and the establishment of White Supremacy. The knowledge needed to invent the gun required the stolen mathematical science of Africa, the mass metal technology of Africa, and the metal mining technology of Africa. It was not until after the Greeks were allowed into Africa, did the Caucasians gain access to these technologies. The Egyptian priests were very guarded about their technology knowledge because of the oath of secrecy in the mystery systems to withhold if from the "Greek Boys" (immature culture) as they were called by Ancient Africans. At first

Africans gave the death penalty to strangers (stealing, lying, barbaric Caucasians) that came to their country or colonies. It was not until 500 B.C. did they let foreigners such as the Greeks into their universities. Their studies amounted to a college preparatory course. They did not have enough intelligence to understand higher African knowledge. Greeks such as Plato, Socrates, Hippocrates, Praxagorus, and Pythagoras studied in Africa. In any case, the mercantile system in Africa and trade with Pacific basin countries spread the wealth, technology, philosophy, spirituality, culture, health practices and medicine of Africa to Europe (also called "World Island" as Africa and Asia are connected by Sinai, Asia and Europe are connected by this land created on that island has 85% of the world's population).

The wars between the Christian tribes and Muslim tribes, better known as the Crusades, stimulated trade between Africa and Europe. Venetian merchants traded with the Muslims because they controlled many countries. Portugal and Spain (1400) were beginning to feel the economic drain caused by the Venetian control of the commerce and herb drug markets. They attacked the peninsula and started an invasion of Africa on the Pacific Ocean side in 1415. These two allies were defeated in their invasion of Morocco. Their individual invasions near the Cape of Good Hope soon brought them reports of the countries on the Atlantic side of the Sahara. Venetian sea control and trade control caused the Italians to invade Africa. The powerful Italian clans were economically starved and hope to create an economic base and food and herb trading in order to profit from the pandemics and hungry population of peasants. Italy joined forces with the Portuguese and Spanish to break the Venetian control. Their plan was to invade the coastal African countries. This would cause the Venetians to extend armies and ships along the coast and create a large network that would weaken their (Venetian) ability to protect established markets. Therefore, they joined the forces of Portugal and Spain began to exploit the gold and herb dry goods and food markets of Guinea. In due course, they used the Indian merchants to buy commodities for them. They bought herbs from Asia at prices below the market rate of the Venetians. Thus, the Venetians were unable to produce enough capital to control and protect their markets in Africa. Venice fell as the controller of the herb market.

The Portuguese invaded Africa around 1445 and colonized the Cape Verde Islands as a port for trade with Mali. The Portuguese penetrated further into Africa for dry goods, food, technology, treasures and medicinal herbs and in 1471 invaded the Gold Coast. By the 1480's, they had invaded the Congo, by 1488, they rounded the Cape of Good Hope and by 1497 to 1499, led by Vasco de Gama, they established markets in India. In 1517, the Ottoman Turks had invaded and conquered the Maghrib except Morocco. The Turks were based in their Egyptian colony. The Turks tried to seize the herb, food and dry goods market from the Portuguese but were defeated (between 1400 and 1500). However, in 1571 a combined Christian fleet of European mercantile adversaries defeated the Portuguese at

Lepanto. Merchants began to trade more with the European controlled African coastal ports instead of using the ancient trade routes of the Sahara.

The European merchants traded mostly with the Asians, Americas, and coastal African colonies. The dense African forests made further trade for medicinal herbs, treasures, sugar and dry goods, extremely difficult. The monks had extracted the technology needed to adapt vegetation to the Americas and this knowledge coupled with the earlier extraction of technology, culture and scientific knowledge by the Greeks, Romans and other nations lessened European dependence on African herbs. In addition, the African forests and lands had been reduced to deserts and wastelands by the Romans and succeeding invaders, so the African monopoly of herbs and food plants was no longer a viable market. Consequently, the economic wealth that could be gained from the market of chattel slaves became enticing. The human plantation system was tested and tried on the offshore islands of West Africa. The kidnapped Africans were mixed with different African cultures with different religions and languages. Slaves that spoke the same language were separated and re-mixed with Black prisoners of war. Oftentimes, if slaves spoke the same language, their tongues were cut out. Some Blacks would starve themselves rather than become slaves and were force-fed with two spoons attached to one handle (the oral forceps). One spoon contained food and the other spoon contained hot coals. A slave had a choice between swallowing food or swallowing hot coals. Black men, boys, women and girls were raped by male and female heterosexual and homosexual European enslavers. Black prisoners of war captives were branded and treated like any other animal of burden. Many were forced to perform dehumanizing tasks and sex acts for the amusement of the slavers. The Black Africans who were teachers, musicians, bookkeepers, navigators, physicians, scientists, and skilled laborers were separated and sold at higher prices or killed in order to further the White Racist myth of Black inferiority (See White Racism Addiction). The European White Racist psychosis of White Supremacy (superiority) has caused much of the scientific advancement created in Africa to be destroyed. However, the African medicinal herbs and holistic diagnosis and treatment knowledge has survived because the European race would have vanished without it. In any case, the slave plantation system was indirectly first perfected with plants. The word itself "plantation" indicates this. On a "plant" plantation, plants are enslaved, domesticated (hybridized), tamed, made nutritionally docile, placed in an alien artificial plant civilization, made to breed out of breeding cycles, made to create plant social systems (hybridized seeds) in alien environments and the plant leaders are destroyed. For example, the more lively seeds are the first to leave the plant while the weaker, less strong seeds stay attached to the plant. It is these seeds that are picked and replanted. It is the weaker aberrationalized seeds that are capable of growing in an alien environment. Thus, the seeds that further the domesticated (man-altered) system are furthering a species of nutritional limited and weak plants that nature was trying to eliminate. In the human plantation system the physically strong and rebellious Black slaves were killed and the educated Blacks of the upper class elite were killed in order to propagate the European psychosis of "all niggers are slow, dumb, ignorant, thieves, uncivilized, savages, and wild sexual animals." (See White Racism Addiction, Anatomy, and Psychology). The plantation system and European mercantile system merely shifted from one non-human item (herb, food) to another non-human item—Black African slaves. The immorality of Caucasians was kept intact by their psychological illusion of White Supremacy supported by White Racism.

The Spanish participated in the Black slave, herb, food, and dry goods markets in North America. They traded slaves across the Atlantic to the West Indies while the Portuguese merchant traders exported kidnapped Black prisoners to Brazil and South Americas. The European slave plantation system could not work in America with native Americans because the Indians were slaughtered by Caucasian invaders, starved due to food shortage, died of European diseases, ran away, did not have the technological skills or agricultural knowledge of the Africans and did not produce enough labor to make it profitable. The slave system was growing too rapidly and their population was too small (12 million killed by European Smallpox disease). Consequently, the Europeans could not feasibly transport the American plantations to Africa's slave labor; so, they transported the African slave labor to the colonized Euro-American plantations. Enslaved Africans, with agricultural skill, technology and labor controlled by Caucasians with a psychosis (White Supremacy) and the stolen land of Americas provide the wealth that produces today's multinationals. If you follow the Caucasian money trail, it will lead to money obtained by the blood of Africans. The fact that conservative estimates state that between 50 and 75 million Black lives were murdered due to slavery and an additional inestimable millions to dis-eases is not a moral issue to Caucasians or the descendants who have the hereditary blood money. The fact that European disease caused massive amounts of deaths killing entire villages is of no moral consequence. The fact that many slaves were killed by slave rustlers (thieves) in many raids of slave caravans, plantations and slave ships arouses no moral issues. Many times, ships packed with slaves were sunk in the battles between slave traders and slave rustlers. Later in history, Caucasians would rustle (steal) each other's slaves, rebrand them, cripple them, kill them or use the Underground Railroad (runaway slave network of people).They would steal each other's slaves and give them to the underground railroad. This was a slave owner's method of reducing or getting rid of his competition. This would cause low crop production, increase the price of crops or increase the price of slaves with special skills. The Underground Railroad was just another way for Caucasians to economically terrorize each other and steal each other's slave livestock along with the help of other slaves' and with the underground's freed Blacks' support.

The foods, herbs and medical science of Africa rescued the European from the Dark Ages and stopped their population decline. The morality and mental illness (White Supremacy) of the Caucasians is overlooked because of the condition of European countries is overlooked. Europe was land poor, resource poor and labor poor. However, they write a feel good history and distort their cave man mentality and present it as civilized and cultured. If they were developed and civilized, they would not have had a need for African land and African peoples whom they called slaves. More information on slavery can be found in *The Masters and Slaves* by Gilberto Freyre and *Slavery* by Nathan Glazer, as well as a host of other books.

THE HERB CONTROLLERS

The need for a scientific medical system and herbs in Europe was caused by continuous uncontrollable outbreaks of pandemics. There was not enough knowledge of herbs or diseases to save the European peoples. Botanical history reveals that there were approximately 235 herbs on the island of Cos in Asiatic Turkey. However, Hippocrates, the Greek father of medicine, was only skilled enough to use less than thirty. He had no knowledge of either psychology or anatomy and did not know blood circulated in the body.

Hippocrates' African knowledge was rejected by his culture and was not used until the late 1800s. Churches capitalizing on the people's fear of dying from dis-ease, advertised for customers by saying they had the original Saints' artifacts. The churches were gathering false relics and bones in order to attract members and amass fortunes during the Middle Ages. This started rivalries between churches. The cathedral in Cologne obtained the skulls of the Three Wise Men of the East in order to attract new members with monies. In competition, the Church St. Gereon produced relics of St. Gereon and the bones of a whole band of martyrs in order to get new customers (members) with monies. Then, another church had an entire cemetery of bones taken from graves and placed in the church and called these bones the bones of saintly martyrs. The eleven thousand bones of so-called female virgin martyrs helped faith healing and raised a fortune, despite the fact that some of the bones belonged to men. The church was using ignorant superstitions and sensationalism to get customers (religious members). European science could not save the dis-eased and dying population, so the church used these devices to attract and cure dis-eased people. They did not save anyone but preyed on the people's money, food supply and land. Soon the churches did produce a legitimate way to help such as herbalist. The church and its monk/herbalists were to play an important part in the invasion of Africa for herbs, vegetables, fruits and knowledge.

The monks helped to develop methods for the adaptation and hybridization of African herbs to the European and colonial climates by grafting and crossbreeding plants. Their knowledge of herbology, agriculture and horticulture was eventually used by the European farmers and this also caused the herbal exploitation of Africa to end. Monks wrote books about herbology, horticulture and medicine like *De Laudibus Divinae Sapientiae* by Alexander Neckham, an Augustinian monk and Abbot of Cirencester. He mentions many African herbs and medicinal fruits in his book. In another book, *De Naturis Rerun,* Neckham mentions essential African herbs for health. Another monk, Walafrid Strabo, a Benedictine, wrote *Hortulus* in which he mentions tropical herbs of African origin and tells how to cultivate them in the European climate.

The African hothouse principle for speeding the growth of plants was adopted by the Romans. A German Dominican monk of the Thirteenth Century by the name of Albertus Magnus in his book, *De Vegetablibus,* describes the Roman's use of this process. The Europeans, in a desperate need for plant foods and herbs quickly adopted this process. The church, in forming a power elite, hid and stored an abundance of herb books and holistic diagnosis and treatment books. They did not reveal this information to the public.

The Romans were engulfed in a variety of superstitions and ignorant practices before the invasion of Africa by the Greeks (332 B.C.). Greek physicians with African knowledge charged the Romans fees for services. The Romans were very pleased with this and considered the Greek doctors to be experts. Actually, Greek doctors did business similar to hustlers and their practices were experiments to learn at the Romans' expense.

After the fall of the Roman Empire, the Arabs collected the herbal medical writings and holistic diagnosis and treatment methods of Galen other Greek physicians. Greek medicinal knowledge was usurped from Africa. This is pointed out in *From Ancient Africa to Greece* by Henry Olela. Avicenna, a Black Moor Muslim physician distilled much of Imhotep's African knowledge and wrote *The Canon of Medicine.* With the fall of Rome and the herbal trade, advances in medical science in Europe began to increase.

The Middle Ages started (perhaps about 700-800 A.D.) and was followed by the Renaissance, which started about 1200 A.D. This corresponds to the time European-African trading started. Europeans needed the African medicinal technology and agricultural sciences because of the famine, food starvation and diseased state of their primitive civilization. The state of their civilization is filled with signs of a civilization on a death path.

The cities in Europe were densely populated. They had no sewage drainage. The houses and streets were filled with accumulations of garbage and filth. Rats were everywhere; the air was foul and offensive and houses were open cesspools infested with flies, black smoke from animal lard candles and wood, rats, human feces, roaches, and other insects. Infections were widespread as European cities became submerged in a pool of disease. The middle ages was one of the worst eras for European women. These women were blamed for sins and labeled as witches if they did not menstruate. Clitorises were removed, and many women were burned as evil witches. Some women were dropped on the floor or couch in order to speed up the delivery of children. Aside from this, they were often used as servants in hospitals. For example, the Hotel Dieo, founded by Saint Landry, a Bishop in France in A.D. 641-649 used women. The old women were physically abused, younger women raped and they were generally the female waste of society (homeless, crippled, diseased, etc.) or whores. Yet the hotel was called "a place for God's hospitality" which was later reduced to the word hospital. The women who worked there and the midmen had to endure rats and air so offensive that a sponge soaked in vinegar held before the nose was the only way to endure the place. It had four to six people in a bed and the sick often slept with the dead. Sick men, babies, children, pregnant women and the dead were often in bed together.

In contrast, the African Escalapius Temples were a model hospital system founded and used under King Zoser of the Fourth Dynastic era in Egypt. In these temples, Escalapius (Greek for Imhotep) African medicine was taught and used successfully for dis-eases.

Surgery was also successfully performed. The earliest pictures of Africans performing surgery are in Memphis, Egypt and it dates at least 2000 B.C. Surgery was not performed during the European Middle Ages. They were performing dissections of the human body. These dissections were usually elaborate rituals with invited guests. The physicians sang chorus and performed readings from Galen while body parts and organs were removed. A seal of the university was stamped on the corpse and a music concert followed the dissection, coupled with a banquet and theatrical performances. This same process was later used with lynched slaves. In addition, the church required the head to be removed from the corpse before dissection because the head was considered the seat of God. (*Fabrica* by Andreas Vesalius, 1543).

Europeans were rapidly becoming an endangered race. The population was declining due to many factors. The cesspool cities combined with the nutritionally imbalanced diet caused pandemics. Pandemics are diseases that strike an entire country while epidemics merely strike a portion. Pandemics were recorded as early as 96 to 1890 A.D. In the cities, pandemics resulted in violence; looting; heterosexual and homosexual rape of boys, girls, men and women; fear; and a short lifespan of twenty years. Houses were filled with dead bodies and the streets were filled with a continuous stream of funerals. Farmers infected with dis-ease neglected their crops. This created food shortages in the cities and rural areas. Farm populations abandoned the land and moved into the cities creating more food shortages and ghettoes of death.

Pestilence and plagues slowly degenerate the body. Because of pestilence, the European population was slowly decreasing. Since the dis-eased and starving population of Europe was weak from pestilence, a plague would strike (plagues struck intermittently and there would be a recovery period between plagues) while the Europeans were recovering from a plague, there would be another occurrence of pestilences.

The pandemics, plagues and diseases which afflicted the Europeans were leprosy, venereal dis-ease, typhoid fever, dysentery (diarrhea), cancer, diphtheria (which killed the young), tuberculosis (which struck entire families), anthrax (which killed people and animals), appendicitis (which caused death through ruptured appendices) and mental illness

Europeans and their cultures were wasting away due to pandemics. An example of a pandemic is a pestilence, which affected 400 people out of 1,000 and two deaths could result, while a plague affected 1,000 people out of 1,000 people and resulted in 800 deaths. Of the remaining 200 people that lived after the plague, a pestilence such as influenza would strike the majority of 200 remaining people, leaving twenty people alive. The Bubonic Plague struck Rome, in 68 A.D., 77 A.D., 125 A.D. and 164 A.D. In 180 A.D., it almost completely destroyed the armies in Rome, Italy. The Romans were defeated more by dis-ease than outside forces. Their initial attraction to Africa was for luxury goods such as ivory, gold, copper, silk, jewelry and dry goods. However, soon their focus was forced to shift to the medicinal herbs and food as a means of saving themselves. Herodotus, an early historian who visited Africa, stated that ancient Egypt was the healthiest country and was filled with physicians. The need for medicinal herbs and food in European countries became very obvious. On the continent of Europe pandemics continued to strike even as late as 1836, 1847, 1889 and in 1918 the plague almost destroyed Europe. With each plague and pestilence, the European mercantile system escalated its profits by controlling herbs, food, magic cures, health knowledge and technology. The clans controlled Caucasian countries. The rulers of clans ruled countries. When their profits increased due to economically exploiting the poor and fearful population, they would increase their military control over the poor. When the poor grew food, the armies would take it in order for the clans to stay in control.

The Europeans were besieged by dis-eases and violence as well as lack of foods and herbs. Every advance the poor made to get out of poverty and diseases, the clans would attack them with their military and seize the food and land for taxes. This maintained the clan's wealth. Hippocrates swarmed the Europeans that fired food (cooked food), pastry and a predominantly animal flesh diet was the cause of constipation and all the dis-eases of European culture. In contrast, the healthy Africans had a diet of primarily of whole raw foods and used herbs and holistic natural remedies. Coprolite studies, which examined the intestines of the mummies, revealed bee pollen, raw food, coarse fibrous vegetables, and mummified bodies free from constipation. Despite the knowledge of Hippocrates about constipation and filth causing diseases, the plagues and pestilences were given religious and superstitious significance. The plague struck England intermittently from 1300 to 1676. Marseilles, France was devastated by plagues. The populations of France and

England were struck by cholera, smallpox, syphilis, diphtheria, typhoid, typhus, rickets and tuberculosis. This helped stimulate the Caucasian food plants and herb trade.

Pestilences and plagues strike women the severest. Men were demanding that all fertile women increase their breeding in order to hold the population in numerical balance against the increasing death rate, which was decreasing the population. Generally, there should be one live birth for every death. Pandemics caused deaths to increase rapidly and the women had to increase breeding. In order to increase breeding, the women had to violate the natural human breeding cycle, which dictates that a female has one child every three to five years. Abstinence of sex during the three-year breastfeeding period had to be violated. The increased birthing resulted in weaker offspring and caused the deterioration of the female reproductive organs. Consequently, whenever pandemics struck, the heaviest burden fell upon women. Women were forced to bear three times as many children. The result of this was an increase in the death rate of birthing women. For example, five women die for every 1,000 children born, the mortality rate for birthing mothers is five. Female death rates increase as the number of previous live births increase. Many children died because the mother's death was caused by pandemics while pregnant. There were many birth defects, miscarriages, mental illnesses, stillbirths and retarded children. Many children were abandoned because the mother was too weak or sick to care for them.

The plagues and pestilences left a trail wherever Europeans traveled. Plagues struck lower Egypt in 1542 and spread up the Nile and into Asia Minor. These plagues struck because the Egyptians were under constant Caucasian attacks and did not have a stable agriculture due to Caucasian attacks. The Europeans traveled along the coast and pandemics followed them. They traveled into the interior and plagues followed them. When they reached Constantinople, their plagues were killing 5,000 to 10,000 people daily. The massive death toll was evidence of a need for herbs, food plants and medicinal knowledge. European plagues were carried to Greece, Italy, Gaul, and to the Rhine. It took 15 years for the Europeans to spread pandemics throughout their travel routes. Europeans carried these plagues into Africa. As a result, food shortages developed due to the death of diseased farmers. This further weakened the health of the invaded African countries and helped the Europeans to become conquerors. European plagues, famines and internal violence disrupted the food supply and the African cultures' protective mechanism. Europeans used their dis-eases as weapons to conquer. The herb trade was controlled by the Venetian Republic from the Ninth to the Fifteenth Century. They defeated their nearest competitor, the Genoese, and remained in control of the herbs until the Portuguese challenged them.

In 1453, the fall of Constantinople disrupted the Eastern food, dry goods and herb trade. This interruption caused a shortage of foods and herbs and an increase in the herb prices. The scarcity of herbs caused herb merchants to sell herbs at a greater price. Only Venetian merchants could afford to buy from distributors and retail to the public, thus helping the Venetian herb trade develop a monopoly.

The Portuguese and Spaniards, using African maps astrology and navigators, searched for a cheaper market for herbs and food plants and journeyed to India. Portuguese merchants, led by Vasco da Gama, circled the Cape of Good Hope and sailed to Calcutta. They reentered the herb trade with cheaper herbs and undersold the Venetians. This ended the Venetian control of the seas and drug trade.

There were many battles fought on the seas between rival herb and food plant merchants. Many ships full of valuable life saving herbs were sunk. Many valuable herbs were destroyed on the land so that other competitors could not obtain them for sale. There were counterfeit herbs sold and dispensed that caused the Europeans to feel herbs were worthless. In any case, the Portuguese ships loaded with dry goods and medicinal herbs docked in Lisbon and caused the merchants of the Rialto to panic for fear of attack or destruction of their herb traffic monopoly.

In 1600, the herb trade shifted to various nations. Fierce sea and land battles were fought to gain control of herbs. Finally, the Dutch emerged as the controllers of the herb trade. The Dutch stockpiled herbs in Amsterdam, Holland in order to inflate cost. They stockpiled the herb nutmeg in Amsterdam for 16 years. They did not sell nutmeg until after it was soaked in limewater for three months. This soaking prevented the buyers from growing the herb from the seed. Stockpiling of valuable herbs caused increased death rates for the Europeans and increased the wealth of the merchants. The Dutch also controlled mace and clove.

The English gained control of the herb trade in 1800. This would be during a time that plagues devastated the population causing a desperate need for herbs, food and knowledge. *Natural History* by Pliny (Gaius Plinius Secundos), a Roman historian, points to many of these events.

Today, the herb trade is falsely referred to as the spice trade. The source of this herb knowledge always pointed to Africa. Despite the fact that herbs were introduced, in Europe, by the Egyptians, Greeks, Romans, Arabians, and Indians, the source of the oldest medical science remains African. The European monks learned herb and food crop hybridization and adaptations from African priests. This adaptation of herbs slowed down the invasion. However, a land and a people were culturally assassinated and utterly destroyed in the wake of the European path for racial survival.

The Spanish tried to enter the herb market. They sent a government sponsored expedition led by Columbus to find a cheap herb market in India. However, he got lost and landed in Hispanola in 1492. Columbus failed in his attempt to reap some of the vast wealth in the herb trade. He did bring a Native American Indian on his return trip as a token gift for the Spanish government, but the Native American died. Queen Isabella and

King Ferdinand of Spain are credited with the sponsorship of Columbus' expeditions, which were actually invasions that were romantically written about.

DRUGS AND EUROPEANS

The herb knowledge of the Europeans was unevolved and lacking in healing application. Apothecaries (today called drugstores or pharmacies) complained that counterfeit manure was being sold by herb traders and that the manure that was authentic was adulterated by traders. Manure was a popular remedy in the absence of African herbs and holistic diagnosis and treatments. Cardinal Richelieu, on his deathbed, drank horse manure mixed with Caucasian wine as a medicinal cure. *Natural History* by Pliny listed human manure, urine and menstrual blood as medicines used by Europeans. Menstrual blood was believed to kill insects and calm storms at sea.

The Europeans imitated the fossilized plant or crystal treatment systems of Africa, instead of using natural crystals. They used the crystallized waste of the liver or kidney. In other words, they used gallstones and kidney stones. These stones were called Bezoar. Charles of France was presented with a Bezoar stone and he was very proud of it. The Bezoar stone was believed to possess curative powers.

Usnea was collected from the skull bone remains of the skeleton of criminals who had been hung in chains. Usnea is the moss scraped from the human skull. It was an official remedy and was listed in the European pharmacopoeia (present day drug chemical formula book). Usnea was carried by all respectable apothecaries. The pharmacopoeia listed the sole of an old shoe worn by some man that walked extensively. The sole would be ground and taken internally for diarrhea (dysentery). Hangman's rope was used for an external medicine. It was ground and applied to sores and bruises. Supposedly, this healed sores. Wounds were surgically treated and most victims died from the wound treatment, not the wound. A male going to a physician for wound treatment had fears of death and homosexual rape. In fact, the Hippocratic oath forbade physicians from seducing females, males, freemen and slaves. (Incidentally, all Caucasian physicians were males during this period of time. Most were homosexuals). Aside from having wounds, many soldiers had syphilis and respectable physicians would not treat them for the venereal dis-ease.

The natives of Haiti used the herb, Guaiacum or Hollywood, for the treatment of mucous discharge symptoms (colds, flu). The Europeans invaded Haiti for Hollywood and they eventually controlled the herb in the herb wars. Sassafras and sarsaparilla were other African herbs marketed during the drug war. However, sarsaparilla is primarily an alterative, diaphoretic, and is used for skin dis-ease. During the 16th century, this trailing vine was used in Europe. Today, the roots are used in steroid chemistry as they yield a progesterone related chemical. Sassafras is similar to sarsaparilla and the two are usually used together. However, the medicinal herbs were basically ineffective for treatment of the mucous forming diet of Europeans, which caused the disease to remain unchanged.

The venereal dis-eases of syphilis and gonorrhea are contemporary pestilences. Gonorrhea is the mucous discharge from the genitals and sexual intercourse is blamed. Caucasian science associates problems with sex as caused by the female and her original sin, which caused the decline of man. Sexism names these dis-eases and implies that women caused disease. Venereal disease is associated with morality and the female Venus. Morality measures right and wrong and is applied specifically with venereal dis-ease only. All dis-eases are immoral (wrong) in the body. No disease is more moral (right) than another dis-ease. The morality of the human body is health. However, morality is applied to venereal dis-ease because of its association with female sexuality. Females were sexistly treated in books such as *Essay Upon Whoring* by Bernard Mandeville (1660). However, African science reveals a proper perspective on dis-ease.

Venereal dis-ease is a holistic dis-ease caused by a weakened condition of the entire body and the degeneration of the sex organs. Usually, water (mucous discharge) is given off in the body whenever an organ, organ system or body section is weak. Water acts as a solvent for elimination of waste. Water comes whenever a cut, burn or bruise traumatizes the body. For example, a burn, sore or cut produces pus (water). Pus is a liquid band-aid. When the body is overloaded with toxins, water is caused to come and is discharged from the nose. This is called "catching a cold." A sick individual cannot "catch health" from a healthy person nor can a healthy individual "catch a cold" from the sick. Ironically, you are healthy, then you catch a cold, then you are sick for a few days and get rid of the cold. The conclusion from this is if you stay sick, you can get rid of disease. This is stupid. Besides, you cannot catch the weather—catch "cold," catch "partly cloudy," catch "hot," catch "snow," or "rain." It is stupid. Diseases, such as a cold, is the body getting rid of disease. Eating a candy bar, hot dog or pickles, etc. cause disease, not a cold. Be that as it may, the mucous discharge dis-eases of gonorrhea is a pestilence caused by undernutrition, improper food combinations, poor diets and excessive sex. These dis-eases are not found in any animal kingdom except the human kingdom. Caucasian scientist accused ancient Egyptians of having syphilis because they associated deformities of bones and the marks left upon mummified bones as being derived from syphilis. These marks have occurred postmortem (after death) and were caused by insects and fungus. The same type of marks have been found on the bones of cave bears. Again, animals in their natural environment and following their specific bodily defined diet and following their mating season (sex cycle) do not have venereal dis-eases. This dis-ease is a holistic illness and contemporary pestilence. The book, which gave the dis-ease its name, is *Syphilis Five Morbus Galicus* by Girolamo Fracastro (1530).

European countries were at a medical loss in solving their pandemics, African herbs, diagnosis, and treatment knowledge was too complex for them to understand and use. The Caucasians made attempts to apply African medical science to the their population. Mithridates VI, king of Pontus (c. 115 - 63 B.C.), was an early pharmacologist. The Caucasians' Pharmacological knowledge was derived from Egyptian herbal pharmacology and chemistry. The Greeks were the first Caucasians to steal the information and adulterate it. Egyptians had a complex system of allopathic, homeopathic and naturopathic usage of herbs and plant drugs. The Greeks used the allopathic system because it is more static and tempered than the naturopathic system. The naturopathic system is based upon the African culture. It is a fusion of the past, present and future, a fusion of time, distance and space, the Male and Female Principles, astrology and the cycles of living substances and the elements. In the period after the Thirteenth Dynasty, the Egyptians' medical systems was partially adopted, distorted and used by foreign cultures. In approximately 500 B.C., Greek physicians such as Hippocrates, studied in Egypt. Upon the Greek conquest, Egyptian medicine began to decline and the Caucasians replaced it with their culture's interpretation of healing. The Caucasian system was economically based. The practitioners formed a secret society and took an oath not to give holistic health knowledge to patients. The oath is called the Hippocratic Oath. Their medical system is filled with mythology (theories, fantasies), rituals and ceremonies, superstitions and the language of medicine but without the healing of medicine.

Preceding the invasion of Alexander the Great (before 332 B.C.), Egyptian medicine was labeled as the primitive practice of ignorant savage Africans and by the time Alexandria was founded, the remains of African medicine were considered totally backwards. The Caucasians had colonialized the concept of medicine and their medicine was the most respected. Their White Supremacy psychosis had defined White medicine as supreme and Black medicine as stupid. At the time of the Middle Ages, African medicine had been basically usurped and the African knowledge of surgery, diagnosis, acupuncture, massage, prescription dosages and schedules had been claimed by the Caucasians. Europeans regarded African medicine as their discovery and rewrote and propagandized history to exclude African medical science, nutrition and medical universities. They eventually named African medicine "holistic."

Mithridates was versed in Egyptian medical science. He attempted to convert all the knowledge into an easily understood linear logic system. The allopathic poison drug formulas he derived were tested on African slaves before being used on Europeans. Mithridates would administer his poisonous experimental compounds on slaves and then try his antidote. This caused him to kill many slaves in the name of science. He focused his experiments on snake venoms and brought all types of poisonous herbs and poison antidotes from Africa in order to research. Mithridates died before he could find an antidote to the poisons. Mithradaticum was the name he applied to the antidote compound; later its name was changed to theriac. Theriac contained from thirty-seven to sixty-three ingredients. A principle ingredient of this life-sustaining compound was the flesh of vipers. Snakes, such as the viper, are immune to their own poisonous venom. He used the Nubian homeopathic system and believed he could cause people to have the snake's immunity quality. Theriac was a primary cure-all for all types of dis-eases until the 1800s. The preparation of theriac was guarded by Renaissance city officials to prevent the adulteration of its healing value. The name theriac was colloquialized to treacle. Treacle was disproved to be of healing value and its use was discontinued. Subsequently, the term treacle was applied to molasses. Treacle and molasses were given to European young children as a tonic. So it follows that today, molasses has been given a high nutritional and curative value based upon its history. However, its high sugar content nullifies its nutritional value and like all types of sugars, it causes a nutritional drain, kidney damage, diabetes, high blood pressure, arthritis, reproductive problems, hyperactivity and addiction. It would be safer to use Dandelion Root, Alfalfa and Yellowdock as a nutritional replacement.

The Egyptian medical science as contained in the volumes of medical books written by Imhotep, who was born in 1827 B.C., was acculturated and distorted by Hippocrates. In the Alexandria University, expansive African herb usage and holistic medicine was taught and reduced to a level that the Greeks could understand and use. In due course, the Roman medical science included many plant drugs and herbs. The African Egyptian science was contaminated by the Assyrians, Saites, Greeks and Romans and these combined civilizations brought a perverted use of the multitude of herbs, foods and plant drugs. The Caucasians began to equate all medicinal herbs as regenerators, life extension, curatives, sex stimulants and digestive herbs. This was primarily caused by the Caucasian civilizations' short lifespan (twenty to thirty years), venereal dis-eased mucous discharges, skin eruptions (smallpox), and the constipating diet that they had. Today, Caucasians follow the static Over-The-Counter (O.T.C.) drug prescriptions usage as if it is a religion. These O.T.C. drug dosage levels do not take into account the biochemical make-up of an individual or whether the individual is a slow or fast metabolizer, the hormone cycle, the diet, whether you have a male or female or child's metabolism, nor the race of the consumer. Each race has a unique biochemistry, genetic code, digestive flora composition and blood cell ratio (i.e., crystallizes differently). The O.T.C. drugs do not consider the diet as a cause of the symptoms (so-called dis-ease) of a dis-ease or the astrological influences or spiritual stressors.

Galen transmuted the distorted system of African medicine into his system and this further acculturated and distorted African science. Galen's system was an attempt to use the Egyptian mystery healings system. He, like other Caucasians, used herbs and defined them as good for digestive problems, sexual diseases, and mucous congestive diseases.

Dioscorides was a field surgeon in the army of Nero. He accompanied the army on many invasions of countries for precious crystals, treasures, technology, food plants, metals and medicinal herbs. Dioscorides collected and compiled the herbal information of Africa. His book was the first European material medica — medicinal dictionary. The book was an attempt to provide cures for the many pestilences, plagues and eliminate barbaric medical practices. Filth, ignorance and barbaric behaviors was the cause of the European population's rapid decline. Many of the substances in his work were the basic medicines used later during the Renaissance. In his book, the domestication, cultivation, collection, storage, preparation and dosages were given for both African herbs and indigenous European herbs. His system was combined with the esoteric healing and medical superstitions of the Crusade era up to the Seventh Century. It is erroneously viewed as primarily a religious herbal system and is called galenicals (after Galen) and vegetable simple (herbs). Today, those same herbs have been scientifically researched and verified as having medical healing properties. Caucasians began using herbs extensively, though not wisely (e.g., Valerian, relatively harmless, used to manufacture valium, very dangerous).

Galen followed the African system of elementals. In this system, the elements of air, earth, fire and water are defined as the primary composition of the body. Elements have qualities- air's quality is dry, earth's quality is cold, fire's quality is hot, and water's quality is wet. The health of the individual is based upon a balance of the elements. A dis-ease state is caused by an imbalance between one or more of the elements. This system requires a holistic understanding of the interrelationship between the spirit, mind and body as well as the Male and Female Principles.

A disease cure was caused by the character and quality of the illness and the character and quality of the elemental cure. Galen used African science's cyclical laws, which were based on the rhythms of the earth, air, water and fire and astrology combined with the cyclical nature of humans. This indicates that the methods of Hippocrates were less elaborate and based upon observations and linear logic while Galen's were based on adulterated African Maat logic.

The Galen acculturated Afri-centric system required several thousands of herbs, foods and plant drugs (i.e., opium) in treatment application. In one prescription, various tropical edible plants and fruits were used in combination with herbs. Today, this approach is labeled an organic whole foods natural diet (unprocessed foods). Medicinal herbs, natural vitamins and minerals and exercise are called holistic treatment just as it was in Galen's distorted Afri-centric treatments. During the Roman Empire's era of power, the physicians prepared and stored their own herbs and hid their knowledge in a mystery system. The professional doctors used a distorted version of

African medical science. Folk doctors who sold and administered medicine to the poor were in competition with the professionals and the Pope (used faith healing). Valuable herbs, medicinal foods and plant drugs (i.e., opium) were primarily controlled by rich merchants. The multinational rich merchant clans owned ships and priced medicine at a price that was too high for common folks. The local apothecaries (drugstores) of the poor were then controlled by retired prostitutes, salesmen with bogus remedies and the poor themselves.

The apothecaries were the only place where venereal dis-eases were treated. Physicians of that time did not want to demean their respectable reputation by treating venereal disease. In the Eighteenth Century, the hospitals in Vienna refused to treat venereal disease. They would hire a man who was not a physician to treat venereal disease twice a year.

Apothecary owners during the Middle Ages attended fairs and sold the latest medicinal herbs from Africa, pigs kidney stones, grave yard dirt, menstruation blood, magic spells, blood letting knives, dead insects and mostly non-medical items. Furthermore, apothecaries in Europe were like today's health food stores, they sold groceries, herbs, purgatives and cosmetics. During the Fourteenth Century, Europeans began to adopt the medicinal herbal (make-up face painting on acupressure meridians) practice of the old age Egyptians. However, they did not have an understanding of how herbs were applied to acupuncture meridian points and assumed face painting was strictly a cosmetic application. In the African acupuncture treatment system, herbal essence, oils, resins and pulverized leaves, flowers and roots were placed on acupuncture points of the face or body that related to internal organs. (See Face Chart). For example, red clover was rubbed on the cheek for blood purification. In Caucasian culture, making the cheeks rosey red is a symbol of fertility and is considered sexy.

Purgatives (laxatives) were a dominant drug in England. This was due to the constipating diet of cooked and/or raw animal flesh and pastry, which was greasy, salty and undigestible, and very, very few vegetables. If a small quantity of vegetables were eaten, they were overcooked in the fat (grease) blood, pus and mucous (called essence) of cooked animal flesh. A diet such as this is constipating and dis-ease forming. The meals were eaten too late in the day or too close together to allow the stomach to empty. It takes four hours for food to leave the stomach and another four for it to leave the intestines. Their scavenger diet and practice of eating scraps of meat or pastry all day constipates. Snacks eaten between meals causes food to stay in the stomach from 16 to 48 hours and thus constipate. Hippocrates stated that the cause of over 90% of all illness among Caucasians was (and still is) constipation. There are many signs of constipation such as halitosis, a tongue coated, one bowel movement daily or every other day, hemorrhoids, a white mucous discharge in comers of the eye, flatulence (stomach gas), varicose veins, foul smelling feet, mood swings, rheumatism, arthritis, and foul body odors. The Caucasians' constipating animal flesh diet is mentioned in Pepy's Diary. Purgatives were taken along with enemas. Apothecaries (i.e., drugstores, health food stores) of long ago also gave enemas. Today, Caucasians have an industry devoted to constipation, called colon therapists. Colon therapists use machines and herbal medicines for Caucasian constipation. In addition to apothecaries, the barbers (hair cutters) administered enemas and used blood letting as disease remedies. The remains of barbers' past activities are revealed by the symbol of bloodletting—red blood strip dripping down a white pole. The ancient Caucasians believed the evil spirit that caused you to be constipated or catch a cold was in the blood. The barber would cut your vein to make you bleed and release the disease. Caucasians used the blood letting symbol during Christmas. The candy walking stick has a red blood ribbon (dye) wrapped around it.

The Egyptians that switched from their indigenous diet to a diet influenced by others took purgatives and enemas three times a month, based on the principle that food is not needed by the body. In fact, many predynastic cultures were vegetarians. This has been verified by the human jaw bone structure of fossilized bones and mummies. The jaws of vegetarians have a wide arch while the jaws of flesh-eating humans and other animals have a narrow arch.

Egyptians practiced the dietary system on the principle that food is a form of worshipping a holy temple (the body) and it excites and stimulates the body's spiritual, mental and physical energies while the Caucasians believe you attack and prey upon food by eating it. In other words, the Caucasians believe that eating food means a plant cell becomes a human cell. A plant, no matter how primitive or evolved, can never become a human being and a human being cannot become a plant (plant energy excites and stimulates human energy). However, this dietary belief is part of so-called contemporary Caucasian science mythology. It is basically a primitive adolescent cultural belief and not scientific in origin or application. Constipation causes the body to become toxic with waste. This is called autointoxication. The ancient African physicians gave laxatives (purgatives) or enemas as the beginning step in a treatment protocol in order to cleanse the digestive tract of waste. Cellular and/or food waste accumulation causes the defenses of the body to weaken. This weakened bodily condition provides a favorable environment for dis-eases to exist. It takes energy to feed a disease as a disease can be starved of energy and will not survive in the body (fast). This complex African knowledge was totally misunderstood by the Caucasians. In the Caucasian culture's allopathic system, they believe constipation to be a dis-ease. In the allopathic systems, the symptom of the disease is believed to be the cause and the cause of a disease is believed to be a symptom. Allopathic drug medicine is a symptom treating medicine. Constant constipation and the continuous use of irritating and poisonous laxatives causes the intestines to become weak and to lose its ability to function. The allopathic cures became the dis-ease and cause of deaths. The diet or unsanitary conditions was not believed to cause disease. Disease was (and is) believed to be caused by an invisible evil spirit (bacteria). The use of laxatives and enemas began to decline in the later part of the Eighteenth Century because of the increase in tropical African foods, herbs, medical principles and the use of what the Caucasians believed to be a ritual and ceremony called hygiene, science and cleanliness.

In the Sixteenth and Seventeenth Centuries, apothecaries began dispensing African medicinal herbs and teaching their clients how to use them. This caused a dispute between the untrained apothecary owners and the professional physicians who used a superstitious cures and practiced allopathic symptom treatment system. In France, in the Sixteenth and Seventeenth Centuries, the physicians won the dispute over the apothecaries. In England, the apothecaries won the dispute because apothecaries treated people during the plague while physicians abandoned the cities and stopped treating plague victims. The people rallied and supported the apothecaries over the physicians. This decision was eventually reversed as prominent people and the Pope were against the apothecaries and in 1866, this dispute was settled by allowing school-trained physicians to prescribe herbs and superstitious cures.

The European distortion of the sympathy system caused them to treat weapons with ointments. In the sympathic system, a person with a knife wound would wash and bandage the wound and apply healing ointment to the knife. The Caucasians believed the evil spirit in the knife and the evil spirit in the wound needed treatment. Actually, the African sympathy treatment application means that if one member of the family is ill, the entire family is ill and every member is treated. For example, if one member of the family is an alcoholic (husband), the entire family (wife, children) should be treated for the dis-ease of alcoholism because they develop co-dependent addiction. The Greek and other European culture's misunderstanding or ignorance of the African sympathy system is due to scientific bias. In the book, *The Power of Sympathy* by Kenelme Digby (1658) this system is expounded upon.

Paracelsus, one of the leading European doctors used weapon ointment in the sympathy system. He was praised for his medical knowledge and is probably one of the best healers in European science. He did not understand that the cleaning and bandaging of a knife would not help the would to heal. He thought the cleaning and bandaging was a way to release evil spirits that caused the bleeding. The African Hygiene system was completely misunderstood. To Caucasians, cleaning and bandaging were rituals and ceremonies. Hippocrates and Galen would pour boiling hot oil on wounds. Paracelsus' use of cleaning and bandages was a progressive step forward in European medicine.

In the first edition of the Encyclopedia Britannica, Usnea and other nonmedical items are listed as curative medicines. The need for medicinal herbs and a holistic healing science to apply them are obvious from the records of Europeans. Their dis-ease remedies were worthless and could in no way curb the tide of pandemics. Many of the herbal remedies they had access to were covered with superstition and medical ignorance.

The egotism of the Greeks prevented the scientific application of African knowledge. Ancient herbalists and drug practitioners of Greece protected their formulas and created an elitist healing group. They created evil stories about herbs to keep their patients from growing them and treating themselves. Rootdiggers or herbalists (called Rhizotomoi) were the inventors of curses on herbs, ghosts that haunted herbs and spirits that protected herbs. Some of their tales of caution can be found in *Enquiry into Plants* by Theophrastus written in the Fourth Century B.C. Many gods and spirits associated with herbs are useful. For example, the ancient Chaldean civilization developed herbal medicine and holistic treatment system. Their god of healing was EA. Prayers were made to EA and these prayers included the names of treatment herbs such as Fleabane and St. John's Wort. The prayers to EA were actually prescriptions for treating disease.

The storing of herbs was dangerous because the early Europeans lacked the knowledge for proper storage. In fact, many dis-eases were caused by this lack of knowledge. For example, St. Anthony's Fire was caused by the improper storage of rye kernels (*See Medical Miracles.*) The heads of the kernels stored in dampness caused an enlarged blackhead to form on the kernels. When these kernels with black heads were eaten, it caused diseases. A plague was started by the consumption of rotten rye. This conclusion was reached by The Duke of Sully France in 1630. His discovery came after the plague killed thousands of Caucasians.

SCIENTIFIC METHOD OR DIET

The European static linear approach to science demands a fixed situation. This fixed situation is called a controlled environment. The African scientific approach however is based upon an unfixed environment, cycles, a mixture of the spirit, mind and body as wholistic, astrology, Male and Female Principle, Maat, etc. In other words, a continuous change of the individual's mind, mood, state of consciousness, internal organs, body and spirit is taken into account. This is called the holistic internal (body) environment and is viewed as one. Similarly, man and his environment are considered to be part of one (Holistic) great spirit, which is too complex to be fixed by Europeans. Controlled observation or an unnatural observation are used in Caucasian science. The effectiveness of treatment is measured by controlled groups to be observed. One group is controlled and given treatment while the other group is uncontrolled and given no treatment. It is assumed that the medicine given the controlled group made them well. If the person gets sick and died from the treatment then it means they died of disease complications and not from the treatment. The person may get well regardless to the treatment. However, these possibilities are not taken into account in Euro-centric medicine. Therefore, it follows that any European proof of drug treatment has too many unforeseen variables and is subjectively interpreted, not objectively interpreted. In other words, the scientific conclusion based upon controls is whatever they want it to be.

Today, the scientific method as used by the United States Government has set the "Recommended Daily Allowance" of vitamin, mineral and protein standards. It recommends 5,000 I.U. (International Units) of Vitamin A based on research that uses the European scientific methods. This recommendation is also based on their scientific method theory (fantasy, fairy tale science) that over 5,000 I.U. of vitamin A will cause liver damage. However, the Hunza people eat over 14,000 I.U. of A in the form of dried apricots. They eat approximately 100,000 I.U. of Vitamin A in foods. The Caucasian scientific method is used to keep the ill from achieving health. It is a military tool used to manipulate and control disease and health and generate money for the disease industry and pharmaceutical cartel.

The European scientific method is tested on sick people. In that respect, all allopathic (M.D.) doctors are trained on sick people. They study diseased people in order to understand (or overstand) dis-eases, not health. While the African medical system studies healthy people in order to understand the holistic process of health. The objective of medicine is wellness. Therefore, the healer must understand how an individual progresses from health to dis-ease, to treatment and returns to health and then to higher wellness. Ironically, the European system progresses from primary disease, then to a treatment and then returning to a secondary dis-ease condition. This secondary disease condition is usually subclinical malnutrition or an undiagnosed dis-ease level known as "good" health. They believe the absence of disease means wellness. In other words, a car driver that has never had an accident is assumed to be a good driver (healthy). This is not the case.

The Caucasian race has a pathological health state predicated on their historical diets. The Caucasian skin pigment is caused by a fundamental deficiency of minerals. Their blood is infested with white corpuscles (blood cells), waste, and mucous constipation. The white blood cells are high in number because they are needed to defend the body from the dis-eases floating in the bloodstream. In the book *Mucousless Diet Healing System* by Arnold Ehret, published in 1922, the Caucasians' white skin complexion and high amount of White blood cells is proven to be caused by the sickly condition of the Caucasian race. The European system never define the cultural the health standards they use to establish health. Consequently, the scientific method is at best is a misused and abused cultural ritual and ceremony of their science mythology and not founded on scientific principles. Their treatments use synthetic inorganic minerals (dirt) as medicine.

The mineral substance treatment for dis-ease was introduced as a means of overcoming the shifting control of herbal drugs. Many specific herbs were being controlled by various European countries. In addition to this there were counterfeit herbs sold. Herbs were secretly stockpiled. European merchants would destroy African herbs, burn villages, and murder natives who grew the herbs (herbalists). This was done in order to keep the herb growth whereabouts a secret. They hid herbs to produce scarcity of herbs. European economics is based upon scarcity, not abundance. An herb such as Quassia kills worms and is used as a febrifuge and laxative. This alone made it important in European diets. It is also good for dandruff, itchy scalp, and it is especially good for blondes. It also poisons fish and is used by fishermen in order to catch fish. An African slave by the name of Quassia withheld the information about the herb's identification from the Europeans. His herbal secret cost him his life. The secret of its medical properties was taken from him in 1756. The Dutch began stockpiling the herb Quassia in Stockholm and sold it in Europe. The drug merchants used many tactics to create herbal scarcity in order to over price herbs and get larger profits. Their tactics caused medical science to use non-herbal remedies. They started using minerals. A leading doctor of the time, Paracelsus, strongly promoted mineral dis-ease treatments. Although this was an improvement over other Caucasian remedies, it had its drawbacks because many of the minerals (such as mercury) were poisonous.

Mercury was used internally and externally as a drug for syphilis and other dis-ease. Antimony or Stilbium was another poisonous mineral used. A medical book such as *The Triumphant Chariot of Antimony* by Basile Valentine published in 1604 helped popularize antimony. This mineral was known to be poisonous as monks died while using it to stop emaciation during fasting. Thus, it was named "anti-monk" or antimony. Tartar Emetic was taken by Napoleon while he was a prisoner on the island of St. Helena. He had a digestive illness, and a dis-ease of the stomach. Napoleon became ill from the poisonous mineral treatment. After this painful experience, Napoleon refused the treatment of learned physicians. Obviously, the need for a safe medical system was needed.

Europeans were trying to arrive at a system or substance that would give health. Health and the saving of their race from dis-eases was an overwhelming problem. The invasion of Africa for lifesaving herbs caused an oversight of the reality that health is based upon a healthy diet, a holistic culture and where food is considered medicine and medicine is food. Herbs are not the real medicine. Herbs primarily give you time to establish a healthy diet. Herbs are a short-term medical device used to adjust the fluctuating health states of the Africans. Food was the main medicine in African's health not herbs. Other cultures verify that it was not medicine but rather a combination of diet and health knowledge that sustain Africans.

A high fiber diet such as those researched and validated by the Hunza people in the Himalayan mountains produces an average lifespan of between 100 to 200 years. Their diet has no oils, bleached Caucasian flour, Caucasian rice, sugars or fried foods. Furthermore, they have a whole food diet (not partial foods, processed) of natural fruits, vegetables, seeds, nuts, spring water, grains, no cow's milk, and no eggs. They consume very little animal flesh and are often vegetarian. More than that, other colored peoples on a whole foods natural organic diet, such as Australian aborigines and African natives have equally long if not a longer lifespan. The ancient Africans must have had a longer lifespan because their diet was the highest in nutrient content and they practiced spiritual health and social health by using Maat.

The Hunza diet is not as rich in wild plants (undomesticated) as the ancient Africans. The ancient African diet was not only the same as the Hunzas but very much improved because of the complex variety of tropical plants, medicinal herbs and the higher evolved health system and holistic Maat culture. The Africans lived well over 200 to 300 years in age. The use of the Hunzas as a correlation for age of raw food diet Africans indicates that the slaves brought to the Americas were between 200 and 300 years of age. Hunzas live well over 100 years on a diet of inferior quality as compared to the massive variety of organic foods used in the Africans' diet. The diet included wild plants and a wholistic use of the environment (See Metals, Crystals, Music, Colors).

The Europeans with a lifespan of 20 years (30 years of age was considered an elderly person) assumed that the slaves were their age or younger. The Caucasians used their cultural standard of age to measure the Africans' age. They recognized that the Africans were the healthiest people, but did not equate that the higher nutritional diet and holistic health standards would produce ages of 200 to 300 years. Today, any race that adopts the junk food diet has poor health, degenerative diseases (Cancer, AIDS), reproductive problems, a life of dis-eases, and a short lifespan (65 years of age is the average). The obvious relationship between diet and lifespan is overviewed in *The Missing Link* by Dr. Jay Hoffman.

A SCIENCE MISGUIDED
(A.D. 800 to 1800)

9th to 11th Century
The Caucasian invasion of Africa for healing herbs, vegetables and fruits began early in history. Emperor Charlemagne demanded tropical fruits for his garden. Some of the African fruits were figs, peaches, plums and pears. *The Capitulate de Villis Imperialibu,* written in 812 by Charlemagne, also indicates that his country actively exploited Africa for herbs, which they called spices or seasonings, such as celery, poppy, parsley, parsnips and other roots of plants. These plants have a medicinal curative effect on the body. Once the Caucasians started using these herbs, it caused Caucasian invasions to capture the source (Africa) and gain the herbal curative knowledge. This caused various Caucasian clans to set up a sea mercantile system to obtain these herbs. The invasion forces funded religious

orders/monks to come to Africa and steal the information technology. The monks were the first invasion force of clan controlled Caucasian countries. The clan's businesses used monks to help establish the sea- merchant commerce industry.

The monks and their monastic groups used African agriculture technology to save France and Italy. These monk/priest/herbalists used African devices and knowledge to implement drainage of the lowlands. The African irrigation helped rid the area of foul water that attracted the malaria carrying mosquitoes. Their African agricultural knowledge did not come from Europe as the Caucasians would drain marshes and stopped malaria pre-Roman (malaria outbreak in 8th and 9th Centuries) and the epidemics of the Renaissance, Assyria, India, China and Babylon. If the Caucasians had the knowledge, there would not have been malaria epidemics.

Agricultural knowledge was derived from Africa by the Caucasian priest (many were homosexuals). The European church insisted that their priests should travel to Africa. The priests said they were saving the pagan Africans, but they actually were saving Europe. They brought the agricultural knowledge back to Europe. African farming techniques spread throughout Europe. The Popes of the Cistercian order in the Fifteenth Century asked the African-trained priests to come to Campagna di Roma Italy and get rid of malaria by using their newly learned African technology.

In 1085, monks at Charteuse, near Grenoble, in France were using African hybridizing and grafting techniques to adapt African fruits, vegetables and herbs for consumption. Charteuse was a splinter group that used the Carthusian Order of the Orient and African herbology and agriculture sciences.

The White Supremacy psychosis of the church and Caucasians caused them to develop species of African herbs that had Caucasian flowers. At Norwich, a monk garden was planted by the sacristan called Saint's garden. In the garden were roses and lilies. Their white flowers indicated purity and holiness. In fact, many African names for plants were changed by Caucasians to the female title "lady." Lady meant a pure virgin saintly Caucasian woman. Herbs, such as Our Lady's Slipper (orchid), Lady's Fingers (Anthyllis Vulnerarira), Our Lady's Thistle (ribbon, grass), Our Lady's Tears However, and Lily of the Valley indicate purity (White Supremacy). Violent battles, in 1545, between the Caucasian tribes that were labeled as Catholics and Protestants, completely destroyed the herb farms (so-called garden) at Abbey of Mailras in Eaton Hills, near the Tweed River in England. In due course, the medicinal herbal farms (gardens) were completely destroyed and this put an additional shortage on the herbs needed to combat dis-ease.

German monks also used African technology to hybridize, graft and domesticate medicinal herbs, fruits and vegetables. Monks from Citreaux, France also hybridized and grafted herbs, vegetables and fruit. The herbal informational network between monks of various European countries was shared because they were in the same religious order and had homosexual bonds between them. The homosexual cults and secret societies bonded tribes together as clans. Clans, in different European countries fight each other and these fights are erroneously labeled as between countries.

The Saracenmic School of Medicine was widely known by the Arabics. The European countries from the Eight to the Twelfth Centuries had tribal wars, cannibalism, food shortages, famines, barbarism, pestilence and plagues, and no time for higher learning. Whatever literature existed was in the hands of elitist groups and among the Moors and Arabs. Aside from this, the majority of Caucasians could not read or write and thought the world was flat. It was not until the Norman conquest of Angleland (England) in A.D. 1066 that the European civilization mimicked and copied the African social system and developed monasteries and cathedrals. The Benedictine monks developed agriculture, herbology, horticultural and medicinal herbal modalities patterned after African systems.

The earliest medical school in recorded European history was in the 11th Century and was called Salerno. This school was modeled on the Imhotep-type schools called Escalapian Temples. These schools had monk/priest/herbalist teachers, as did all the early schools. Most of their teachers could not read or write. Actually, the Caucasian healing schools amounted to tribal initiations into herbal and spiritual witchcraft cults, known today as schools of medicine, not as cults. Today, the process uses information, ritual and ceremonies called memorization and tests. They issued degrees for skills in the ability to memorize and repeat information. However, these healing schools cure nothing, they just practice the medical cult. In any case, the first Salerno instructors were Black Moors from Arabia and of the Jewish faith. A decree by the Lateran Council, in 1139, forbade the monks from acting as doctors and wearing beards. The church did not want the monks blamed for causing deaths or associated with African civilization or the African Egyptian practice of shaving, which meant purification of the soul. More than that, the practice of medicine and spirituality was developing into two separate cults. The Greeks, mainly Hippocrates, separated his African hygienic system from the church's faith healing. The church was hiding healing medical books in monasteries to keep the people ignorant and sick and to hold on to their power. The church was a religious terrorist group that had wealth, military influence and control over whether a person would go to heaven or hell and they had herb farms and control over disease cures. They withheld the books of Galen for over 200 years then translated them into Latin and made it a sin against God to disagree with Galen.

William the Conqueror, son of Robert Normandy, was treated at Salerno. There were books written about Salerno, one of which was *The Metamorphosis of Ajax* by John Harrington, published in 1596. It was a translation of the medical textbook titled *Regimen Sanitatis Salernitanum*. This book was written in verse (poetic) as all early medical books were. It listed bleeding as a cure for sexual passion dis-ease. European medical science took other drastic extremist postures. The book is the first account of toilet use among Europeans, as *ajax* means toilet. Before that time, Caucasians would defecate and urinate inside their house or cave because they feared animal attacks and had no idea of sanitation.

One of the first European healing books, that used distorted African medicine, was written by a Dominican monk by the name of Albertus Magnusor Albert von Bonllstadt (1193 to 1280). This book was written on midwifery, African electromagnetic herb forces (auras) and medical applications and was considered a modern technology. It was far advanced over the Caucasian health books. This informative book has been distorted and titled *White and Black Magic.*

13th Century

In the 13th Century, the European medical science was still isolated among the monks and a select few. Galen, an early physician, taught in European medical schools. He taught the new modern science of anatomy of human beings. It was based upon superstitions, science mythology—theory (make believe) and ignorance. Galen's teachings revealed that the human breast-bone was segmented like the apes, the liver had many lobes like the hog, the uterus had two horns like a dog, and the hipbone was believed to be flared like the ox. This European anatomy belief was considered scientific until 1543 when Vesalius, a Belgian, proved that the hipbone was not flared. Galen's error in anatomy was attributed to evolution. The Caucasians believed that the hipbone had changed from being ox-like to its correct anatomical shape due to Europeans wearing tight pants. The Church said Galen's theory about the ox bone hip was Godly and should not be changed or protested. Caucasian medical ignorance did not help produce cures for plagues but rather caused diseases and added to the death toll.

The book *Anatomy* by Andreas Versalius was written in 1316 and was published in 1487. In the book, Versalius had had the correct drawings of the human body. He was tormented by medical men, the public and the church because it was widely believed that it was against God. It did not support superstitious ignorance. The book's information was not released until 1543 because the church hid it. Versalius was mentally abused and persecuted by the experience of trying to teach correct anatomy. He was driven insane and died of insanity.

The presence of Europeans in Africa caused a spread of the Bubonic Plague. Plagues spread to Greece, Italy and throughout Europe. By 1348, the plague had struck the Venetian Republic. In due course, they established the first quarantine of forty days based upon the forty days of a Black African biblical figure named Moses. He stayed in the desert (incidentally, quarantine is derived from Italian and means forty days). Be that as it may, the Venetians were stimulated to find herb cures to save the Republic. Their cures for plagues were not effective. One of the cures for the plague was the execution of Jews as an appeasement to God to stop the plague. This was really a device designed by the nobility and merchants to get rid of their Jew creditors. The Jews (Black moors) were trying to collect debts of large sums of monies from the Caucasian kings. Their death was the King's device to get rid of his bills. The plague caused the society to deteriorate. Violence, riots, and looting of the king's wealth were rampant. The kings and rich merchants were willing to finance invasions of Africa to get wealth and power and develop a military to protect their wealth and to get herbs to cure the "Black Death." Plagues were called the "Black Death" because of the dark areas formed by the minute blood vessel hemorrhages, caused by the dis-ease. The broken vessels blacken the white skin of Caucasians.

The plagues caused twenty-five million deaths in Europe. This can give a vague correlation to the death toll of Africans. This does not include deaths from pestilences, accidents, violence and venereal dis-ease. The many plagues in London from 1349 to 1666 were recorded in the *Journal of the Plague Year* by De Foe. Many people were persecuted, executed, tortured and branded as plague spreaders. Interesting to note the plague doctors used an imitation of the African medicine men masks. They would fill the mask with aromatic purification herbs to protect themselves. The Europeans acculturated these African masks and made them to resemble the beak of ducks. The doctors were called quacks because their masks looked like a duck's beak. In due course, the masks were called a European invention. Historical records indicate that the earliest use of a medical protective mask in recorded history occurred in Africa.

14ᵗʰ Century

The plagues, lifestyle, pestilence of venereal dis-ease and lack of herbs, resources and food caused a peculiar dilemma in Europe. They needed to find a source of medicinal knowledge and herbs. The venereal dis-eases were rapidly making the continuance of their race doubtful. Their future could only be in the immediate invasion of Africa for drugs, herbs, resources, technology, cultivatable land and healing foods.

Gonzalo Fernandex de Oviedo made one of the earliest European records of the under-nutritional Caucasian diet that caused a so-called tropical disease. He was raised in Spain among the pages in the palace of King Ferdinand and Queen Isabella. He was in Barcelona, in 1493, when Christopher Columbus returned from Haiti. He stated that Columbus' men on the voyage had Bubas or Yaws, better known as syphilis. Their diet on the ship's voyage was the typical Caucasian diet of mucous-forming foods and grains with the addition of salted flesh. The Italians passed the syphilis dis-ease to the French. It appeared in France, Germany, Switzerland, Holland and Greece in 1449. Vasco da Gama carried it on his ships to India in 1498, the Europeans brought it to China in 1505, and by 1569, it was allegedly smuggled into Japan. Since the Caucasian sailors on ships were men, it was probably spread due to homosexual activities. The Caucasian Jews and Mohammedans (Muslims) who were driven out of Spain by King Ferdinand and Queen Isabella after the conquest of Granada carried the dis-ease (pestilence) to Africa.

The Baron Gros (a painting) now in the Louvre, entitled "Les Pestiferes De Jaffa" shows Napoleon touching pus sores and the syphilis of his soldiers. This dis-ease was ultimately blamed on the French by many other European countries.

The European invasion was also stimulated by the travel of Mansa Musa. He was an African Islamic emperor of Mali and in the 14th Century B.C., he went on a religious journey to Moslimized Mecca. Emperor Musa carried many exotic fruits, plants, medicinal herbs and health practitioners along with warriors and displays of his vast wealth. He also carried a very large quantity of gold on his pilgrimage, which caused the price of gold to fall in Egypt. The accounts and reports of his pilgrimage reached Europe and on the first European map of West Africa in 1375, they labeled Mali as "Lord of the Negroes." The health of these Africans and the curative herbs of the physicians stimulated European interest in Africa.

The herbs that the merchants were selling on the international market were becoming too high. The fall of Constantinople stopped the Eastern trade and caused an even higher increase in herb prices. Consequently, another method of getting herbs was needed and was found with a machine called the printing press.

The advent of printing speeded up the exploitation of Africa for herbs food plants, technology, land and human resources (labor). The herb usage and treatments became easily available through books and notices. Printing also increased the spread of information about Africa's herb grafting, hybridizing, agriculture and treatment systems. In 1476 to 1477, Caxton brought printing to England. Consequently, many sacred herb books, treatment applications, holistic medicine science (mystery systems) were translated and printed in various languages. Books written in Persian, Cuneiform, Arabic, African languages, Latin and Greek were made available to the very few Caucasians who could read and elitist groups. Consequently, African sciences started the age of information technology and the space age, which is based upon African astrology.

William Turner collected herbal information and holistic medicine science from Germany, Holland, Italy and Switzerland. He wrote *Libellus De Re Herbaria Novus,* in 1538. His work indicates that these countries possessed African herbs that they obtained in the herb wars.

There were books that revealed herb medical use and medical ignorance. Accordingly, *Fabrica* by Andreas Versalius, in 1543, delineated the dissection of corpses in amphitheaters accompanied by music, singing, poems, dances and a play.

The use of books and herbal domestication techniques of the monks helped to escalate the invasion. Oddly enough, the books and information system of monks also slowed the invasion because they eventually learned to acclimate and domesticate herbs on farms (called gardens). Consequently, once the herb was obtained and domesticated, the traveling and invasion by many different Caucasian tribal groups was reduced by large multinational clans. These clans eliminated all small groups. Their philosophy was "get big or get out the slave trade." These large clans had large modern armies (guns and cannons) that terrorized and exterminated competitors.

15ᵗʰ Century
The holistic knowledge of African medicine was not easily accepted in 15ᵗʰ Century Europe. Europe was very sexist in addition to being racist, and their resistance to knowledge was based on many superstitions. They rejected Hippocrates' hygienic system in 640 B.C. and did not actually accept it until 1900 A.D.

In 1513, Eucharis Roslin of Worms, at the request of Catherine, the Duchess of Brunswick, wrote a book on midwifery. The book, *The Garden of Roses for Pregnant Women and Midwives*, contained dietary suggestions and stated that pregnant women should not eat garlic and pepper. It advised that the diet should include beans, peas, lettuce, rice, almonds and hazelnuts. This diet was actually taken from the African medical writings. The herbs and foods mentioned were not indigenous to Europe.

The oldest record of natural childbirth is in the Temple of Esneh in Africa. These records reveal that the best position for giving birth was in the squatting position. Further, the midwives had a court or entourage of assistants similar to the European marriage entourage of the bride and brides' maids. The diet for pregnant women was delineated in the Ebers Papyrus of 1550. It contained fertility recipes and formulas for contraceptives, such as the insertion of a lint tampon soaked in acacia and inserted in the vagina before intercourse. This makes the vagina acidic and kills the sperm. Furthermore, the Berol Papyrus of 1350 B.C. describes a method of determining the fetal sex of a child. In this method, the first urine of the day of the mother is used to moisten a small bag of barley and another small bag of wheat. If the barley sprouts, the sex of the unborn baby is a girl and if the wheat sprouts, it is a boy. If there is no germination (sprouting), the woman is not pregnant. This ancient African test was verified as 80% accurate in 1933 by Dr. Manger. The sprouting of the barley or wheat is caused by the estrogen in the urine. The papyrus mentioned the use of auras as a means of detecting pregnancy and fetal sex. The diet has an effect on gender. A highly acidic diet and acidic herbs eaten for a period of time before sex can cause the conception of a boy while an alkaline diet and herbs causes the conception of a girl. A diet very very low in natural sugars can cause abortion.

Imhotep's medical writings (Eber Papyrus) have the oldest records of biological conception. His writings mention a garlic douche for cleansing.

The Petri Papyrus of 1850 B.C. mentions contraceptive herb formulas. According to the Ebers Papyrus, the ancient African women used contraceptives such as the diaphragm. The Ebers Papyrus also mentioned indicators of detecting the imbalance of hormone levels in women. They were the excessive amount and shape of hair around the mouth or chin (decreased estrogen) and the hair shape around the uterus. Vaginal hair in a triangular shape indicates excessive male hormones. Incidentally, the first story (myth) about a bird bringing a baby to the mother came from Africa. The myth symbolized the godhead and the Ibis (a crane like bird) was that symbol. The Europeans distorted the myth and used the bird called the stork. In any case, the papyrus describes the chewing of Black Cohosh for menstruation problems, menopause symptoms, depression and nervousness. The medical papyrus information was severely needed in Europe. Multinationals (rich clans), secret societies (rich clans) and religious organizations (rich clans) that controlled the armies and wealth stopped the information from being widely used and accepted. Because it would jeopardize their power and ability to manipulate and control the peasants (citizens). These clans disguised themselves as European countries in order to tax the peasants and use them as armies for the protection of their empires. The clans told the peasants that their country was terrorized or their country had to fight a war or that the savage Africans needed to be civilized. This kept the peasants emotionally attached to a country (the clan).

In the early medical science, European males were forbidden to participate in births because females were sinful and cursed. Consequently, 1522, Dr. Wertt of Hamburg put on a woman's dress in order to attend a birth and make a case study of labor. He was discovered and burned to death as punishment. Ironically, Eucharis Roslin wrote his book on birthing and never witnessed a birth because his male purity could be exposed to the curse of women. It was believed that menstruation was a curse. In fact, the word menstruation means purging the body of sin. Ironically, all males are birthed by so-called sinful females and yet they considered themselves pure.

The types of ignorant devices were many. Sir Unton, ambassador to Queen Elizabeth in the court of Henry IV, on March 1, 1595 used combinations of herbs for diseases. As a further precaution for his dis-ease treatment, he tied a dead pigeon to the side of the chest of his sick patients. His patient had mucous congestion of the lungs (pneumonia) caused by a constipating diet and generally poor hygienic health standards.

Paracelsus was the leading medical doctor during the 15th Century. He was born in Switzerland and in 1493; he went to Africa and studied the African treatment modalities (Exoteric). This was during the period of the Dutch invasion of Africa. He introduced many scientific African health concepts and tools to Europe. However, the Caucasians did not accept African science and thought it was witchcraft. They still used their superstitious rituals for disease treatments and resisted scientific African disease definitions. In 1580, thousands of children and old women with diseases were killed as witches. This was sanctioned by the religious leader, Pope Innocent VII. Ironically, 15th Century Europe, besides lacking science knowledge also had no handkerchiefs, nightgowns, toilets, or forks. The introduction of these African gadgets and accessories caused many negative social and religious attacks. The newly introduced accessories caused problems. Sir Charles Bill in his book the *Bridgewater Treaties* written in the 15th Century, expounded on the crisis focused on the African table fork. In the reign of the early Stuarts, the fork was introduced as an instrument to assist in the act of eating. Africa had many cooking utensils while the majority of the European people resisted the fork because it was viewed as a sad and uncalled for innovation to be cast upon the physiological mechanism of the fingers. The church viewed it as a direct interference with God. It was reluctantly accepted by Caucasians. However, a drastic change was needed to save the dis-eased European population.

The Genoan Jewish mercenary, Christopher Columbus, observed the herbal smoke treatment system when he invaded Hispanola—the never reached America. On his second invasion, a monk/herbalist, Ramon Pane accompanied him in order to gather new information about herbs that could save the Caucasians from disease. In 1502, the aromatic (smoke) and herbal incense treatment system was introduced in Italy and Spain. Again, the new treatments met with resistance. Smoke eaters (smokers and herbal incense) were threatened with the death penalty.

The French were also trying to uncover the African health sustaining information and cures. In 1850, French medical schools used Egyptian mummies as learning vehicles. They grounded up mummies and ate them as medicine and a sex stimulant. However, the Caucasians needed more than mummies to save their race.

The European invasion of Africa for herbs and food stimulated other invasions. Christopher Columbus, established African routes, which were used by the Portuguese when they invaded the African coast and the Indies. Portuguese Admiral Pedro Alvares Cabrial invaded South America seeking goods and herbs. He baptized that part of South America as Vera Cruz on April 9, 1500. Today, it is known as Brazil. The natives resisted the invasion by the Portuguese. However, the superior weapons (guns and cannons) and the spread of European dis-eases caused the defeat of the natives. By 1530, the invasion was basically complete and the Europeans copied the natives' living style, customs, herb medicine and a part of their diet.

The vast variety of equatorial edible plants and medicinal herbage were not identified by the natives for the European invaders. This led to a search to find a key to the identification of these valuable herbs. This search ended with the kidnapping of Black Africans and the importation of them as human technology (slaves) in South America. Many of the African herbalists, scientists, agriculturists, craftsmen and administrators maintained their religions, African accents (i.e., Negro dialect), and social structure.

However, the technology that the Europeans needed was that of the health practitioners. The health practitioners had knowledge of the medicinal herbs and their use for treatment. Because, the Brazilian climate had foliage that is related to that of Africa, it was logical to get the Africans. These kidnapped African herbalists and holistic doctors identified herbs for the natives, European conquerors and the herb merchants.

The Portuguese merchants indoctrinated the natives and Africans in their religious cults. The missionaries bought, sold and owned slaves. The Jesuits and Franciscan missionary monks began to practice African technology on herbs and to use plant domestication to Brazil. From Brazil, they were exported food plants, herbs and African information technology through other missionaries and monks.

The Portuguese became wealthy and their wealth motivated herb merchants to invade South America. First, the British came after the medicinal and edible plant foliage of the Amazon, then the French, then Spaniards and the Dutch. These invasions to control resources and food plants caused the ruin of land and killed many natives and Africans. They were exploiting plants such as the herb Taheebo (Pau D'Arco), which is used for cancer, yeast infection and other severe dis-eases; the herb Guarana a stimulant; Sarsaparilla that is used for a low sperm count, arthritis and to rid the body of waste; the herb Jatabo, which is used for diabetes and other herbs such as Gergelim. They exploited the cash crops of cocoa and rubber plants.

The medicinal herbs found in Brazil by Africans were used by the Inca Indians. Some of the herbs that were identified were the Urucum plant, which is used to repel insects and acclimate the body to the tropics, for the protection against dis-ease, and the herb Casca De Anta that is used for the digestive tract dis-ease such as diarrhea. The Curate herb was used in warfare as a weapon. It is a muscle constrictor that can cause paralysis of the muscles of soldiers. It was put on the tip of arrows. When the tip of the arrow punctured the skin, the sap of the herb would immobilize the victim. However, the herb most sought after was the Rhubarb (laxative), which was combined with Sarsaparilla to cure the European syphilis pestilence. Without the African knowledge of herbs, the Europeans would not have survived the climate. It was Africans who identified the Camerara herb that was used for inflammation of the sebaceous glands caused by the hot tropical climate of South America and Africa.

The history of the African presence in the Americas, especially Brazil, predates the European invasion. Relics of African cultures have been found which date back to 8000 B.C. The current Black natives Tupi-Guarani date back to 500 A.D. This tribe was present when the Europeans invaded Brazil. The book, *Brazilian Herbs* by Antonio Bernades, gives a distorted account of this invasion.

African plant food was needed to keep the Caucasians alive while they searched for knowledge and tropical foods. They only wanted to be healthy in order to seize other peoples' resources and land. Health was motivated by a need to be Godly or humane (not humanist) to their fellow colored and African heathens.

16th Century

In the 16th century, the effects of plague, pestilence, medical ignorance, and the lack of foods and medicinal herb drugs persisted. The selective rejection of African medical knowledge still persisted. In this respect, the lives of many prominent figures were endangered. Many of them died of causes that could have been prevented had they used the African knowledge to which they had access.

King Charles II, in 1685, died of a blood clot. His diet was poor and his health status during his life was questionable. The medical prescription used allopathically as a last minute to save King Charles from death included African herbs and knowledge. He was prescribed herbs, such as violets, fennel, thistle, licorice, chamomile, rue, angelica, mint, sweet almond, cloves, melon seeds, nutmeg and anise. In 1600, King James died of malaria. This same illness can be traced to Alexander the Great who died in Babylon of malaria complicated by alcoholism. Alcohol means spirit. Alcohol was believed to be an unpleasant spirit of a higher evil able to rid Alexander's body of the lesser evil spirit that caused the dis-ease. In contrast, alcohol in the form of herbal wine was used as an antiseptic to wash wounds in Ancient Africa. Subsequently, its use in Europe was first medicinal then it later became a social beverage drink that caused alcoholism. The abusive use of alcohol affected King James I so badly that he could not walk until he was six years old. This was attributed to the bad milk of his wet nurse who had a normal (for her time period) diet. Her diet was constipating and she was an alcoholic. Subsequently, this was one of the primary motivations to seek superior milk and influenced the Caucasian colonials to use Black African slaves as mammies (wet nurses). Health and life remained a questionable dilemma in Europe.

The Portuguese ruled the herb trade in the 16th century and were attacking other herb merchants' cargo. They were destroying valuable medicinal information and herbs during sea battles. For example, the Peruvian Count Chincha, in 1632, used an African herb to cure himself of malaria. This herb possessed the curative ingredient quinine. He, egotistically, named the herb Cinchona in honor of himself. Some countries had curative herbs but were hoarding them to create scarcity. They did this to protect their own physical survival, and to assure economic high profits from their sale. Many ships carrying legitimate and fake herbs were sank at sea. There were other cures based on myths and superstitions that were in use.

In the 16th century, many popular European remedies were parts of animals. For example, Unicorn Horn sold for as much as $10,000 in Europe. Many (in fact all) of the horns were fake or counterfeit and came from cattle or even rhinoceros and other African animals. These counterfeit horns were another market ("black market") for herb merchants. The bone of

Luz was sold. This bone was believed to be the indestructible nucleus bone of the human body. It was similar to the seed from which all bones of the human body grew. Accordingly, it was in some way connected to the rib of Adam being the Luz bone for women. Another curative European remedy used to purify the body and prevent future disease was the imitation of the African mummification. A child at birth was mummified, so-called wrapped in swaddling clothes. The wrapping was applied on the child and the child was salted over the entire body. This prevented movement. These wrappings of bandages were removed once per day for several months. In due course, over half the children treated this way died within their first year of life. Galen, the famous European doctor, used mummification for medical mythological reasons. In the original African mummification process, herbs were used to purify the body. The internal organs were removed. Then the body was soaked for 70 days in a salt and herb solution. Afterward, the body was coated with gum resin (oil from a medical plant) and wrapped in swaddle (bandages). Finally, the corpse would be placed in a sarcophagus (coffin in shape of the human body with a face resembling the deceased). Actually, this first coffin would be placed into several coffins each larger than next The result would be a coffin the size of a garage for a car. The Caucasian mummification technique applied to living children did not halt dis-ease. Children were still struck by plagues, pestilences, and venereal dis-ease. Children continued to die from fevers or puerperal infections between 1652 and 1862. The Caucasians blamed the puerperal infection on bad weather. Today, this mythology is followed as "colds" are blamed on bad weather. It was thought that a cold wind from the moon caused "colds." Ironically, the cure for puerperal infections was the washing of the hands. This simple dis-ease cure of midmen and/or midwife's washing their hands before and after births or treatment was first recorded in ancient Africa over 2,000 years before Europe discovered it.

In the 16th century, in Germany, it became a requirement that each house would have an outhouse (toilet). It became law that pigpens were to be cleaned. Previously, the European houses were filthy cesspools of human manure and urine, scraps of meat, menstruation blood, rats, foul odors, roaches, lice, fleas and the pigpens were cesspools. Both of these cesspools contributed to a dis-eased country. Ambrose Pare, a French doctor, departed from using medical myths as science. He used more herbs and less mysticism than Hippocrates and Galen. Pare used the African technique of herbs on wounds followed by partial mummification (wrapped affected part with bandages). He did use pulverized African mummy powder as a medicine. However, this was widely practiced by Europeans.

In the 16th century, the potato became a popular food. The herb and food plant merchants found the potato easy to transport, but were unable to create scarcity as the potato can grow in most types of climates and soils. Potatoes were used as sex stimulants and rejuvenation of life by Europeans. Roasted coffee beans were believed to be a curative herb almost equal to the potato. Coffee or Kaffa is the Providence in Ethiopia where the coffee bean came from. In Constantinople, in 1554, and in London in 1652, coffee houses were established where coffee sold for high prices such as thirty dollars a pound. Tobacco was a lesser-received herb by the Turks. They imposed the death penalty for using tobacco and any aromatic herbal treatments. In fact, the emperor of Russia ordered that "tobacco drinkers" should have their noses slit and then be properly whipped and deported to Siberia. These plants such as the potato, coffee and tobacco were exploited and their medicinal properties obscured. Consequently, their introduction in Europe as miracle herbs was just part of the advertisement campaign by herb merchants. A vast collection of medical knowledge was usurped from Africa in the 16th century. Knowledge stolen from Africa was the foundation for the European Golden Age and all future advancements of the Caucasian civilization.

The archives of Africa were stripped and the information was taken to Europe as new scientific information that was developed and discovered by Caucasians. However, each discovery can be traced to Africa. J. A. Rogers in his books *World's Great Men of Color, From Superman to Man* and *100 Amazing Facts About the Negro,* fully documented the rape of Africa for knowledge. A few of the great European scientific finds are childish. For example, the discovery of gravity. It is assumed in the discovery that for over 4,000 years Africans did not know that an object would fall on their heads. It is unbelievable to assume that the builders of the pyramid did not know about gravity or the speed that a falling object can travel. Yet, ancient Africans calculated a star that passes over the center of the pyramid every 50,000 years. Another great scientific European find is that matter is transformed and not destroyed. In this find, Einstein ignores that for over two million years Africans would eat and have a bowel movement (manure evacuation). Supposedly, the ancient Africans never associated the defecation or urination of food (matter) was the result of what they had eaten previously (transformation of food). From this European scientific perspective, it is assumed that African's chewing (mastication) food (transformation of matter) never considered that they were transforming energy. Sobeit, Galileo and Einstein are great men in European science. They are considered childish and primitives compared to African scientific advancements. Europeans obtained knowledge from Africa and this knowledge seems to have mysteriously been born as European knowledge in the 16th century. During the 16th century, Pare founded orthopedics and massage; Magellan discovered the world could be circumnavigated; Galileo discovered falling bodies; Paracelsus discovered chemotherapy; Versalius discovered human anatomy; Copernicus discovered revolution of the planets around the sun; and Fracastaro named the mucous disease syphilis. These discoveries did not overshadow the Caucasian need for African herbals, food and methods of domesticated plants.

The Treatise of Fruit Trees by Ralph Austin (1653) gives definite instruction for the pruning, grafting, setting and domestication of plants. He mentions that he improved on the methods of the fifth, sixth, and seventh centuries. There would have been no need for adapting plants unless they came from a different climatic country such as Africa. The exotic tropical African medicinal fruits stimulated an interest in importing them. However, the people in Angleland (England) dis-ease causing diet, which was primarily flesh and they were not interested in massive fruit or vegetable consumption unless it could stop dis-eases. The French and Dutch had farming methods for tropical African fruit trees, these plants could stop starvation and dis-eases. Books that provided ways to adapt African plants were translated by Leonard Mascall in 1572. The books of knowledge were useful but the need for cures caused drastic measures. Plagues and pestilence were still prominent.

Plagues caused the deterioration of European social structure and affected the rich merchants with landslide profits. Merchants sold herbs and foods at higher prices (more profit). In London in August 1665 during a one-week period, 171 children were born. However, there were 5,568 deaths and 4,237 of the deaths were caused by the plague, as reported in *"Bill of Mortality"* for the week of August 15 to 22 in 1665. "Bill" was an early European name for newspaper. The people running from plagues looted and destroyed property. These people were often ambushed and killed as carriers of the plague. This was reported in a 1625 pamphlet called *"A Rod for Run-Aways"* by Thomas Deekes. Aside from this, many myths surrounded the plague. Pepys in his *"Diary"* reported that a comet appeared December 1664 before the plague struck. King Charles II was reported to have witnessed the sighting of a comet before the plague struck. In previous histories, events occurred to give mystical meaning to plagues. For example, before the plague of Justian in 543 A.D., the harvest failed and there was an earthquake that preceded the coming of the plague. Nonetheless, plagues brought further dis-ease to the land.

The European cultures' need for food caused them to use the quick growing method. The quick growing method was used in Africa in areas where towns, cities, or other building structures were to be established. Cultivation is the name of the quick crop growing method. Cultivation without rotating crops will destroy the land. It does not matter how shallow the land is plowed, plowing kills valuable earthworms, insects and secondary plant life and the soil. In addition, cultivation exposed the land to excessive sunlight, air and water that causes the soil to be drained nutritionally and electromagnetically of its vital elements. The naked lands do not breathe properly, hold moisture properly, nor can the sun's energies be stored by plants for the winter. In this respect, the soil dies or is forced to produce substantially poorer quality plants. Plants enslaved on a plant plantation react just like human slaves. Consequently, it is a constant struggle for nutritional survival. The book, *The Secret Life of Plants* by Peter

Tompkins, addresses the emotional aspects and intelligence of plants. In Africa, plants were respected and studied far beyond today's Caucasian science. In fact, the Europeans from their visits to African cities were aware of the herbs, food and knowledge that they could exploit in Africa.

Many ancient West Africans had complex social systems. The University of Timbuktu was widely known as a higher learning institute that was far more advanced than any institute in Europe. The health of Africans was far better than the Europeans. African physicians possessed higher knowledge. A town such as Benin (in present day western Nigeria) was remarked on by the Dutch in 1602 as being greater than the towns, streets, houses and the King's court of Amsterdam, Holland. In due course, the Europeans seized and destroyed this city and many others during their invasions.

17ᵗʰ Century

The herb market was controlled by the Dutch in the 17th Century. The herb market still had demands for more varieties of herbs because dis-ease continued in European countries. These countries tried to use protection against plagues but they were based on medical myths, superstitions and ignorance. In Geneva in 1743, Jean Jacques Rosseau tells of quarantines being instituted to prevent diseases. Napoleon, on his return from his invasion of Africa initiated a quarantine, in 1795. European physicians believed the spread of dis-ease was caused by open pores after bathing. Consequently, Caucasians stopped taking baths and burned aromatic herbs. The introduction of African soap was considered a modern invention, by the ancient Greeks, and they used oil for cooking and washing. Oil for protection against evil was the purpose of oil baths among Caucasians as cooked animal grease was used for cleansing the body. The African herbal water system was adopted by Europeans. Perfumed herb water essences were used as a protection against evil and to hide the unbathed Caucasian foul body odors. Today it is called "cologne." In many cases, people were persecuted as carriers of the plague or as witches who started a plague. *The Constitution Criminals* by Maria Theresa in 1768 mentions the elaborate machines that were used to torture people to confess to starting a plague. Some of the torture devices were the thumbscrew, the rack, hot oil baths and the burning of body parts with lighted candles.

There were attempts to use the stolen African medical knowledge. The antiseptic principle of African medicine is erroneously claimed to be invented by Joseph Lister. He wrote a book on *The Antiseptic Principle in the Practice of Surgery,* in 1866. This did not alter the sad fact that between 1864 and 1866 that at least 45% of the patients died after minor surgery as well as amputation because antiseptics were not used. The compound fracture operation caused overwhelming deaths and was as dangerous as the Bubonic Plague. The Escalapius Temple or Imhotep medical training system was introduced to nurse. A German by the name of Theodore Fuldner who as a pastor converted his asylum for discharged female prisoners into a nursing school in 1853. One of his famous students was Florence Nightingale (who died from syphilis). The Europeans still used African medicine as a type of superstition combined with their ignorant medical myths. Caucasians used dis-eased animal pus to fight disease. The same animal pus system was first introduced to England by Lady Mary Wortley Montague, wife of the British Ambassador to the Ottoman Court in 1717. At that time, it was called inoculation against cowpox. Later, this filthy septic pus inoculation proved to be harmful and was abolished by an act of Parliament in 1840. In 1754, the Royal College of Physicians issued an official paper against its harmful effects. Oddly enough, European social medical myths, ignorance, and superstitions allowed Edward Jenner to re-institute this same system under a new name of vaccination. In 1798, he wrote *Inquiry Into the Cause and Effects of Variolas Vaccine* and this served to legalize a superstition. Medical ideas and treatments that are morally wrong can never be scientifically correct. It is morally wrong to make a healthy person sick with pus and germ vaccination. It would be better to add to the person's health by giving them a mango or papaya instead of giving them pus. Inoculation or vaccinations were performed by Africans holistically (usage of herbs orally) and unholistically (use of pus topically).

The Nubians were among the earliest recorded Africans to use inoculation. They would have a healthy person sleep with a sick person as a form of inoculation. The Baris of Laluaba inoculated themselves over the heart on the skin area above the left breast. Moreover, the Pouls and Black Moors of Senegambia used inoculation against specific dis-eases such as mucous congestion known as pleuro-pneumonia. The Arabs, Ashantis and Moors in Northern Africa used the direct body contact of arm-to-arm inoculations. The direct body contact system was also used in Senegal for the children. The Dutch learned of these systems during the 17th Century as they controlled the herb market and had made more invasions in Africa. They popularized inoculation in Berne and Switzerland. Other countries imitated the inoculation system. Cotton Mather spoke of inoculations as being practiced in Turkey in his book *Philosophical Transactions* in 1721. Inoculation was a desperate means to save Europe from disease. Queen Mary II of England died of smallpox in 1694. In 1790, a total of 60,000,000 persons died of smallpox. This added strong support for the need to get more herbs and herbal knowledge from Africa— whether holistic or unholistic was not an issue. The search for a way to use the African science of anatomy to save Europe was attempted.

The medical schools in Europe needed corpses to dissect and study. This caused a wave of grave robbing and mysterious deaths and reports of missing people. Grave robbers were not respected and could be tried as thieves if they stole a corpse wearing clothes. Consequently, grave robbers avoided being convicted of theft by removing the clothes from a corpse before stealing it. In 1752, grave robbing was made legal and they were titled Resurrectionists in England. The grave robbers and schools (cults) that dissected corpses were not fully accepted in America by Euro-Americans. For example, no anatomy was allowed to be taught at the University of Pennsylvania in Philadelphia. Furthermore, in New York City, a large protest was organized against doctors performing autopsies. The protesting crowd became an uncontrollable mob and the doctors had to hide in jail to protect themselves against death. This event was recorded as "The Doctors Mob of April 1788." In any case, the study of anatomy helped to elevate the medical knowledge of the body but not of cures or the dietary prevention of dis-ease. In contrast, anatomy was studied for over 4,000 years in Africa.

18th Century

In the 18th Century, the English controlled the herb market. African foods were considered as drug cures.

The herb supply declined in England and the search for more herbs caused the need to invade Africa. England was besieged by European tribes from the north of Britain and from the northwestern coast of Europe. The medicinal herb farms (erroneously called orchards or gardens) plantations that the Romans had previously established in the first century had long died out. Many native tribes of England had become uncivilized and barbarous from the invasions of other European tribes. Consequently, the need to constantly defend life and property caused the herb farms to waste away.

Monks were encouraged to look for herbs not grown in their countries and to procure any information about how to cultivate the herbal drugs. Monks seemed to have knowledge of horticulture and were welcomed to European countries. The monks that came from France and Italy were encouraged to bring seeds, parts of herbs, tropical herbs or a plant when they came to England.

The monks domesticated, experimented with grafting and adapted many African herbs and fruits to the European climate. However, their knowledge of how to control and successfully prescribe herbs was steep in ignorance and lacked the African holistic medical technology.

Europe demanded more herbs from Africa. Consequently, the herb merchants increased their exploitation and invasions of Africa. The Caucasians, in order to keep a healthy army needed pain suppressants for battle injuries and wounds. They needed the dis-ease remedies ancient Egyptians had perfected. They needed the African science of anesthesia and herbs such as Opium, Mandrake, Hash and others. However, the Africans were aware of the individualized dosage and herb ratios needed for the application while Europeans were not. The African scientist employed meditations (called prayers by Europeans) in order to clear the thinking for proper herb dosage and proper diagnosis. The ancient symbol for the invocation of medication was the distorted symbol of Jupiter Rx. Before Europeans gained African anesthetic usage, they would tie, bound and gag patients in pain. This newly usurped anesthetic and antiseptic knowledge did not decrease deaths. The European surgeons did not wash their hands or use antiseptics. They usually waited in the autopsy room before surgery. While they were in the autopsy room, they would touch the contaminated, dis-cased flesh of the corpse. It was not until 1818 that a man by the name of Semmelweis (born in Budapest, Hungary) scientifically reasoned that deaths were caused by the unwashed hands of surgeons. In contrast, African medical scientists were washing before and after patient care over 4,000 years before the Europeans discovered washing hands and antiseptics.

Drugs were used by many health practitioners. In 1879, William Morton of Charlton, a Massachusetts pediatrician, started using cocaine. In the pediatrics medical branch known as midwifery, there was much protest. In contrast, ancient Africans did not use drugs for childbirth. James Simpson wrote the paper, "*Answers to the Religious Objection Against the Employment of Anesthetic Agents in Midwifery and Surgery.*" to defend drug use for birth in 1847. The "Lancet" magazine of May 1853 had an article against drugs for birthing. Today, drug use during birth is acknowledged to have side effects and risk factors. Drug use during birthing did not cover up or satisfy the Caucasian medical need for more information about the African natural birth and drug free systems. In order to save lives, more dissection and more corpses were needed for study in the schools of Europeans.

Many Resurrectionists and illegal markets for dead bodies inspired murders and the stealing of cadavers. For example, in 1827 William Hare and William Burke of Edinburgh, England were partners in the business of killing people to get cadavers. They performed clandestine murders to get dead bodies to sell to medical schools for dissection. Burke would kill people by getting them drunk and then smothering them with pillows. The sound the victim made grasping for breath became known as "burping (burking)." Today, the term is still used and called "burping." In any case, knowledge was needed, and Africa was invaded for its wealth of knowledge.

The invasion of Africa for herbs during the 18th Century included the capture of Black Africans who could teach herbal use. Black women were kidnapped because they were herbalist/cooks and prepared many herbals for the family. Elderly Black females became a source of herbal knowledge and during slavery saved Blacks and Caucasians alike. Before the European invasions, many of the captured Africans who were enslaved were farmers who grew herbs for the African herb trade market. African herbalists became prized slaves along with elderly women and medicine men. The earlier exploitation of herbs use by herb merchants, monks and slave traders had drained the African continent of its human resources. This caused the new European arrivals to Africa to assume that Africa always existed as a backward country. It was backwards because it was culturally raped by explorers and made undeveloped. Actually the exploitation of the land by

Greek (332 B.C.) and Roman (201 B.C.) cattle farmers, the exploitation of the land by abusive cultivation, the rape of the books and herbal science, coupled with the slaughter of over 75 million Blacks because of the slave trade, added to the never estimated deaths caused by the Caucasian diseases brought to Africa. Many Africans became culturally destabilized due to the constant inmigration because of European attacks. Before they could gain strength to fight the Caucasians, they had to retreat to barren areas. Eventually, the African original cultural structure fell apart. These factors are but a few of the reasons why Africa appeared uncivilized and backwards to Europeans. Aside from this, the Europeans had a distorted evaluation of African culture and knowledge because the Caucasians were illiterate, had a limited vocabulary and had a barbaric primitive culture whose society was based upon "The Law of the Caves" mentality. The Caucasians had a fictionalized idea of Africa and a false over glorified image of European culture itself. In that respect, a view of the European scientific method can reflect upon this youth culture that crystallized itself in the 18th Century.

The ancient African scientific method would never validate the Caucasian practice of eating a brave man's heart as a means of acquiring bravery. Further, the African scientific method cannot validate the eating of an owl's brain to make an individual wise or the eating of a lion's heart to acquire the wisdom of a king. Today, this animal organ flesh eating is called the glandular extract treatment by Caucasians. These ancient Caucasian beliefs and practices are supported by their science and continue today. They eat cow's liver capsules, pancreatic capsules and other animal flesh as dietary supplements. The eating of dead animal corpses' internal organs can excite human internal organs in a negative or positive manner. European science indicates that animals as well as transplanted human organs are rejected by the recipients. So it follows that the nutrients of a glandular extract excite a person's organ's defense to reject the animal's organ thus it is believed to increase health and immunity. By the way, the liver is the most toxic and most waste-filled gland in an animal's body and should not be eaten. Eating animals' eyes to improve human sight cannot be validated by the European scientific method. If this were: so, then the animal flesh eaters should have the best of health by eating every gland, organ and piece of mucous and feces that are found in an animal's corpse. Yet, from eating meat, they do not have superior health and are still diseased. The meat eaters' logic assumes that animal flesh is medicine. In any case, the thought distortions of Caucasian cultural psychosis causes their medical science to maintain their superstitious caveman mentality. The short lifespan of Europeans 200 years ago (20 years of age) combined with dis-ease, pestilence and plagues caused this superstition to have an ever-increasing lifespan.

Ancient Caucasians used bloodletting to cure dis-eases. Physicians of the Seventeenth Century promoted blood transfusions for curing dis-eases and rejuvenation. Ancient Caucasian Jews believed that a dying man who had sex with young girls could be rejuvenated and avoid death. This did not work. Ponce de Leon searched for magic youth-giving herbs and the fountain of youth. Mohammed selected one wife of seven years of age and another of eight years of age to restore his deteriorating health. Another Caucasian belief was wearing an animal skin could give you the powers of that animal and cure of dis-eases. None of these practices can be scientifically validated and yet they persist. They persist because White Supremacy is a psychosis. This psychosis generates and creates the inability to see or understand reality. It creates supportive psychoses. The Caucasian gadgets and machines have changed and the Caucasians assumed that they have changed. Machines, computers and science do not make people healthy. People make people healthy.

The Euro-Americans and Europeans still have plagues and pestilence. For instance, a plague struck America in 1900, occurring in San Francisco. The Federal government and local governments argued that the plague did not strike. Yet, they used all the prevailing methods to stop a plague. They killed millions of rats and well over 20 million squirrels that carried the disease. However, they denied the existence of a crisis. Today, the same crises exist in the human health arena, the diet is synthetic and nutritionally poor and causes diseases. Caucasian medicine is controlled by the pharmaceutical clans and it operates as a business.

THE ORIGIN OF HEALTH AND MEDICAL TERMS

The terms, names, labels and health words used in anatomy, biology, chemistry and the sciences are culturally based. Words expose a culture's life blood and are what keeps the culture's heart pumping. Culture is people. People are their words. The Caucasians' original words and terms contain their true feelings, emotions, behaviors and state of mind. The Caucasian's dictionary gives the origin of the word (etymology) and then deliberately omits the original meaning. The dictionary civilizes (modifies) their words by omitting the historical crude behaviors and thoughts that defined the word. Caucasians civilized their words, but not the culture that defined the words.

An examination of a "word's" original journey in vocabulary is an examination of culture in motion. For example, "Nigger (Niger)" referred to Africans captured around the Niger River. It became transformed by slavery and colonialism and made derogatory by Caucasians. Essentially, "words" are neutral. It is people that make them "good" or "bad." People change then the word changes. Changing a "word," shortening it, making it longer, spelling it backwards, adding or omitting letters or altering words in various ways does not change the nature of the people that gave birth to the word. Words transmit and translate culture. They are conscious and subconscious symbols of the nature of a culture. The ancient Caucasians clearly attached their naked feelings, emotions and knowledge to their "words."

The terms and words about the body (anatomy, physiology, etc.) are steeped in Caucasian ignorance, superstitions, and myths and reveal the Caucasians' true nature. The ancient (original) words reflect a primitive understanding of life. The ancient words' usages are the foundation of Caucasian life. Their "words" may take on various new meanings. However, it takes an advanced spiritual and emotional vocabulary to keep pace with a "words" movement through time. People change words. Words do not change a people. The Caucasians' emotions are naked and refuse to become a part of the new changes in word meaning. More than anything, Caucasian behavior indicates that people are words, words are not people.

The terms and words used in the health field have their origin in the primitive Greek and Roman culture's stories (mythology). Words usurped and stolen from the ancient African Egyptians, such as Aset (Isis) variations are Venus, Diana, Princess, Madonna, Donna, Mary, Menu, Minerva, Ceres, Juna, June, Ma, Mama, etc. These words connect the Caucasians to their invasion of Africa, colonialism and slavery. If their culture is as civilized and advanced as they claim it to be, they would not have stolen African words.

The ancient Caucasians' limited vocabulary caused them to spell words backwards in order to create new words. For example, in mythology, Oedipus means a boy who wants to have sex with his mother. Spelled backwards, it is Supideo. Supideo means a girl who wants to have sex with her father. Electra (Electricity) means a father who wants to have sex with his daughter. Electra spelled backwards is Artcele. Artcele means a mother who wants to have sex with her son. These words were used to label the incest customs of Caucasian culture. The words did not create the behavior, the people did. The original (ancient) words mirror the culture.

Words can be seen clearly if the Caucasian culture is seen clearly. The ancient Caucasians' health and diseases were manipulated and controlled by their own ignorance. They did not know blood circulated in the body, did not practice hygiene, did not bathe, did not know the heart pumped blood, believed the world was flat and had no concept of zero (0). They used bones and sticks for counting; the bone and stick symbols are called Roman numerals (i.e., IV, X, III) Their expanded stolen vocabulary (words) did not advance their knowledge or culture.

The ancient Caucasians lived in caves and their feet were dirty, filthy, and dark from grime. The primitive Greeks called the feet "tarsal" after the mythological god Tartaros who lived in the dark grimy gloom. The claws or teeth of animals were tied on to shoes. This indicated that the wearer was a good hunter, powerful and/or in control. The wearing of tassels on shoes has replaced the claws. The word "tassal" indicates that primitive feelings are still in Caucasians.

Shoes among the ancient Caucasians were associated with sex and Aphrodisia (Aphrodite). In mythology, the god Zeus sent a bird to steal the shoe of Aphrodite. In ancient Caucasian culture, when a father gave his daughter's shoe to a man or woman, it meant that they were given permission to rape his daughter. Remnants of this custom are found in the children's story *Cinderella*. Cinderella's shoe was found by a Prince. Once he put the shoe on her foot, he was allowed to have sex with her (marry her). The red shoe of the character Dorothy in the story *The Wizard of Oz* subliminally expresses that Dorothy has come of age (sexually active). Sex, as a gift, was associated with shoes in Caucasian culture. Originally, Christmas gifts were put in shoes then in contemporary times, the shoe was replaced with socks. Caucasian's primitive sexual feelings are still attached to the shoe. For example, the pointed toe and high heels on their shoes are symbolic of the penis. The word "tassel's" ancient meaning and the sexual custom involving the shoe helps to expose the nature of the Caucasian. The following examples of ancient (original) words' definitions reveal more about the Caucasian.

The Pectoralis chest muscle's name is derived from the mythological Picus (Peco) who had a hairy coat. Picus was the servant god of Saturn. The chest of Caucasian men is very hairy (Picus). The primitive Caucasians called the chest Picus. This word eventually evolved to Pecus, then Pectoralis.

Urine is derived from Urea. The gods Kronus/Crown (Fire) and Rhea/Urea (Water) had a daughter named Dementia (Demented). The birth of Dementia was a loss for the father. Boys were valued above girls and girls were often killed at birth because they had no social importance. Dementia means loss, failed, etc. A mind that has lost its ability to function properly is "demented." Accepting the original meaning of Dementia exposes the emotional and intellectual foundation of Caucasian thought.

Sacrum (flat sack) or tailbone was called the flat brain by primitives. The ancient Caucasians believed you had a round brain (skull) at the top of the tree (vertebral column) and a flat brain (skull) at the bottom of the bone tree (vertebrae). Vertebral (twist) column (tree) or back bone means "twisting tree."

The "Anus" is the hole between the buttocks, which evacuates manure (bowel movements). The word Anus is derived from Roman mythology's Temple of Ianus (Anus), which had two cheeks/faces (two buttocks). Anus meant "the hole between two cheeks (Anus)." The ancient Caucasian simply referred to it as "the hole of two cheeks." Anus was not and is not a medical term but a social word for "the hole of two cheeks." Today, Anus may seem like a medical term but it is more of a social term. It is not an advanced word but a crude word from a crude people. It is an "icon" word that glues Caucasians to their ancient culture.

The word "Semen" is derived from the primitive Greek's mythology (belief) about Dionysis (the son of Zeus). Dionysis (wild orgy god) ate his wife Semen/Semele in order to give birth. He ate Semen and stole her unborn baby. Dionysis sewed the baby (put semen) into his thigh (buttocks) and gave birth immaculately. Immaculate Conception means without a "wolf (lupus), wolf-man = wo-man" (self-fertilized). This myth provides the primary spiritual rationale for the Caucasians' perversion of semen swallowing and ejaculation in bowel movements in rectum of the buttocks activities in homosexuality and homosexuality rituals in secret societies, occult groups, brotherhoods, orgies, sororities, fraternities, etc.

The word "queer" is derived from Roman mythology's Quere/Quirites. Romulus (Rome) was the homosexual brother of the homosexual Remus. Romulus formed the male homosexual city of Rome. Incidentally, in Rome, the thieves, liars and criminals were forced to live on a hill of the city called Capitol Hill. The ruling senators and congressmen of the United States of America work in a section called Capitol Hill. The male homosexual city's population was becoming extinct because it had no women. Romulus devised a scheme to get women to breed with the homosexual men. He invited the men and women from another city called Sabines (means cave) to come to a festival. At the festival, the Roman homosexual men raped the Sabine women. The husbands of the raped women became angry. In order to avoid a war, Romulus promised that his men would marry the raped women. Romulus' and Sabines' peoples eventually united and called themselves the "Queers (Quere/Quirites)."

Rhomboideus back muscles that resemble a hill or Christmas (pine) tree in shape. Rhom/Rome was established on a "hill." The "Id" part of the word Rhomboideus means the demon nature of the man's mind. "Id" also means primitive uncivilized dark thoughts or "idiot" mentality. Rhomboideus means "the demon hill on the back."

Plantaris (Plant) muscles of the feet touch the ground. Things that grow in dirt were called "ground things (plants)" by primitive Caucasians. The foot, because it touches the dirt, was called "the ground (plant) bone."

In mythology, Nessas (Nesa, Neva, Navel) raped Deianeira (Hercules' wife). He told Deineira to use the blood caused by her rape and/or menstruation blood on Hercules as an aphrodisiac. The blood was believed to restore fertility. A child's umbilical cord (rope) bleeds when cut. When the baby's umbilical cord heals itself, it is renamed the navel. The navel (umbilical cord) was once in the sea (amniotic fluid) of the womb. Navel (Navy) means "the sea rope."

The disease Lupus is associated with females. Lupus was the female wolf that nursed Rhomulus and Remus. Lupus means wolf (wolf-man = wo-man).

The lower leg bone (shin) is called the Tibia. Tibia (Thethy) was a mythological god that lived in Olympus. The Tibia bone was believed to grow from the sacrum (flat brain). Sacrum (Sacred) was believed to be the home of the gods. The gods gave birth and created Tibia.

The Ileocecal valve is inside the intestines and located where the small intestines joins with the large intestines. The valve prevents liquid food from the large intestines from going back up into the small intestines. The valve is inside the intestine, which processes liquefied digested food. Iolas (Ileos) was the brother of Hercules. Iolas protected Hercules by killing Hydra, the three-headed crab monster who lived in the watery swamp. Hydra means water (i.e., Fire Hydrant). Ileocecal means "protect from swamp (manure)."

The Sternum (breast bone) is the stern that guides the boat made of bones. The ribs are shaped like the frame of a wooden boat. The Clavicle (key) bone of the chest connects to the boat and the shoulder bone. The shoulder has the Tricep (three heads) and Bicep (two heads) of the crab monster Hydra. Ileo (Iolas) cut off the crab monster's heads in the Delta (Deltoid) swamp. This prevented Hercules from being trapped (Trapezius) in the swamp (Delta). The "bone boat (chest)" traveled along the coast. Therefore, the muscles in between the ribs (frame of boat) are called "Intercoastal." The "Scapular (shoulder blade)" was believed to be the bone sale of the boat.

Inguinal (groin) ligament (rope) was believed to be the groin ropes that tied the leg and hip together.

Phalanges (Phallux) means penis. The fingers were believed to be penis-like with a bone inside. The penis-like bones grew from the carpi (fruit/flower) petal palm of the hand.

Pyrrhea is the inflammation of the jaw and tooth joint. In mythology, the Pyrrhea people had fire. This enabled them to survive the flood of the earth. Zeus told Poseidon to flood the earth. Prometheus helped save some people from the flood by giving them fire (Pyrrhea). Zeus punished Prometheus (promiscuous = disobey) for saving people. He took him to Caucus in order to destroy his body. Caucus means body.

The primitive meaning of Caucasian words reduces the range of their intelligence. It is similar to taking a rope and tying a dog to a tree. The dog's range of motion is limited by the tree's roots (word origin) anchored in the soil (culture). Words such as Brachioradialis arm muscle means a branch of a limb of a bone tree; Zygomaticus face muscle means a yoke that holds the jaw; Orbicularis Oculi is a series of words combined. "Orb" means mouth, "cularis" means sack (bag), "oculi" means eye. The combined words mean "the mouth sack of the eye." Abdomen is derived from "ab," which means "away from," "domain" means house. The combined words mean "muscles that grow away from the belly's house." Serratus (teeth) anterior (front) muscles means the tooth-like front muscles. Petellar (leaf) ligament (rope) means the knee leaf (cap) with ropes, etc.

Psychology is derived from the word Psyche. Psyche means butterfly. Wings, such as those on Butterflies were associated with Furies (Eriyas) who is the goddess of retribution or vengeance. The Caucasians believed their mind to be filled with hidden demons or primitive untamed desires.

The mind was believed to have a wing of "good" and a wing of "evil." They believed the battle between good and evil make the mind fly (think). Good seeks vengeance against evil and causes the mind to think (pros-cons).

Caucasian words broadcast their culture. Their words are connected to primitive rituals, ceremonies and customs. Words are icons that keep a culture glued together. Icon is a derivative of Iron. Iron (Icon) was their primitive classification of races. The Iron Race was uncivilized and only knew how to crudely survive. The Bronze Race was a race of criminals. The Golden Race was the race from the land of the Golden Sun (Africa) where the land had plenty food. The word Icon" reflects the Caucasian understanding of their own culture (Iron Race/Age) and others' cultures. An "icon" picture symbol nonverbally helps ideas to "survive" and live without defining the spoken or written word. Icons are symbols commonly thought of as being limited to computer technology. It is a social term.

Words ancient (original) meanings and subliminal subconscious Caucasian meanings are obvious when you take their ancient words as ancient words. For example, in primitive Roman mythology, the god Numa (Month) arranged the gods of the months in an order. Janus (January) was the god of Peace; Mar (March) was the god of war; and Feb (February) was the god of death. February is Black History Month—the month of death. The Caucasian words and definitions have to be understood from their ancient meanings and origins. Take Caucasian words for precisely what they once meant, then refer to their contemporary meaning. The contemporary meanings wander away from the ancient meaning. However, they still have their ancient beginning or else the word itself would not exist. In other words, take their words for what they mean—take their word for it.

Ancient African words were created holistically (spirit, mind, body) and mixed with the concept of the past, present and future as one. For example, the African word "Maat" means the same thing as it did over a million years ago. Caucasian words change in order to reach a more perfect definition. The original Caucasian terms and words truly mirror the history of their health and culture. Their words are not merely grammar, they expose the nature of Caucasian people.

HEALTH AND MEDICAL TERMS

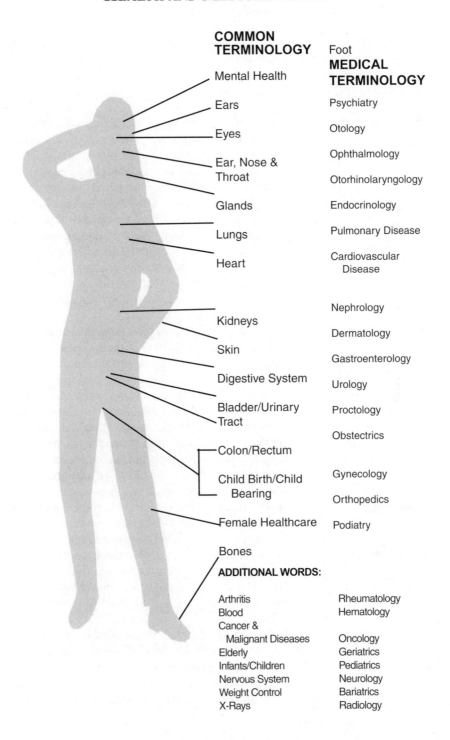

COMMON TERMINOLOGY	MEDICAL TERMINOLOGY
Mental Health	Psychiatry
Ears	Otology
Eyes	Ophthalmology
Ear, Nose & Throat	Otorhinolaryngology
Glands	Endocrinology
Lungs	Pulmonary Disease
Heart	Cardiovascular Disease
Kidneys	Nephrology
Skin	Dermatology
Digestive System	Gastroenterology
Bladder/Urinary Tract	Urology
Colon/Rectum	Proctology
Child Birth/Child Bearing	Obstectrics
Female Healthcare	Gynecology
Bones	Orthopedics
Foot	Podiatry

ADDITIONAL WORDS:

Arthritis	Rheumatology
Blood	Hematology
Cancer & Malignant Diseases	Oncology
Elderly	Geriatrics
Infants/Children	Pediatrics
Nervous System	Neurology
Weight Control	Bariatrics
X-Rays	Radiology

HERBS
(A complete listing would be beyond the scope of this writing)

These herbal drugs and many more were fought over by European drug traders. They helped to stimulate the invasion of Africa. Four hundred years ago, they were used to cure many dis-eases. Today, they are forgotten or used as so-called spices and seasonings.

Aloe/Aloe Vera   An herb of the cactus plant tribe. It was controlled by the sultan and it was sold by the King of Socrota to England in the 17th Century. The records of the East Indian Company verify this trading. The invasion of the herbs' habitat of south and east Africa caused ecological damage and destroyed lives. Aloes are used as laxatives, bitter tonics, vermifuge, and emmenagogue.

Agrimony   This herb has an astringent effect. It contracts and hardens tissue. It strengthens and tones the muscles of the body. It allows fluids to pass more readily through the kidneys and is regarded as a diuretic.

Basil   For diarrhea, digestive disorders, and urinary tract inflammations. Basil wreaths have been found in ancient Egyptian burial chambers in the pyramids. This African herb was used as an expellant of the placenta (afterbirth) and menstruation pains. In the 15th and 16th Centuries, the Venetians, Portuguese and Spaniards fought battles over this herb and many Europeans were killed. It was very important in the combining formulas of nutmeg and clove. In addition, it is used to extract poisons from insect bites.

Boga Bark   It was used in Africa (Nigeria and the Congo) as a relaxant. European-Americas use it psychotropically. It is used to stop addiction.

Calumba   For digestive problems, skin dis-ease and to expel worms. It is a stimulant, nervine and laxative. This African plant grows in Madagascar, near the Zambezi River, Mozambique and East Africa.

Chamomile   Used as a tonic and stimulant.Egyptians combined this herb with olive oil, used it for massage, and rubbed it on sore muscles. The Romans learned of this medicinal herb and used it for massage, venereal dis-ease, nervous disorders, as well as a hair rinse for blondes, and for alcoholism treatment.

Camphor
The Arabian herb was used for bruises, nervousness headaches and to lessen sexual desires. The Romans and Greeks did not learn of this herb's use.

Cinnamon
The Arabian drug and herb trade was not limited. They controlled the herb cinnamon. They were the principle merchants that sold the herb to the Phoenicians, Greek and Romans. It has been found in African tombs. Cinnamon was used for embalming and for spiritual enlightenment. Aside from being a germicide, stomachic, and antispasmodic it was used for uterine hemorrhages and as a sex stimulant.

Celery
Used as a carminative and for respiratory conditions. The Greeks and Romans learned of this herb and used it as a sex stimulant. Additionally, the seeds (Smilage) were used for protection against witches and evil. European herbal use of celery lasted until the 17th Century.

Clove
Aside from being an antiseptic, astringent, and stimulant for the circulatory system. It was fought over during the herb and drug trade. The Venetians controlled clove and sold it in England for its curative value. The Arabians competed with the Venetians in marketing this herb. Other countries such as the Portuguese and Dutch fought sea battles, much blood was spilled and many merchants were killed in the wars to control cloves.

Coriander
This African herb is used for digestive and skin dis-eases. The historian, Pliny, reports that it was used in Egypt by physicians to treat dis-eases. Europeans used it to treat the pestilence called St. Anthony's Fire. It was controlled by the English drug merchants.

Cumin
This African herb was used for digestive disorders, inflammation, and soreness. The Egyptians used it as a remedy for colic, flatulence, and skin dis-eases.

Eucalyptus
Used for respiratory dis-eases, skin dis-eases, and inflammations. Africans used this tree to prevent malaria. Wherever it was planted, fever, dis-ease, and mosquitoes disappeared. The seed

was much sought after by the early French and
Romans. A German botanist and African
invader, Baron Ferdinand von Muller in the
18th Century brought this plant to Europe. It is
one of the largest trees.

Fennel
This African herb was used for digestive disorders, inflammations, and skin disorders. The
Egyptians used fennel and it was reported in the
papyrus with extensive preparation, dosage and
herb combining formulas. This particular
papyrus was destroyed when the Alexandria
library was burned. European traders learned of
this herb. Egypt and Dutch traded with it.

Frankincense
A purifier. It was used for religious purposes.
When Constantine the Great declared
Christianity the official religion of the Roman
Empire, the burial ceremonies in which the herb
was used, were discontinued and was replaced
by cremation. Thus, religious use of this herb
for funeral rites and mummification was halted.
This herb was marketed by the Arabians in the
4th Century.

Gotu Kola
This herb is used to increase circulation, mental
powers and for memory. In ancient Africa, elephants were followed and it was noted that they
ate this herb. It was used and found to be good
for memory.

Herbane
This African herb is used for stress and nervous
conditions. It has a narcotic effect and is a pain
reliever.

Henna
This herb is used for inflammation of the skin.
Ancient Egyptians used it as a dye for fingernails. Mummies have been found with Henna
dye on fingernails. It was used to dye the navel
and breast of ancient Egyptians. Caucasians use
it as a hair dye.

Horsetail
Used for respiratory and skin dis-eases in
Africa. The Romans learned of it, used it as a
food, and ate horsetail sprouts.

Hyssop
A diaphoretic and is used for digestive and skin
dis-eases. The Persian Blacks used it as a purifier.

Kola Nuts
Used as a cardiac tonic and beverage by ancient
Africans. Caucasian Americans copied the beverage tonic drink and called it coca cola. They
copied the ancient African flower essence (dew

water) dis-ease treatment system and called it dew water (Mountain Dew was originally a treatment for disease).

Licorice
Licorice is used as a demulcent, emollient, laxative and hormone (estrogen) regulator. The Greeks and Romans used it. Writers such as Dioscorides (Greek), Celsius and Scribamus Largus (Roman) mentioned it. Hippocrates learned of it from the Africans and treated diabetes and dropsy with it. Licorice was stored in King Tut's tomb (Tutankhamen).

Lime
This tropical fruit found in Burma and Africa is used for liver disorders. The Jewish slave trader, Christopher Columbus, traded with it in the East Indies.

Mandrake
This African herb is used for liver dis-eases and inflammations, varicose veins, ulcers, and used as a narcotic. The Egyptians used it to cleanse the female reproductive system and for surgery. The Arabians called it the devil's apple. The Europeans used it as a sex stimulant and for casting out demons.

Marshmallow
This African herb is used for inflammation, a diuretic, a demulcent and a laxative. It was used as a food during times of famine in Egypt. It was adopted by the Greeks, Assyrians, Chinese and Romans. Historians Pliny and Dioscorides wrote about it.

Marjoram
This African herb was used for pain, bruises and arthritis. The Romans learned of it and used it to increase thinking.

Mastic
Used as a diuretic and for respiratory disorders and as a stimulant. Africans used it as a varnish for wood in boats and furniture.

Myrrh
Used for skin dis-ease, brushing teeth, circulatory problems and as an antiseptic. The Egyptian papyri of 2,000 B.C. mentioned its use. Myrrh was used as an aromatic (burned as incense) in the temples of Isis, the Egyptian Goddess of Love.

Olive Oil
Used for digestive problems and for skin disorders. Ancient Africans used it for massage, machine oil, soaps, ointments, salves, plasters, liniments and hair oil. The monks brought it to America in 1796. Ancient Greeks, Romans, and

Assyrians learned of it from Africans and used
it.

Oranges   A fruit used for stomach and spleen disorders.
Drug merchants brought it to America in 1565.

Opopanax   This plant was used in northern Africa as a fixa-
tive. The Greeks learned of it and used it for the
same purpose.

Parsley   Used for urinary tract dis-ease and the nervous
system. The Greeks learned of it and used it for
the same purpose.

Papaya   Used for pancreas dis-ease and digestive problems. Today, an ingredient of the fruit (papain
enzyme) is injected into animals before they are
slaughtered. This causes the flesh to decompose
and be tender.

Peppermint   Peppermint was cultivated by the Egyptians and
used as medicine. Hippocrates, who as an
Escalapian (Imhotep), learned of its effective
usage by studying African science. Peppermint
usage was adopted by the Greeks and Romans
as reported by Pliny.

Peony   Used for respiratory and female reproductive
dis-eases. In the European Middle Ages, it was
used as a protection from witches. The Greeks
also used it as a food flavoring.

Periwinkle   Used as an astringent, and for hemorrhages and
toothaches. In southern Africa, it was used for
pancreas dis-eases such as diabetes. Today,
Europeans are using it for cancer.

Plantain   This ancient African fruit is in the banana plant
tribe. It is used for skin dis-eases, inflammation,
varicose veins and digestive disorders. The
Europeans learned of it in the Middle Ages and
used it for female reproductive dis-eases. It was
believed that wherever the English took posses-
sion of the soil of Africa, a plantain would grow.

Pineapple   Used as a general tonic, digestion and for wasting dis-ease. In the 16ᵗʰ Century, the Portuguese
controlled this fruit medicine and sold it to India
and St. Helena.

Pyrethrum   This herb is from North Africa and was used as
an insecticide. Today, Caucasians use it in many
commercial insecticide products.

Rose   An astringent. Used for female reproductive
complaints, skin diseases and for urinary tract

Saffron

disorders. The Europeans learned of it from Africans and used it during the Middle Ages. An anodyne and diaphoretic. Used for female reproductive disorders and as a carminative. Ancient African royalty used it as a dye. The Greeks and Romans learned of it and used it to scent baths and halls.

Sage

Used for asthma and is a vermifuge, astringent and expectorant. Sage was used as a hair rinse to soften hair and soothe the scalp. Europeans used it to hide the flavor of spoiled meat. The Romans used it for muscle pain and soreness. Today, Caucasians use it to flavor food.

Sandalwood

Used for inflammation, indigestion, skin disorders, respiratory dis-eases, and fevers. King Solomon's temple was built of sandalwood. The Burman Empire used it as a purifier.

Squil

This herb is a diuretic, emetic, expectorant and is used for respiratory inflammation. The Egyptians used it for heart dis-ease in 1500 B.C. The Greeks and Romans learned of it and used it for the same purpose.

Tragacant

Was used for mucous congestion and as a demulcent. Africans in the areas of Asia Minor and present day Iran used this herb. The Greeks learned of it in the 4th Century.

EUROPEAN DIS-EASES DEFEAT ANCIENT AFRICA

The European *"disease invasion of Africa"* caused massive deaths and weakened the strength of Africans to fight off the invasions. Rome, during its Golden Age (6th Century), had dis-eases and plagues. These disease epidemics slowed down the Caucasian conquest of many countries and limited the travel of dis-eased Caucasians. Caucasian plagues spread into Africa. Where Caucasians traveled they brought poor hygiene, food crop exploitation, hunger and disease. In 542 B.C. the European disease of the Plague spread to the Nile then to Asia Minor. European dis-eases followed their invasion route along the coast and reached Constantinople, killing an estimated 10,000 persons daily. The total figures for the dis-ease deaths of Black Africans are beyond estimation. Plagues generally reverse themselves. They travel forward with Caucasians, then travel back to the ports with Caucasians, which doubles the plagues' killing power. The European invasion routes thus escalated the dis-ease death toll of Africans. The Plagues were in Greece, Italy, and Gaul to the Rhine taking 15 years to travel the European inter-tribal trade routes. It took over 50 years for the air to clear from the foul stench of decayed bodies. The European dis-eases in its path killed millions of Blacks.

In the 14th Century, over 25 million Whites died in Europe from plagues and the plagues ceased because it ran out of White victims. However, the plague did not run out of Black victims, in Africa, so it killed many more Blacks than Whites. The plague of 1348 caused deaths of Blacks in Africa. The Dutch brought plagues during their invasion. Again, the rich get richer and the poor died when over 100,000 diseased Roman Catholic Church members marched to Rome and less than 10,000 survived the march. The church confiscated the riches of the dead marchers. Those that survived the march were blamed as the cause of the plague and were burned or murdered. The moneylenders of that era were various tribes, Jews, rich individuals and Church. The Church label their creditors as plague carriers and had them killed in order to get out of debt and then confiscated the riches of the dead Jews. These ancient European Christians used faith healing, prayers, incantations, charms, animal and human sacrifices to stop the dis-eases without success. Faith healing was crude and superstitiously based. Moreover, the early Christians stopped using the hygienic rational African approach to health that was taught at the Escalapian Temples. The Greek system of Hippocrates was abandoned, as rampant hunger, dis-ease and famine turned neighbor against neighbor.

The diseases were carried on the high seas and on slave ships and the death toll of the invasion routes of Africa were massive. Historian Pliny relates that during the war with the Teutons in the first century after Jesus the Christ, the invading Roman Army was nearly exterminated on the Rhine River banks by scurvy.

Portuguese invaders of Africa also carried dis-ease in the 15 and 16th Centuries. In fact, they killed themselves with their self-inflicted diseases. Vasco da Gama usually had from 6 to 12 healthy sailors left in his crew after journeys. This was caused by dis-eases killing his crew. The remaining sailors were either dis-eased or had scurvy as in 1497 when he invaded India. Spaniards carried smallpox dis-ease and pellagra to Africa. The total African deaths due to this dis-ease have not been estimated. However, it must have been approximately 4 million. In 1735, Gasper Casal, a physician at the court of King Philip of Spain described the dis-ease as rose disease. They also brought smallpox to New Mexico in the 16th Century, causing the death of 32 million natives.

Smallpox is a self-inflicted dis-ease, which was recorded in Europe in the 10th Century. Historian Macaulay denoted that smallpox was always a constant disease, causing deaths and plagues among Europeans. In 1628 it was in London, Queen Mary died of it and in France Charles IX's nose was scarred by it and it appeared as if he had 2 noses. In addition, the Europeans brought the dis-ease with them when they invaded America as the colonists had it. In 1700 there were 6 smallpox epidemics in Boston.

In 1793, Yellow Fever killed 10% of the population of Philadelphia. In correlation, Africans must have had a similar population decline due to European dis-eases. Again, the invasion route was also the dis-ease route as Asiatic Cholera came with the Europeans to the Americas, to Quebec, then to the Great Lakes, then to the Upper Mississippi, then New York where over 10,000 Whites died. The Native American and African deaths were equally high for these same dis-eases and were not recorded because Africans were considered the same as livestock animals. Incidentally, Blacks drove the hearse carts of plague victims. In fact, they were the only people at White funerals as Whites (including relatives and priests) would not attend funerals for fear of getting the dis-ease.

The number of European dis-eases caused by the poor hygienic practices, lack of soap and clean water use, famine and hunger is beyond count. However, the diseases of a wealthy king with good doctors and the best European diet can reflect the health of the White peasant. Louis XIV of France is recorded as having smallpox at 9 years of age, venereal dis-ease at 11 years, then typhoid disease, measles at 25 years, intestinal parasites (worms), rotten teeth and abscesses, gout at 44 years, dislocated elbow at 45, hemorrhoids operation at 48 years, then malaria, kidney stones and hardening of arteries. He died of gangrene of the leg. This indicates the general health (dis-ease) status of the European population.

Venereal dis-eases were transported to Africa and wherever Europeans invaded. In fact, the Puritans that first arrived in America had syphilis and accused each other as the sinners. It nearly caused the Plymouth Rock (Puritans) to disband. In fact, the syphilis carriers in European history are very extensive: Catholic Pope Alexander VI had syphilis, Henry III of France, Emperor Charles V, Ivan the Terrible of Russia, Herod King of the Jews, Henry VIII accused Cardinal Wolsey of giving him syphilis by whispering in his ear and he made whispering a crime which carried the death penalty. In James Savage's *Diary 1826,* he mentioned that syphilis could be the result of blameless manners (immorality). Moreover, gonorrhea was a prevailing cause of death and its origins are lost in antiquity. However, dis-ease and man-created famines depopulated Africa.

European dis-ease, famine (lack of food) and hunger played a major role in the European invasion of Africa. In many battles with Africans, it was European disease that killed Africans and won the battle for the Europeans. Dis-eases caused Europeans to be constantly in fear of death; while famines caused them to be in constant fear of starvation. The lack of natural and human resources and the small land area of the Caucasians was a prime factor for the invasions.

Europe consists of the combined tribes of the Soviet east and capitalist west. No other tribal region on the earth's surface has existed on the continuous dependency on Africa for human resources (slaves), knowledge, natural resources, medicinal herbs and edible plants. Geographically, the Soviets are Europeans, aside from their obvious membership in the

Caucasoid race. Europe has 4% of the earth's surface, Caucasoids are 6% of the world population and they have historically been dis-eased, predatory militaristic thieves and cultural cannibals who romantically call themselves explorers.

Europe (named by African Queen Europa) has always existed in one form or another of hunger and disease from its cavemen beginnings to the Feudal period. Europe was divided into large estates of 16,000 acres. White slaves (called serfs) suffered hunger and dis-ease under the control of lords. (*Historia Economica y Social De La Edad Media* by H. Pirenne).

European dis-eases caused a population drain. It left vast areas of farmland vacant and caused land to be exploited for food, which caused barren land and famines. Caucasians were in perpetual hunger and fear of death from dis-ease. And Africa's attraction was the absence of hunger and disease.

The oldest documentation of forced hunger in African is the "Stele of Famine." It was discovered over a granite tomb at the first cataract of the Nile. This famine devastated Egypt during the reign of Tosorthrus. During this famine the Nile did not flood for several years and massive starvation occurred. The Europeans' geopolitical land control caused starvation in Africa despite it being four times the size of the United States (11,500,000 square miles) with a scant Black population to feed. There is an over-abundance of fertile land to feed its population. Aside from this, the large water supply of the Congo, Zambezi, Nile and Niger rivers can keep the land fertile for food. Africa has the richest supply of natural resources, all of which are directly or indirectly controlled by European land barons.

The majority of the land is in the Torrid Zone and the land is either equatorial jungle or tropical desert both of which are difficult to artificially control. This caused the Europeans to search for other land areas and other means to exploit existing land and people in Africa.

Europeans were after quick-growing crops. These quick crops necessitated artificially controlling the land (cultivation), resulting in soil nutritional deprivation, which caused food nutrient deprivation, which resulted in causing diseases to become rampant.

The pandemic stricken Europe seized all types of African herbs and European tribes were in vital need of medicinal herbs so much so that they used plants of any type (medicinal and non-medicinal) seeking disease cures. They resorted to eating all types of leaves, roots, plants, and trees in a blind effort for medicinal herbs. They also practiced tribal (collective) hibernation. Entire tribe collectives (villages) would spend 4 to 5 months with limited physical activities accompanied with long periods of lying down. They would drug induce artificial sleep. (*Histoire de l'Alimentation Vegetal* by A. Maurizio).

The exploitation of the land of Africa for quick easy profits and Caucasian imported diseases caused Africa to weaken. Thus, the European invasion was quickened and devastated a land and its people.

The European tribes that invaded Africa for ivory, gold and herbs were initially the Portuguese, later the Spanish, French, English, etc. It was the English that began the plantation colonies. The plantation farming system requires destroying the naturally occurring plant balanced flora and fauna and the destruction of the natural food crops' ecological systems.

In contemporary time, land exploitation was caused by the Aswan Dam built in 1902. This established year-round irrigation resulting in nutrient-poor soil. However, this dam killed the soil because rich mud from the interior no longer came to the farmlands, and year-round cultivation destroyed the existing fertile soil. Aside from this, the European geopolitical structure caused the land provided by the dam to be devoted to mono-crops (cotton and sugar) and no food crops to feed the Africans, which created forced hunger. The European mono-crops temporarily stopped hunger and improved health but in due course caused vitamin deficiencies and soil destruction. Consequently, this allowed the European invaders time to focus on building wealth, while destroying African peoples and land.

European invaders committed all types of land and people abuse. Romans invaded Africa and killed the Africans with weapons and with the dis-eases they carried and they overworked the soil for grains and herbs. The great olive orchards of the Atlas Mountain slopes and forest were destroyed for wood, which Caesar and the Romans used to build egotistic luxurious palaces and boats. They stripped the land which caused an end to the food supply needed to feed them as well as the Africans. This, combined with dis-eases, caused an end to Roman power in North Africa. The Romans caused desert to replace the fertile land, leaving vast areas of barren soil. Aside from this, they destroyed animal balance and annihilated the elephants of the Atlas Mountains for ivory.

These primitive cultured Europeans not only exploited Africans but also exploited each other on stomachs full of African foods.

In France, the merchants exploited the hunger crisis by mixing grains with non-foods. The devotion of vast amounts of land to grains resulted in killing the land and peoples. The Europeans' diet of high grain content is not a necessary factor for proteins as many African cultures, as well as Eskimos, exist without bread. In any case, bread (and its many forms- pastry) is a good stable for Europeans. Bakeries were besieged during famines and bread sold at high prices. The price of bread kept it out of reach for most poor and most of them died (the rich got richer and the poor die). Aside from this, the bread was usually bitter, burnt, and full of clay. This resulted in inflammation of the gastro-intestinal tract and throat and brought on constipation accompanied with stomach pain.

Famine and so-called overpopulation are not natural causes that produce starvation. Caucasians control the land and therefore cause and control famines and starvation.

The false notion that there is not enough land to feed the European is a barbaric lie. The planet earth has plenty of land. The Earth's oceans covers 71% of the surface, leaving 29% land. This land surface is estimated at 56,000,000 square miles. Of that surface, grass plains are 20%, 32% is desert, 30% is forest and 18% is mountain. This leaves 25,000,000 square miles of agricultural land or half of the land surface (minus desert and mountain land). Yet, the conservative United States Department of Agriculture estimate leaves 8 acres per person. Further, it is estimated that only 2 acres are required for each individual (based on animal flesh diet, less land is required for vegetarian diet). The problem of starvation rests in the European geopolitical structure- who controls the land controls starvation and dis-ease. There is 50% arable land (farm land) on the planet and only 10% is used for food crops.

The world population did not produce starvation. Starvation is produced by land exploitation. This exploitation is a result of governments, businesses, and individuals that control vast amounts of land, which contribute to a shortage of individual ownership.

Soil erosion is not producing starvation. Soil erosion is an earth cycle. Soil erosion is part of soil inter-mixture and balancing, which has always kept soil in harmony. This is similar to our skin as the soil is the earth's skin. Our skin is constantly replaced in our taking in food and evacuation of waste process. Further, soil erosion would have destroyed China 5,000 years ago. The Yellow River Valley in China is the cradle of their culture. This river carries away approximately 25,000,000 tons of soil to the sea yearly. According to Western theory, the Yellow Valley should have disappeared 5,000 years ago. However, nature created and maintains soil balance on this planet despite European science mythology (theories), gadgets (technological machines—computers) and land exploitation.

It is European military land control, hunger, disease, poor hygiene and uncleanliness that caused one-crop diets such as cereals.

Cereals (fruit seeds) served as the dietary prime food for the ancient Chadean, Indian, Mayan, Chinese and Egyptian. This food allowed large population growths in the valleys of the Euphrates, Tigris and Nile. This resulted in a large accumulation of wealth for the Egyptian few.

Africans primarily ate uncultivated seeds that had vitamin and mineral values far higher than domesticated cereals. However, when the European domesticated cereal-based diet is used by Black Africans, dis-eases arise. This occurred among Africans in the Belgian Congo once they were forced to abandon sorghum, cassava, millet, etc. Their population decreased by 50% due to European-forced hunger, and the dis-eases produced by poor diets and poor hygiene. When the conditions are created to cause people to die, the Europeans called it genocide. Caucasians have created social and nutritional conditions that cause Africans to die or live in a dis-eased state.

The recorded famines between the 10th Century and the Renaissance number over 400. Europe had 22 famines in the 13th Century alone. Legal and illegal human flesh markets developed as cannibalism increased in Europe and hunger and dis-ease were the norm. Moreover, there were over 20 famines between the *11th* and 12th Centuries (see *The Famines of the World* by C. Walford). These famines caused Europe to invade Africa for food.

The usage of Africa for food, plants and medicinal herbs in the 16th Century decreased famines in Europe. However, for the most part European famines continued and starvation and dis-ease producing diets and habits continued. England had its worst famine in 1586. France, around Blois, had a famine, which caused people to eat the field grass like cattle, they chewed on roots, brushes and thistle, hoping to save their lives. Furthermore, in the 17th Century, famines caused children to suck the bones of dead humans in cemeteries and adults lay dead on the roadside with mouths packed with half-chewed grass. (*Hunger and History* by E. Prentice).

Hunger in Africa was primarily created by the dehumanizing European invasion of Africa and the European dis-ease carriers, forced inmigration, which destabilized the food supply, culture and colonial merchants. Their European one-crop culture was unable to feed their economics (*Hunger* by Knut Hamsun).

Western (European) science has not mastered human hunger. For example, this inability continues today as Western Science killed many starving people in Nazi Germany's concentration camps. In the camp of Bergen Belsen in 1945 the Red Cross and Allied Medical men orally fed predigested food and used intravenous injections to feed those in the last stages of starvation. The result was torturous death and the victims thought it was another form of torture. Later, they found skim milk to be the safest food to curb starvation. Aside from this, human milk is the better choice to combat starvation, but European dependence on lower animal milk (goats and cows), instead of human milk, prevails. Ironically, the massive amounts of people to die during the two major European tribal battles (so-called World Wars) were due to dis-eases and starvation not battles. In addition, the vast majority of the deaths during the Russian Revolution were caused by starvation of 17 million dis-eases, which resulted in over 25 million deaths.

The Europeans, during their tribal war called World War I, had technical domination of food and the land that it grew upon. Further, during their World War II they had biological domination of food and land. Currently, they control the land with synthetic chemicals and their military. Hunger and dis-ease is the most obvious underdevelopment of European cultures. It clearly indicates that they cannot satisfy the fundamental element of life-food!

In observing Africans, the Europeans failed to note cyclical food crop planting, varied plants and food combinations and hygienic care.

Black African Arabs introduced a nutritional diet high in fruits, herbs, vegetables, and food mixtures into the Iberian Peninsula, Asia Mirror and to the Romans, Portuguese and Spanish. Former Professor of Nutrition at the School of Public Health, Santiago, Chile, Dr. Sanila Maria, verified the nutritional benefits of this African diet. The merits of many plants in the African diet are being rediscovered by Europeans.

The palm was brought from Africa to Brazil because its vitamin content helped stop blindness, retarded growth and other dis-eases caused by faulty European nutrition.

The Black Arabs caused Spain to be the best fed country during the Middle Ages. Arabs living there used varied plant agriculture of fruits and other edible plants. The herb farms, so-called gardens and orchards of Andalusia's Moslem Spain, provided medicine, vitamins, minerals and proteins, which kept Spain well nourished. These African Blacks grew dates, almonds, oranges, figs and pomegranates and a complex mixture of African plants. (*La Penisule Iberique Au Moyen - Age* by L. Provenal and *Historical Geography of Europe* by W. G. East).

The North African Berber populations lived largely on vegetables. They ate semolina (in the form of couscous), wheat and barley, olive oil, dates, figs and small quantities of camel milk and animal flesh of goat and sheep and used herbs. Incidentally, the fig is closest to human milk in nutritional value while dates are good for building strong bodies. Europeans have always remarked on the superior physiques of the Berbers. And yet they ignored the vast dietary food combining system and medicinal herb systems of these Africans.

The Blacks who stay close to their original societal structure diet are nutritionally balanced. They abide by their holistic culture and keep tribal organizations and the diversified crop rotation farming system. Further, these Blacks rotate crops by burning out small areas in the forest for agriculture, thus shifting soil nutrients for their crops. They cultivate plantains, bananas, cassava sprouts, medicinal herbs, yams, potatoes, millet, corn, rice sorghum, oleaginous and indigenous plants of the forest. This predominantly vegetarian diet is nutritionally complete. Six tribes using this diet in Kenya were examined and not a single case of tooth decay was found (*Nutrition and Physical Degeneration* by N. Price).

The Blacks of the Belgian Congo have a highly acculturated nutritional diet. It is dominated by large amounts of tropical fruits, medicinal herbs and green leaves. They are dis-ease free on their diet. ("L" *Alimentation Au Congo Beige* by Bigwood and Trolli). The physique of Blacks varies according to the soil, vegetation and the areas of the African continent on which they live. Africa has natural regions such as the savanna, semi-arid steppes, subtropical, rain forest and desert.

The rain forest is on both sides of the equator. It has thick and massive vegetation that is mostly impenetrable (excluding the Amazon basin). The forest vegetable diet lacks a balance of nutrients and may cause small bone formation (Pygmies). Pygmies characteristically have achondroplasia, a variety of bone deformities and prognathism. The Black population, not forced into nutritionally lacking regions by Caucasian created social and cultural factors, have healthy physiques.

The diet of Blacks was drastically altered wherever the plantation system (one-crop or mono-crop) was used for exploiting herbs (so-called spices) and foods. Blacks abandoned their own land to work on the European cocoa plantations on the Gold Coast and the peanut mono-crop of Senegal. Their massive plant domestication caused the soil to become ruined especially in the Louga region and Cayor. This inadvertently caused damage in the Sudan as laborers abandoned their own farms and land of the Sudan to work in Senegal for the Caucasians, so, during the Sudan rainy season, African labor was not available to protect their own farm land and widespread erosion resulted. Further, the forced hunger of Blacks caused massive deaths in the Black population of the Congo and the 1920 Belgian Governor General M. Lippan stated that abandoning salad for rubber (black gold) caused the deaths.

The White racist depiction that the slaves were lazy and mentally slow is erroneous. Laziness and below normal mental capabilities were caused by a lack of proper food nutrition, and this further verifies that Africans forced to abandon a nutritionally food-rich variety and concentrate on the limited diet of Caucasian food crops become ill. They (Africans) had physical and mental lethargy (slow, lazy, shiftless nigger behavior) because of a poor diet. The slowness was a slavery resistance behavior. European experts of the United Kingdom's Committee on Nutrition in the Colonial Empire study indicated that the slow, lazy, shiftless nigger behavior is a lethargy caused directly by a European controlled mono-diet coupled with the European dis-ease contamination.

The limiting of one crop or a few types of plants on a plantation causes the soil to lose nutrients. This translated into a nutritional drain and subclinical malnutrition for the Blacks that must survive on the plantation's food crops.

The human infestation of parasites (worms) is created by a soil lacking nutrients such as calcium. Calcium stimulates the nitrogen-fixing bacteria, which stimulates proteins in plants. Soil erosion causes the nitrates to be washed away. Iron deficiency due to soil abuse occurs. Aside from this, worm infestation can be cured by including proteins and iron in the diet. However, the mono-plant crops (mono-animal crops) and land abuse causes 80% to 95% of Blacks living on such soil to have worms. Worms cause a nutritional lost which results in a pint of blood being lost daily. It is estimated that people such as the Chinese are raising an intestinal worm population equal to furnishing food for 400,000,000 Chinese. Consequently, disease and hunger are caused by land exploitation and undernutritional diets. The Europeans were constipated, worm infested, diseased and hungry.

The European invaders limited the African food supply and used the farmland of cash crops. This control of mono-crops limited the diet and was dis-ease forming, causing the Africans' health to become weak and deteriorate, the European hygiene and unsanitary behaviors were poor. Caucasian invaders and colonizers did not treat human waste by composting it with vegetables or use carbolic acid, which neutralizes its small pathogenic organism. The non-decomposed human waste would be washed into the drinking water of insects and animals would use the bacteria infested water. The African natives and invaders would drink the water. The Caucasians forced their constipating diet on the Africans, causing their health to become too weak to ward off dis-ease. The Caucasian heterosexual and homosexual raping of African women, young girls and young boys and the forced increase in breeding of Africans caused sex organ deterioration, resulting in venereal dis-ease. African society was unstable and weak because of the attacking Caucasian invaders. Social unstableness and an unstable food supply caused a poor diet and forced hygienic deterioration, further resulted in diseases among Africans. Hunger became normal. The White racist taboos and murders of African health practitioners (witch doctors) caused Africans to stop using their medicine and switch to allopathic medicine. This increased their health deterioration and dis-eases.

Europeans lacked medical knowledge. Their population declined because of diseases, famines and wars. The European civilization was living in caves 25,000 years ago and 500 years ago used human sacrifices for diseases. Hippocrates started using African medicinal art in 640 BC He separated Greek primitive medicines from the Church and used the hygienic system. His treatments were not widely accepted until late 1900. In the 2nd Century A.D., Galen revived Hippocratic medicine. However, the Christians rose to power and this religion spread eastward to China until the 7th Century. The Christian Church used human sacrifices and faith healings, and forbade the use of African hygienic or rational treatment. For example, a man with tuberculosis would be told to fast, pray, repent of sins and prepare to die. And, he would die. This medical ignorance and mythology was exported to Africa during the invasions. Oddly enough, in the 16th Century, Hippocrates' use of the African rational system of healing was revived by Paracelsus. He burnt Galen and Avicenna's books and stated there was no one more knowledgeable before him and that his beard had more knowledge than Hippocrates. He believed the myth that there is a synthetic chemical for every disease and made no association with hygiene and cleanliness. The Caucasians' militaristic predatory clans, mental and physical illnesses, ignorance, medical mythology and superior weapons allowed them to force generations of Africans to have diseases, famines, hunger and destabilized societies.

Section 18

Enlarged Charts and Pictures

EYE CHART
(Sclera = Whites)

Right

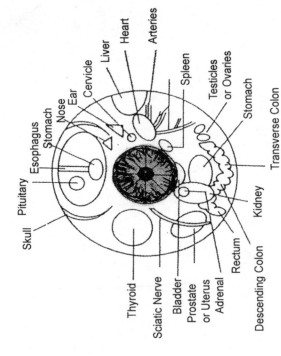

Left

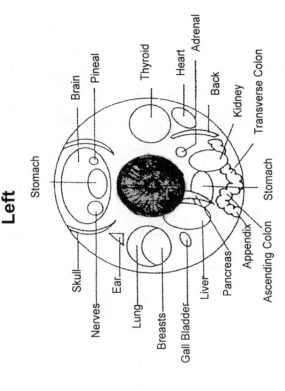

Hand Chart

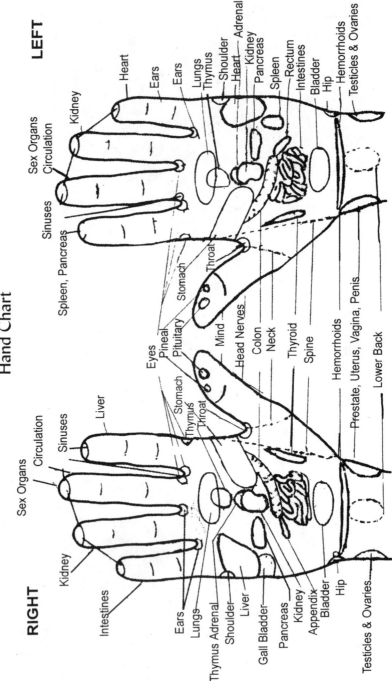

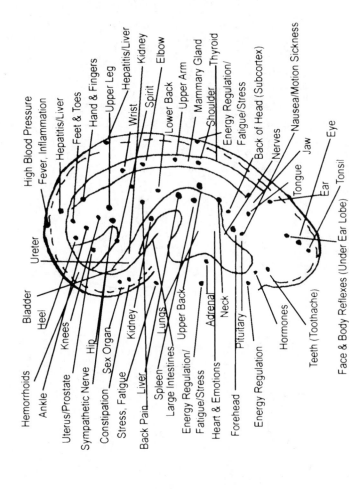

Ear (Auricular)
Acupuncture Points

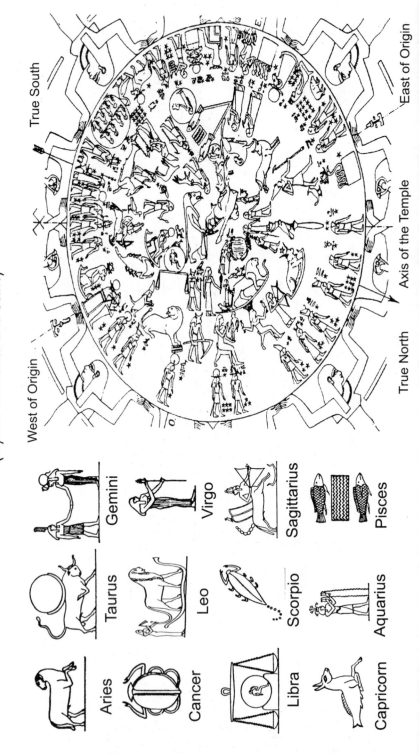

Tentyra Temple Curcular Zodiac—World's Oldest Zodiac
(Cycles of Plants and Stars)

Aries, Taurus, Gemini, Cancer, Leo, Virgo, Libra, Scorpio, Sagittarius, Capricorn, Aquarius, Pisces

True South, East of Origin, West of Origin, Axis of the Temple, True North

Sexual Matching
(Do not confuse with Personality Matching)

SEXUAL TYPE MALE / FEMALE		COMPATIBLE		TYPE OF MATCH	COMPLIMENTARY	
Type One Warrior March 22 to May 12	Aries ♈ Taurus	**Type Seven** Visionary January 28 to March 2	Aquarius ♒ Pisces ♓		**Type Two** Innovator May 13 to July 3	Gemini ♊ Cancer ♋
Type Two Innovator May 13 to July 3	Gemini ♊ Cancer ♋	**Type Three** Leader July 4 to August 24	Cancer ♋ Leo ♌		**Type One** Warrior March 22 to May 12	Aries ♈ Taurus
Type Three Leader July 4 to August 24	Cancer ♋ Leo ♌	**Type Two** Innovator May 13 to July 3	Gemini ♊ Cancer ♋		**Type Four** Idealist August 25 to October 15	Virgo ♍ Libra ♎
Type Four Idealist August 25 to October 15	Virgo ♍ Libra ♎	**Type Three** Leader July 4 to August 24	Gemini ♊ Leo ♌		**Type Five** Organizer October 16 to December 6	Scorpio ♏ Sagittarius ♐
Type Five Organizer October 16 to December 6	Scorpio ♏ Sagittarius ♐	**Type Six** Counselor December 7 to January 27	Capricorn ♑ Aquarius ♒		**Type Four** Idealist August 25 to October 15	Virgo ♍ Libra ♎
Type Six Counselor December 7 to January 27	Capricorn ♑ Aquarius ♒	**Type Five** Organizer October 16 to December 6	Scorpio ♏ Sagittarius ♐		**Type Seven** Visionary January 22 to March 2	Aquarius ♒ Pisces ♓
Type Seven Visionary January 28 to March 2	Aquarius ♒ Pisces ♓	**Type One** Warrior March 22 to May 12	Aries ♈ Taurus		**Type Six** Counselor December 7 to January 27	Capricorn ♑ Aquarius ♒

FEMALE AND MALE EMOTIONAL CYCLES

	1	2	3	4	5	6	7	8	9	10	11	12	13	14	15	16	17	18	19	20	21	22	23	24	25	26	27	28
1. JANUARY	1	2	3	4	5	6	7	8	9	10	11	12	13	14	15	16	17	18	19	20	21	22	23	24	25	26	27	28
2. JAN/FEB	29	30	31	1	2	3	4	5	6	7	8	9	10	11	12	13	14	15	16	17	18	19	20	21	22	23	24	25
3. FEB/MAR	26	27	28	1	2	3	4	5	6	7	8	9	10	11	12	13	14	15	16	17	18	19	20	21	22	23	24	25
4. MAR/APR	26	27	28	29	30	31	1	2	3	4	5	6	7	8	9	10	11	12	13	14	15	16	17	18	19	20	21	22
5. APR/MAY	23	24	25	26	27	28	29	30	1	2	3	4	5	6	7	8	9	10	11	12	13	14	15	16	17	18	19	20
6. MAY/JUN	21	22	23	24	25	26	27	28	29	30	31	1	2	3	4	5	6	7	8	9	10	11	12	13	14	15	16	17
7. JUN/JUL	18	19	20	21	22	23	24	25	26	27	28	29	30	1	2	3	4	5	6	7	8	9	10	11	12	13	14	15
8. JUL/AUG	16	17	18	19	20	21	22	23	24	25	26	27	28	29	30	31	1	2	3	4	5	6	7	8	9	10	11	12
9. AUG/SEP	13	14	15	16	17	18	19	20	21	22	23	24	25	26	27	28	29	30	31	1	2	3	4	5	6	7	8	9
10. SEP/OCT	10	11	12	13	14	15	16	17	18	19	20	21	22	23	24	25	26	27	28	29	30	1	2	3	4	5	6	7
11. OCT/NOV	8	9	10	11	12	13	14	15	16	17	18	19	20	21	22	23	24	25	26	27	28	29	30	31	1	2	3	4
12. NOV/DEC	5	6	7	8	9	10	11	12	13	14	15	16	17	18	19	20	21	22	23	24	25	26	27	28	29	30	1	2
13. DECEMBER	3	4	5	6	7	8	9	10	11	12	13	14	15	16	17	18	19	20	21	22	23	24	25	26	27	28	29	30

Put the number that coincides with your emotion on the date it occurs. You may have to use a different color pen (red, green, etc.). At the end of two or three months, you will see an emotional pattern (cycle). This will be your emotional cycle (Personality Cycle).

KEY

1	Anger	18	Mistrustful
2	Anxiety	19	Talkative
3	Cramps/Pain	20	Spend too much money
4	Cheerful	21	Want to fix things for people
5	Depressed	22	Menstruation
6	Energetic	23	Back Pain
7	Food or Snack craving	24	Sexually Aroused
8	Forgetful	25	Swelling
9	Headache	26	Tenderness
10	Hopelessness	28	Water gain/Retention
11	Impatient	29	Weight gain
12	Insecure	30	Lack energy
13	Insomnia	31	Nervous
14	Irritable	32	Moody
15	Lonely	33	Jealousy
16	Worried	34	Tend to cry
17	Want to sleep	35	Stressed

Additional Categories

36 _____
37 _____
38 _____
39 _____
40 _____
41 _____

The Three Layers of the Uterus

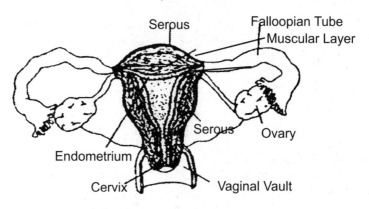

Serous

Falloopian Tube
Muscular Layer

Serous   Ovary

Endometrium

Cervix   Vaginal Vault

The Various Types of Fibroid Tumors.
Fibroids can grow anywhere, including on the ligaments of the uterus.

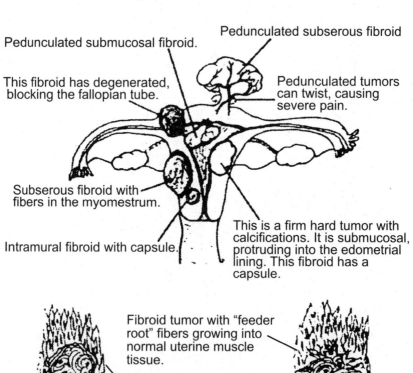

Pedunculated subserous fibroid

Pedunculated submucosal fibroid.

This fibroid has degenerated,
blocking the fallopian tube.

Pedunculated tumors
can twist, causing
severe pain.

Subserous fibroid with
fibers in the myomestrum.

Intramural fibroid with capsule.

This is a firm hard tumor with
calcifications. It is submucosal,
protruding into the edometrial
lining. This fibroid has a
capsule.

Fibroid tumor with "feeder
root" fibers growing into
normal uterine muscle
tissue.

Fibroid tumor with capsule.

Food Effects on the Body's Acid/Alkaline Balance Chart

Most Alkaline	More Alkaline	Low Alkaline	Lowest Alkaline	Food Category	Lowest Acid	Low Acid	More Acid	Most Acid
Baking soda	Spices/Cinnamon	Herbs (most)		**Seasonings**	Curry	Vanilla	Nutmeg	Jam/Jelly
Lime Nectarine Persimmon Raspberry Tangerine Watermelon	Cantaloupe Dewberry Grapefruit Honeydew Loganberry Mango	Apple Avocado Blackberry Cherry Lemon Papaya Peach Pear	Apricot Banana Blueberry Grape Orange Pineapple Raisin, currant Strawberry	**Fruit**	Date Dried fruit Fig Guava	Plum Prune Tomato	Cranberry Pomegranate	
Burdock Daikon Lentil Onion Sea vegetables Taro root Yam	Broccoli Endive Garlic Ginger root Kale Kohlrabi Parsnip Parsley Mustard greens Sweet potato	Bell pepper Cauliflower Collard greens Eggplant Mushroom Potato Pumpkin	Beet Brussels sprouts Chive Lettuce Okra Squash Lettuce	**Vegetables**	Chutney Rhubarb Spinach	Chard	Carrots	Carob
				Beans	Fava beans Kidney beans String beans	Aduki beans Lima beans Navy beans Pinto beans Tofu White beans	Chickpea	Soybean
				Legumes			Green pea Legumes (other) Peanut Snow peas	
Pumpkin seeds	Poppy seeds	Almonds Cod liver oil Primrose oil Sesame oil Sprouts	Avocado oil Coconut oil Flax oil	**Nuts / Seeds**	Canola oil Grape seed oil Pine nuts Pumpkin seed oil Sunflower oil	Almond oil Safflower oil Sesame oil	Pecan Pistachio	Brazil nut Hazel nut Walnut
				Sprouts				
				Oils				
				Grains	Amaranth Brown rice Kasha Millet Triticale	Buckwheat Semolina Spelt Teff Wheat	Corn Oat bran Rye	Barley
				Cereals				
				Fowl	Wild duck	Goose Turkey	Chicken	Pheasant
				Meat **Fish** **Shellfish**	Fish Venison	Elk Shellfish Lamb	Mussels/squid Pork Veal	Beef Lobster
		Quail eggs	Duck eggs	**Eggs**	Chicken eggs			
				Dairy	Cream Yogurt	Aged cheese Cow/goat milk Soy cheese	Casein Fresh cheese	Ice cream Processed cheese
		Green tea	Ginger tea	**Beverages**	Kona coffee	Black tea	Coffee	Beer
	Molasses	Rice syrup	Sucanal	**Sweeteners**	Honey Maple syrup		Saccharin	Cocoa Sugar
		Apple cider		**Vinegar**	Rice vinegar	Balsamic vinegar		White vinegar

Selected Readings

Abrahamson, C. and A. Pezet. *Body, Mind and Sugar.*
Abrams, M.D., Albert. *New Concepts in Diagnosis and Treatment.*
Afua, Queen. *Heal Thyself for Health and Longevity.*
_____. *Sacred Woman.*
Agillar, R. A. *Estudios sore las Auithaminoses y Las Perturbaciones del Crescimento en los Ninos Avitamonosicos.*
Airola, P. *How to Keep Slim, Healthy and Young with Juice Fasting.*
_____. *Sex and Nutrition*
Akers, Keith. *A Vegetarian Sourcebook.*
Amen I, Ra Un Neter. *A Holistic Guide to Family Disorders.*
_____. *Nutrition, Herbal and Homeopathic Guide to Healing.*
_____. *Optimizing Health Nutrition.*
Anderson, Henry. *Helping Hand (Guide to Healthy Living).*
_____. *Organic Welness (Fasting Technique).*
Andoh, Anthony. *The Science and Romance of Selected Herbs used in Medicine and Religious Ceremony.*
Ani, Marimba. *Yurugu.*
Arklinski, L. *Crystal Power.*
Arrnah, Ayi Kwesi. *The Healers.*
Ashby, Dr. Muata. *The Kemetic Diet.*
Ashanti, Kwabena PhD. *Psychotechnology of Brainwashing.*
Austin, Ralph. *The Treatise of Fruit Trees.*
Awadu, Keidi Obi. *The Conscious Rasta Report.*

Baerlein and Dower. *Healing with Radonics.*
Bailey, A. *Esoteric Healing.*
Baker, Douglas. *Esoteric Anatomy.*
Bailey, Peter. *The Harlem Hospital.*
Ballentine M.D., Rudolph. *Diet and Nutrition.*
Barnes, Carole. *Melanin: The Chemical Key to Great Blackness.*
_____. *Melanin: Protective Intoxicant Capabilities in the Black Human and its Influence on Behavior.*
Beddoe, Dr. A.F., *Biologic Ionization as Applied to Human Nutrition.*
Beddoes, Thomas. *Hygiea or Essays Moral and Medical on the Causes Affecting the Personal State of Our Middling and Affluent Classes.*
Benjamin, H. *Better Eyesight without Glasses.*
Bernades, Antonio, *Brazilian Herbs.*
Best, C. *The Physiological Basis of Medical Practice.*
Bicknael, F. *Chemicals in Food and in Farm Produce: Their Harmful Effects.*
Bigelow, J. *Earth Energy.*

Birket-Smith, K. *The Eskimo.*
Boericke, W. *Pocket Manual of Homeopathic Material Medical.*
Boyd, William, *Genetics and the Races of Man.*
Bragg, P.C. *The Shocking Truth about Water.*
Brena, Stephen. *Yoga and Medicine.*
Brothwell, Don and Patricia. *Food and Antiquity*
Brown, Dennis, M.D. and Pamela Toussaint. *Mama's Little Baby.*
Butler, Samuel. *Erewhon.*

Carrington, H. *Save Your Life by Fasting.*
Chaitow, Leon. *Amino Acids in Therapy.*
Chapman, E. *How to Use the 12 Tissue Salt.*
Charters, S. *The Bluesmen.*
Cheatwood, Kiarri, T.H. *To Save the Blood of Black Babies.*
Chirimunta, Richard Rosalin. *AIDS, Africa and Racism.*
Chissell, John T., M.D. *Pyramids of Power (Ancient African Centered
     Approach to Optimum Health).*
Choundhuri, N. *A Study on Matura Medical.*
Ciccone, Diana. *Heal Thyself Cookbood for Natural Living.*
Clark, L. *Color Therapy.*
Clarkson, R. *The Golden Age of Herbs and Herbalists.*
Clements, H. *Kidney Disorders.*
_____. *Nature's Cure for Painful Joints.*
_____. *Nature's Cure for Arthritis.*
_____. *Sexology* by.
Coon, C. *The Story of Man, From the First Human to Primitive Culture
     and Beyond.*
Cost, Curtis. *Vaccines are Dangerous.*
_____. *What is Safe in the Age of AIDS: If You Only Know What they
     Aren't Teaching You.*
Cott, A. *Fasting: The Ultimate Diet.*
Crawford, R. *Plague and Pestilence in Literature and Art.*
Cress Welsing, Frances. *The Cress Theory.*
Coon, CS. *The Races of Europe.*

De Foe, *Journal of the Plague Year.*
De Foe, D. *History of the Plague, 1722.*
De Graft-Johnson, J.C. *African Glory.*
De Lery. *Voyage Av Bresil.* 1556.
Deimel, D. *Vital Foods and Visual Training.*
Densmore, E. *The Occult Causes of Dis-ease.*
Densmore, E. *How Nature Cures.*
Dextreit, R. *Our Earth, Our Cure.*
Dichter, B. *Handbook of Consumer Motivation, The Psychology of the
     World of Objects.*

Digby, Kenelme. *The Power of Sympathy,* 1658.
Dimiscio, W. *Never Catch Another Cold.*
Diop, C. *The African Origin of Civilization.*
Donsbach, *Glandular Extracts.*
Dorchester, F. *Muscle Action and Health.*
Douglas, N and P. Slinger. *Sexual Secrets.*
_____. *Sexual Secrets.*

East, W. G. *Historical Geography of Europe.*
Ehret, Arnold. *Mucousless Diet Healing System.*
_____. *Mucousless Diet Healing System.*
Ellis, Havelock. *Man and Woman.*
Engels. *Conditions of the Working Man in England.*
Enti, Albert A. *The Rejuvenating Plants of Tropical Africa.*

Fattner, A. *The Truth About AIDS: Evolution of an Epidemic.*
Ferguson, Elaine, M.D. *Healing, Health and Transformation.*
Fielding. N. *Homo-Sexual Life.*
Fowler. *The Science of Life.*
Fracastro, Girolamo. *Syphilis Five Morbus Galicus.* (1530)
Fredericks, C. *Eating Right For You.*
Freyre and Gilberto. *The Masters and Slaves.*
Fuller, Neely, Jr. *The United Independent Compensatory
    Code/System/Concept: A Textbook/Workbook for Thought, Speech
    and/or Actions for Victims of Racism (White Supremacy).*
Fulton, Alvenia. *Radiant Health through Nutrition.*

Gaer-Luce, Gay. *Biological Rhythms in Human and Animals.*
Ganong, W. *Review of Medical Physiology.*
Garten, N. *Health Secrets of a Naturopathic Doctor.*
Geddes and Thompson. *Evolution of Sex.*
Glanville, S. R. K. *The Legacy of Egypt.*
Glazer, Nathan. *Slavery.*
Goldsmith. *The Deserted Village.*
Goss, Paul, Dr. *Forever Young.*
_____. *The Rebirth of Gods.*
Graham-Bonnalie, *Allergies.*
Gregory, Dick. *Dick Gregory's Natural Diet for Folks Who Eat with
    Mother Nature.*
Gruner, O. *The Canon of Medicine.*
Guthrie, K.S., MD. *Regeneration for Women.*

Hall, Gregory. *Overcoming Anemia.*
Hakim, Rashan Abdul. *Basic Herbs for Health and Healing.*
Hamsun, Knut. *Hunger.*

Harley, G. W. *Native African Medicine.*
Harrington, John. *The Metamorphosis of Ajax,* 1596.
Hatonn, Georges C. *The Last Great Plague upon Man: AIDS Related Murder Tools.*
Heape. *The Sexual Season of Mammal.*
Heindel, M. *Occult Principles of Health and Healing.*
Heinerman, J. *Herbal Dynamics.*
Hills, Hills. *Supersensonics.*
Hoffman. Jay. Dr. *The Missing Link.*
Horlan, Jack. *The Origin of African Plant Domestication.*
Hotea. *The Secret of Regeneration.*
Hotema, H. *The Science of Human Regeneration.*
Howell. Dr. *The Status of Food Enzymes in Digestion and Metabolism.*
Huepser, W and Conway, W. D. *Chemical Carcinogensis and Cancers.*

Ignatius, Doctor. *How to Select and Combine, Fruits, Vegetables and Tubers through their Color Powers.*
_____. *Spiritual Nutrition.*
Ilza, V. *Yellow Emperor's Classic of Internal Medicine.*
Inglis, B. *Drugs, Doctors and Disease.*

Jackson, M and T. Teague. *The Handbook of Alternatives to Chemical Medicine.*
Jaffrey, K. *How to Fast.*
Jevons, W. *Principles of Science*
John, Yvonne. *The Guyanese Seed of Vegetables, Seafood and Desserts: The Vegetarians and Food Lovers Paradise.*
Jones, Del. *The Invasion of the Body Snatchers.*
Jones, J. *Prejudice and Racism.*

Kadans, J.M. *Encyclopedia of Fruits, Vegetables, Nuts and Seeds for Healthful Living.* West Nyack, NY: Parker Publishing Company, Inc., 1973.
Kallet, A and F. J. Schlink. *100,000,000 Guinea Pigs. Dangers in Everyday Foods, Drugs, and Cosmetics.*
Kellogg, J. *The Awakening of Woman.*
Kenyatta, J. *Facing Mount Kenya.*
Kervan. *Biological Transmutations.*
Kirban, S. *Health Guide for Survival.*
Kloss, J. *Back to Eden.*
Kohman, Eddy, White and Sanborn. "Comparative Experiments with Canned, Home Cooked, and Raw Food Diets" (1937). *Journal of Nutrition* 14:9-19 [1937].
Kondo, Zak A. *Vegetarian.*
Kropotin. *Mutual Aid, A Factor of Evolution.*

Kyte, C. Wolde. *Caribbean Medicine.*

Lambscher, B. *Sex, Custom and Psychopathology: A Study of South African Pagan Natives.*
Laversen, M.D. M and S. Whitney. *It's Your Body.*
Leadbeader, C. *The Chakras.*
Longwood, W. *The Poison in Your Food.*
Lorenz, K. *Studies in Animal and Human Behavior.*
Lorraine, Keefa K. *Claim the Victory.*
Lust, J. *The Herb Book.*

Mayer, M.D. K. *AIDS Fact Book.*
Michio, K. *How to See Your Health; Book Oriental Diagnosis.*
Mickey, Karl. *Health From the Ground Up.*
Miller, F. *Eating for Sound Teeth.*
Mindell, Earl. *Vitamin Bible.*
Morgulis. *Fasting and Undernutrition.*
Morrison, L. *The Low Fat Way to Health and Longer Life.*
Moyle, A. *Chronic Bronchitis.*
Muhammad, Elijah. *How to Eat to Live: Volume I and II.*

Napheys, G. *Physical Life of Woman.*
Neckham, Alexander. *De Laudibus Divinae Sapientiae.*
Newton, N. *Maternal Emotions.*

Osier M.D., William. *The Principles and Practice of Medicine.*
Ostrander, S. *Astrological Birth Control.*
Olela, Henry. *From Ancient Africa to Greece.*

Paul, B. *Health, Culture and Community.*
Peter Frank, Johanna. *Mediziniche Polizei.*
Pearson, D. and S. Shaw. *Life Extension.*
Pfeiffer, C. *Mental and Elemental Nutrients.*
Pookrum, Jewel, M.D. *Vitamins and Minerals from A-Z with Ethno-Consciousness.*
Popper, K. *The Logic of Scientific Discovery.*
Powell, Alfred "Coach". *Message in a Bottle.*
Prentice, E. *Hunger and History.*
Price, N. *Nutrition and Physical Degeneration.*

Quick, C. *Sinusitis, Bronchitis and Emphysema.*

Raleigh, A. *Woman and Superwoman.*
Ramazzini, B. *Treatise on Diseases of Tradesmen.*
Robertson, Diane. *Jamaican Herbs.*

_____. *Live Longer, Look Younger with Herbs.*
Rogers, J. A. *World's Great Men of Color.*
_____. *From Superman to Man.*
_____. *100 Amazing Facts About the Negro.*
Roll, I. *Rolling the Integration of Human Structures.*
Royal, P.C. *Herbally Yours.*
Roslin, Eucharis. *The Garden of Roses for Pregnant Women and Midwives,* 1513.
Royal, P.C. *Herbally Yours.*

Shelton. *The Hygienic Care of Children.*
Sneddon, R. *Nature's Cure for Gastric and Duodenal Ulcers.*
_____. *Nature's Cure for Varicose Veins and Ulcers.*
Steven, E and Ashley Montagu. *Anatomy and Physiology.*
Shahani, K., J. Uakil, A. Kilara. "Natural Antibiotic Activity of Lactobacillus Acidophilus and Bulgaricus II. Isolation of Acidolphilin from L. Acidolphilus." *Cultured Dairy Products,* J 12(2): 8, 1977.
Shelton, H. *Fasting for Renewal of Life.*
Smith, J. *Proper Food of Man.*
Sneddon, R. *Nature's Cure for Gastric* and *Duodenal Ulcers.*
Sneddon, J. *Natural Treatment for Liver Troubles and Associated Ailments.*
Speech, K. *The Gurdjeff Work.*
Staugh, R.A. *Health Teachings of the Ageless Wisdom.*

Taber, C. *Cyclopedia Medical Dictionary.*
Thienell, G. *My Battle With Low Blood Sugar.*
Tobe, S. *Liver Ailments and Common Disorders.*
Thwaite, Cowper. *A Textbook of Gynecology.*
Theophrastus. *Enquiry into Plants.*
Tompkins, P. *The Secret Life of Plants.*
Tompkins, P. and C. Bird. *Secrets of the Soil.*

Virby, L. *Hygiene Philosphique.*
Valentine, Basile. *The Triumphant Chariot of Antimony.* 1604.

Waite, A. *Alchemists Through The Ages.*
Walford, C. *The Famines of the World.*
Walker, N. *Colon Health.*
Warmbrand, M. *Overcoming Arthritis and Other Rheumatic Diseases*
Wason, Betty. *Gluttons and Gourmets.*
Weiner, Ph.D. M. *Getting Off Cocaine.*
Weiss, P. *Beyond Reductionism.*
Wensel, L. *Acupuncture for Americans.*

Westermack. *History of Human Marriage.*
Whitehoose, G. *Every Woman's Guide to National Health.*
Wiancek, D. *The Natural Healing Companion.* The Complete Natural
    Medicine Reference CD-ROM.
Wiley, M.D. H. *History of Crime Against the Food Law.*
Williams, R. A. *Textbook of Black-Related Diseases.*
Williams, R. *Nutrition Against Disease.*
_____. *Textbook of Black-Related Diseases*
Williams, R. A. *Diseases.*
Wilson, Amos. *Awakening the Natural Genius in Black Children.*
_____. *Blueprint for Black Power.*
_____. *The Developmental Psychology of the Black Child.*
Wright, Keith T. *A Healthy Foods and Spiritual Nutrition Handbook.*
Wright, J. *The Coming Water Famine.*

Index